HNO Praxis heute 21

Springer
Berlin
Heidelberg
New York
Barcelona
Hongkong
London
Mailand
Paris
Tokio

Practical Procedures in
Aesthetic Plastic Surgery

Practical Procedures in

Aesthetic Plastic Surgery

Tips and Traps

Foreword by STEVEN M. HOEFFLIN

With 510 Illustrations and 46 Color Plates

Springer-Verlag
New York Berlin Heidelberg London Paris
Tokyo Hong Kong Barcelona Budapest

Tolbert S. Wilkinson, M.D., F.A.C.S.
Institute for Aesthetic Plastic Surgery
One Oak Hills Place
1901 Babcock, Suite 200
San Antonio, TX 78229
USA

Library of Congress Cataloging-in-Publication Data

Wilkinson, Tolbert S., 1937–
Practical procedures in aesthetic plastic surgery / Tolbert S. Wilkinson.
p. cm.
Includes bibliographical references and index.
ISBN-13:978-1-4612-7598-5
1. Surgery, Plastic. I. Title.
[DNLM: 1. Surgery, Plastic—methods. 2. Face—surgery. 3. Breast—surgery. 4. Abdomen—surgery. WO 600 W687p 1994]
RD119.W535 1994
617.9'5—dc20
DNLM/DLC
for Library of Congress 93-41835

Printed on acid-free paper.

Production coordinated by Publishing Network and managed by Karen Phillips; manufacturing supervised by Gail Simon.
Typeset by ATLIS Graphics, Mechanicsburg, PA.
Color separations and printing by New England Book Components, Hingham, MA.

9 8 7 6 5 4 3 2 1

ISBN-13:978-1-4612-7598-5 e-ISBN-13:978-1-4612-2594-2
DOI: 10.1007/978-1-4612-2594-2

Foreword

THOSE WHO KNOW DR. "T" WILKINSON ARE NOT SURPRISED BY HIS individualistic, creative thinking and "straight Texas style shooting" approach to teaching. His long-term editorship of *Technical Forum* has allowed him to draw upon the innovative contributions of plastic surgical experts and the free flow of important procedural commentaries.

Describing the intricate art and science of plastic surgery in writing is a formidable challenge. My congratulations to him for meeting this challenge. The importance of exchanging critical commentaries from plastic surgery experts cannot be overemphasized. The text departs somewhat from traditional writing by frequently drawing upon the critical but subtle capsule comments and anecdotes of others. Characteristically, small personal pearls of wisdom and helpful tips are often exchanged at meetings, but many are seldom published. The importance of their publication here is its obvious wider exposure. This is certainly well done in this text, which applies a wealth of special emphasis on the practical technical detail of standard and new procedures. This is especially helpful when new, innovative procedures or modification of old procedures may lack wide-spread evaluation and rapid feedback

The chapters on facial procedures, fat grafting, and adjunctive procedures are especially instructional. Good results can be obtained by combining small, multiple procedures, i.e., cheek augmentation, fat grafting, liposuction, and combined peeling with a standard rhytidectomy. You will find that the consistent attention to detail allows the surgeon to easily follow step-by-step through various procedures. The very innovative footnote-style commentaries of many experienced plastic surgery experts add tremendously to understanding the true value of various procedures.

It is obvious in his writing that Dr. "T" places special emphasis on searching for the truth in evaluating new procedures, attempting to avoid the inaccuracies and exaggerations that often accompany such techniques. This fine text is an excellent guide to performing both standard and new aesthetic procedures. My congratulations to Dr. Tolbert Wilkinson for a very important and useful contribution.

STEVEN M. HOEFFLIN, M.D., F.A.C.S.

Contents

PART TWO *The* Body

Color Plates

1

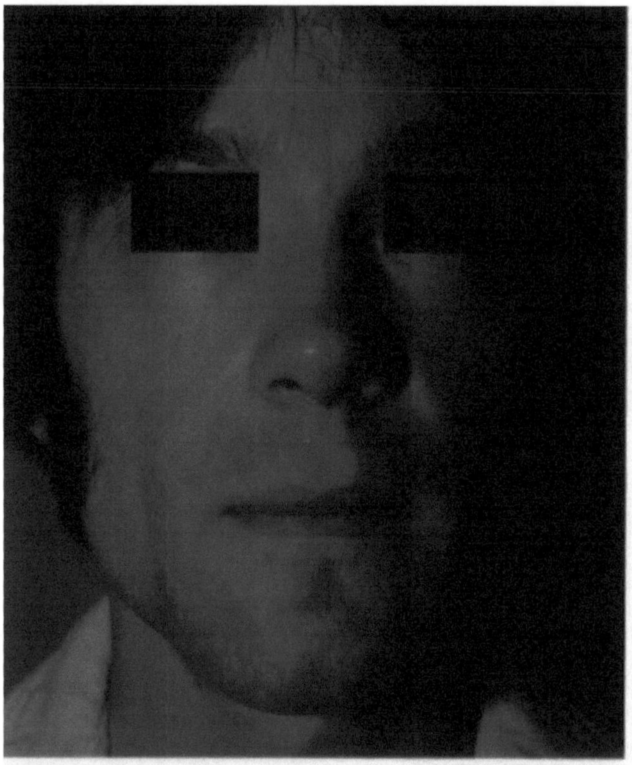

2

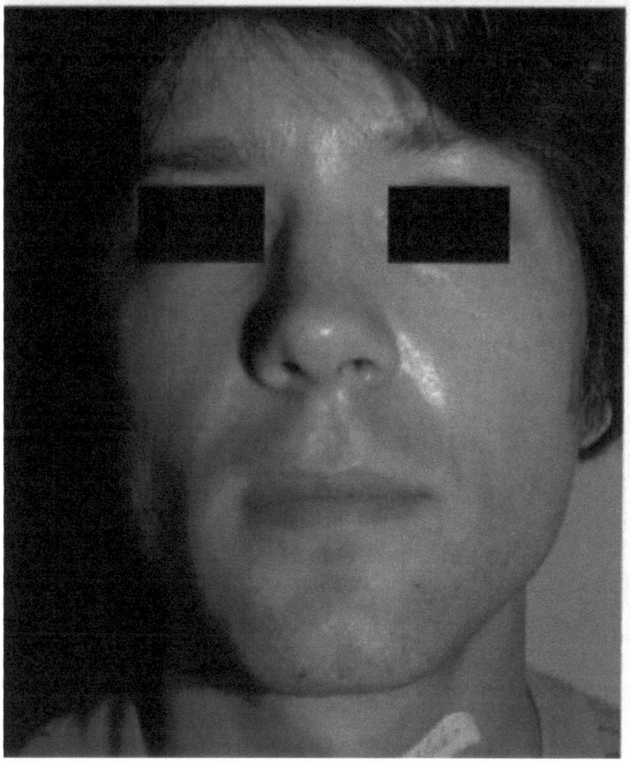

3

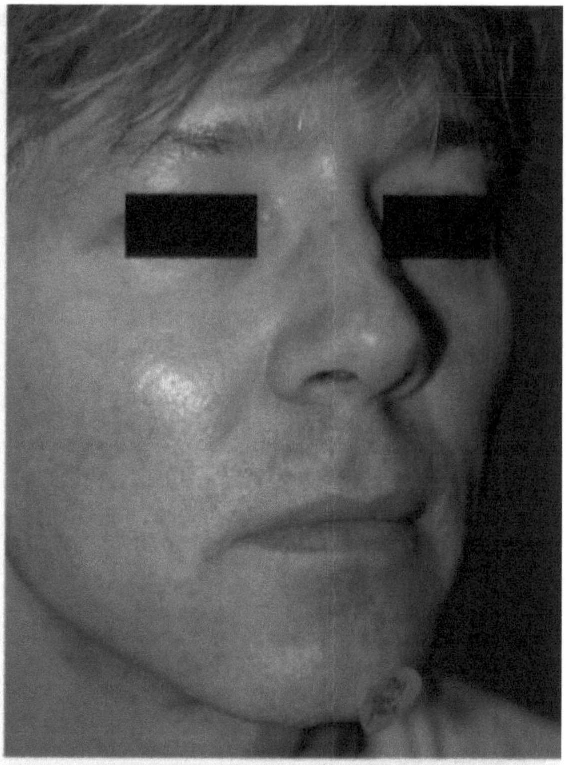

4

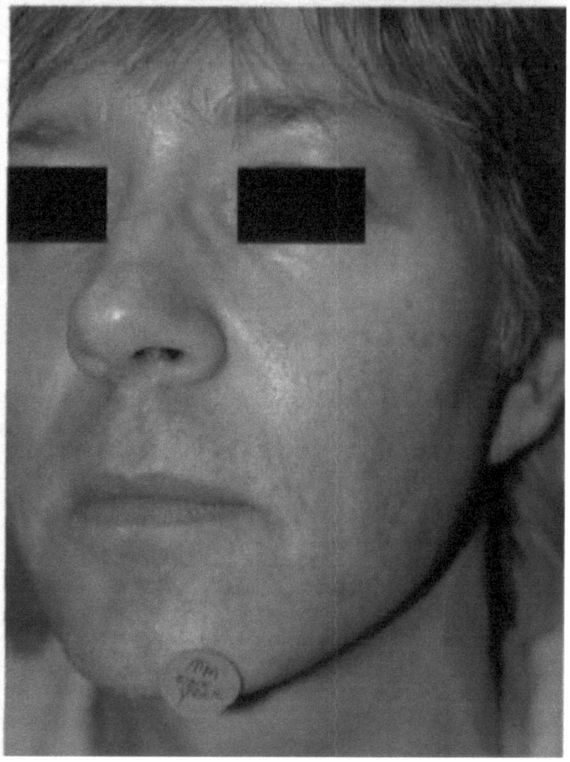

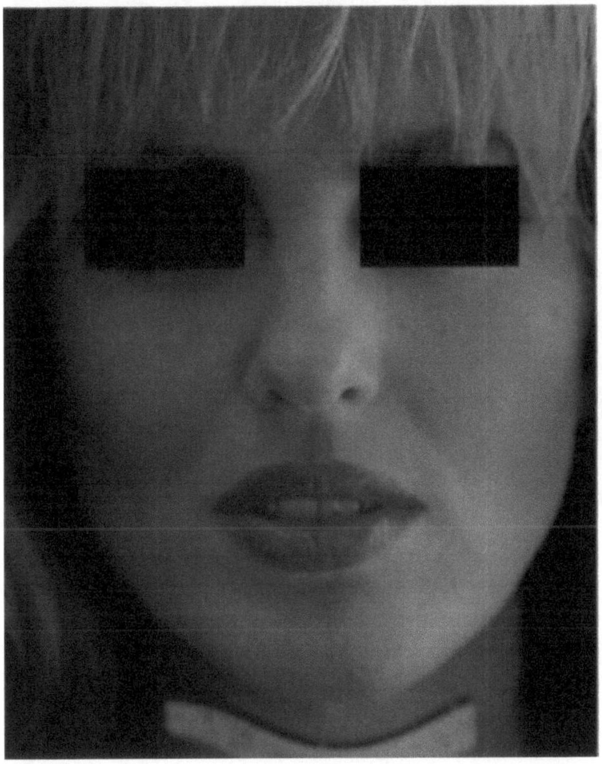

5

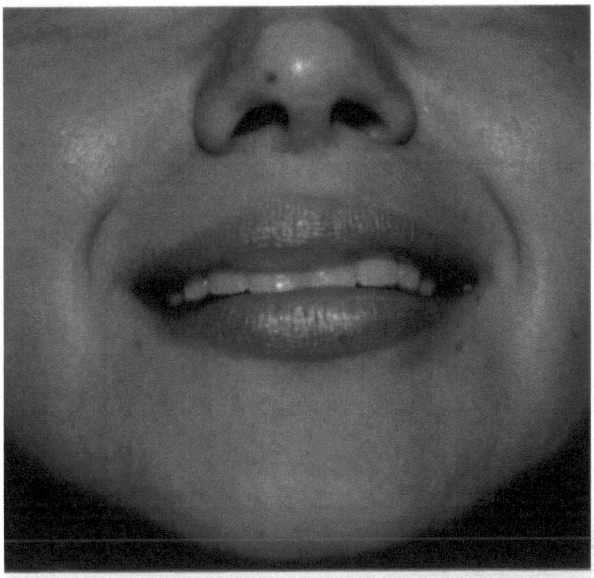

6

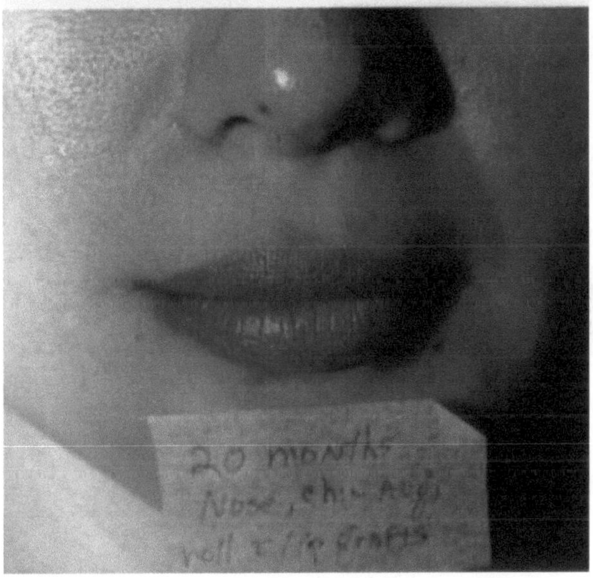

7

Figures 1–5. The degree of fullness and amount of visible vermillion are determined by the extent of lip undermining and advancement. As the years pass, the lip fullness becomes even more prominent, probably as a result of dependent tissue edema. This typical "Texas Girl" is shown preoperatively in 1984 in Figures 1 and 2 and postoperatively at the eighth year in Figures 3–5.

Figures 6–7. An unusual complication of the lip roll procedure is the "double-lip" deformity, similar to that which occurs naturally in a few young women. The patient asked for greater fullness of the lower lip and moderate fullness of the upper lip. The dissection was stopped at the "wet-to-dry" vermillion junction, leading to the development of this "double-lip" folding with her smile (Figure 6). Correction was with fat grafts placed in tunnels beneath the fold. The corrected appearance is shown at 20 months in Figure 7.

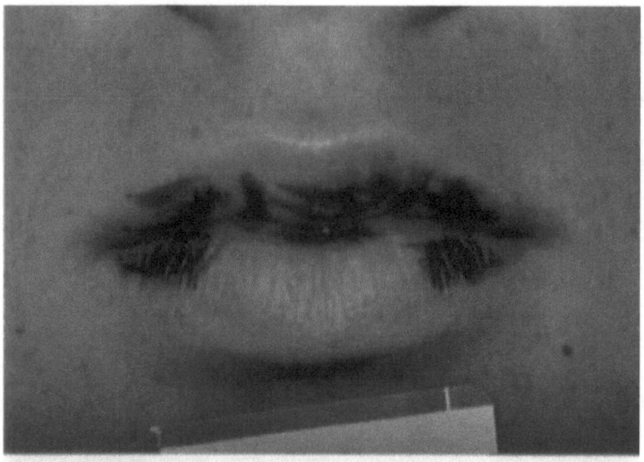
8

9
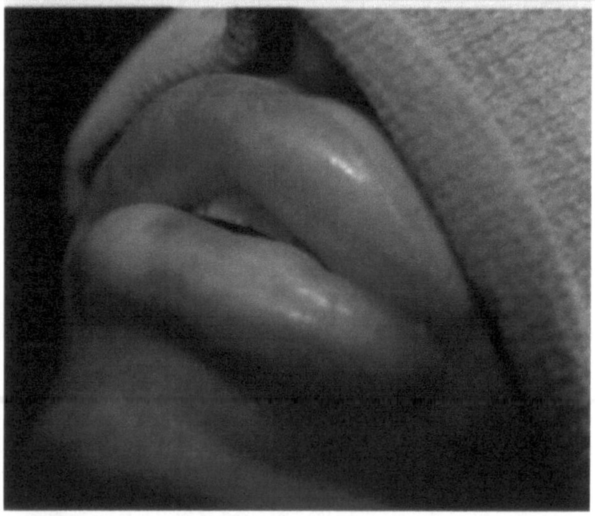

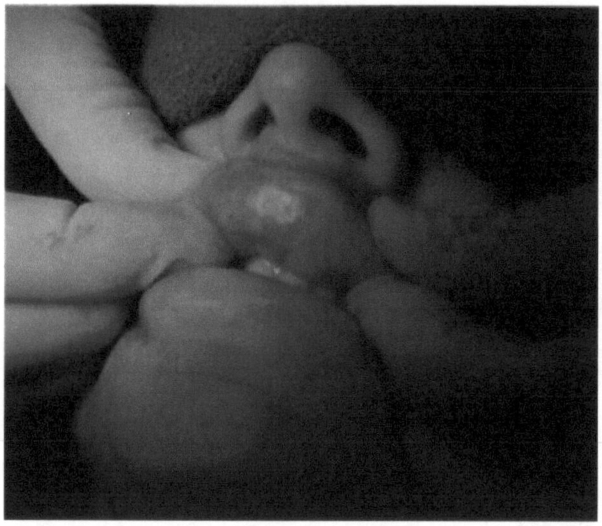
10

Figures 8–14. In patients with adequate lip vermillion who request the "full-lipped" appearance that is popular with professional models, concentrated autologous fat grafts alone provide the enhancement. The patient shown in Figure 8 already has adequate fullness in the center of the lower lip. The multiple tunnel technique is tailored to fill the areas marked in blue. For a fully augmented appearance, overcorrection by more tunnels is required (Figure 9). As a final adjustment, more tunnel fat is moved toward the center (Figure 10) to achieve the desired result (Figures 11 and 12). By contrast, patients who possess only marginally adequate vermillion (Figure 13) are enhanced by an upper and lower "lip roll" procedure. This degree of enhancement is more commonly requested (Figure 14).

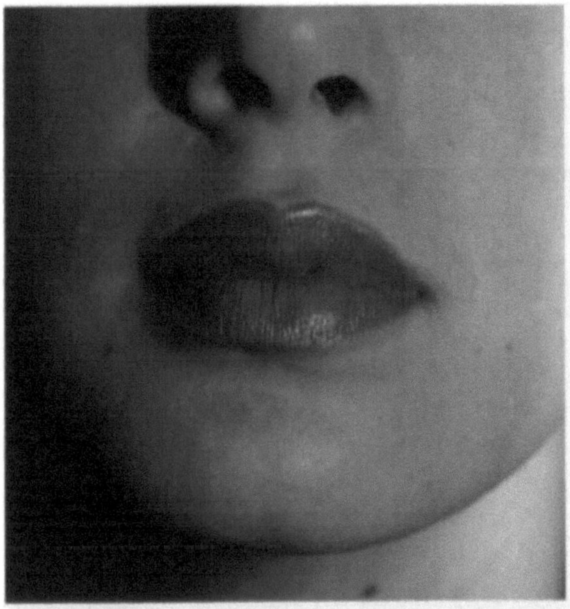

11

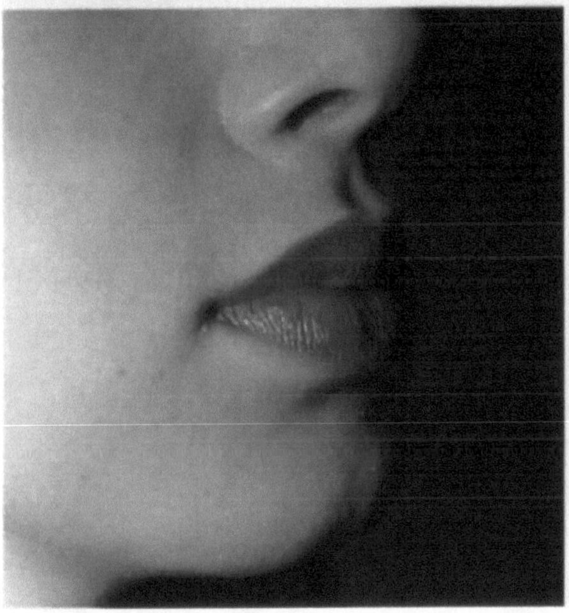

12

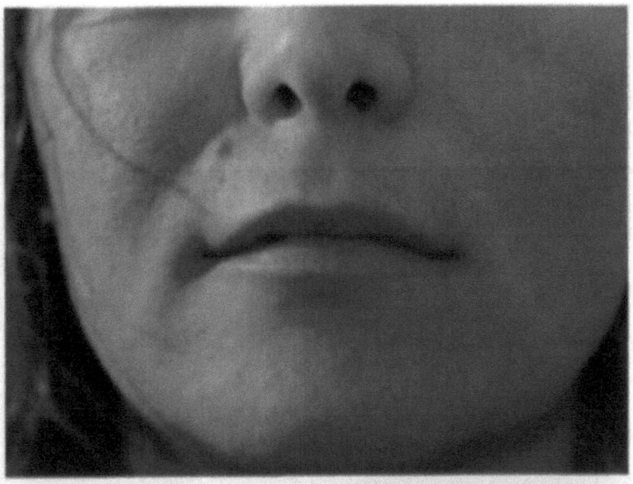

13

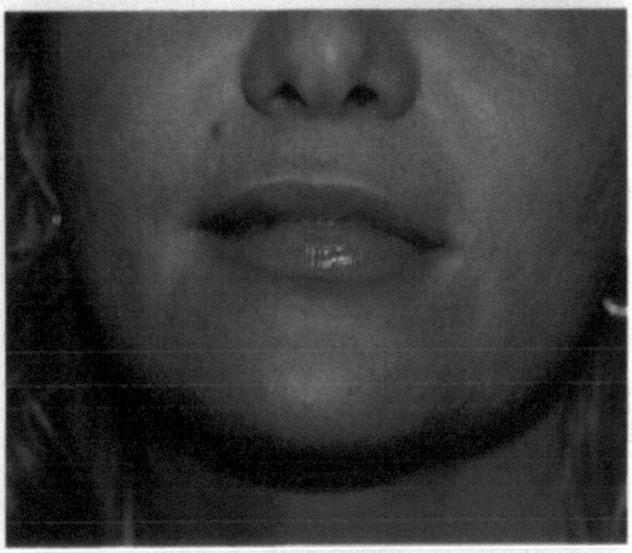

14

15
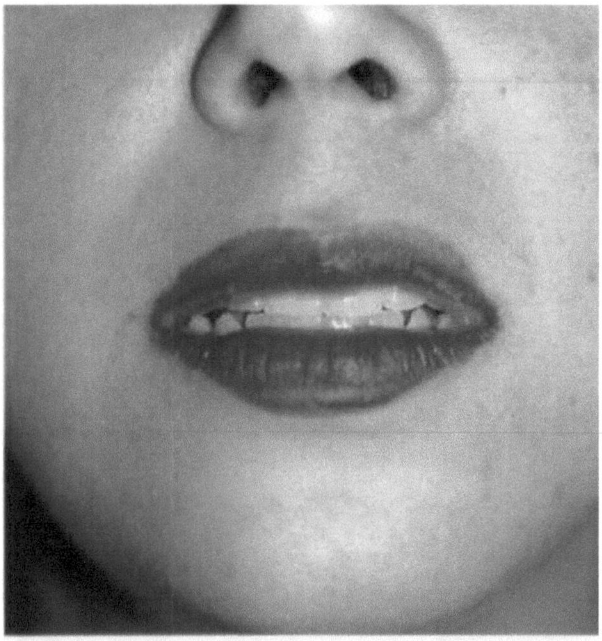
16
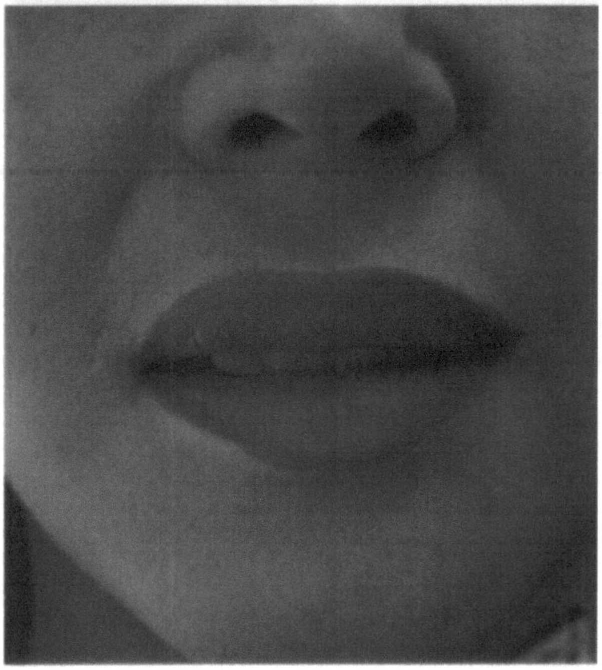

17
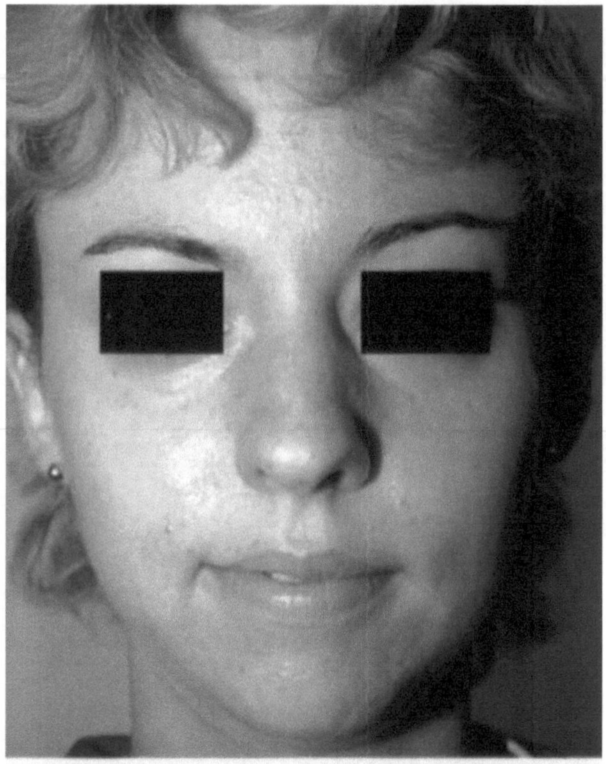
18
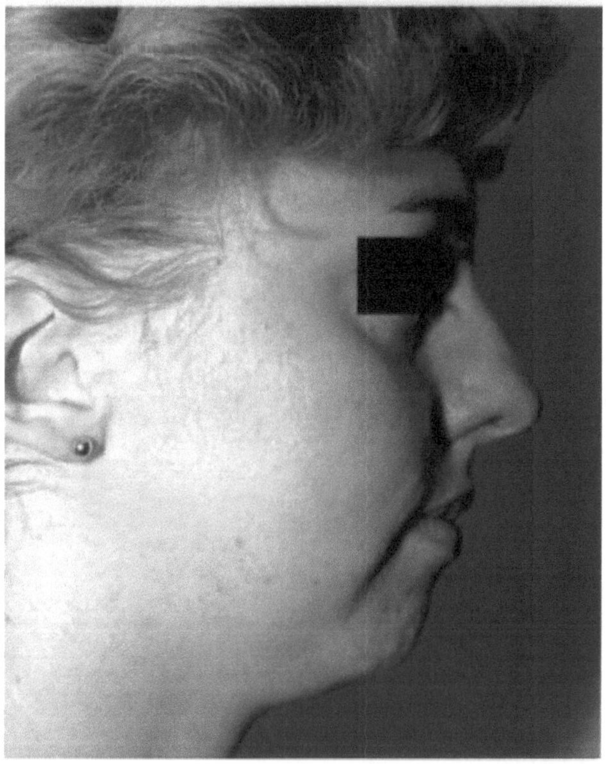

Figures 15–16. For patients with little visible vermillion (Figure 15) who request the "mega-lip" fullest enhancement, a combination of the "lip roll" procedure and fat is used. Fat tunnel grafts are placed submucosally and in the orbicularis muscle to achieve the desired fullness (Figure 16).

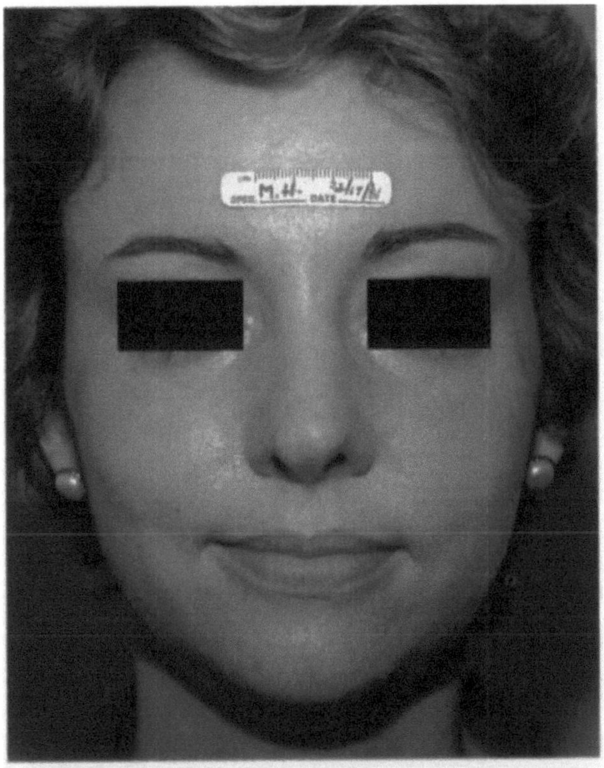

19

20

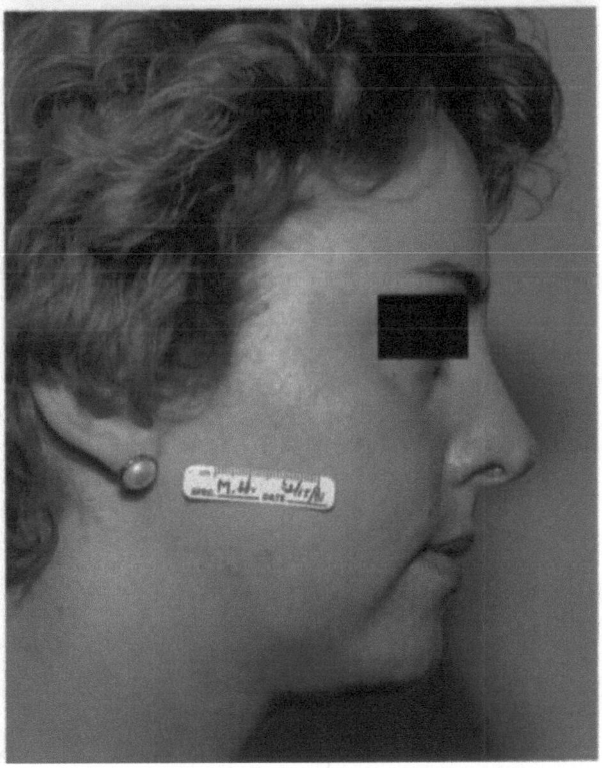

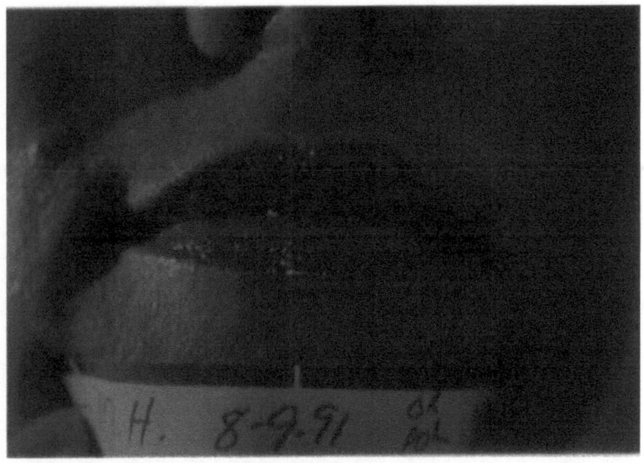

21

Figures 17–23. Combining procedures in young adults often includes understanding changes in desired self-appreciation. The first patient (Figures 17 and 18) chose a rhinoplasty and a silastic chin augmentation in 1980, which created the desired improvement (Figures 19 and 20) shown in these 1981 photographs. Adding cheek liposuction, a submental "tuck," fat grafting for lip enhancement, and filling the nasolabial groove added further improvement in 1990. Continued skin care added to the natural and "fresh" appearance depicted in 1991, one year postoperatively (Figures 21–23).

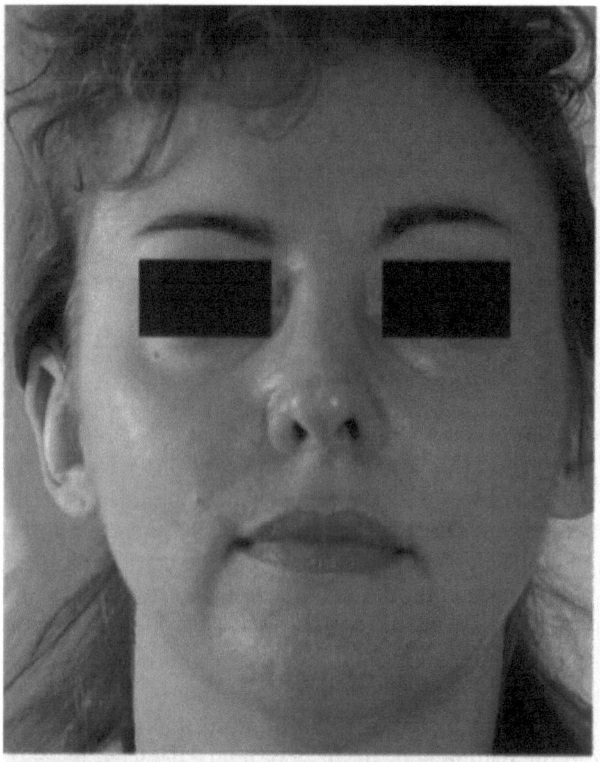

22

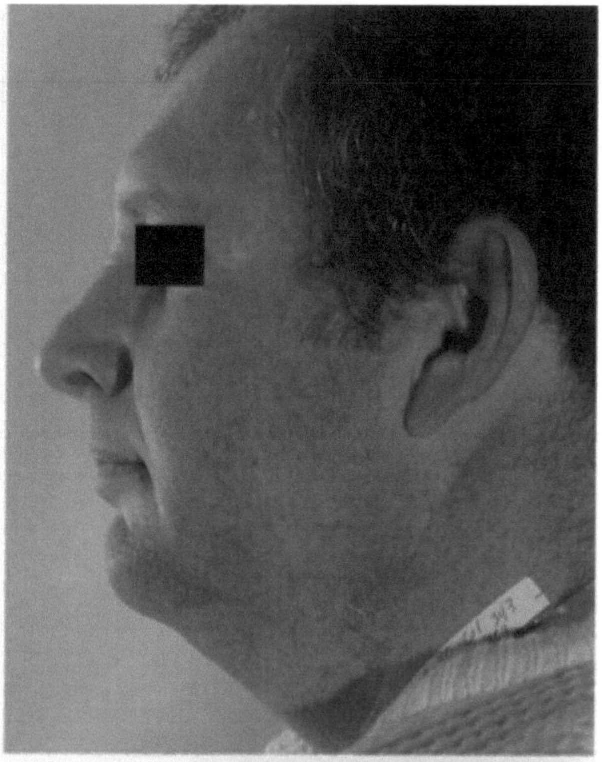

24

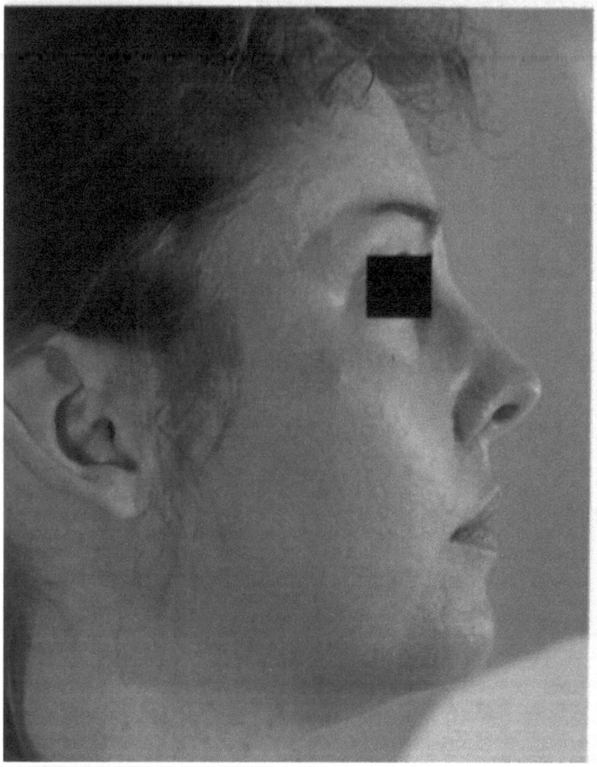

23

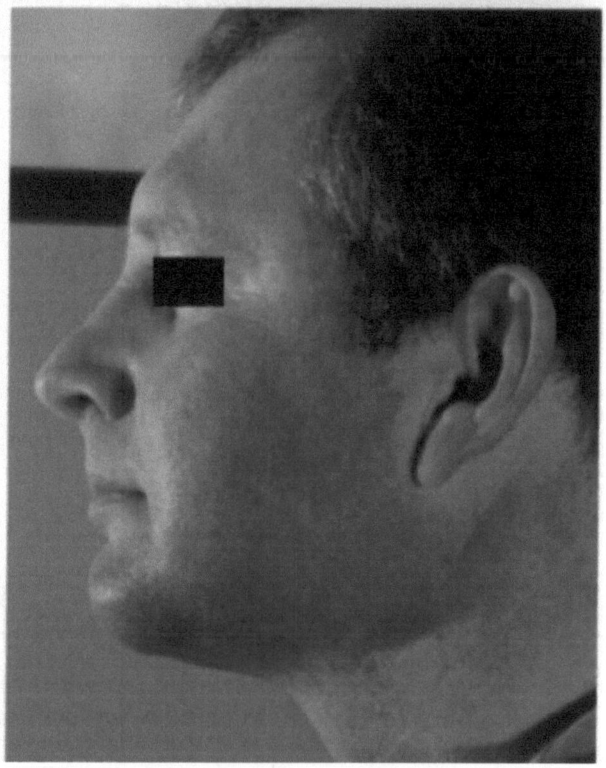

25

Figures 24–25. The submental "tuck" and jowl liposuction in combination give a more natural jawline in males (Figures 24 and 25) than either procedure alone in patients with this degree of laxity. No skin excision or superficial lipocurettage was performed, but his chin was enhanced with the multi-tunnel fat grafting technique described previously for lip enhancement. At one year, it appears as if he had a silastic chin implant, but the effect was achieved with fat grafting alone.

Figures 26–27. The "classic" positioning of malar silastic implants provides even greater improvement with time. A young woman is shown preoperatively in 1980 in Figure 26 and in 1990 in Figure 27.

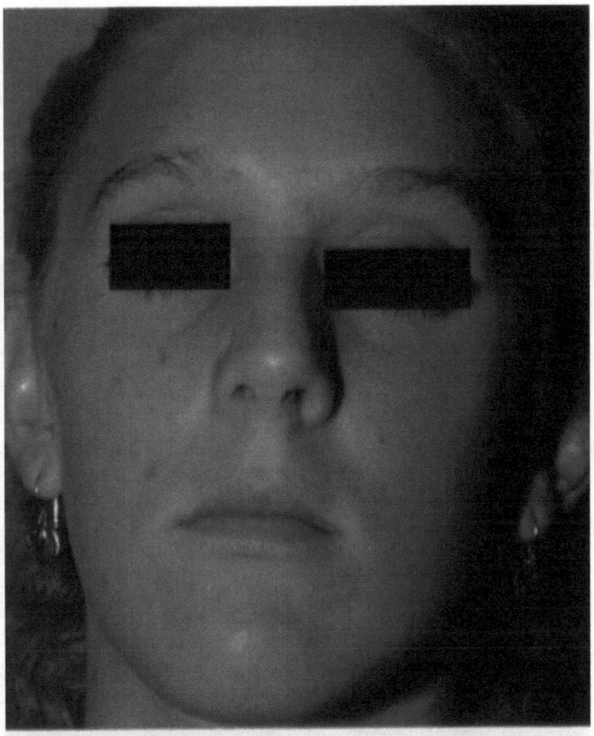

26

27

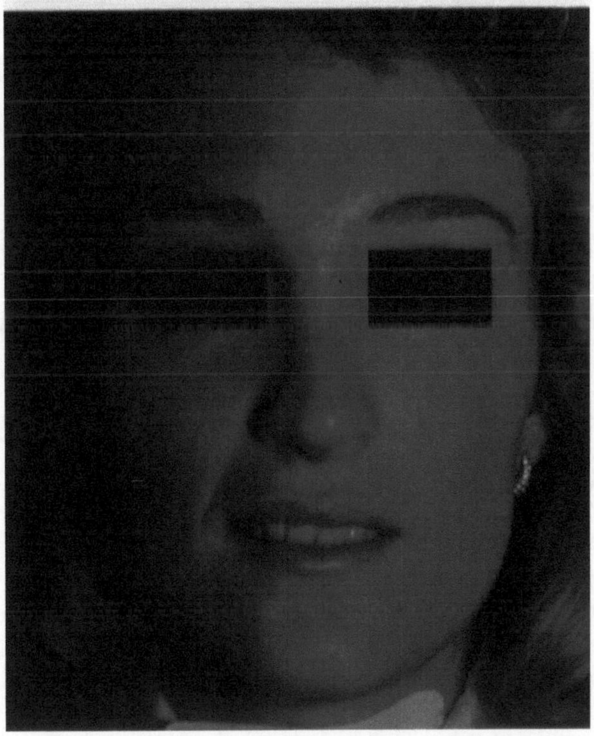

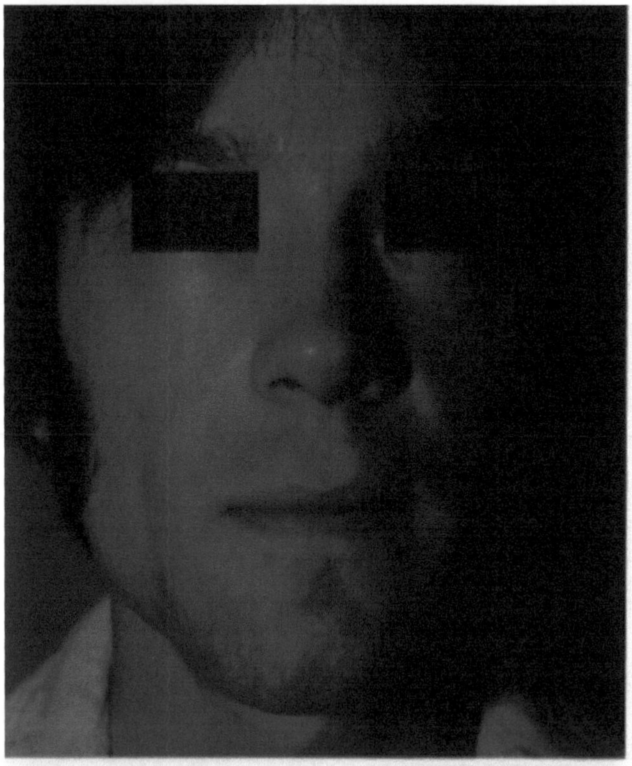

28

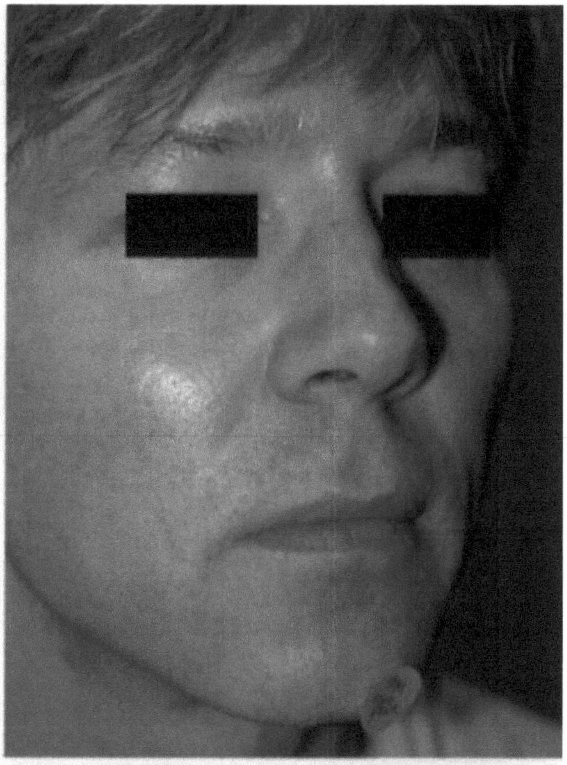

30

29

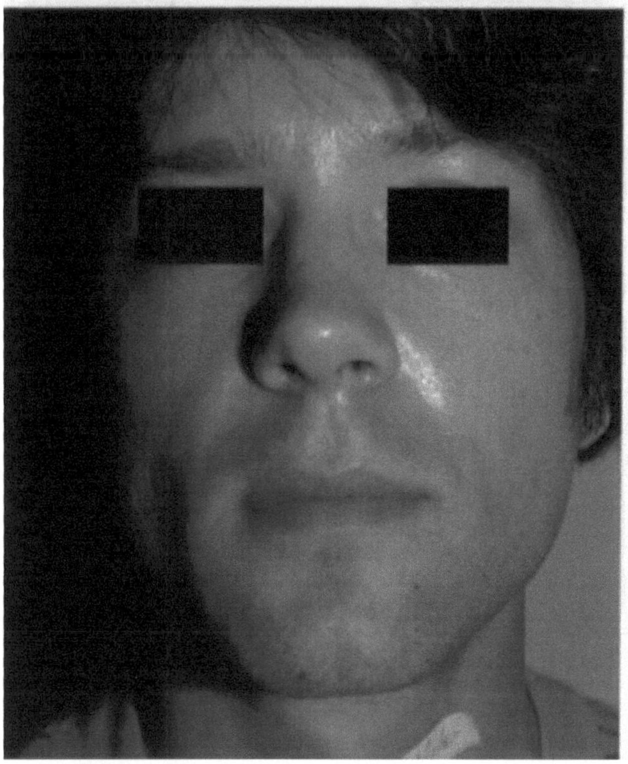

31

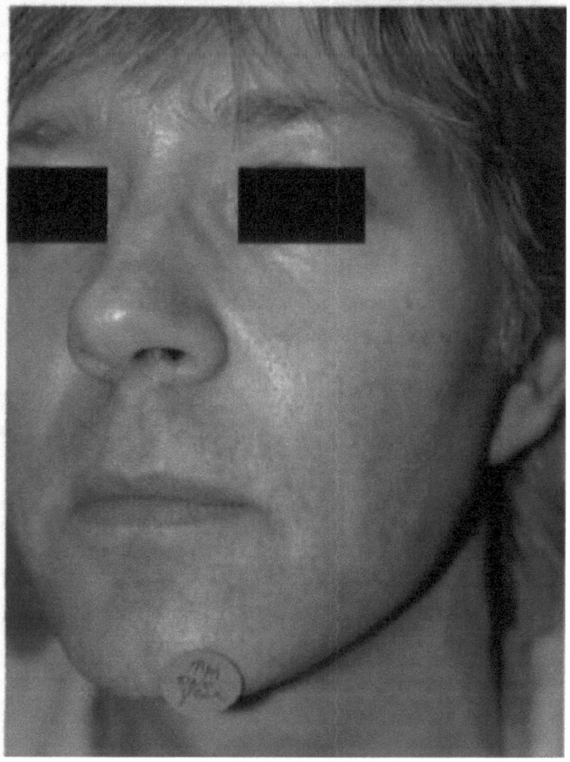

Figures 28–31. Fat grafting in combination with malar silastic augmentation gave a pleasing result in a patient who resented his "Rock Star" facial appearance (Figure 28). The initial corrections were with a "½ face lift" procedure in 1982 (Figure 29). The final correction, in 1992, was with secondary mid-face skin tightening, "shell" type malar implants, and fat grafts to the triangle below, between the malar implant and the jawline (Figures 30 and 31) plus an ongoing Retin-A/glycolic acid program and Micropeels.

Figures 32–35. This young adult with acne and severe sun damage initially requested only a filling of a deep glabellar frown line. Figure 32 shows the undercorrection that was achieved by fat grafting in the undermined area. Corrugator thickness and attachment were also disrupted from the same hairline stab wound as described in the text. Further correction involved local anesthesia and a second minor fat graft. The patient holds the ice-cold "Cryoglobe" (Medical Cosmetic Services) on the area (Figure 33) before a local anesthetic is painlessly injected.

Contrast the skin quality and facial lines in the black and white photograph taken one and a half years earlier, with the appearance in color (Figure 34). She had just completed a series of 40% glycolic acid "aesthetician's peels." Figure 35 shows the improvement in skin "rejuvenation" achieved six months later. The deep glabellar line is still corrected at two years.

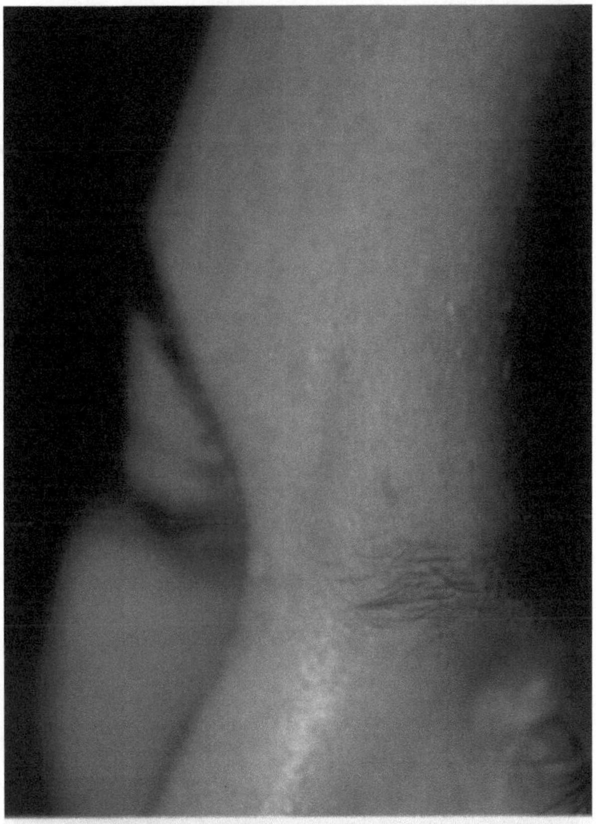

32

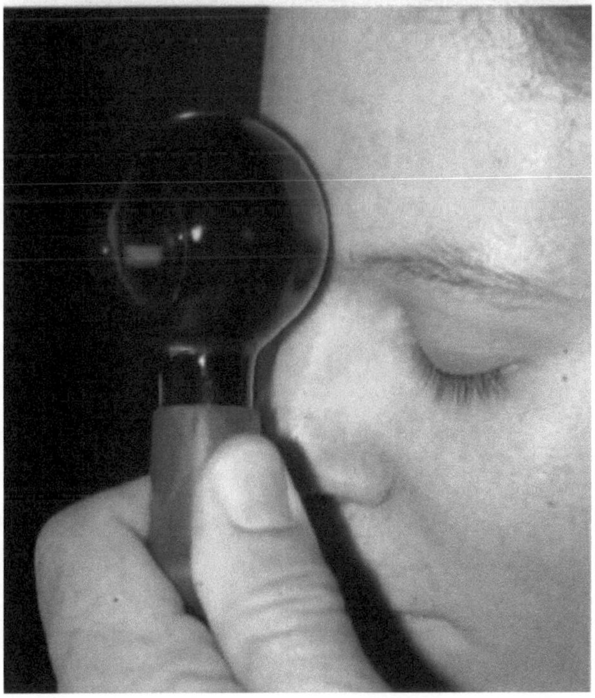

33

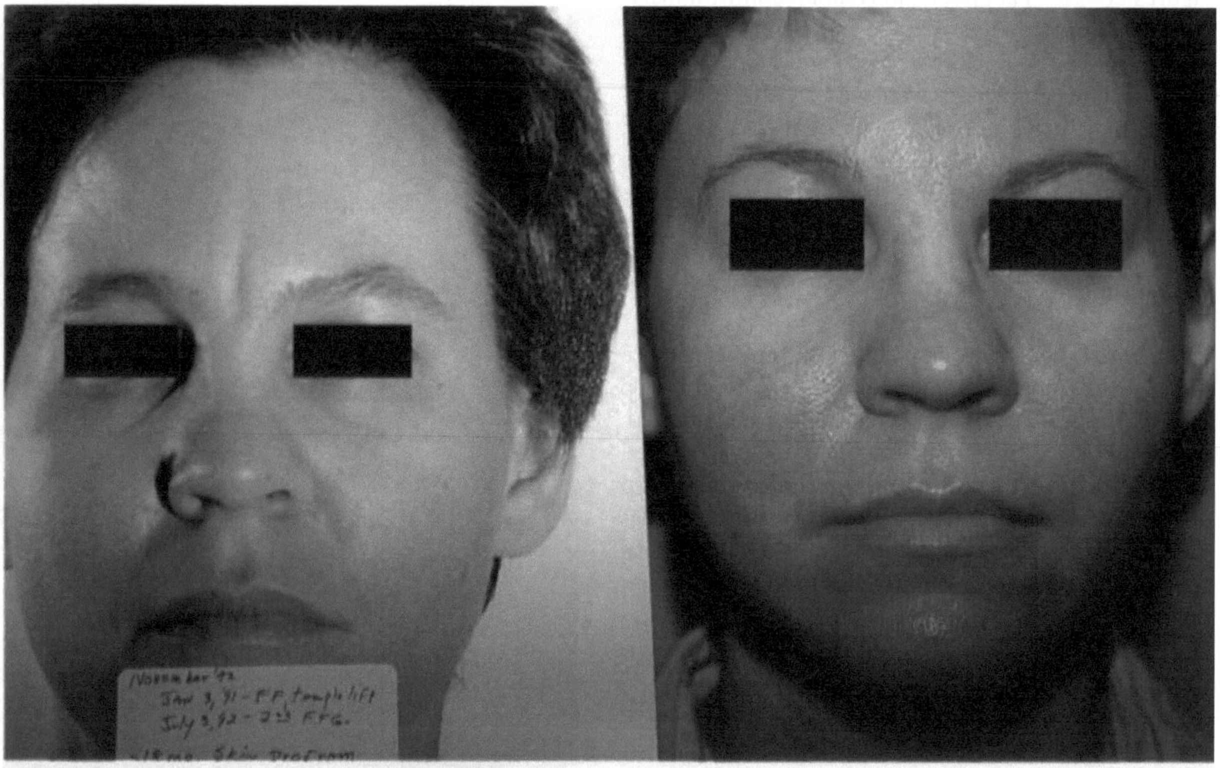

34

35

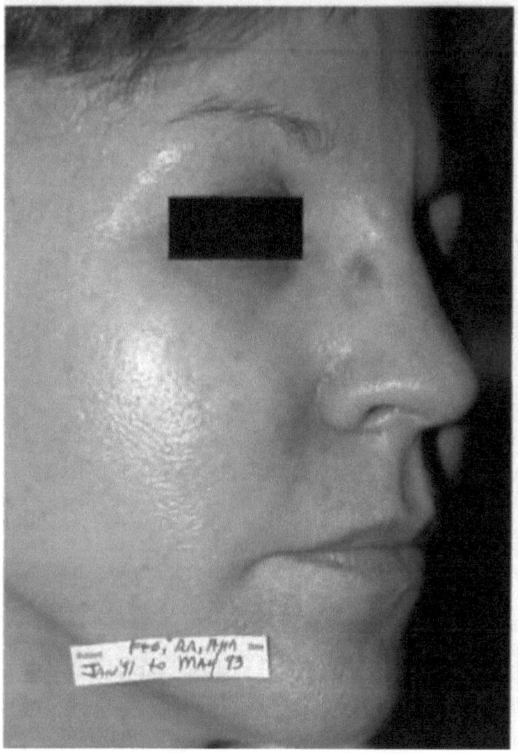

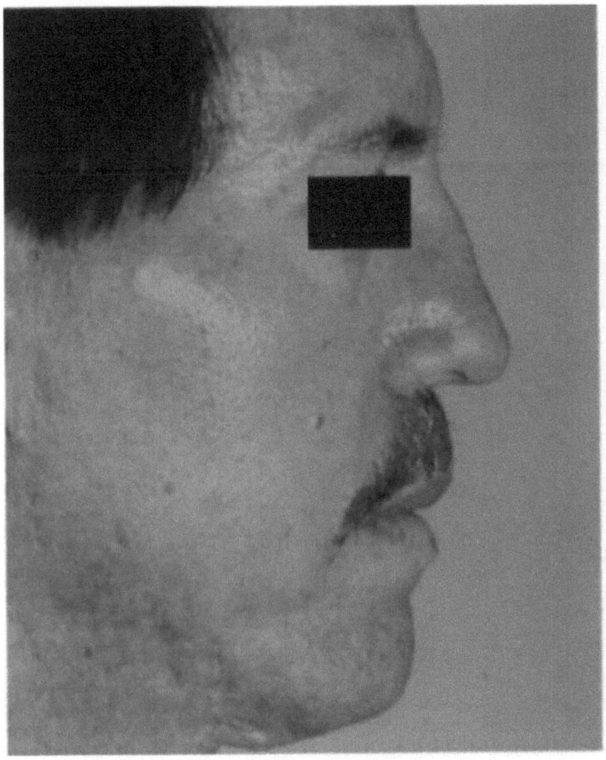

36

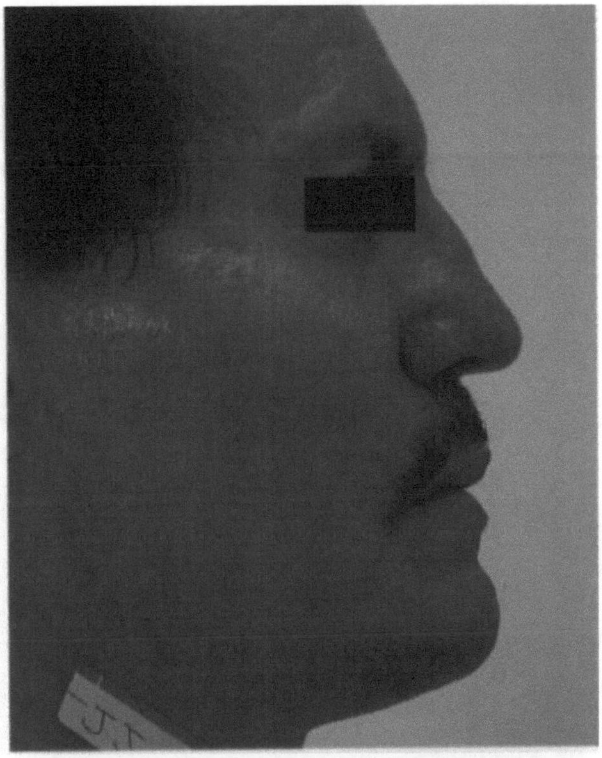

37

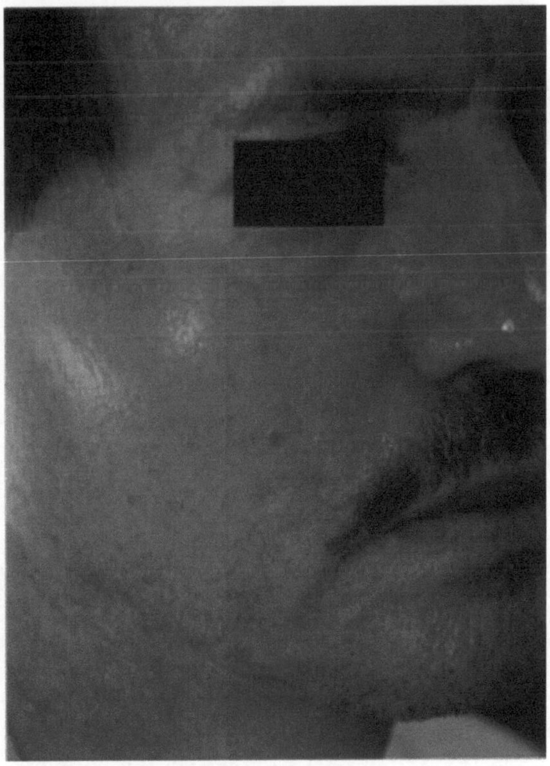

38

Figures 36–38. For the adult acne patient, fat grafting beneath acne-scarred areas and skin stretching offered by malar and chin augmentation sclastic implants are complemented by a vigorous "home program" of Retin-A and glycolic acid. Contrast the shadows and oiliness of this patient's skin in the preoperative black and white photograph in Figure 36. We choose black and white photographs to fully illustrate the lines and shadows so that each patient may appreciate the progress they have effected under our direction.

At two years, the daily application of glycolic acid and Retin-A creams, and several 40% AHA "aestheticians peels," have significantly altered the skin texture (Figures 37 and 38) without skin bleaching. Male patients are even more intolerant of white patches than female patients. Notice also the tightness of skin beneath the chin. No skin excisions have been performed.

39
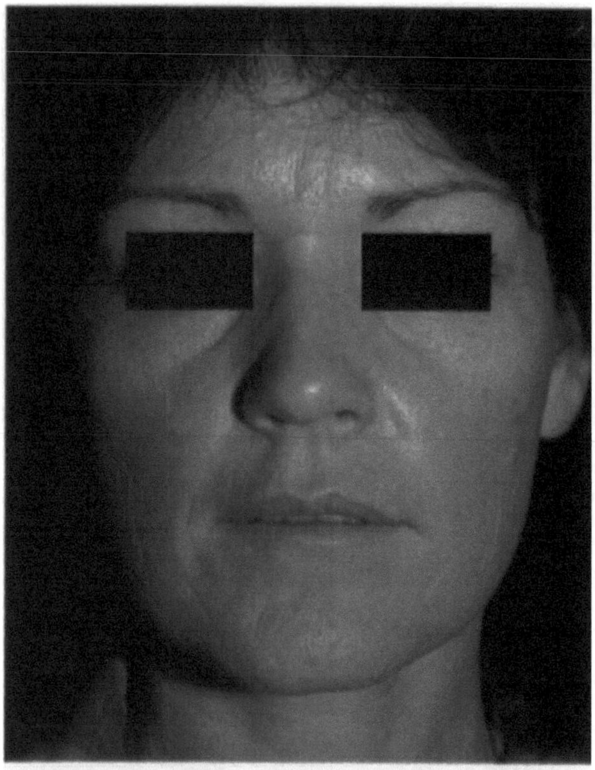

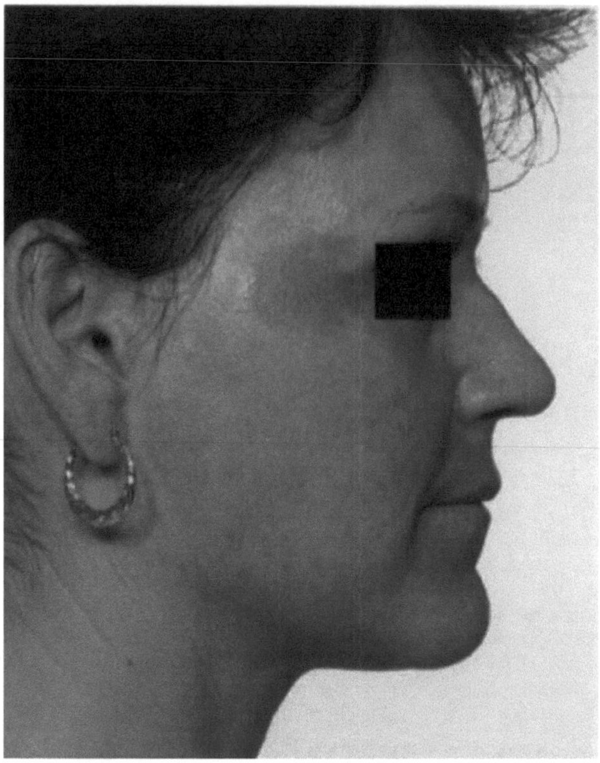
41

40
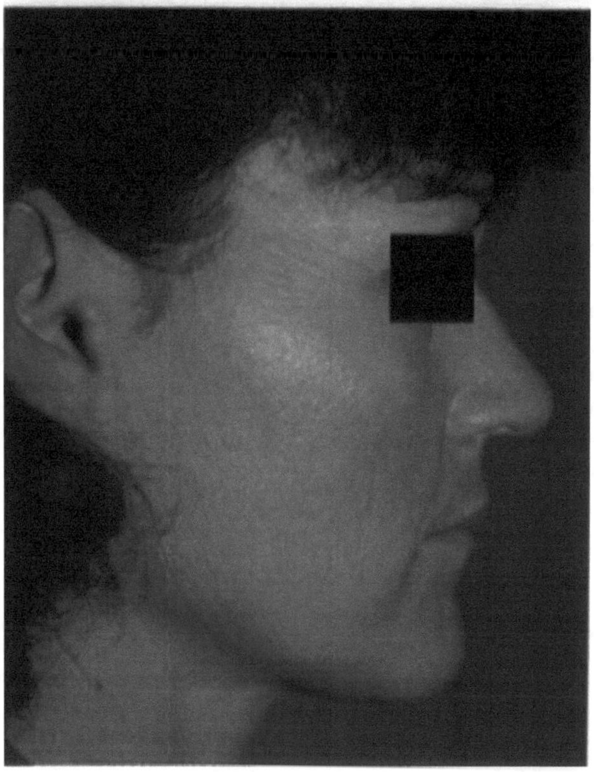

Figures 39–45. Before becoming aware of the advantages of TCA, we used spot peels of Baker's Formula phenol diluted by one-half with saline to limit the depth of the peel. A severely skin-damaged young woman is shown preoperatively in 1985 in Figures 39 and 40 and with color corrective cosmetics ($GlamouR_X$) applied at the tenth postoperative day in Figures 41 and 42.

Unfortunately, even the lesser concentration of phenol can create spotty bleaching (Figure 43). The only help we can offer is our ongoing glycolic and Retin-A program, and a blending TCA peel to minimize the contrast. The improvement shown in the 1992 photos in Figures 44 and 45 is acceptable when complemented by a minimum of makeup applied under the instruction of our medical aesthetician.

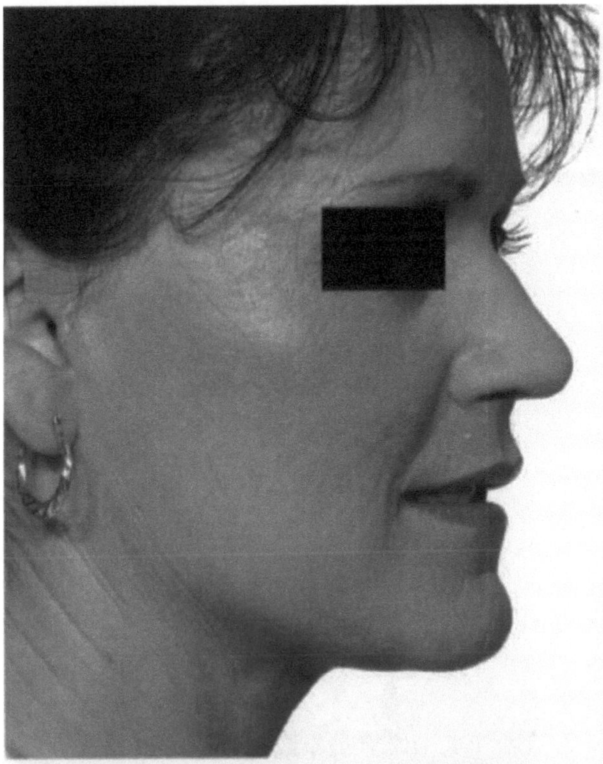
42

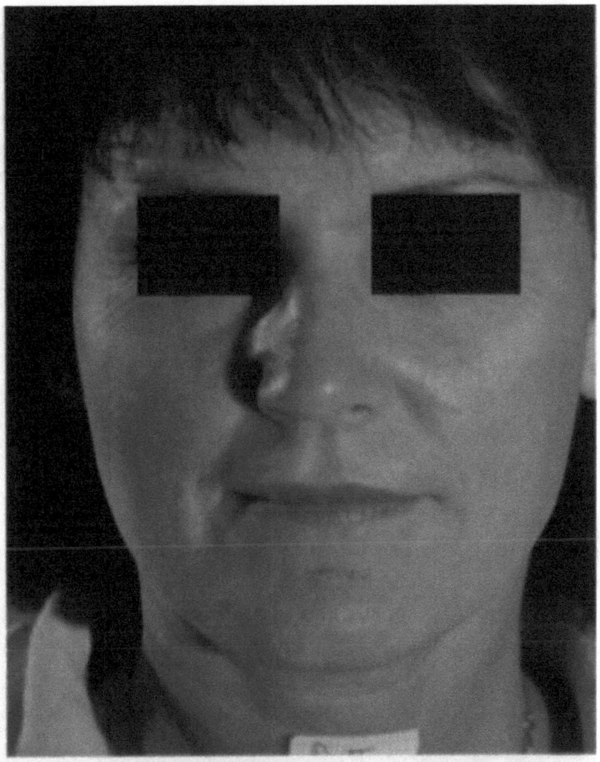
44

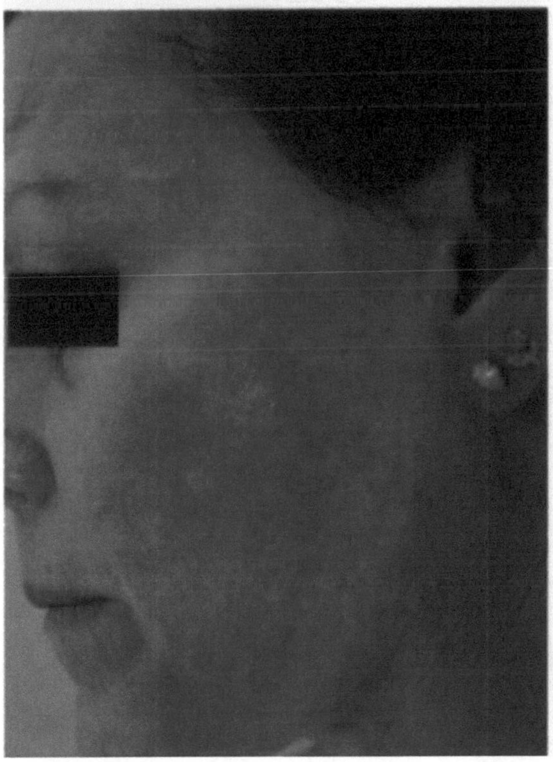
43

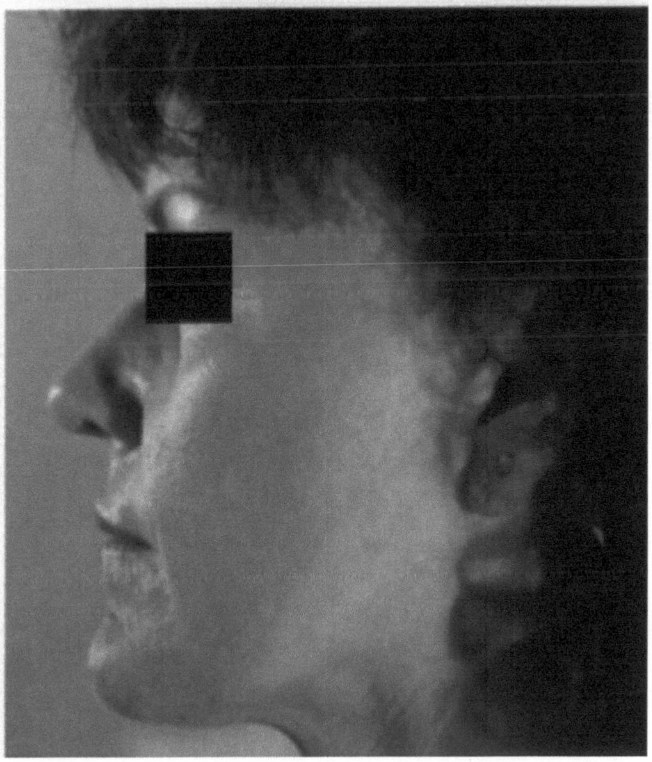
45

46
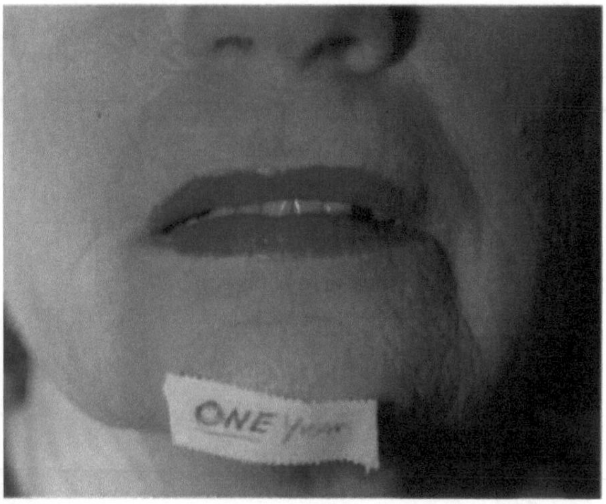

Figure 46. Correction of facial rhytids without skin bleaching is a breakthrough improvement in surgery of the ageing face for patients who have deeply wrinkled lips. After correction, the plump, natural-colored appearance is shown at one year. Undermining and fat grafting the vertical lines and the white roll area, light scalpel-edge abrasion of rough spots, and a 35% TCA lip peel with an occasional "touch-up peel" consistently produce this satisfying result.

Introduction

TECHNICAL DETAILS AND INDIVIDUAL APPROACHES TO THE PREvention or correction of problems occupy much time in the world of plastic surgery. This text addresses those issues and reviews my personal experience in evaluating new techniques. With the help of contributions from some of the best minds in plastic surgery, I emphasize herein what we used to do and how we have changed those outmoded techniques and philosophies, and I detail the problem-solving methods that have contributed to the evolution of our specialty. The emphasis here is on technical expertise. Therefore there is not an overabundance of pre- and postoperative photographs. The presentations are limited to aesthetic surgical problems that are "hot topics."

We plastic surgeons are dealing with a generation of healthy people who have an intense interest in self-improvement and in eliminating what they deem personal deficiencies—educational, mental, medical, personal, and physical. Our patients are becoming as critical of our work as we are ourselves, and they are often knowledgeable about technical details. They therefore appreciate the concern for the restoration of a natural appearance and reject with us the artificial "operated on" look of many of our earlier efforts.

My hope is that the reader will learn from my experience, my mistakes, and my attempts to duplicate efforts of others—and in turn contribute to the next edition of this text, which will continue our mutual quest for perfection.

It is a fact of life that tissues heal in an unpredictable fashion, and sometimes body parts react in an undesirable way. The nose, for example, perversely tends to return to its original shape; and stress, gravity, fibrocystic disease, pregnancy, and normal male-female relationships affect the size, shape, position, and comfort of the breasts.

Although rejecting the unhealthy demand for super-thinness (the "social x-ray" described by Tom Wolfe), we do have a healthy appreciation of a body habitus, both male and female. Liposuction was not a good procedure at first but has now become an integral part of many surgeries. Removal of nonresponsive fatty deposits and reinjection of fat to soften or correct contour deformities has replaced unsafe practices. Discussed here are the planning for less obvious scars, limiting incision lengths, and hiding incisions. My correspondents and I discuss the wishes of our patients for corrections that fit within new bathing suit styles, requests for fuller lips or higher malar prominences, and clear, youthful skin. I emphasize adjunctive programs that have become widely important, particularly skin rejuvenation programs. α-Hydroxy acids, "refresher" peels. The use of tretinoin (Retin-A), and skin care are integral parts of our office regimen.

The successful plastic surgeon sees patients treated years ago. We hope this book will stimulate you to look critically at your results, evaluate them with the current knowledge, and apply the lessons that have been learned through years of experience. We also discuss "reoperations," so the new results conform to the more recently accepted standards of excellence. These evolving concepts may be new to some of the readers, and there are problems yet to solve.

Humor is important in our specialty. We cannot change society, and we cannot change men and women. The group will always envy the individual with the new Cadillac, the diamond ring, the beautiful skin. Modern women still care as much for their families and home life, but they are equally involved with their appearance, their health, and their well-being.

It has been often said that, "Men grow distinguished, but women grow old." Not so. We are now helping men get back into the job market with a natural rested appearance achieved by face lifting, nose surgery, fat grafting, and skin rejuvenation. A patient may be highly motivated, whether male or female.

In the chapter on skin rejuvenation we emphasize the use of glycolic acid, and Retin-A, sunblocks. Moisturizers substitute for makeup in male patients. For female patients, the moisturizer plays a secondary role to Retin-A/chemical peel-compatible makeup. Our role in modern plastic surgery is aesthetics as well as the overall appearance and well-being of the patient. The days are long gone when we concerned ourselves only with the structure of bone and soft tissue.

Do not expect a long list of references with each chapter. There are a number of good plastic surgery textbooks that can provide such references. This book is concerned with hands-on experience and notes the contributors by name. Ideas and approaches to problems are summarized. Do not hesitate to call on the contributing surgeons: They are more than willing to discuss techniques with you—what they are doing and how they do it.

Be aware that in a few years much of what we discuss here will be as obsolete as the "old techniques" to which we refer. Plastic surgery is a dynamic, changing specialty. We are able to achieve what we and our patients want with greater accuracy despite Mother Nature. We improve on "old" procedures. When we discuss the "internal" repair work hidden under the skin in face lift or breast lift, the procedures are not new, just improved.

A cardinal rule is to avoid overdoing or overcomplicating operations. The new chemical peels, open rhinoplasties, breast surgery without major scarring, even the simplest hair transplants are discussed here. My particular interests lie in lip enhancement, eliminating age lines, fat recycling, and restoration of the aging face. Emphasized are avoidance of the "stigmata" of the rejuvenated face: the white lips, pulled-down earlobes, overly tight cheeks, "surprised" forehead without expression, and so forth.

A decade ago we were leery of any technique that came from South America, France, and Switzerland, the lands of "no complications, no problems." Now we have opened our eyes to brilliant surgeons from many countries, and with this recognition have improved our standard plastic surgery procedures and achieved results of which we could only dream.

Do we have happier patients? Perhaps. We certainly are happier with ourselves and our abilities because we have learned to listen to our patients' complaints and made an effort to correct the problems they see. Two examples come to mind. The most brilliant breast reductions and breast reconstructions, when viewed by a layman, are quite different than when viewed by an academic surgeon. Can we not reconstruct, rebuild, or reduce without lengthy warnings about the "trade-off" of scars and deformity? Yes, we can. The story of the Mexican plastic surgeon who was asked if he was bothered by lawsuits comes to mind. "Yes," he said, "I had one such patient. She came into my office threatening to sue me." "What did you do," we asked? "I called my brother-in-law, the chief of police, and that was the end of the problem." We do not have that privilege in the United States, and the improvements in our techniques certainly do not guarantee against dissatisfaction and malpractice suits. However, if we feels better about ourselves and our technical capabilities, that is a step in the right direction.

"My heroes have always been cowboys." The same sense of adventure motivates my other heroes, those brilliant and innovative plastic surgeons from the generation slightly ahead of me as well as my contemporaries and those who are pushing hard from behind. The list is endless, but I must single out a few of my "heroes," beginning with my professors: Francis X. Paletta, Kenneth Pickrell, and Nick Georgiade. They made enormous contributions to my understanding of the basic sciences and aesthetic plastic surgery. The men I call my contemporaries and friends, such as Mario Gonzales-Ulloa, Jose Guerro-Santos, Ivo Pitanguy, Rex Peterson, and Gene Courtiss, are the new generation of "old timers" (a title that has been directed at me more than once and firmly rejected). Cowboys are daring, and credit must go to the cowboys of my plastic surgery generation: Adrien Aiache, Luis Toledo, Shel Rosenthal, Greg Hetter, Gus Colon, Steve Hoefflin, Peter McKinney, Mark Mandel, Mark Rubin, Ewaldo Souza-Pinto, Bruce Connell, Alan Matarasso, Oscar Ramirez, and Hilton Becker. For those of you I neglected to name, accept my apologies. Also, my two older brothers who were role models. Charles, my oldest brother who is a general, vascular & chest surgeon, and Harold, the chairman of the Neurosurgery department at the University of Massachusetts.

Lastly, I must recognize my wife, Suzanne Wilkinson. Our clinic struggled with postsurgical makeup and skin care for 10 years before I asked her to take up the difficult task of designing and manufacturing cosmetics specifically tailored to the plastic surgery patient. For the candidate and the chemical peel patient, she designed programs of preoperative skin preparation and postoperative maintenance that we describe here in detail. She has also supported me in my travels, lectures, and writings, and has indulged me my beloved sport, polo. Thanks, honey!

PART ONE

The Face

Introduction

THE FIRST CHAPTERS IN THIS SECTION ADDRESS THE TECHNIQUES and philosophies on which modern aesthetic surgery are based. All surgeons concerned with aesthetics must change with the times, which means changing the results to accord with patients' wishes as well as adopting new techniques and new approaches to old problems.

In the idealized face, the skin quality should not show the effects of wind, weather, sun damage, and aging. The chapter on facial rejuvenation addresses the techniques of multilevel peels, fat grafting, and alternatives to face lifts. Such alternatives may involve approaching the midface descent with malar augmentation, stretching crumpled skin with a contoured prosthesis, or simply plumping the area with a series of staged fat grafts.

The idealized face has a smooth contour, a masculine or feminine chin that is prominent but not overly so, and a smooth jawline. The chapter on the submental tuck addresses the role of liposuction which, in combination with the traditional platysmal resection and plication, produces dramatic improvement. The changes in cheek contour, which are individual choices, reflect the changes in the prosthetic materials. I advocate Silastic contoured prostheses for most patients with emphasis on their obvious advantages over other materials and other shapes and forms.

I address also the position, size, and contour of the lips. The aging process withers the lips, whereas youthful lips are full. We can create this effect with a number of techniques. The surgeon chooses the technique depending on the patient's wishes and desires. We do not waste time discussing the "Paris lip"—the illegal, unsuccessful attempt to create a full lip by injecting collagen material in the tissues. The same lip can be created with lip roll procedures or fat grafting, or a combination of the two.

The "elegant eyelid" involves contouring and elevating the lateral eyebrow. The currently available choices of submuscular, subdermal, or transconjunctival blepharoplasty are herein contrasted with traditional techniques. Today our approach frequently involves a trichloroacetic acid peel to the bridge of the nose, forehead, crow's feet areas, and eyelids. Even with submuscular blepharoplasty, this technique would have been dangerous with the level V Baker Gordon formula phenol peel.

The contrast between a "manly look" and a feminine one, particularly when it involves eyebrow position and the depth of the eyelid fold, is addressed.

Selective use of the open technique for rhinoplasty can be helpful. Emphasis must be placed on the patient's choice of shape, size, and configuration. Some surgeons seem fixated on tilted tips or high dorsums which may well satisfy certain individuals, but one must be prepared to create a shape that fits the patient's face and personality. Furthermore, following the lead of surgeons with extensive experience in ethnic rhinoplasty, I attempt to put this subject in perspective and add a few of my own preferences and precautions.

Another particular interest of mine has been the secondary face lift—achieving a natural appearance with hair in all the right places and hidden incisions. The technical points of placing incisions around the tragus, rotating hair upward or downward in the "double opposing rotation procedure," and methods for ensuring that an earlobe hangs free (and is reduced in bulk) are discussed. Techniques to reduce tension in certain areas and provide extra tightening in others are important considerations when creating a natural face lift.

Whether to risk over complicating a procedure or taking on additional risk is a sobering question. My preference is to avoid extended dissections. For example, I believe that one can create a natural face lift with a lesser procedure and certainly with a low risk of annoying complications. I discuss the patients with midface descent who can benefit from skin rejuvenation, chemical peeling, and the so-called midface lift. Suction and fat grafting add elegant touches and should become part of the plastic surgeon's armamentarium.

In the chapter on breast surgery, most of the discussion involves choices and techniques in breast augmentation and mastopexy, with a subsection on a particular interest of mine, circumareolar breast reduction, mastopexy, and internal repair of the postaugmentation breast. The differences in life style of the West and the East, as well as personal choices by women determine placement of the incision as well as the ultimate size, shape, and projection. I try here to cut through the maze of statistics and self-aggrandizing promotions to provide you with the best information on aesthetic surgery of the breast.

The illusion mastopexy, with a minimal incision, creates a breast that is quite natural but more "mature." We borrow heavily from the experience of Erol and Brazilians in an effort to eliminate the T scar during reductions and mastopexies. You will become familiar with the "Texas Diamond," the "Toledo triangle," the "double Benelli stitch," and a concept of social and therapeutic brassieres.

The chapter on abdominoplasty is interesting. The changing times are reflected in patient requests for shorter incisions and French line closures. With increasing use of liposuction, certain technical maneuvers must be undertaken to ensure that the closures are without tension lest the blood supply be compromised. Liposuction plays an important role, and my preferences for particular techniques and approaches are described along with simple ways of protecting the flap and creating a new umbilicus with a minimum of fuss.

Regarding the subject of liposuction: Most of the discussion focuses on how superficial suction works, how to prevent problems, and the value of fat regrafting for treating the condition called "cellulite."

In the chapter on miscellaneous subjects I touch briefly on a number of areas. They include buttock and pectoral augmentations. Also discussed are helpful hints for running an office surgical center.

My hope is that this book, with its collection of comments from outstanding surgeons as well as my personal prejudices and experiences, will prove useful to you. I hope that it will stimulate you to share your experiences with me—with an eye on a later edition.

1 Facial Rejuvenation

FACIAL REJUVENATION HAS RADICALLY CHANGED. IT INVOLVES new ideas about "bone structure" changes (malar, extended chin, angle of the mandible implants), soft tissue enhancement (lip "rolls" and grafts, facial liposuction, fat grafts), and the trichloroacetic acid (TCA) peel preceded and continued with a controlled Retin-A program. Protection from ultraviolet rays is incorporated into cosmetics, and compatible components are added to sunscreens and cosmetics.

The chemical peeling technique is different as well. We do not go so far as to say there is no place for phenol peels. Even with the changes that have been incorporated—no tape, antibiotic ointment only, and less aggressive skin cleansing—the basic problem of the toxicity of phenol to melanocytes remains, resulting in white, sun-sensitive faces or, worse yet, a white perioral ring in a normally pigmented face. It is easier to avoid this problem altogether by using TCA or other "new" peels.

Spurred by sensational media descriptions and offerings of expensive training courses in skin rejuvenation, the combined efforts of plastic surgeons, aestheticians, cosmetologists, and dermatologists have produced a logical, progressive regimen of skin rejuvenation that involves Retin-A (tretinoin), skin cleansing programs, and a combination of alphahydroxy acid, various strengths of phenol, and TCA peeling solutions, often supplemented by superficial dermabrasion.

Treating Severe Skin Damage

Severe skin damage can be caused by unsupervised use of Retin-A, a topical compound that induces thickening of the collagen and elastin content of the dermis. The first step in facial skin rejuvenation is a safe but effective treatment regimen with Retin-A. It involves counseling by trained personnel and close supervision to avoid the problems that might result from, for example, the fact that it is incompatible with certain sun blocks, moisturizers, and ingredients in common cosmetics. Hence the use of Retin-A and chemical-peel-compatible protective makeup is taught to patients in our clinic. The skin care products we use are specifically designed for use with Retin-A and the chemicals used on peel patients based on our 20 years of experience.

In essence, the patient begins with the use of minimal concentrations of Retin-A or 9% α-hydroxy acid cream (or both) at infrequent intervals and gradually progresses to daily applications from the clavicle to the forehead hairline. Non-PABA (paraaminobenzoic acid) sun blocks are incorporated in all facial products to protect the rapidly changing surface of the skin. Patients are then allowed to progress to stronger concentrations of Retin-A. After a period of about 6 months each patient is evaluated as a possible candidate for a "mix and match" chemical peel with or without dermabrasion.

The ultimate in skin rejuvenation involves techniques of fat grafting to elevate depressions, eliminate acne scars, and reduce wrinkle lines, combined with new techniques of skin care and chemical peeling. For whatever reasons, our practice is shifting more and more toward facial rejuvenation, which works hand and glove with facial cosmetic surgery. Fat grafting plays an important role.

Chemical peeling no longer has to be an "all or none" phenomenon. The Baker formula (5 ml phenol, 4 ml distilled water, 3 drops croton oil, 5 drops hexachlorophene) is effective, but its safety margin is narrower than many desire. Added to this problem is the longer recovery time and the occurrence of skin whitening. Other dermatologists have used various formulas for what was termed a "light peel" to freshen the skin temporarily; these peels do not remove pigment to the same degree.

State of the art methods today allow choosing the depth of penetration and the chemicals necessary to support that decision. The key to achieving rejuvenation, however, is preparing the skin with Retin-A, which must always be used with care. Our in-house program's success is reflected by the number of patients who continue to use Retin A.

We have found through trial and error that a minimum of 2 weeks of Retin-A pretreatment is necessary to achieve the desired effects of a "mixed peel" (TCA/dilute phenol peel, two formulas on the same face). The Obaji technique is one of many ways of preparing the skin, but only one formula (50% TCA) is used with that method. I propose a less risky approach: We prepare the skin in the operating room with alcohol, not acetone, for a less "stripping" effect. We initially apply 35% TCA to the areas that need "freshening" but do not use it for deeper areas of dark skin coloration. For those areas, we use a single application of dilute Baker's formula phenol. Deeply pigmented spots and the white roll area of the lip are treated with full-strength undiluted Baker's formula.

Surgeons vary their approach to the skin preparation, but we generally agree that TCA alone is insufficient in certain areas. Although dilute phenol works best in most cases for problems of the upper lip, lower eyelid, and crow's feet area, fat grafting plus repeated 35% TCA peels is a better technique in these patients.

Our success with lipografts was inconsistent in 1986. Tunneling with a 16 gauge needle produced incomplete release of deep fibers, and the fat was literally "injected" under pressure into a compressed space. The procedure sometimes helped, but usually it failed.

A spatula-like dissector was the answer. Using the flat "rhytid dissector" (Byron Medical), we are able to elevate the deep dermis safely and create a tension-free spot for careful placement of concentrated lipografts in the lip, "marionette" area, and facial lines. We have now achieved a 95+% success rate; and scores of patients have good to excellent fat grafts that have lasted more than 7 years. In the older patient, fat grafting simply elevates vertical lip lines and facial creases so a deep peel is not required to achieve smoothness.

The key to success is to increase the safety margin. It is far better to come back and touch up an area with peel solution than it is to risk a hypertrophic scar or whitened area. Postoperative steroids and hydroquinones are prescribed for the 30 days following the peel and grafting, and the Retin-A program is resumed later but at a much slower pace with lower concentrations. Retin-A is much more effective after a "mixed" peel than after a single-solution peel. These techniques are simple maneuvers and can largely be controlled by an aesthetician.

Skin Rejuvenation Technique

Rejuvenation of the skin involves more than just a chemical peel and covering makeup. Skin rejuvenation requires specially trained medical cosmetologists or aestheticians who understand the skin and how to care for it. It is part of the surgeon's responsibility to be knowledgeable about the concepts involved in Retin-A and α-hydroxy acid programs and to be thus able to adequately care for patients with TCA peels, mixed peels, and dermabrasions. It is not uncommon for patients to ask: "What do I use after surgery?" The following general guidelines can help avoid many posttreatment problems.

1. With selective use of color correctors, Retin-A, and skin-peel-compatible makeups, patients can appear in public within 10 days of any

surgery or chemical peel. The exception is the patient who has had a level five peel with Baker's formula.

2. Preoperative consultations relieve patient anxiety. Patients should learn about color selection, covering makeup, and long-term skin care; and they are assured that someone will be caring for them after their surgery.
3. Each new patient should be placed on a Retin-A regimen with gradual progression.
4. The overriding rule of a Retin-A program is "don't peel, don't burn."
5. Each patient sets his or her own pace for progression of the Retin A regimen. Some patients reach third level (0.10%) in 6 months, and others achieve this goal in 6 weeks. Second level (0.05%) is the highest concentration some patients' skin can tolerate.
6. The glycolic acid creams (e.g., α-hydroxy, glycolic, or lactic acid) are useful. First, they instantly smooth the skin, so the patients are not discouraged by the slow progress of the Retin-A treatment. Second, they facilitate penetration of the Retin-A, thus producing a stronger effect. The "micro-peel" program is very helpful.
7. The chemical peels that involve TCA and other combinations depend on skin preparation, and Retin-A is the key.
8. There are a number of ways to prepare the skin for peeling. There is no secret formula or magic potion.
9. A minimum of 14 days of skin preparation with Retin-A and α-hydroxy acids allow one to achieve the desired effect of a chemical peel without the drawbacks of the early phenol peels. There is little discomfort or "down-time." Most importantly, skin color is preserved.
10. The aesthetician can advise patients about their progress from first- to second- to third-level Retin-A, how often they should use α-hydroxy acid creams, and when a "micropeel" booster may be added.
11. The 35% α-hydroxy acid peel is the "aestheticians' peel." We call it a second-level peel, and it is a good "jump start" for the skin care patient. The surgeon does not have to be present or perform second-level chemical peels. It is done by the aesthetician as are "Micro-peels".*
12. For third-, fourth-, or fifth-level peels, the physician must be the one to apply the chemicals.
13. Preparation of the skin before the peel is important for determining the depth of a peel. Jessner's solution and acetone are skin strippers; however, because TCA may penetrate deeply, medical grade alcohol is

*Micropeel™, Biomedic Clinical Care, 8757 East Viade Commercio, Scottsdale, AZ 85258.

a safer agent to use. For certain areas, an additional TCA application may be needed for a slightly deeper peel.

14. TCA is not like phenol. Once phenol is applied—in either its dilute form or its full-strength Baker formula—it stops working. The depth of peel, then, is increased only by inducing maceration; we once used waterproof tape for this purpose. The depth of penetration of a TCA peel depends on volume and repeat application.
15. The eyelids may be treated with TCA using a Q-tip. For deeper peels on the cheeks, apply pressure on the skin using a 2 × 2 gauze. The endpoint is uniform frosting.
16. Aftercare is essential. Steroid creams, hydroquinone (Eldoquin) bleaches, or both are used before and after the TCA peels to prevent problems of hyperpigmentation.
17. Full-strength Baker formula phenol may be used on the white roll of the lip or to bleach an exceptionally dark spot. If a slightly deeper peel than TCA is needed, use dilute "half-strength" Baker formula. (I prefer repeated applications of TCA to achieve a higher than 35% concentration in areas that were formerly treated with "half-strength phenol formula.")
18. Start aloe vera based oil applications 3 to 4 days after a TCA or mixed peel. Add a topical steroid and possibly skin bleach to the regimen shortly thereafter.
19. Initiate the Retin-A program 30 days later. Begin with the least concentrated formula, i.e., 0.025% Retin-A, three times a week maximum. Warn the patient to progress slowly to avoid developing skin burns.
20. As with any facial surgery, Solu-Cortef 100 mg IV or methylprednisolone (Medrol Dosepak) orally helps to reduce the swelling and return the patient more quickly to normal activities.

Five Levels of Chemical Face Peeling

Little attention was paid to chemical peeling before Tom Baker and Howard Gordon introduced the Baker formula. Plastic surgeons had noted that flash burn patients healed with attractive skin; they also noted that skin that had been kept out of the sun, for whatever reason, did not seem to age. Unfortunately, there was little communication between us and our dermatology colleagues.

We once told patients that chemical peels were useful, but only for patients who were older and who did not plan to engage in outdoor activities. The phenol/croton oil formulas we used are what we would now call a level five peel, the "all or none" method. These techniques were effective, but complications were frequent. We peeled the entire face as far as the jawline, leaving the patient with a brown neck, hands, and so on. Even worse was the practice of using the Baker formula on the upper and lower lip. These patients had a white zone that was obvious and difficult to cover with makeup. The patients had not anticipated such a result. Clyde Litton, another pioneer, pointed this out.

Chemical face peeling must be considered a selective procedure. The first level of peeling is with a closely monitored, graduated regimen of tretinoin application. This drug is used to prepare the skin for chemical peeling, but it has a rejuvenation effect of its own if carefully applied. Unfortunately, it can also damage the skin if it is applied too frequently, in too great a concentration, or in conjunction with certain common cosmetic ingredients that sensitize the skin.

Retin-A and α-hydroxy acid creams thicken the deep dermal layers and induce epidermal turnover, which we call *first level peel.* Products with glycolic acid are used in our "home program" along with tretinoin.

Second level peel is accomplished with a 35% glycolic or lactic acid solution. This "rapid exfoliation" is the aesthetician's peel. Medical cosmetologists use this peel once a week until at least five to ten ultralight peels have been done. The acid is neutralized within 1 to 3 minutes by spraying with water. An office technician must be trained in medical cosmetology so the peel is not allowed to become too deep and is not performed too frequently. In "micropeels," we use 30% glycolic.

A

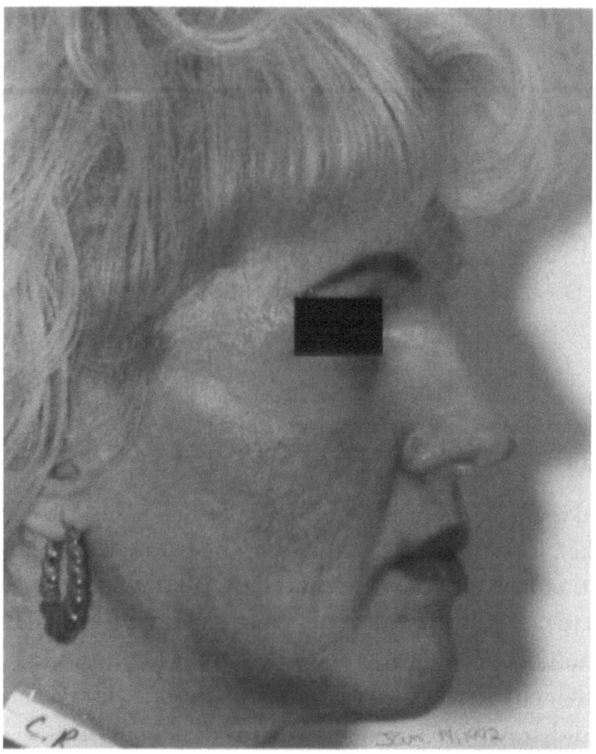

Figure 1-1. Facial rejuvenation. This patient, who lives on a yacht in the Caribbean, did not have time to prepare her skin with Retin-A. Her midface acne scars were worse on the right. Two years before these pictures she underwent a mixed peel with dermabrasion; fat grafts were applied to the glabella, nasolabial line, lips, and under the acne scars; and then a single touch-up was done with a TCA peel. She then undertook 18 months of AHA and Retin-A applications with sunscreens.

Third level peel is done with 35% TCA. This concentration provides as good a result as 50% TCA but without the risk of the more highly concentrated acid. Use of 35% TCA, though, is undertaken only after the skin has been adequately prepared by at least 2 weeks of Retin-A application.

Fourth level peel is the "mixed peel," for which one may use stronger applications of TCA in certain areas, dermabrade over the peel in an acne scar area, and use either dilute Baker's formula phenol or full-strength phenol for its bleaching effect in certain zones. For example, one may use a lighter peel (35% TCA) over most of the face, a heavy peel on the lip edge (Baker's formula), and dilute Baker's formula for crow's feet or for hyperpigmentation of the lower lid. Diluting Baker's formula simply provides a safety margin in that a single wipe can accomplish everything required without the risk of over-peeling the area.

Fifth level peel is done with standard Baker's formula. It is an all or none procedure.

In contrast to TCA peels, Retin-A and α-hydroxy acid skin care require progressive maintenance programs. They comprise excellent enhancement techniques for the plastic surgeon's practice but are certainly more complex than simple peels.

B

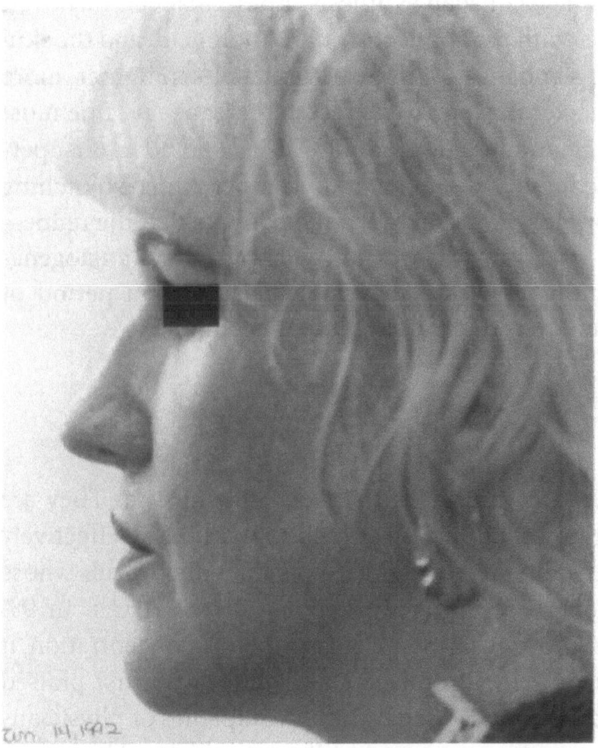

C

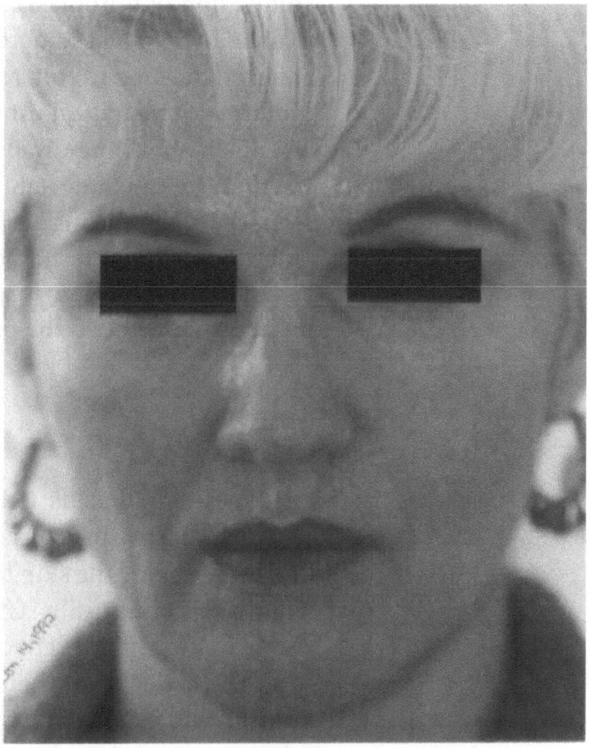

Level I Peel

The topical solution Retin-A was designed for superficially peeling the acne patient's skin in order to clear blocked pores and reduce the bacterial count. A side result was a miniature "chemical peel" effect, as Retin-A peels away epidermis. Inevitably, it was recommended to patients without acne as an alternative to facial chemical peeling. It is not an alternative, but an active agent for skin rejuvenation. When it was first used tretinoin application was uncomfortable, as many doctors handed the patient a prescription and said simply, "Try this." Patients had to choose their own concentration limits by using the product to the point of tolerance.

According to dermatologists, retinoic acid has anti-aging and anti-cancer potential. It stimulates deep dermal collagen synthesis, epithelial turnover, and elastin fiber ingrowth. Superficial furrows even out with a supervised program, and fine lines may disappear entirely. With long-term use, even deep wrinkles become "less prominent." One unpleasant side effect is increased sensitivity to sunlight, requiring the use of protective sunscreens.

Clinically, retinoic acid increases blood flow in the microvasculature, improving skin color. The skin's "reactivity to stimuli" is also enhanced, and desquamation of the horny material of the follicles is promoted. The improvement of skin turgor and reduction of fine wrinkles are brought about by the stimulation of fibroplasia and new collagen synthesis. Epidermal cell turnover, which slows with age, increases with the application of retinoic acid, and the skin appears thicker and fuller. This enhanced skin turnover results in lighter, more uniform pigmentation. Actinic keratoses may regress and disappear. One must ask, then, about the disadvantages of using tretinoin. With sporadic, unsupervised usage, uncomfortable redness and scaling and even permanent blotching may result. Physicians were originally instructed to tell patients that the redness and stinging was "desirable"—the drug was working. These signs of angiogenesis and new collagen formation, however, may take place over a period of months, not days, so the patient need not suffer while it is ongoing.

Level II Peel

α-Hydroxy acids (AHAs) are fruit acids that smooth the skin. They are useful to plastic surgeons because they allow tretinoin to work more effectively and thus prepare the skin for a peel procedure quickly, even in individuals whose skin is thick and oily. Glycolic acid is the work horse of the AHAs. In 9% concentration, it is an effective morning at-home cream; in 40% concentration, it is a once-a-week "aesthetician's peel." Problem: The doctors who first praised glycolic acid patented it so it could not be used by other companies or physicians who want to work with stronger concentrations or different vehicles. This patent has been overturned, so AHA is widely available now.

α-Hydroxy acids have been used alone to accomplish light chemical peels. In the modern era, these super-light peels are considered level II peels, which means that they can be safely applied by a trained medical cosmetologist and are not considered medical procedures regulated by state medical examiner boards. As noted above, we have used AHA peels as part of our home therapy program and also offer them to patients as a "jump start" to their therapy. A series of AHA AHAs. Our program uses a regimen of once-weekly applications of 9% glycolic intervals.

α-Hydroxy acids are found in food, e.g., glycolic acid in sugar cane, lactic acid in sour milk, malic acid in apples, citric acid in fruits, and tartaric acid in grapes. In low concentration, as is used for the home program, the AHAs diminish corneocyte cohesion but do not destroy the epidermis, as do the stronger concentrations. Major complications have occurred with peels described in the dermatologic literature, such as those performed with 50% to 75% AHAs. Our program uses a regimen of once-weekly applications of 40% glycolic acid, which is neutralized with water as soon as the patient reports intolerable burning. Although this method is safe, an even safer method is to use dilute tretinoin and AHA cream until several weeks after completion of the last "aesthetician's peel."

Dermatologists often perform a 70% glycolic acid peel that involves the lower layers of the epidermis and the upper papillary dermis. The peel is then repeated at 1-month intervals.

Our method is similar to the glycolic acid treatment program in which 50% to 70% glycolic acid is applied to the face every few weeks. I would warn against the risks associated with that regimen, however. It has been stated that an experienced physician, before applying glycolic acid, can prepare the skin with Jessner's solution or acetone to "improve the peel." Glycolic acid creams or gels have been proposed for twice-daily application between treatments. My consulting aestheticians believe that this regimen is too harsh. A gentler regimen we use for rapid progress is the Micropeel (shaving the epidermis plus a 30% AHA peel). The aesthetician should have the leeway to advise patients regarding the frequency of application, when to resume Retin-A use, and about other factors that can keep the surgeon and the aesthetician out of trouble. I am not familiar with the pyruvic acid peel, other than it is a medium-depth peel that has a high potential for side effects.

The AHAs may be summarized, for our purposes, as follows.

1. They have no known toxicity and no photosensitivity.
2. They can be neutralized by water (a necessary factor; otherwise they continue to exert their effects).
3. Glycolic acid is a midstrength AHA. Over-the-counter lactic acid has little effect. Pyruvic acid, though, is a "drug from hell": scars, exploding bottles, and so on.

4. Low AHA concentrations dissolve the dead cells' "glue," and the patient then sloughs *sheets* of cells, as with a TCA peel.
5. Bleaching agents and Retin-A are more effective after AHA peels, and after TCA peels.
6. The effectiveness of 70% glycolic acid is similar to that of 35% TCA—but it is more risky. Do not use it. Rapid exfoliation is advantageous when the solution's concentration is only 35% and can be quickly neutralized when the patient feels pain.
7. Acetone scrubs may be responsible for scarring with AHAs. Use alcohol for preparing the skin.
8. "Frost" refers to the dermal damage done by AHAs. There has been little research about the depth of peel with AHAs, but we do know that there is some danger when using AHAs for chemical peeling. Individual variation is reflected in how quickly the peel "goes deep" (i.e., produces scars, white spots, or worse).

Levels III and IV Peels

Preparing the skin with Retin-A in a carefully graduated program allows us to obtain new, younger-looking, tighter skin in facial rejuvenation patients with a minimum of chemical peel application. Plastic surgery must be open to new ideas. Hence we have recognized the need for aestheticians who are trained in medical matters. These professionals can advise the patient taking Retin-A about gradually increasing the strength of the drug, excluding the use of products that interact unfavorably with Retin-A, and how to live with its effects prior to chemical peeling. When the skin has been prepared with Retin-A, it has more elastin and a thicker collagen base. One can then obtain a smoother surface using a variety of methods, including level II "rapid exfoliation" with glycolic acids, peels with TCA (level III), or the "mix and match" choices of dermabrasion, TCA, and dilute phenol (level IV). Even skin pores respond to the latter regimen.

A "light" chemical peel (level III) is performed with 35% TCA or even 10% TCA without taping. The 10% solution is used on the neck, so there are minimal color changes but some skin tightening. The 35% TCA is the major component of the "mix and match" protocol and is used on most of the face. Phenol is reserved for the deep lines, dark spots, or edge of the lip. Phenol is applied either as the full strength Baker's formula or a dilute version of it. We mix equal amounts of saline with equal amounts of Baker's formula for a half-strength phenol solution.

It has been essentially true that pores look worse after chemical peeling, but there are new thoughts on the matter. What do you tell the patient who comes in

1-2 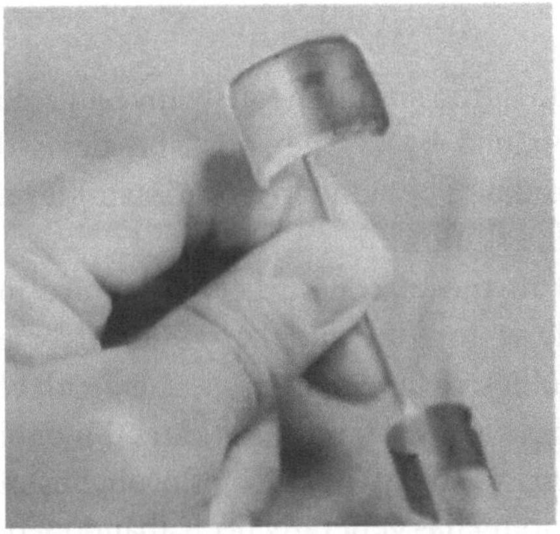 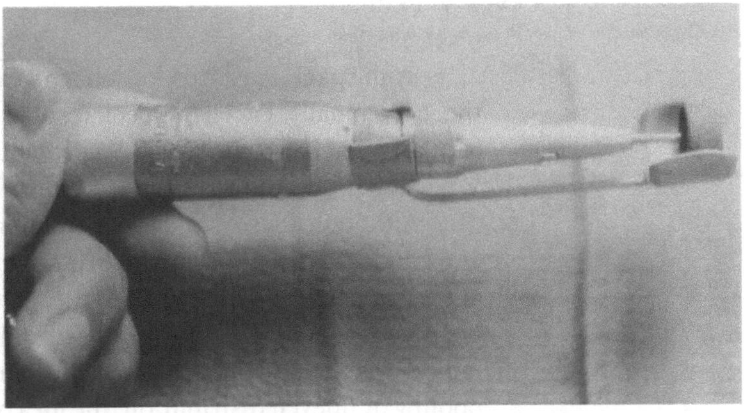 1-3

Figures 1-2, 1-3. Can you get AIDS from dermabrasion? It seems likely that there is a hazard if blood products are splattered from an AIDS patient into the surgeon's conjunctiva during a face lift. The device shown in Figures 1-2 and 1-3 has been available for some time. It fits easily on a variety of "hand engine" dermabraders. Two types are shown: a wide one (**Fig. 1-2**) and a narrow one for narrow brushes that are used for touch-ups on fine lines (**Fig. 1-3**). Clipped on, it keeps the debris from spraying upward. With practice, there is no loss of visualization of the area on which you are working. Also, wear a clear plastic eye protector.

with prominent pores and deep wrinkles? First, a light chemical peel with TCA can tighten the superficial portion of the skin, making the pores appear smaller. It also eliminates fine lines. A deep peel, which tightens the deep dermis, stretches the pore; hence a light peel results in smaller pores.

Retin A thickens the dermis by adding collagen and elastin, which improves the appearance of skin pores. Do you stop there? No. The aesthetician trained in medical cosmetology can certainly perform a 40% glycolic peel, steaming, and pore sebum extraction—the processes most often used to empty pores in acne patients. This technology can be applied to the older patient as well.

The technique is as follows. Each new patient undergoes a consultation that includes advice on sun blocks, skin cleansing, and the value of facials. The regimen begins with 0.25% tretinoin applied on alternate days or three times per week. The aesthetician explains the details of application and if one should use small amounts in problem areas on the alternate days. The patient sets the schedule for progression until he or she can apply this concentration of tretinoin 7 days a week without peeling or burning. At this point the aesthetician determines that the patient may progress to a higher concentration. The only responsibility of the surgeon at this point is to determine when (or if) the patient is ready for a light or regular facial peel. (We use TCA for the peel more often than phenol and obtain more rapid recoveries and more natural, less depigmented facial skin.)

Level V Peel

Tom Baker, Howard Gordon, and Clyde Litton simultaneously investigated the occasionally excellent peel results obtained by lay persons and devised formulas that have gained wide acceptance today. The standard solution for level V peeling is referred to as the Baker formula solution.

Although these peels were discussed in the plastic surgery literature in 1961 and 1962, wide acceptance did not follow until the mid-1970s. The debate at that time was whether one should apply adhesive tape to increase the depth of the peel or should leave the area open and apply a powder after 24 hours. Thymol iodide was the powder of choice and remains so today. Because of problems of pooling or uneven distribution, the idea of taping has generally been abandoned. Topical antibiotic ointments are now applied immediately following the Baker formula application. Unlike with TCA, the method of application is relatively unimportant. With TCA, a deeper penetration is achieved with a different means of application, such as substituting gauze squares for cotton tip applicators. If certain areas require a deeper peel using TCA, the skin is rubbed with the wet gauze square rather than brushed.

In our practice, level V peeling is reserved for a few patients with pale extremely wrinkled skin who have no desire to participate in outdoor activities. Because of the bleaching and subsequent skin sensitivity involved, these candidates should be clearly advised to expect a lifetime of occlusive and protective makeup.

Integrating Use of AHAs and Retin-A into a Surgical Practice

"The times they are a' changing." Patients expect full service, and we can certainly provide it with the help of medical aestheticians and the innovative teaching courses currently available to plastic surgeons. A number of us have been working to incorporate into our specialty the knowledge flowing from our dermatology and aesthetician colleagues as well as from other plastic surgeons who have moved beyond standard chemical face peeling.

First, skin care and facial rejuvenation home programs can be offered to *all patients,* ranging from those being treated for breast reduction or trauma to the mother who has come in with a child with a cut finger. Trained aestheticians can be employed on a part-time or full-time basis, with the surgeon generally overseeing the process—commenting on the improvement and perhaps adding a suggestion or two. The process is as follows.

Each new patient is advised extensively on the risks and advantages of the use of tretinoin and how AHA creams can be used in conjunction with them.

Explain it this way: "If you want good teeth when you are 65, you brush them everyday. If you want trouble-free, fresher, more youthful skin without extensive wrinkling, use this program." There is no charge for this advice. Emphasize that tretinoin and AHA usage must be complemented with compatible moisturizers and makeup that do not contain common irritants. Our clinic uses the GlamouRx system, which includes makeup, foundations, moisturizers, and lipsticks with no PABA, lanolin, perfume, or alcohol. They can be used by the postoperative patient as well as the preoperative candidate.

The aesthetician then starts each patient on 0.025% tretinoin two or three times a week and guides them as they progress to daily and then twice-daily application. This regimen begins the process of replacing the damaged deep skin collagen with simultaneous formation of elastic fibers. The 9% alpha hydroxy acid cream is used each morning or twice daily. Glycolic acids such as AHA simply smoothe the skin. Depending on sensitivity one patient may use a cream twice a day, others only twice a week.

After this period of treatment, one of two approaches may be used. Many of our colleagues immediately schedule a chemical peel after a 2- to 4-week preparation. Retin-A is the key to success, but you may want to add topical steroids and hydroquinone (bleaches) during the preoperative period. We generally use them both pre- and postoperatively to avoid the hyperpigmentation that occurs in some TCA-treated patients.

Our approach is to give the patient 3 to 6 months of tretinoin and AHA applications, after which they decide if they want to undergo the peel. Mixed peels means that one may use dilute phenol for the lip edge or to bleach a spot, but the work horse is TCA. If the peel is undertaken, several days after the peel the patient begins applying an aloe-vera-based oil to the peeled area. Essential Oil (GlamouRx) is our choice. If the redness seems to be excessive, we follow Steve Hoefflin's advice and begin twice-daily applications of 1% Hytone. This cream based steroid is tolerated better than an ointment-based preparation. The aesthetician must watch to see if hyperpigmentation appears; if it does, either an AHA with iodoquin, 4% hydroquinone (Eldoquin Forte), or 8% hydroquinone is added to the regimen.

It is best to wait 3 to 4 weeks before starting Retin-A. We advise beginning with 0.025% Retin-A three times a week. The concentration is then slowly increased until the patient is ready to resume what we call "third level" treatment. This progression from 0.025% to 0.05% to 0.01% Retin-A is patient-controlled.

Unlike some of our dermatology colleagues, we baby our patients; we use less harsh solutions and do minor touch-ups at intervals as needed. This tender, loving care approach pays off in many ways. Patients also appreciate consultations on color selection, powders, bases, lipstick, and color coordination as well as the aloe vera approach to smoother, more comfortable skin. Hence the advice offered above is offered once more: Do not try to do it yourself. Hire a medical

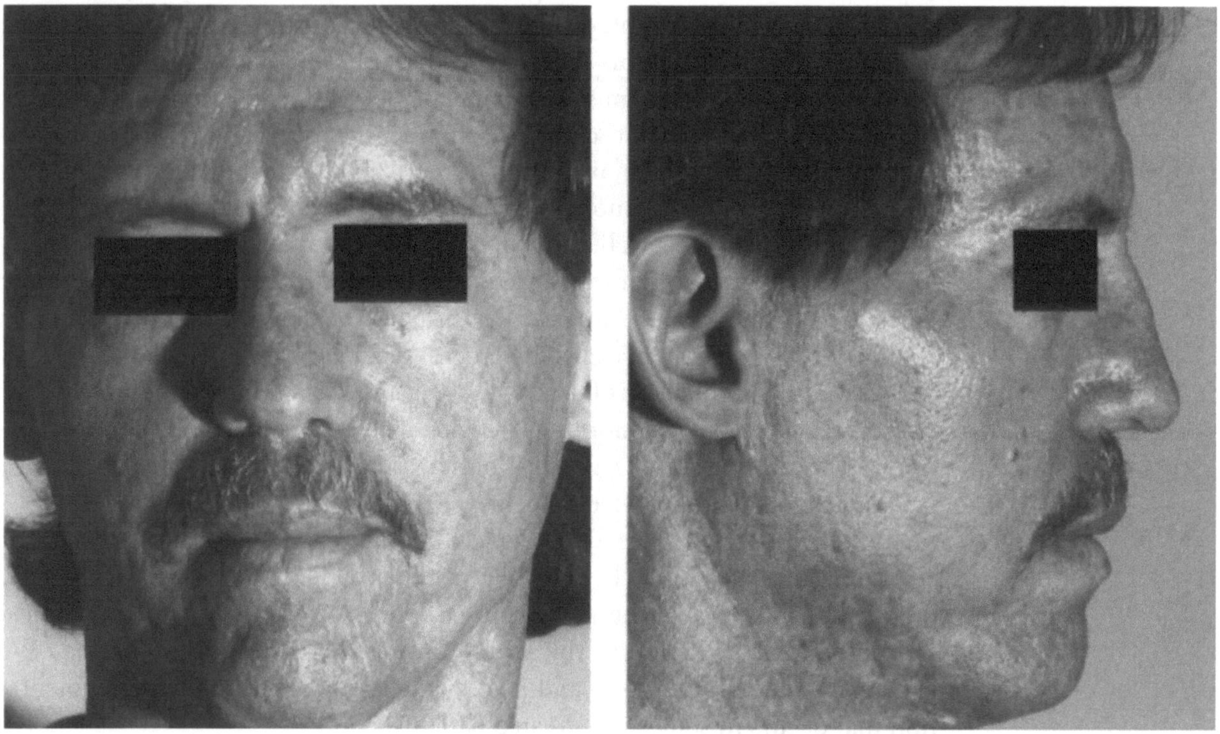

A B

Figure 1-4. This man underwent facial rejuvenation with tretinoin and α-hydroxy acids (AHAs) followed by fat grafting. His oily, acne-scarred skin is shown preoperatively in 1990 (**A,B**); the end result is shown 2 years later (**C–E**). It took approximately 10 months for the texture of his skin to change with our graduated program of tretinoin and AHA creams. In 1990 we surgically added malar augmentations in the "classic position," thereby elevating the nasolabial groove to a certain degree and giving the patient the "look" he wanted. Fat grafting was done in the glabella, the nasolabial areas, and throughout the chin in the acne pits. A second minor fat graft followed in 1991 (**C**). Note in the 1992 photographs (**D&E**) the smoothness of the skin and its contours. Note also that the Retin-A regimen has tightened the once baggy skin underneath his chin. A chin augmentation helped somewhat, but the change in skin quality is a result of tretinoin. Needless to say, he is pleased with his new skin condition, his comfort, and his new facial appearance.

In men, blepharoplasty alone is employed on most occasions without elevating the eyebrow. This patient had complained of a "menacing" look that might have been helped by an eyebrow elevation, but it would have been a drastic change and would have been detrimental to his profession.

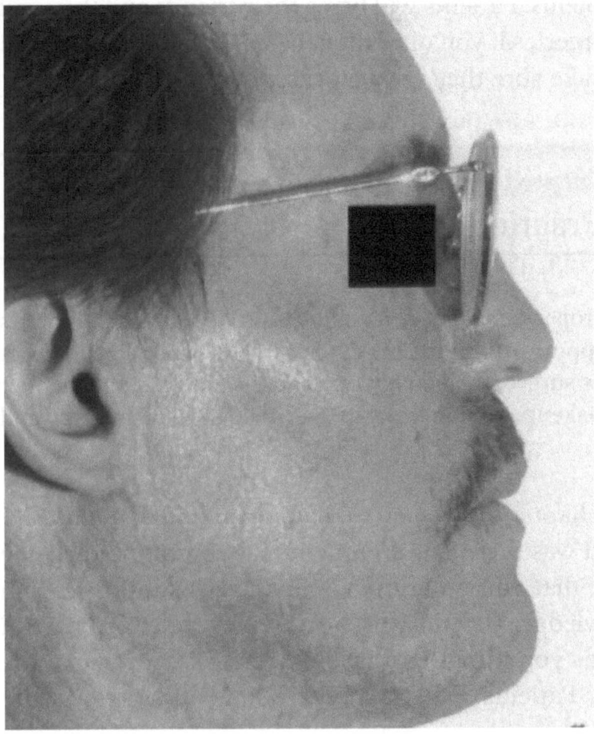

C

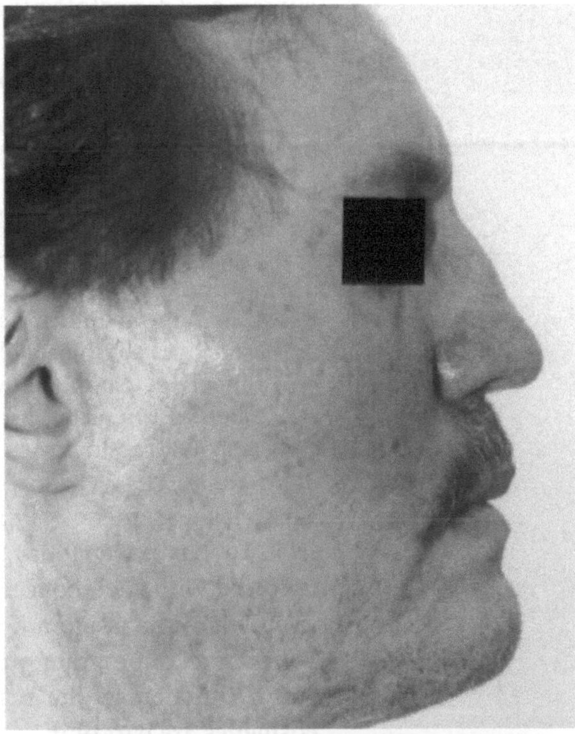

D

E

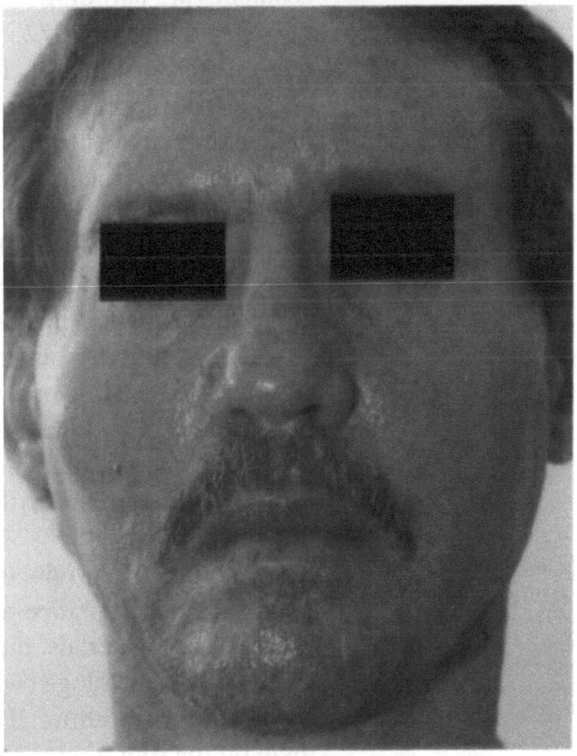

aesthetician who has been trained by a company that specializes in plastic surgery and dermatology problems. Patients will bring their friends and they will be happier with their other surgeries if you offer them beneficial program as well as the backup personnel to make sure they are well cared for.

Cosmetics as Part of a Surgical Practice?

> The surgeon's office is a proper atmosphere for discussion of fears and anxieties and for establishment of rapport with a member of the surgeon's staff. I believe it is important that the aesthetic surgeon personally give approval of each patient after she has completed her makeup session as a further evidence of interest and aesthetic sensitivity.

That closing sentence of my chapter in *Symposium on Surgery of the Aging Face* from 1976 is as true today as it was then. The argument that you cannot become involved with such concerns, that you do not have time, lacks substance. You simply have to assign a knowledgeable and trustworthy person to this part of your aftercare program, just as you might entrust someone else to remove the sutures hidden in the scalp. Patients expect aftercare, and in our specialty cosmetics are part of it.

Beginning in 1972, we realized that patients were uncomfortable with referrals to outside agencies for aftercare cosmetics and were reluctant to pay outside fees for preoperative skin care counseling. We began an inhouse service of demonstrations that has endured to this day. We had the same problems with cosmetics as we had with other products: Once a particular brand name was demonstrated, you would find that it had been discontinued or was not available in the stores in the area. There was also the problem of oversell. Even when we sent patients to a department store with a list of the items they needed by brand name and sequence, they were still sold material they did not need.

The solution is an inhouse program that is not costly and that can be administered by someone who has been trained not only in cosmetic application but in the care and feeding of the postsurgical patient. The rules and requirements for makeup after chemical peels, facelifts, blepharoplasties, and so on are radically different from those the average beauty store operator encounters during training.

We use the products of Medical Cosmetic Services and Biomedic. The financial and acceptance results have been spectacular judging by the constant reordering of materials. Furthermore, patients enjoy the privacy and services of a personal cosmetologist who understands their feelings and the biodynamics of their surgical procedure. If the surgeon supplies the products and they can obtain them on the spot, that is even better. This is the basic premise behind MCS and the Biomedic organization. We buy the products from them wholesale and sell them to the patients retail. We hire our own aestheticians, paying them to be available for preoperative consultations and postoperative makeovers. The profits from the retail sale of the products more than cover the wholesale costs and all the salaries.

Beware of companies that claim their products are unique. The basic ingredients of practically all cosmetics are the same. The aim is to eliminate those ingredients that cause allergic reactions or skin irritations, and this process is undertaken only by applying the products to surgical patients, each of whom predictably reacts differently. Most of you have seen patients who suddenly could not tolerate their own cosmetics after a face lift, blepharoplasty, or chemical peel. The products sold as "private label" cosmetics are the least expensively produced, and their quality may be far below that to which your patients are accustomed. Another consideration is the cost of private label products. According to our consultants, had we accepted the offer of one company to affix our name to the labels we would have had to buy more than 100 jars or bottles of numerous products. Yes, we would use the moisturizers, bases, and oils, but it would take several years to use that number, even if we gave it away. The cost would have been compounded by the capital tied up on the shelves and possible by deterioration of the product.

Lastly, the "care and feeding" of the skin in these patients is an art in itself. Beware of anyone who simply wants you to recommend or sell cosmetics in your office. Talk with companies who offer training programs for your personnel and who offer you the products at wholesale costs rather than retail or "10% off." Having cosmetics available as a service in your office is a good idea. Properly managed, it is a productive as well as profitable venture and can be an important form of practice enhancement.

Choices Available for Facial Rejuvenation

The young patient who wants to refresh her face can use several approaches. Our patients begin with what we call the home program, a regimen of gradually increasing tretinoin application, compatible sunblocks and moisturizers, and the addition of AHA creams each morning. The AHA cream simply removes the upper stratum corneum and allows tretinoin to be more effective. The patient also may choose to bypass this part of the procedure and undertake it later. These young women may choose the half face lift, malar or chin augmentation, or fat grafting; or they may progress rapidly to the mixed peel abrasion.

A recent patient illustrates these choices. A young lady had previously undergone dermabrasion predictably resulting in deep scarring and deep pigmentation, but her facial contour reflected that the mid-face and malar zone had not developed. We talked about redoing the rhinoplasty and elevating the

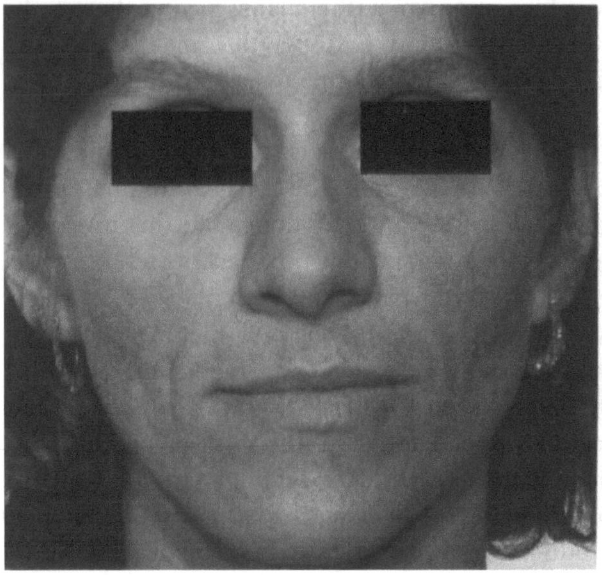

A

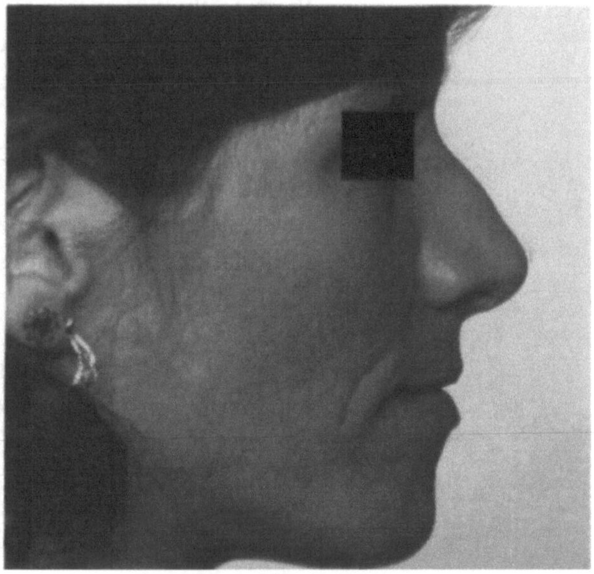

B

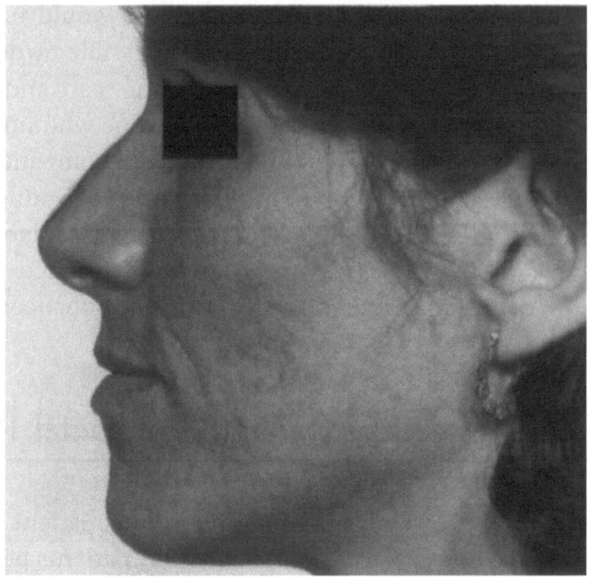

C

Figure 1-5. Role of chemical peels and fat grafting in an acne program. At the end of this chapter is a copy of the office information sheet that we give to our acne patients so they understand the role of each component in a multidisciplinary approach to their problem. The aesthetician's role involves facial cleansing, opening of pores, steaming, and supervising the tretinoin and glycolic acid regimens. The plastic surgeon's role is to minimize color loss by employing fat grafting, the "mixed peel" technique, and frequent light peels during the postoperative period. Each program is tailored to the individual's needs and requirements and may involve a period when the patient does not use tretinoin or glycolic acid and a period during which there is rapid progression of the program.

(A–C) Preoperative appearance of a young woman in 1988 prior to fat grafting. Note the deep acne pitting. **(D & E)** Same patient in 1991 following a mixed peel abrasion. TCA (35%) was used with spot abrasion on each cheek. The fat grafting was not repeated (our cameras were stolen around this time so the lighting does not match). **(F & G)** Same patient in 1992 following a recurrence of the acne. She is now scheduled for a second light peel and will resume the Retin-A regimen. Note the improvement in her lip contour that has resulted from lip roll and fat grafting procedures performed a year earlier and the persisting correction of the nasolabial and forehead lines from 4.5 years previously. This type of patient fights a continuous battle against acne, and the surgeon must maintain good rapport with these patients so they continue to improve the quality of their skin. The TCA touch-up peels are usually applied with light pressure and without anesthesia in a clinic examining room. The patient may resume using makeup the next day. The objective is to continue to smooth the skin and correct the irregularities brought on by persistent acne without compromising the color of the cheeks or face.

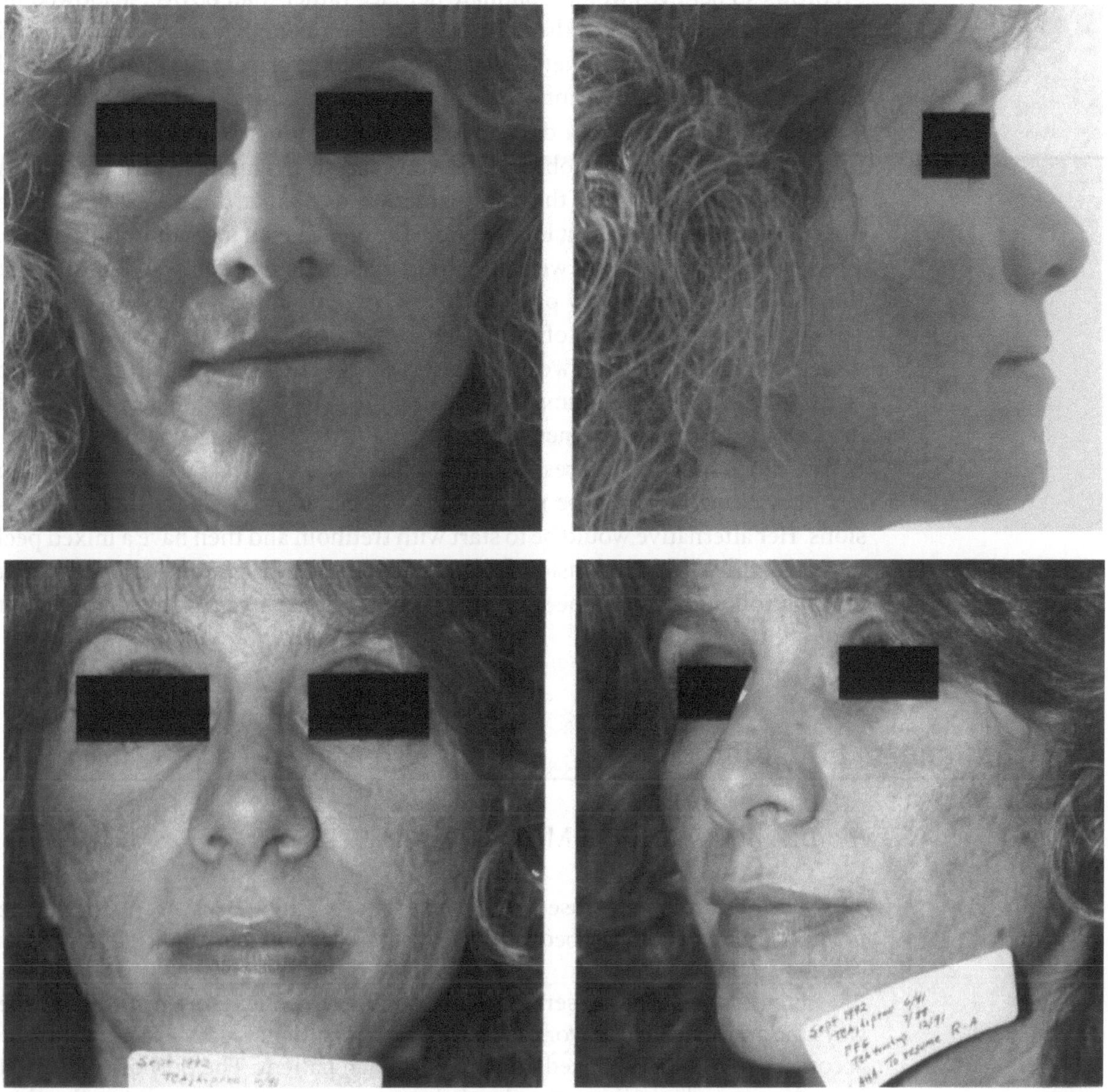

D E F G

eyebrows so her eyes would dominate her face rather than be overshadowed by her forehead descent. We also talked about feminizing her nose, which would make her eyes more prominent. We then came to the crux of the matter. She had had early aging with descent of the neck and lower cheek, white areas due to scarring incurred by a prior dermabrasion, and a flat malar and zygoma zone.

Her first choice was obvious. She needed to begin an AHA and Retin-A regimen to remove some of the dark pigment and equalize these areas with those that had permanent pigment loss. Second, the area of scarring required elevation. We have had good success with undermining and then placing fat deposits, but this method would be only partially helpful. We discussed several approaches: The half face lift would offer the chance to build up soft tissue directly underneath that zone, and we could insert a large shell-type malar prosthesis to cause further stretching. Simply stretching the skin with my fingertips showed her that a marked improvement in shadowing and contouring would be affected. Because the other scar depressions were closer to the nose in the area we would not undermine, it would be reasonable to place fat grafts under those depressions. Her alternative would be to start with tretinoin and then have a mixed peel perhaps without dermabrasion because of the already present color loss. Fat grafting could be done at the same time to puff out the area, and a malar implant could be done safely too.

Comments and Commentary

Viewpoint: Melissa Stoltz, Medical Aesthetician

The discovery and use of anti-agers is exciting. Because of them, the medical aesthetician has become an integral part of many plastic surgeon's practice.

Providing education, services, and products to patients are just some of the ways the aesthetician can work in the physician's office. Treatment services vary according to the specific needs and goals of each patient: The purpose of a facial is to cleanse and condition the skin before surgery and to recondition the skin after it has gone through surgical trauma.

Maintaining the quality of the skin has been incorporated into these services with the use of cosmetic peels. α-Hydroxy acids (AHAs) have long been praised for their skin-smoothing properties. Glycolic acid, a form of AHA chosen because of its molecular size, applied topically in high concentrations causes epidermolysis. This property provides an alternative for treating seborrheic keratoses (commonly known as age spots), actinic keratoses, and verrucae vulgares, all of which lesions involve distinct epidermal hyperplasia as well as retention of stratum corneum.

Facial wrinkles can be modified with the application of this topical peel. The daily home application of lower concentrations produces outstanding results. The length of time the peel solution is left on the skin by the aesthetician is governed by skin type and the strength of the solution. Home skin care is discussed with the patient, including the use of tretinoin for long-term tightening and firming.

Within the framework of an aesthetic surgical practice, the medical aesthetician offers a team approach that ensures the best possible results for the patient. Being the communication link between patient and physician, the aesthetician educates the patient about the recommended programs.

The aesthetician can bring new patients to a plastic surgeon's practice. This form of marketing is one of the main ways to expand a practice. Aestheticians make presentations to business women's organizations, social and health fairs, and continuing education programs. The ability to communicate with people is thus important for the aesthetician. To set up the recommended regimen, the patient and aesthetician discuss and schedule the required office procedures at a one-on-one consultation.

Selecting the specific skin care for home use is important for reaching the desired result. This decision is also reached during a consultation, usually at the initial patient visit. It is the aesthetician's responsibility to keep the surgeon informed of the patient's progress by making notes in his or her chart.

The procedures in which the aesthetician is involved are the treatment of skin health and appearance. The acne patient, for example, usually begins treatment with a series of deep pore cleansing facials along with a topical antibiotic. We also recommend and prescribe tretinoin as an aid to this particular problem. The patient would be instructed to begin on the lowest concentration of the drug, applying it two or three times weekly and then gradually increasing the strength and the number of applications to every night. After the pustular activity has subsided, we address the scarring that often accompanies acne. A series of glycolic acid peels would be administered. Different levels of these peels are beneficial, depending on the skin type. The depth of the pigment changes on the surface usually determines the strength of peel used. A 40% peel applied no less than once weekly and no more than three times weekly in increments of 2 to 5 minutes each can effectively minimize the appearance of darker scars. We also recommend the use of glycolic acid (available in Derma-Gly products) to be used at home. The Derma-Gly Peeling Gel (2% hydroquinone and glycolic acid) aids in lightening acne scars. The quality, texture, and smoothness of the skin are greatly improved with this combination of treatments. Benefits continue with bimonthly visits for a peel. The patient is now ready to see the doctor and move forward with any surgical procedures desired.

Making quality skin care available to patients to achieve their goals is essential. The Derma-Gly skin care products that contain glycolic acid comprise a varied treatment line that effectively treats conditions ranging from severely wrinkled, sun-damaged skin to oily skin with large pores. It works well with tretinoin. For the patient having cosmetic surgery, skin quality is a major concern. Incorporated into a preoperative service, patients may be given products and an introduction to such services as facials, peels, and makeup applications. These services are greatly appreciated and well accepted.

A B C D

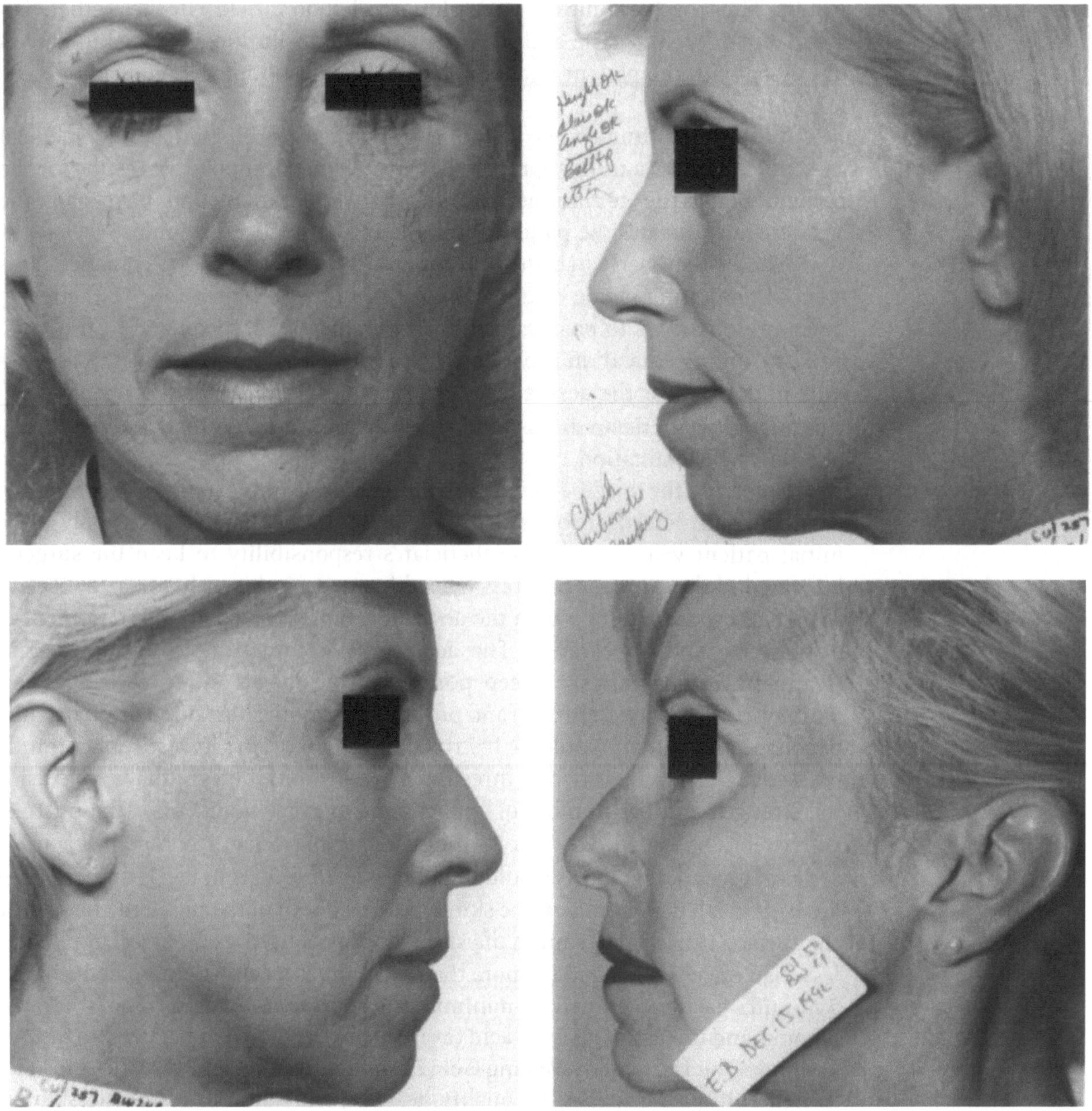

Figure 1-6. Serial improvement: rhinoplasty, lip fat augmentation, TCA peels. Many patients choose to have progressive facial enhancement, which may involve structural changes such as rhinoplasty and fat grafting, with subsequent chemical peels after long-term application of α-hydroxy acid (AHA) creams and Retin-A. **(A–C)** This patient, shown in 1988, had had a previous blepharoplasty with scars that were high and in the "unacceptable zone." We successfully undermined and stretched this area, moving the scars down to the normal fold zone. We simply redraped the skin of the lower lid. Today, we would consider submuscular tightening with a simultaneous TCA peel. **(D–F)** Same patient 3 years later. The only remaining problem is the quality of her skin, which has responded slowly to our home program. Note that the lips are fuller, and the nasolabial shadows have disappeared.

When planning the next procedure, she requested

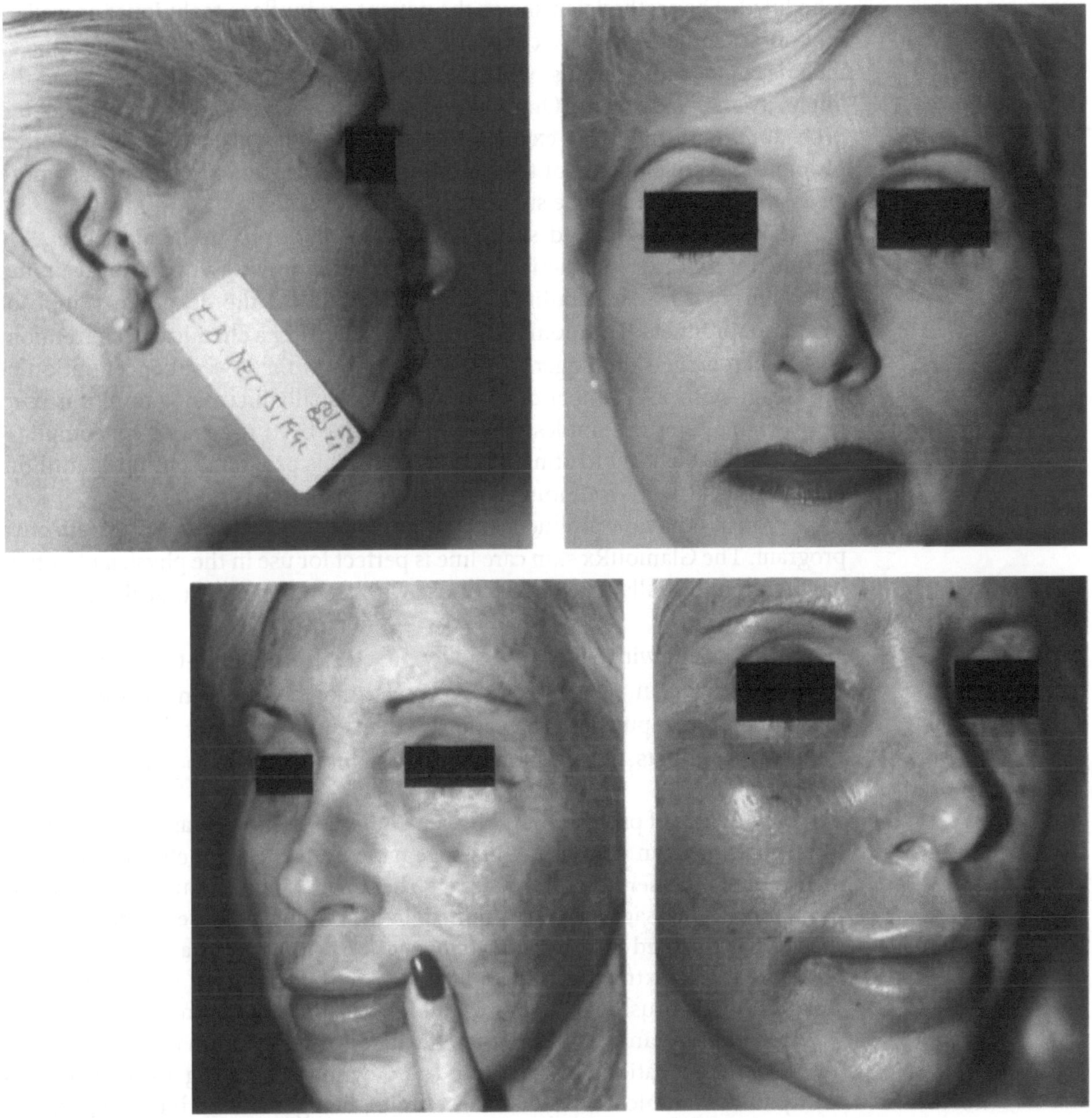

E F H

that we add a small amount of fat to her lips because she desired an even greater improvement, and we planned to add a small amount as well to a few spots along the nasolabial zone. Our major procedure was to be a full-face TCA chemical peel.

When applying TCA peels to the entire face and eyelids, we use a cotton swab around the eyes but apply vigorous pressure in the areas that require greater penetration. On the sixth postoperative day, these areas have not yet separated the coagulum. At this point we prescribe a collagenase cream, which rapidly removes the crust; hence the patient can meet the makeup team for covering and protective makeup instruction by the eighth or ninth day, returning her to the usual schedule of chemical peel patients. **(G&H)** Note the improvement in skin quality, which will be further improved upon resumption of Retin-A and AHA use.

Beginning at 5 to 10 days after surgery, a complimentary make-over is scheduled. The aesthetician shows the patient camouflage techniques as well as how to accentuate the new contours. Thirty days after operation the services include rejuvenating facials, which speed the healing process and improve the longevity of the surgery. Other services may be suggested according to the procedures performed. For example, use of a nose guard after a rhinoplasty often promotes severe clogging of the pores, in which case an exfoliating, deep pore cleansing treatment may be suggested.

For severely wrinkled skin, our surgeon performs a chemical peel. My treatment services, as aesthetician, would include applying a hydrating, calming mask during a facial. Paraffin is an excellent aid for the deep penetration of treatment products. Tretinoin is then prescribed. After a chemical peel, tretinoin is a "supercharged" anti-ager. Treatment begins at the lowest concentration of the cream, with the number of applications gradually increasing until it is used every night. After the mildest concentration has been used with no complications, the middle level treatment is instituted. This program continues until the patient is using 0.1% tretinoin cream on a permanent basis.

Proper skin care products ensure minimal irritation during this effective program. The GlamouRx skin care line is perfect for use in the physician's office, having been specially formulated for use with tretinoin and surgical procedures of any kind.

The patient with oily skin usually benefits from a long-term relationship with an aesthetician. Most oily skin is prone to clogging and acne, so the first step is to loosen the impurities. The patient is then educated about the proper use of home care products, the function of these products being to soothe and promote healing.

The choice of professional skin care equipment is important. A comfortable facial chair that can double as a massage table is an excellent choice. Our office incorporates the services of a massage therapist. Liposuction patients benefit from proper massage and are trained in techniques to use at home. More specifically directed at facial skin rejuvenation is the use of a steamer to relax pores for easier extraction and to facilitate detoxification of cellular tissue. A facial and body brush machine is useful for effective exfoliation and cleansing.

Most importantly for the aesthetician who wishes to maintain a satisfied clientele are education, an open mind to new ideas, a caring attitude, and the ability to communicate. Beyond these traits, being a skilled businessperson is essential. The aesthetician and physician's talents complement each other, ensuring an optimistic outlook about the future growth potential of our work.

Miscellaneous Observations

1. According to Howard Gordon, the phenol peel appeals to most surgeons: It may be done with no extensive preparation and no long aftercare.

Gordon has stated that the same results can be obtained with TCA but that the procedure is more complex. He likes to treat and tell them goodbye!

2. Retin-A is the key to successful peels, but Retin-A is fraught with hazards if it is not used properly. It has been reported to produce dark, pigmented burns, for example, that are difficult to correct.

3. Accutane (isotretinoin), the anti-acne drug, has caused enough cases of scarring even 2 years after a patient has used it, to make one wary. Accutane has a reputation as an excellent anti-acne drug but with some serious side effects. One that is emerging is the risk of atypical scarring in peel patients, even years after discontinuing the drug. One patient developed bizarre stellate scars 4 months after a successful peel when Accutane was taken. There are only a handful of such cases, but most occurred in patients who had had TCA peels (even as mild as 25% TCA).

4. Permanent scarring can result from TCA as well as from phenol. The worst case I have seen was in a patient who had deep second and third degree burns due to TCA. Apparently, no one remembered that TCA could be neutralized with ordinary tap water. Our suggestion is to use 35% TCA (rather than 50% TCA) for the peel because it provides a margin of safety. Even if you must touch up areas at a later date, it is easier than trying to deal with a scar.

5. The Obaji technique does work, but so do all other techniques that involve TCA or "mixed" peels. Our objections are unethical claims of zero complications, scars, and toxicity. (There are reports from Southern California that the Obaji technique is producing some failures, and that such failures are not rare occurrences.) See also Observations 23 and 24.

6. The choice of agent for preparing the skin for a peel is a personal one. Some surgeons believe that alcohol is better than ether or acetone. The bottom line is to cleanse the skin in order to achieve a uniform peel. Some advocate antibiotic ointment for the first 24 hours, but this practice deepens the peel. Others use Vaseline and still others antibiotic powders. Some use Jessner's solution to clean the skin and débride it before the peel.

7. For African American and Oriental patients, the basis of treatment is the same: a slow Retin-A program for up to 3 months. One method is to dilute Retin-A with facial cream and then slowly increase the concentration. Some allow these patients to peel with Retin-A, but we do not. The desirable end result is a thicker, more elastic skin that will respond to a lighter peel. Resuming Retin-A is then the key to continuing the improvement. African American patients do show lightening of the skin, but the color slowly returns after a TCA peel. Use 4% hydroquinone to prevent darkening, and treat with 8%.

8. A practical suggestion: Solar Shield manufactures the sunglasses a number of surgeons give to their patients after blepharoplasty. These lightweight

plastic glasses presumably prevent ultraviolet light from striking the area of surgery. We believe this use is not particularly important, but the glasses do shield the area from dust and dirt. Solar Shield also makes a clear variety of glasses that sells for about $8. We have used them ourselves in the operating room when performing dermabrasions. They are relatively comfortable, inexpensive, and convenient. In this era of the AIDS epidemic, it is well to wear protective glasses.

9. There is still some inconsistency regarding the effect of peels in terms of lightened skin on the neck and chest. One cannot help but be impressed by the number of patients with "skin inconsistencies" after phenol peeling and even after deep TCA peeling that are used for illustration cases in textbooks. In one text, photographs of an attractive young woman whose neck was treated with 50% TCA, showed post-peeling "inconsistencies." It was chilling to see the large areas of depigmentation, hyperpigmentation, and areas that were dead white, on her chest and the back of her neck.

TCA in higher concentrations can be as problematic as phenol. As already stated, my approach is to use 35% TCA for all cases and dilute the solution by half when treating the neck or chest, areas that are unpredictable. Once there is skin bleaching, there is no recourse.

Other patients have been reported whose faces were treated with Baker formula phenol and whose necks were treated with 50% TCA. Again, there were marked contrasts between the skin tones and colors. Perhaps it is better in some patients to minimize the correction attempted.

One of my personal rules is to never peel a man's face with phenol, but others have no such hesitation. Certainly, the patient himself contributes to that decision. For example, in Texas a weather-beaten face is attractive and "natural," whereas pinkish, multicolored skin is not!

10. We often have patients who report unfortunate experiences with Retin-A. Two recent patients had been to a physician who had given them full-strength Retin-A in gel form. They applied it and immediately began to peel and burn. One patient now has permanent hyperpigmentation. Use of full-strength Retin-A without proper sun protection "begs" for just that type of sun damage. Retin-A strips the skin and makes it more vulnerable. Had an aesthetician been consulted, a graduated program such as the one we offer would have been undertaken and these problems avoided. By the time the patient is using full-strength Retin-A, at least 6 to 8 months have passed and the subdermal tissue has responded, making it less vulnerable.

11. Does proper use of Retin-A diminish or erase the "permanent tan" marks left by poorly planned peel treatment? Probably, but it takes some time. Many of the solar spots on the face and hands can be induced to fade over time. The lesson: Do not simply hand out prescriptions for Retin-A. Consult with an aesthetician to map out the proper regimen for the patient.

12. In an effort to explain a series of complications associated with phenol chemical peels, three plastic surgeons conducted experiments in rats and managed to confuse the issue completely. One author had seen "five patients who developed hypertrophic scarring at the lateral limits of chemically peeled areas." (I have never encountered this complication). The scarring should have had nothing to do with undermining the adjacent tissue for a rhytidectomy. Is it not possible that the chemical peel solution pooled in this area? Perhaps under the tape? My guess is that the tape was applied over wet peel solution and thus trapped the fluid. Alternatively, too much solution may have been used; a high concentration of phenol would create that problem.

13. Richard Albin wants to make it clear that the scarring complications encountered in TCA peeling occurred with *35% TCA* and "a sparing application." He also did not rub or abrade the area, as some surgeons have suggested. He believes that the Dow Corning silicone sheets as well as triamcinolone injections are useful for controlling scarring. The latter certainly is.

14. The Scanlan Company (St. Paul, Minnesota) has a line of skin markers in 10 colors. Why would you want 10 colors? One reason is that if you are planning to perform mixed chemical peels you may want to outline the areas for dermabrasion, liposuction, and fat reinjection using different colors. You may want to draw in each color for different structures in the nose. The only thing wrong with this concept is that you cannot use these markers preoperatively, as they wash off. That characteristic is a plus because you can outline your plan on the patient the day before, and he or she can wash off the colors before leaving the office. I prefer to do the drawings on the face before the patient enters the operating room in order to save time and to save our surgical marking pens.

15. A dermatologist wrote, in a letter to the editor of *JAMA*, "We explain to patients that they must tolerate erythema and peeling for up to 3 months to repair their severe UV-induced skin damage." Nonsense. A graduated program of skin care protection and slowly increasing concentrations of tretinoin allows one to achieve the same beneficial results without patient pain, peeling, and dissatisfaction. Four years ago few of our patients stayed with Retin-A; now almost all are unduly satisfied. Those who discontinue Retin-A do so because it does not live up to their expectations. Our Retin-A program is an important practice enhancement factor. Patients who are seen for other reasons are offered a complimentary skin care consultation. I simply check off "Retin-A" on the prescription sheet, and the staff does the rest. A gradual program of increasing concentrations and number of applications make believers of many patients. Technical point: Be sure to warn the patients that they will not be able to determine if it is worthwhile for at least 3 months. By then facial and hand skin will have responded, and a pleasing appearance will be evident.

16. How do you induce your patients to use Retin-A without their complaining that you turned them into pink, peeling pumpkins? Prescribe moisturizer and sunblocks along with the Retin-A and use a lower concentration of the drug. Mixing a moisturizer and tretinoin does not accomplish as much as tretinoin applied directly to the skin but at intervals, which are shortened according to tolerance. Whenever a patient asks for Retin-A, we provide a free prescription of minimum strength *only* if they sit down and discuss minimizing skin irritation. The aesthetician sets up a routine of daily moisturizers, sunblocks, and gentle skin cleansing for the morning after the patient has applied a nightly dose, and this regimen continues until the next application. The patients then may progress to more frequent applications. Before we started this program of education about use of the drug few patients used tretinoin more than a few weeks.

17. Having read about the problems encountered with phenol, some of you may be squeamish about using phenol at all. Lightly applied, it may be a good choice for light-skinned people with spotty deep wrinkling. I prefer TCA, of course. For people with coarse darker skins, it is better to deepen the TCA penetration by pressure and use of a gauze square for an applicator—then follow-up with 8% Hydroquinone.

A patient shown in the Color Plates section is an example of what can happen. Overall, the patient shows good facial "rejuvenation." We used 35% TCA over the face and "half-strength" Baker's formula for the dark pigmented zone at her jawline and crow's feet. Examine the last closeup—the unsightly white streak along the jawline is where rough dark skin was treated with the phenol peel. The only choice was to "blend" it using TCA in all the other areas and to continue the AHAs and tretinoin. It helped. If I had applied TCA to these spots the first time, instead of "mixing," this area would not have become so depigmented (although the opposite side and crow's feet areas did not depigment).

18. John Kelleher (Amarillo) also prefers a diluted form of the Baker formula for phenol peels. He noted more rapid recovery with less depigmentation and reasonable "good correction" of fine wrinkle lines. He uses TCA peels after tretinoin preparation as well.

19. "Hot peel" is a phrase dermatologist Mark Rubin uses to describe a combination of methylsalicylate with TCA. The methylsalicylate acts like croton oil with the phenol peels: It makes the penetration deeper in areas where a deeper peel is desirable. The down side? The deeper the peel, the more pigment that is lost. The "augmented TCA" can produce white patches. That result might be good with a "mixed peel" where you want to bleach out a dark area, but it is not a good idea for the average face and certainly not for the darker-skinned individual. Rubin reported that with this method the upper dermis collagen that is formed after the lighter peels seems to be healthy and longer lasting. The elastic fibers that come into the mid-dermis play a significant role as well. The same rejuvenation of the skin can be accomplished without as deep penetration as is done with the standard Baker formula in most individuals.

20. "All you can do is turn back the clock a little. You can't stop the ticking." A great way to describe peels but not necessarily a justification for the transient effect of collagen injections. There may even be a need for double skin testing prior to collagen injections. The only problem here is the rare patient who develops full-blown allergic reactions or even dermatomyositis after the first skin test.

21. We are told that The "secret formula" for the Obaji type chemical peel is as follows: 50% TCA (5 ml), Hibiclens (8 drops), and *Yucca* extract (3 drops). The secret, of course, is "pretreatment." Bill Carter sees numerous patients who had problems with the 50% TCA peel. Thus it is best to use 35% TCA and perform touch-ups as needed.

22. One observer has commented:

> "Any claim of zero complications with the Obaji peel and scarring from this technique is certainly not true." He reviewed a case in which the Obaji peel caused severe scarring about the mouth. Massive doses of Kenalog and Aristospan were injected into these areas. There was an infection and erosion of a previously inserted chin implant. She also developed extreme muscle weakness and was diagnosed at the Scripps Institute with proximal muscle myopathy secondary to the corticosteroid injections!

23. Despite what you may have heard, tanning is not a protection from skin damage due to ultraviolet solar radiation. A study of people in mental institutions, who had never been exposed to sunlight for their adult lives, showed that they have much younger-appearing skin. This fact, along with the report that one drink a day seems to prevent heart attacks (less stress?), must not be overinterpreted. Cheers!

24. Alternative methods for handling the giant hairy nevus in children include dermabrasion. Private practitioners are hesitant to accept the glowing reports of this treatment, but some decided to try dermabrasion and, "It worked beautifully." More than simply "working," the result looks excellent 1 year later.

For these patients dermabrasion should be done during the first 5 months of life when the nevus cells are apparently in the upper layers of the skin. Dermabrasion can result in permanent removal with little risk and without the deformity engendered by skin grafting. After dermabrading the area, pig skin can be used to accomplish four aims. Its use (1) promotes epithelialization; (2) reduces the possibility of infection; (3) eliminates fluid loss, which is essential in an infant; and (4) reduces pain so the child remains quiet during the convalescent period.

It is gratifying to pass along a technique that renders benefit to patients who might otherwise have to undergo more extensive, disfiguring surgery. As for melanoma potential, only time will tell. Because dermabrasion removes great masses of nevus cells, however, only a few nevus cells remain that might undergo degeneration.

25. Can dermabrasion eliminate stretch marks on the thighs or abdomen? No. How about Retin-A? No. Retin-A may speed scar resolution though.

26. In 1992 we began to aggressively treat patients who have upper face sun damage and blepharochalasis. It is safe to perform TCA peel with an upper and lower lid blepharoplasty so long as one uses a skin muscle flap. I use 35% TCA and then employ fat grafting using fat from the eyelids. There is little or no risk and only a slight delay in recovery.

27. Dermabrasion, used alone is no longer acceptable; it is relegated to the resting place of the other dinosaurs of facial surgery. More modern rules are as follows: (1) Use light dermabrasion for rough acne spots after "frosting" the entire face with TCA. (2) Protect the patient with intravenous sedation—ketamine-diazepam (Valium) or methohexital sodium (Brevitol)—and local anesthesia before you start. Do not depend on meperidine (Demerol), as it is too sedating and some individuals react with excitement and resistance, even when diazepam has been given. (3) If you dermabrade, use the wire wheel sparingly. Smooth over with a diamond wheel. (4) Light dermabrasion over a TCA peel and "touch-ups" are preferred to scars.

The Gospel According to Tom Baker

Just when you think you are being innovative, you read an interview with one of the great surgeons and find that he is doing everything you are, and probably did so long before you thought of it. I refer to a "discussion" with Tom Baker in Kottler's book on chemical rejuvenation. The following list contains some rules applied by Baker, and some of his observations I once thought derived from my own insights.

1. Do not perform face peeling on men.
2. Do not use patch testing. "It [does not] tell you anything."
3. Start an intravenous infusion in all patients and use midazolam (Versed) and meperidine (Demerol) or diazepam (Valium) and meperidine.
4. Establish supraorbital, infraorbital, mandibular, and great auricular nerve blocks using Marcaine, for the longer duration.
5. When repeeling, one must use good judgment. (Baker has repeeled, or spot peeled, patients numerous times to obtain homogeneous pigmentation.)
6. Do not perform neck peels because of the problems of hypertrophic scarring. (Baker avoids the neck but says, "They can be peeled safely with TCA.")
7. "The worst cases of hyperpigmentation have been people from Central and South America. I do not see it much in pure Caucasians."

8. "I do not advise patients to stop their female hormones." He does prescribe antibiotics, although "I guess as much [for] my own peace of mind as anything."
9. The patient with a history of herpes must begin a course of preoperative Zovirax. About 5% to 10% of Baker's patients have the herpes virus, so one cannot be faulted for placing everyone on the drug prophylactically.

Supercharged TCA Peels

The program we have used successfully at the Institute for Aesthetic Plastic Surgery involves slow, gradual preparation of the skin without the pain of peeling and redness. The difference in our philosophy is simple. We allow patients to prepare their skin at leisure unless they *want* to be on a "fast track." Then there are two choices: The first is to proceed directly to the 40% glycolic acid peels performed by an aesthetician (rapid exfoliation) on a weekly basis followed by a "home program" of Retin-A and AHAs. For those impatient people, another choice is to use tretinoin for 2 to 4 weeks and then schedule a TCA or mixed peel.

As noted earlier, use of 35% TCA provides a greater safety margin. Nevertheless, some physicians take a totally different approach. They "supercharge" the TCA by adding substances to the formulation to achieve a deeper peel. James Fulton, for example, adds methylsalicylate and 1% Polysorbate as a detergent. The 5% to 10% methylsalicylate causes deeper penetration of the 35% TCA, which Fulton claims is less risky than using a stronger (50%) concentration of TCA. This supercharged formula, of course, is used only for facial areas that require greater penetration. My difference in philosophy is that one should come back and touch up these areas as necessary, letting the subsequent tretinoin program provide the safety net. We ultimately achieve the same rejuvenation.

Areas of Agreement

There are many ways to achieve facial rejuvenation. A few common points are as follows.

1. "Retinization" is essential.
2. The skin preparation determines the depth of the peel. Alcohol cleansing allows lighter penetration, and ether or other skin degreasers allow greater penetration.
3. Antibiotics and often Acyclovir (Zovirax) should be prescribed.
4. The method of application on the eyelids is important. Use cotton

swabs. For areas such as crow's feet that require deeper penetration apply the TCA peel with a 2 × 2 gauze square.

5. Topical steroids and hydroquinones are useful before and after TCA peels.
6. Light spot dermabrasion may be performed at the time of the peel. It makes little sense to wait 3 to 4 weeks before performing light dermabrasion.

Foolishness That Succeeds Is Still Foolishness

A French surgeon recently urged his audience to follow his example in removing the "unsightly scars" of the patient's torso by his "new" technique. This is the same surgeon that told one of my patients that he did not think that silicone implants should be used in the face. He didn't even talk about dermabrasion or any of the techniques that require surgical skill. Here's his solution: a *full body phenol peel!* The audience was *not* plastic surgeons.

Anyone trained in plastic surgery is well aware of the cardiac threat of phenol peeling of the face. Compare the area of the face to the space between the clavicle and the pubis.

Chemical peeling might be useful for removing pigmentation around an areolar scar in a rare case, but it won't affect the scar itself! Burning off the top layer of hypertrophic scar does nothing at all. Topical AHA creams are helpful for body skin changes and perhaps a 15% AHA solution may be worth using in severe sun damaged body areas.

OFFICE INSTRUCTION SHEETS

Derma-Gly Prescribed Skin Care Program: Glycolic Acid

Derma-Gly skin care has been formulated for the entire face and body with glycolic acid, a particular Alpha Hydroxy Acid found in sugar cane.

These products provide the optimal combination of ingredients to make the skin appear softer and smoother.

The substances used are gentle, non-toxic, and help remove the overly-thick outer layers of dead skin, without causing sensitivity to sunlight.

Derma-Gly skin care is formulated to be used in conjunction with the GlamouR$_x$ cleansers, toners, and moisturizers. It may be used with Retin-A as well.

Directions:

Apply to cleansed skin morning and night underneath prescribed moisturizer. May be used as close to the eye as the cheekbone.

How to Combine Products:

The following sequence is the best way to combine Derma-Gly skin care with other products you may be using.

After thoroughly cleansing face or body first apply the Derma-Gly skin care product.

Any other product used, such as RetinA, benzoyl peroxide, or antibiotics should be applied directly on top of the Derma-Gly skin care. Moisturizer or makeup will always be applied last.

Caution:

For External Use Only.

More Good News:

Derma-Gly Rapid Exfoliator Peel is applied in our office by the Esthetician. This highly concentrated formulation accelerates removal of the dead outer layers of skin and enhances the results obtained with Derma-Gly home use products.

Retin-A is a prescription drug that has a mild peeling effect on the skin. It must be used with caution. When used properly, Retin-A can be very beneficial to the skin.

Retin-A was originally designed as a treatment for the cystic acne patient. Through the years we have found that as well as helping to control acne, it has a rejuvenating effect for aging skin.

To experience the optimum benefits of Retin-A, we must first find out if your skin can tolerate it. We have found that this can best be done by using our GlamouRx Prescribed Skin Care Cosmetic Line. GlamouRx treatment products are compatible with Retin-A.

We have provided two non-detergent cleansers, an alcohol-free toner, a Paba-free sunblock with an SPF-15 (which doubles as the patient's daytime moisturizer) along with other treatment products to keep your skin comfortable while using Retin-A.

Usage of Retin-A:

Step 1: Cleanse with prescribed GlamouRx Cleanser.

Step 2: Apply prescribed GlamouRx toner with a cotton pad all over face and neck.

Step 3: Squeeze a pea size amount of Retin-A onto your finger. Quickly smooth the Retin-A over the surface of the skin, being sure not to put it on the lips, corners of the mouth, corners of the nasal area near the mucus membrane, or the immediate eye area. The Retin-A may be used as close to the eye as the cheekbone, however never on the eyelid.

Now relax for ten to fifteen minutes for complete absorption of the Retin-A.

Step 4: Apply prescribed GlamouRx moisturizer.

The Next Morning:

STEP 1: Cleanse with prescribed GlamouRx Cleanser.

STEP 2: Apply prescribed GlamouRx toner all over face and neck.

STEP 3: If you are using the Derma-Gly product, it would be applied next, as directed.

STEP 4: Apply sunblock as daytime moisturizer.

During the first two weeks, Retin-A should be used at night only. Beginning Monday and Friday. If after two weeks there has been no reaction (burning, itching, redness, sensitivity), then you can apply on Wednesday night also for the next two weeks, i.e. Monday, Wednesday, and Friday. You have now been using Retin-A for one month. If you have not experienced any reaction you may now begin during your 5th and 6th week applying on alternating nights, i.e. Monday, Wednesday, Friday, and Sunday. In each of the following two week periods, you may add in an additional night's application.

When you reach the point that you are using Retin-A seven nights a week, if time permits you may begin applying Retin-A in the mornings. At this point you would begin your two-week cycle all over again. Example: You are using the Retin-A seven nights a week, you are now beginning to use Retin-A on Monday morning for two weeks, etc. Once you have reached the point where you are using Retin-A seven evenings and seven mornings with no reaction, you may ask your physician for a stronger dosage or percentage at which point will begin with the original Monday and Friday for two weeks. Continuing the program as stated above.

This program is one that will be beneficial as long as the patient continues. If for any reason the patient stops the program, they would not regress, however no further progress will be made.

Institute for Aesthetic Plastic Surgery

ACNE

The Role of Fat Grafting, RetinA, Chemical Peel, and Dermabrasion (Patient Instruction Sheet)

Acne is a most difficult condition with no known causes and no age limitation. Antibiotics are effective but only temporarily. The traditional methods of "skin sanding dermabrasion" were often unsatisfactory because of pigment changes and texture changes. The efforts of control include the drug, "Accutane" which is prescribed by dermatologists and has serious side effects in some individuals, and the new regimens which we use at the Institute for Aesthetic Plastic Surgery. These programs restore much of the damage and minimize future damage. In any one individual, they may involve pretreatment with RetinA followed by a combined "Level IV" chemical peel-dermabrasion with fat grafting or a simple maintenance program of "Level II" fruit acid peel and good skin care.

RetinA has been used to alleviate the symptoms of acne and improve skin appearance for approximately 15 years. It was approved for this use by the FDA. Subsequent clinical trials had indicated its usefulness in restoring collagen and elastin to sun damaged skin and restoring a more youthful appearance. For the acne patient, both results are beneficial. RetinA will thin the thick upper layer of the skin so that skin appears to be smoother. Its primary effect is beneath the skin with a gradual increase in youthful-appearing collagen ingrowth. After a period of treatment with RetinA, the skin not only appears to be more youthful and healthy but has new blood vessels, new collagen, and eventually, new elastic fibers. The ingrowth of blood vessels is one of the beneficial effects for the acne patients since increases in blood supply help to contain bacterial breakthroughs.

We advise a complete program of skin cleansing, which may include opening of comedones and pustules, occasional topical antibiotics, occasional antibiotics by mouth for short periods of time, and an ongoing program of skin cleansing and rejuvenation.

Patients with acne must avoid makeup and moisturizers that are "comedogenic". This means that certain ingredients in popular cosmetics will plug the pores of the skin and contribute to the formation of pustules. The cosmetics that are prescribed for Institute patients are aloe vera based and do not contain mineral oil. Another side effect of RetinA is occasional sensitization and drying of the skin. Aloe vera based cosmetics and moisturizers help to prevent this from becoming a problem.

Working closely with our office aesthetician, the acne patient will slowly progress from intermittent RetinA at the lowest concentration to more frequent applications. At a certain point, each patient will attempt to use a stronger concentration until the maximum concentration is tolerated without burning, peeling, or discomfort. There is new information that the effects are more permanent than what was once believed.

Acne patients must understand that the control of acne is an ongoing process and that they may not "grow out of it". Although diet has been implicated, there are no definite indications in the scientific studies that the use of chocolates, sugar or other foods play a major role.

Fat Grafting: Because many acne patients have valleys and depressions from previous infections, fat grafting is used as a means of elevation. The fat is obtained from the "permanent" fat that forms around eyelids in certain people or it may be obtained from the abdomen or hips. Fat is concentrated and placed as a graft underneath the depressed areas which has been elevated. For certain acne patients, grafts are placed under the entire midcheek. The effect of this elevation is only a part of the total picture.

Chemical Peel: There are five levels of chemical peel and two are used in acne patients without the requirement of the office surgical rooms. The first is RetinA as explained above. The second is the fruit acids. These light chemical peels may be used on a weekly basis. They strip the skin of the thicker upper layer and allow free penetration of RetinA. There is an instant smoothing of the skin and the pores are unclogged. The benefits are temporary, however, and should be incorporated into an ongoing program with RetinA and day and/or night creams. These Glycolic Acid creams also smooth the skin and must be adjusted to individual tolerance.

Chemical Peel with Dermabrasion: The "Level IV" chemical peel is a Trichloroacetic acid concentration which is used in conjunction with light sanding of the surface of the skin. One may think of fat grafting as elevating the valleys, the Trichloracetic acid peel as a smoother and tightener of the rough surface, and a light dermabrasion as a means of controlling elevations of scar tissue and skin above the surface. This procedure requires a seven to ten day recovery period. It is performed in the office surgical center under "twilight" anesthesia. Nerve blocks are administered during the period of twilight and pain is kept to a minimum. Many patients do not require pain pills. The areas of dermabrasion form thicker crusts than the areas of chemical peel. Aloe vera based oils are prescribed on the third day postoperatively. These loosen the crusts and facilitate healing of the new skin beneath the crust. The peel area crusts will separate more quickly and leave less redness and irritation. Protective makeup is prescribed on the seventh or tenth postoperative day. You can expect to return to normal activity at that time. In the first week, it is advisable to schedule only indoor activities that do not require social contact. Redness of the skin treated with dermabrasion will usually subside in four to twelve weeks, depending on the depth of the dermabrasion. The lighter TCA peels show a quicker recovery period than the traditional heavy depth Phenol or Bakers Formula peels. These "Level V" are rarely used, except in the area around the lip or for dark spots that require bleaching. Tape masks are no longer employed but we may advise topical antibiotics for showering during the initial healing phase. The "Extremely Effective Oil" should be applied liberally as directed.

The lighter chemical peels may be repeated as often as indicated. For the majority of patients, this will mean a second light peel in four to six years. In patients with ongoing acne or more severe damage, a peel may be scheduled on a yearly basis. The second peels can usually be performed in the clinic without anesthesia and do not require the operating room, so there is only a minimal cost.

Our success rate with fat grafts has been impressive in undamaged skin, such as the grooves between the eyebrow or above the lips. Acne patients seem to do as well, even though the tissues are more scarred and, therefore, less likely to be easily lifted to a normal position. Our goal is to improve the appearance as possible. Your cooperation as a patient is essential. Please read all of your instruction sheets carefully and maintain close contact with our office staff during this period. The office is fully prepared and capable of answering most of the questions. Please feel free to call us at (210) 349-4353 for further information or for questions concerning your particular needs.

2 *Fat Grafting*

NO ONE PROCEDURE HAS ADDED SO MUCH REFINEMENT TO facial surgery as autologous fat grafting. Fat grafting, in combination with tretinoin (Retin-A) and α-hydroxy acid programs and chemical peeling, is now state of the art in facial rejuvenation. Fat grafting and fat resection play a role in correcting defects in the nasolabial line area. We no longer have to overstretch the skin in an effort to erase nasolabial lines; we can attack them directly and augment the depression at the same time we reduce the fatty roll outside the nasolabial groove. Although fat grafting does not eliminate fine lines, these lines can be controlled with level II, III, and IV chemical peels. Fat grafting simply elevates depressions associated with these fine lines. We are seeing success even with acne scars.

Pierre Fournier popularized fat grafting in 1986, even though Yves Illouz had discussed the use of fat grafting as early as 1984. American surgeons were introduced to a new technique of "fat injection" in 1986 at the Review of Aesthetic Plastic Surgery meeting. We all tried it, and it generally failed. Multiple techniques were attempted thereafter, using "fat pearls," insulin washes, and other methods of inserting autologous material that would replace dermis grafts. Dermis grafts, such as SMAS or temporalis fascia grafts, certainly are effective, but they resorb in some cases, and cysts may form. Harvesting is a problem, and so we were looking for a simple technique that could utilize tissue readily available from a blepharoplasty or submental tuck. By 1987 the current techniques were in place, and we began to see long-lasting softening and, in many cases, total elimination of facial grooves and lines. With the development of fat-concentrating techniques, including in-line traps, centrifugation, or simple placing of fat from liposuction on a sterile 4 × 4 gauze and then harvesting it for placement, good long-lasting effects have been achieved. Most of our patients have now had good results that have lasted 6+ years.

The important points regarding fat grafting are as follows.

1. Fat grafting is inexpensive and, if properly performed, effective. I was not impressed with the publicity regarding Fibrel. This gelatin material, which is mixed with the patient's blood at a cost of about $200 per injection plus personnel time, has not been effective in the hands of many of my colleagues.
2. Our original failures with the Fournier technique are now understandable. We "injected" rather than grafted.
3. The major change in my technique is that I now completely undermine the dermis so there are no attachments to underlying tissue. This method allows the wrinkle, scar, or depression to be easily elevated and maintained in its new position.
4. Elevating the area is the essential point. The fat is not "injected"; it is gently laid into position to act as a buffer graft to prevent reattachment.
5. Fat cells live long enough to perform their function. It is unimportant whether the fat is still alive at 6 months or has been replaced with fibrotic material. The end result is the same.
6. Undermining instruments, such as the Wilkinson Rhytidissector, or Lobe's (Brazil) nasolabial dissector were developed to allow clean separation of the dermis from the underlying soft tissue. Entry is made at a hidden point within the nose or behind the hairline.
7. Concentrated washed fat may be collected in a number of ways with a number of traps. The hand-held syringe technique (Tulip system) is as effective as the trap technique.
8. When fat is collected with the Tulip system and a relatively large-bore cannula, large portions of fat are preserved without damage. Centrifugation or filtration removes the oils and lidocaine (Xylocaine), allowing one to collect pure, undamaged tissue for reimplantation.
9. For the nasolabial and marionette area adjacent to the oral commissure, one may introduce a stylet within a 14-gauge needle. This instrument can be advanced into the marionette area after the nasolabial fold has been undermined using an intranasal approach. The 14-gauge needle allows easy introduction of autologous fat into prepared, tension-free areas underneath the skin.

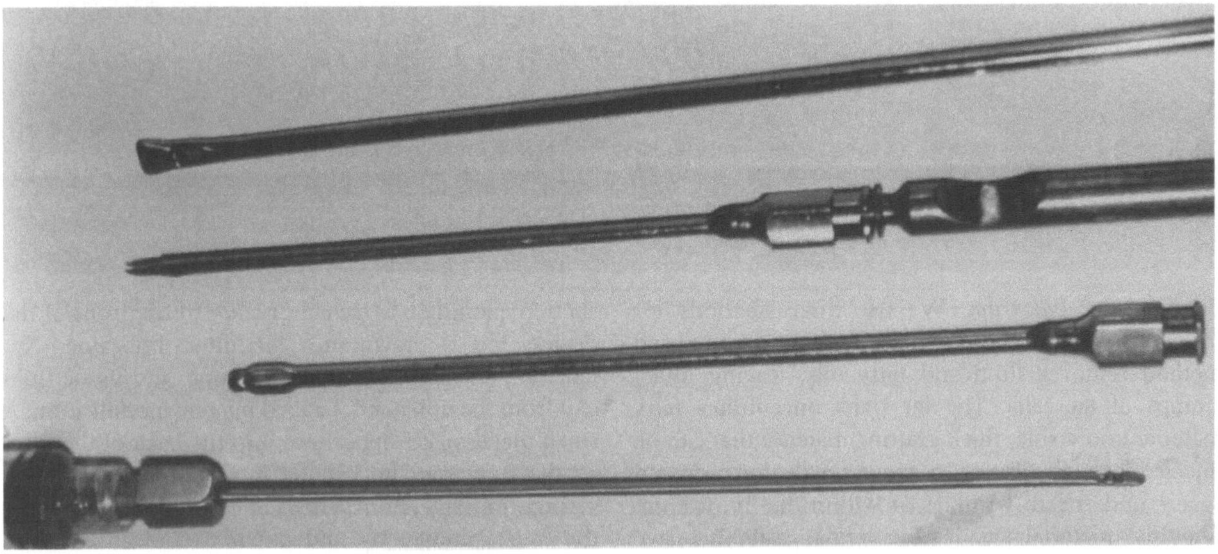

Figure 2-1. These instruments are useful in "fine tuning" a face, particularly one that has irregularities from acne, strange fat deposits, or other generous liposuction. The principle is fairly simple. In flat spots, undermine the dermal attachments and place autologous tissue in the undermined area to prevent reattachment. Concentrated fat works quite well, but you must be careful not to overcorrect by 30 or 40%. In the center of the face one should not overcorrect by more than 20%. We used the top instrument with its rough dissecting point to scrape out scar tissue from the nasolabial line in several ladies. They had silicone, or contaminated collagen, injected into their faces with a resultant hypertrophic subcutaneous scarring. The surface was relatively intact. The serrated blunt tip allowed us to scrape down the dermis and remove the debris with back suction from a syringe attached to the Luer Lok. The same was then used to undermine the entire nasolabial zone and place concentrated fat subdermally to smooth it out. The second instrument from the top is a 14-gauge Trocar that is useful in punching through the inner aspect of the nostril for fat graft deposits in the "Marionette Zone" and nasolabial zone. The third zone is one of several Tulip-type cannulas. Notice the wide open ends that allow you to collect undamaged strips of fat from the periumbilical zone for later regrafting. The Luer Lok version of this cannula may be attached to a Medical Engineering fat trap. The bottom instrument is Luiz Toledo's new aspirator. We found this to be very useful in damaged faces. It's small enough to pass into the tiniest of fatty hillocks in the cheeks, and blunt enough to redirect that fat into small adjacent valleys. Many of our patients examine their faces for such details.

10. For other areas, such as the lip or forehead, a disposable, long, 16-gauge needle is used. It is important that the fat be delivered into the pockets you have created without applying destructive pressure on the injection syringe. Remember: This procedure is fat *grafting,* not fat injection.
11. Lightly abrading the surface of the skin with a No. 15 blade is particularly effective on the upper lip and forehead. Most wrinkles are surrounded by roughened tissue. This light abrasion provides a level field on which to work. The procedure is quick, adds to the aesthetic result, and does not carry the risk of dermabrasion.

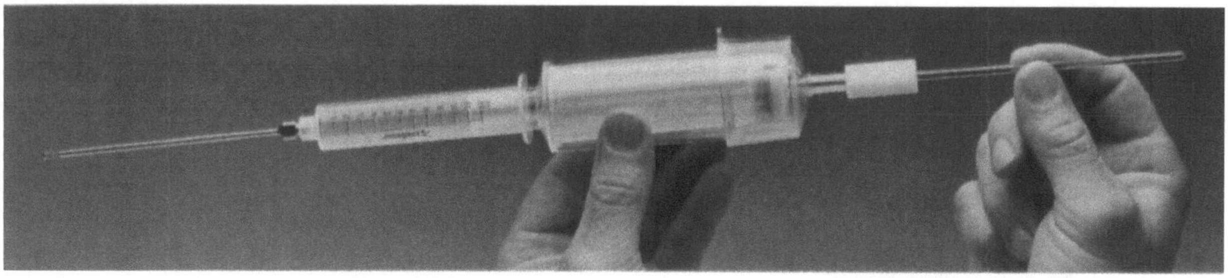

Figure 2-2. *Fat traps.* We use three methods for collecting and concentrating fat for reinjection. Each method removes fluid and fatty oils, leaving intact clumps of fat cells. The fat trap concentrates fatty material into viable, thick grafting material that can be injected through a 14- or 16-gauge needle into prepared spaces underneath wrinkles or within the lip or chin. The thick material acts like the dermal grafts that gave us reasonably good results a decade ago.

The Berkeley fat trap (shown here) is an inexpensive system that simplifies reinjection of fat into the body or face. When fat is collected with the syringe technique, the fat may be filtered or centrifuged or simply drained. With the Berkeley fat trap, however, the suction cannula is attached directly to the front of the device. Fat is drawn into the filter, lidocaine (Xylocaine), and the excess oil, lidocaine, and tissue fluid exit from the other end. I added my one modification: A small metal piece that screws into the back of the filter so the harvested fat can be pumped directly into a syringe for reinjection. When collecting the fat, working the trap's plunger up and down two or three times usually results in 10 to 20 cc of fat. The procedure can then be repeated if more fat is needed. A 2-inch piece of tubing makes a satisfactory connecting device between large-handled cannulas and the trap. These traps are inexpensive and can be discarded at the end of the procedure, although we reuse them several times.

12. No one believes that bathing fat in insulin is helpful.
13. Always overcorrect by 30% to 40%, and be prepared to perform a second fat graft. Among our patients second grafts are required in only 5% to 10%.
14. Do not neglect the saber-like facial lines outside the nasolabial area, even if you are doing a face lift. These lines should be lightly abraded on the surface and deep fat grafts placed underneath the dermis to elevate these areas.
15. One way to view fat grafting is according to its marketing value. If you can take the patient's own tissue without additional cost and use it to achieve a satisfactory result, it is a marketing advantage. For example, all of our blepharoplasty patients are asked whether they would like the extra fat to be placed in the nasolabial area or to enhance the fullness of the vermilion of the lip.
16. In the senile lip, the vertical lines are undermined using a intranasal approach, and fat grafts are laid carefully underneath each wrinkle. The area just underneath the white roll is also undermined, and fat grafts are placed there prior to light abrasion. For most patients, a 35% TCA peel completes the procedure, giving a fuller zone without bleaching.

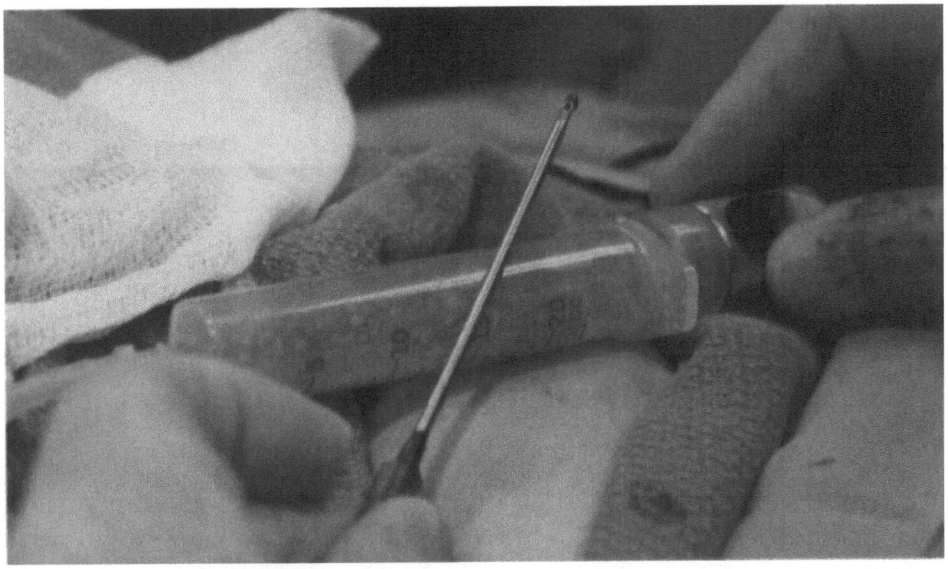

Figure 2-3. Trap used for minor suction procedures. This M.D. Engineering device fits inside a 20-cc syringe. The small holes in the rotation part, which is composed of reusable autoclavable, sterilizable plastic, allows lidocaine (Xylocaine), oil, and tissue fluid to pass through it into the suction reservoir. The trap itself must be sterilized with gas, as autoclaving melts it. A technical point: For the traps shown in both Figures 2-2 and 2-3, the suction cannula should be periodically immersed in sterile saline during the procedure to remove broken fat cells and debris.

17. For both youthful and senile faces, lip enhancement with fat grafting involves multiple tunnels and tension-free grafting rather than injection of fat. Concentrated fat is placed in these tunnels during the withdrawal phase and simply maintains the distortion of the lip. I have a number of patients who have had lip enhancements that remain unchanged even after 5 years.
18. Lip enhancement with fat grafting is most effective in the atrophic, wrinkled, older patient; and these individuals are the most grateful ones. Moreover, the procedure adds only 30 seconds to the rhytidectomy operating time.
19. The big deal about fat grafting is that it is *not* a big deal. According to a recent American Society of Plastic and Reconstructive Surgeons (ASPRS) brochure, one should not expect long-lasting results from fat grafts. Nothing could be further from the truth. If you undermine, overcorrect, and graft undamaged fat, you can achieve excellent results without the problems of dermal grafts in certain facial areas.
20. Fat grafting plays a major role in superficial liposuction. The principles are the same. Small spatula tips are used to undermine the area to break

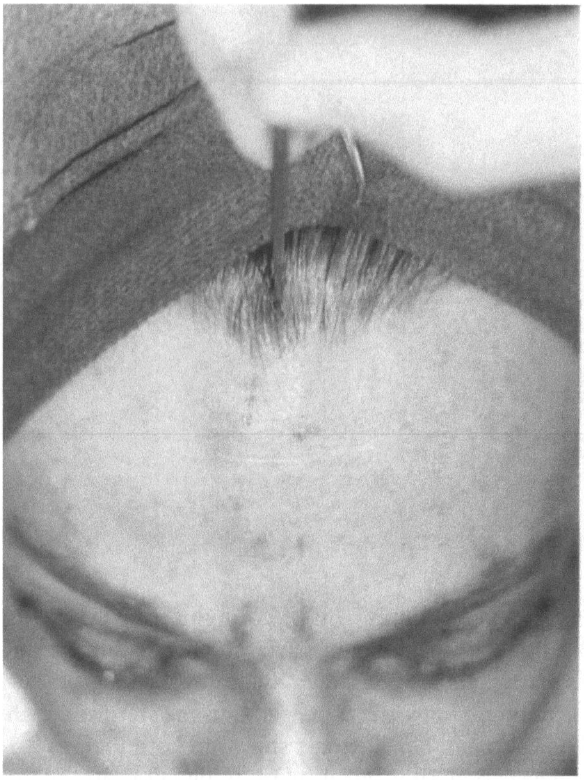

A

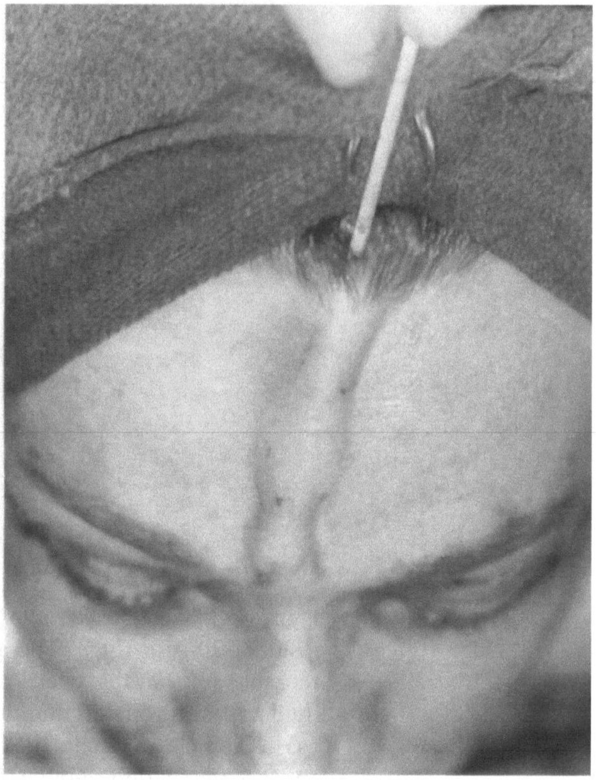

B

Figure 2-4. The key to successful fat, fascia, or SMAS tissue grafts for glabellar lines is undermining. Make the entry inside the hairline (A) and then slide the rhytidissector under the galea until you reach a point just above the folds (B). At this point punch upwardly so the semisharp tip lies subcutaneously. Move the tip up and down against the undersurface of the skin until the lines disappear. Then add a fat graft to keep the skin from returning to its original position. Concentrated fat delivered with a percutaneous 16-gauge needle works well. Some "frowners" require a second or third graft. Placing fat both subcutaneously, into muscle, and under the galea is helpful for deeper lines. Break up the corrugator and separate periosteum, too.

up adhesions, as is done in the face. Concentrated fat is then placed under the dermis to elevate and overcorrect the depressed area, again as in the face. The procedure is as effective as in the face, although one must overcorrect to a greater degree with body regrafting.

Glabellar Frown Lines

Years ago I reported a technique to correct glabellar frown lines. It involved subcutaneous undermining of the frown lines with simultaneous division of a portion of the corrugator muscle. A dermis graft was introduced through a small

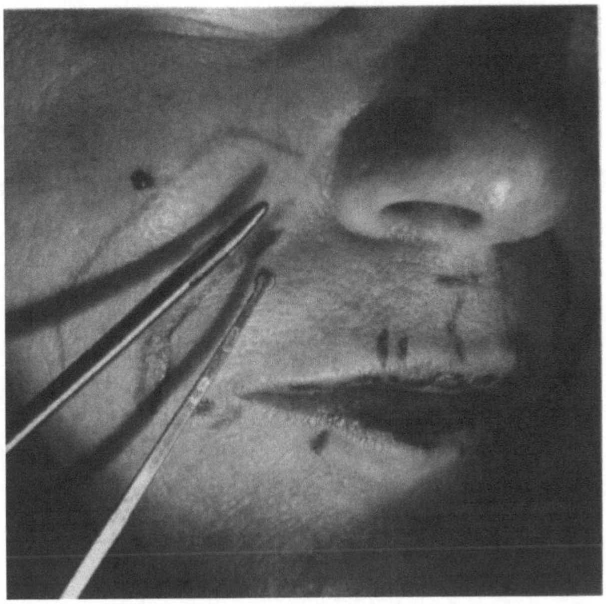

Figure 2-5. This pointed-tip three-holed cannula (left) is a good choice for fat removal in the nasolabial area, and the flat-tipped Wilkinson Rhytidissector (right) is recommended for lysing the fibrous attachments of the fold itself. The pointed cannula passes readily through the fibrofatty tissue lateral to the fold, and the semisharp tip of the underminer easily cuts fibers but is blunt enough to allow a safe rasping motion against the dermis. Note the markings for fat grafting of this senile lip.

stab incision within the eyebrow. Despite meticulous preparation, however, a number of patients developed cysts that required excision; and removing the portion of the corrugator muscle left a few minor but noticeable depressions. The long-term results were good, however: The soft tissue remained elevated, and the depressions were softened (*Annals of Plastic Surgery* 3:341, 1979).

Using today's techniques of multiple-level, 18- or 16-gauge fat "injections," our results in 1986 were mixed. In some patients the glabellar lines remained corrected, whereas in others there was little effect. I thought it was more important to separate the fibrous bands underneath a facial line or depression than it was to "inject" anything, as we had learned from collagen injections for depressed scars on the nose.

Therefore we modified the technique for correcting glabellar frown lines. An 18-gauge needle was introduced from a separate area, and its cutting edge was used to free the soft tissue. The defect was then filled directly with Zyderm or Zyplast (both collagen preparations). The only problem was the rapid and early disappearance of the collagen. Hence we substituted concentrated, undamaged autologous tissue and placed it in an already prepared bed. (These "fat grafts" were thus not injected into a closed space.) It was no surprise to find that the correction percentage dramatically increased. Now we expect a 90% success rate when correcting dimples, grooves, lines, even acne scars using this technique. Failures are corrected with a subsequent fat graft in greater volume.

Jack Fisher pointed out, "The unthinking acceptance of this technique [fat injection] by the aesthetic surgical community is serving to inhibit our pursuit of biologic facts." There is a deserved air of skepticism simply because West Coast

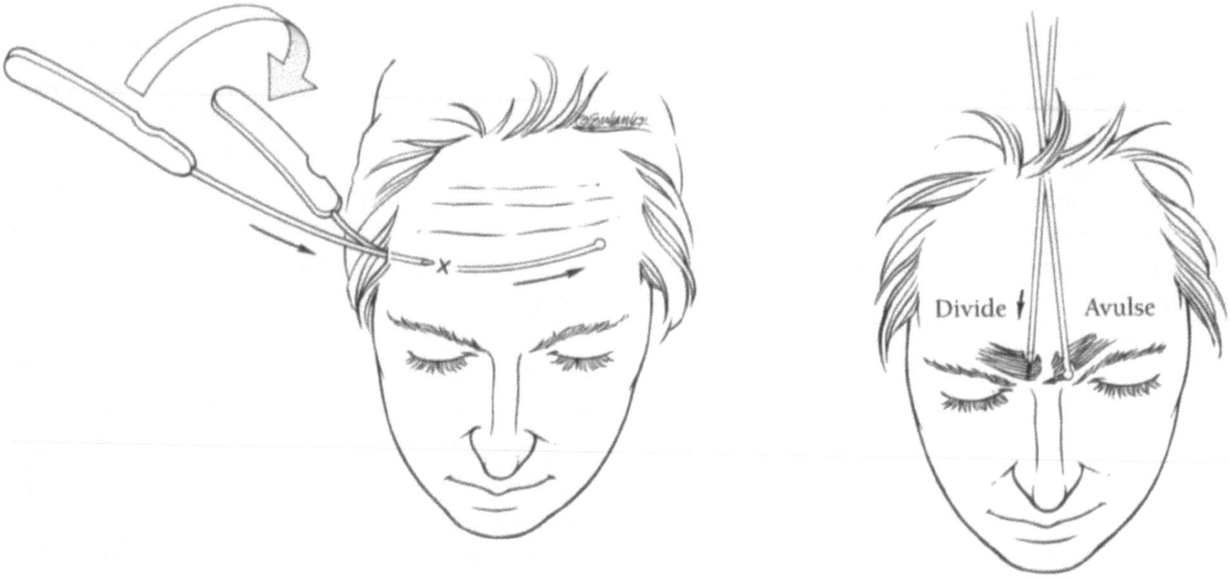

A B

Figure 2-6. Undermining forehead facial lines involves use of a subcutaneous dissector device. A rhytidissector can be modified so it has a longer curve. **(A)** Insert the dissector through the hairline, with the curve pointed upward, then pass it gently underneath the dermis, scraping away the area underneath each wrinkle. Once you reach the midpoint, rotate the handle 90 degrees, so the curve of the dissector now follows the curve of the other side of the forehead; proceed on to the other hairline. Withdraw the instrument in the same way. The width of the tip allows you to separate the area underneath each wrinkle for about 3 to 4 mm. I perform this step at the beginning of facial procedures, so any bleeding that occurs has stopped by the time we are ready to place the fat grafts through direct skin punctures. **(B)** Dividing and avulsing the corrugator muscles and the medial attachment of the orbicularis oculi is easy to accomplish and may contribute to the final result.

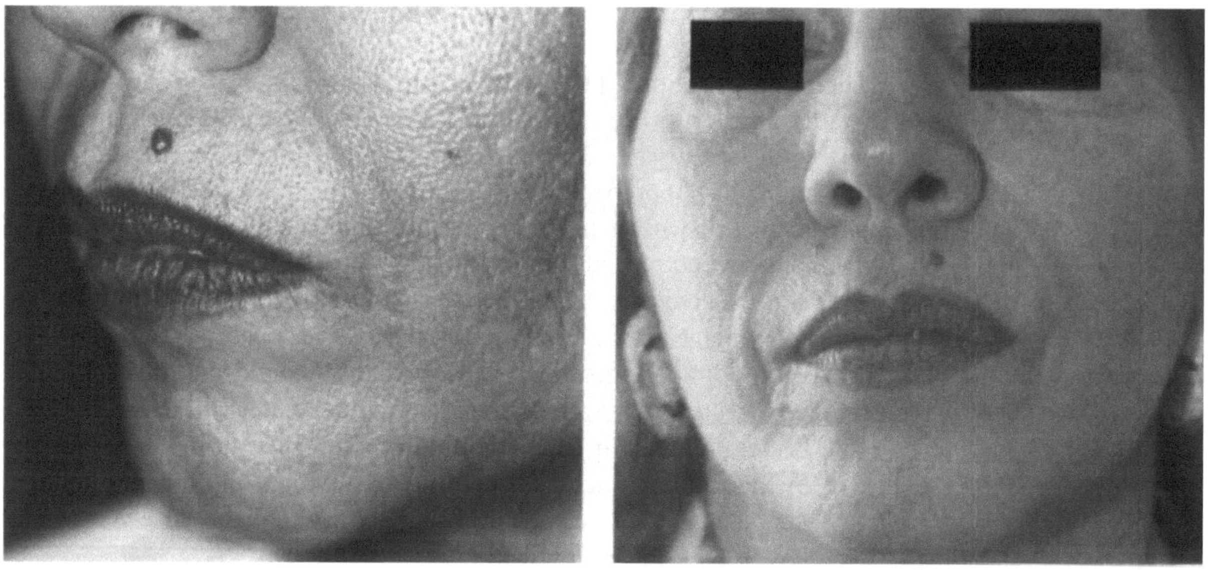

A B

surgeons were so vocal at the initial reporting of this procedure. One also has an inborn skepticism of foreign case descriptions. We recall many rather bizarre presentations over past years. Nevertheless, when one listens and observes, one can see that thinking surgeons from both the aesthetic and the reconstructive side of plastic surgery are pursuing reproducible success in fat grafting and are achieving results better than those mournfully reported by Matt Gleason. We have all heard Gleason's advice: Paraphrased, he said, "If you want to praise fat injection, stop examining your patients after 3 months."

The techniques of undercutting glabellar and nasolabial lines and deep acne scars followed by a two-stage instillation (not injection) of concentrated fat have made believers of many of us. It is true that the dried "creek bed" face of the elderly patient is helped minimally, but there can be some improvement. The best results, as expected, are in young men and women with deep nasolabial folds and few facial aging signs. The same is true for the chronic frowner, but they eventually reform these lines although to a lesser degree. In our experience the lines have remained softer and in many cases absent after a 6 year follow-up.

Touch-Up Procedures

Fat grafts are still somewhat unpredictable. In one of our patients there was resolution of all of the deep facial lines except one spot in the lower half of the right nasolabial fold, which was made more prominent by a thick nasolabial fat fold on that side. He has not had a face lift and does not need one. The answer to his problem was a "touchup" second graft. I use the original Fournier technique. First, concentrated fat is removed from the abdomen. Second, that last bit of wrinkle I undermined a second time by wiggling the tip of a 16-gauge needle underneath it, producing almost the same release as was accomplished with rhytid-dissector as underminers. Another good idea is to use an empty syringe to microsuction the lateral nasolateral fat roll. Passing the 16g needle point back and forth several times while holding back pressure with the fingertips, a small amount of fat is removed, making a noticeable difference. If there is insufficient volume, 2 to 3 cc of thicker fat from the abdomen is added, and placed under the nasolabial line medial to the suctioned zone. I can create smoothness by simultaneous fat removal and fat grafting.

Figure 2-7. This patient is one of four who had had "collagen" injections 3 years earlier, which had left ridges of scar tissue (**A & B**). We planned the correction in two stages. The second stage, dermabrasion, was to be done only if the first procedure was unsuccessful, as it changes the color and texture of the skin. Fortunately, the first procedure was successful.

Using a modified suction dissector on a syringe-lipoplasty setup, the undersurface was scoured using an intranasal approach. The same suction-dissector was used to taper fat and free skin on either side of the nasolabial thickness, following which the space below was filled with concentrated fat grafts. All scar and foreign material was thus excised and the entire area elevated.

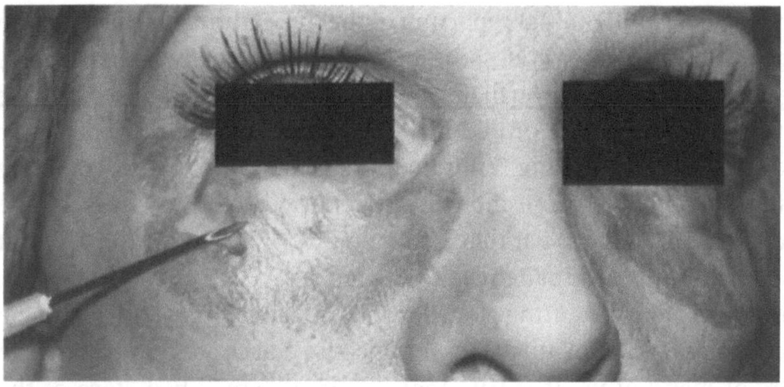

Figure 2-8. Touch-ups. Fine lines, small depressions, and tiny fat bulges after blepharoplasty are approached in the following manner. After local anesthesia, a 16-gauge needle is introduced to aspirate the fat bulge. This fat is immediately transferred to the opposite side where a small depression has been loosened with a cutting motion of a 16-gauge needle. A 35% TCA wipe with a Q-tip completes the procedure.

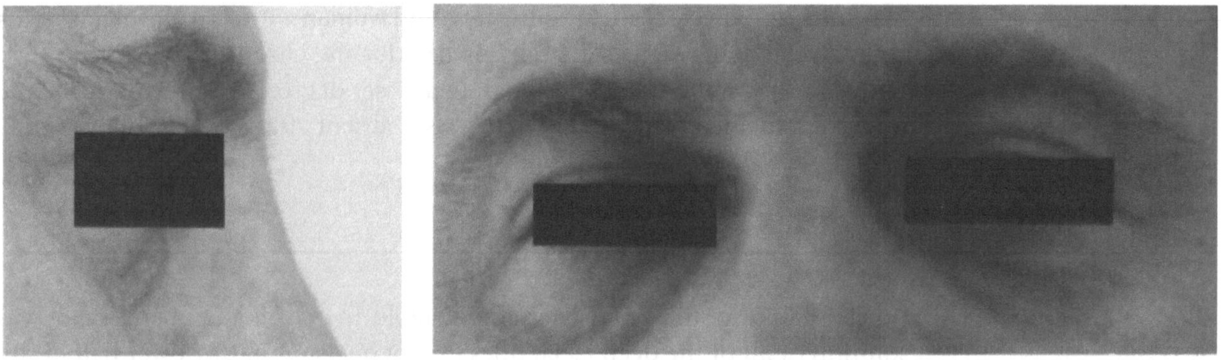

Figure 2-9. Fat grafts for periorbital grooves. This man "wasn't ready" for a blepharoplasty, so I placed concentrated fat in the recessed areas at the lower eyelid edge. Six months later the visible overcorrection was still there, much to our dismay. When the skin was subsequently reflected during a blepharoplasty, there was a neat roll of yellow fat on each side, sitting there as if it had never been transferred.

Questions Regarding the Fate of Fat Injections

Colleagues initially raised questions about fat injections, only some of which can now be answered.

Could the response to a fat injection depend on the type of fat aspirated? No, it seems to make little difference, although many believe that eyelid fat gives better results than fat aspirated from other parts of the body. The aspirated fat works equally well. With eyelid fat, I have had cases of overcorrection that required steroid injections or excision to remove excessive grafted fat. With aspirated fat, one must overcorrect by 40%, less so with eyelid fat.

Does fat from obese individuals produce more edema? No. Beware of the physician who reports a single case! In our clinical experience, it makes little difference whether the individual is fat or thin, but there certainly is a difference if they are over age 65. The surface abrasion technique, a multilevel graft placement technique, undercutting with flat spatula-type instruments, and other mechanical means seem to give fat instillation a better chance of achieving a result that pleases both patient and surgeon.

Fat Metabolism

A few quirky facts may stimulate your interest while contemplating the never-ending battle against obesity and unwanted fat deposits. It seems that obesity is related to cells, not to behavior. It was once believed that obesity was an emotional disorder: People used food to relieve anxiety and depression and then, being fat, became more anxious and more depressed. Studies in animals regarding the methods by which they regulate their eating has led to a new theory—that emotional disorders linked to obesity are the result of being fat and, in fact, are probably caused by attempts at dieting. Diets equal stress. We are asked to believe that stress makes one overweight. I doubt it.

Rats that have twice as many fat cells as usual regulate their eating so their fat cells are the same size as normal rats' fat cells. Because they have twice as many cells, of course, they look fatter. It is different with normal rats. If you excise fat from young rats so they have only half the number of fat cells, they too eat just enough to keep their fat cells a normal size and of course they appear slim. Strange.

If you destroy a part of a rat's brain that regulates its eating, the rat becomes grossly obese, and its fat cells swell to four to five times their normal size. In humans, the fat cells of obese people are much larger than those in normally sized individuals.

Fat cells in once-obese women after dieting are tiny; in fact, they look like starvation fat cells. Such women do not menstruate, their pulse rates and blood pressures are low. Interestingly, these women burn about 25% fewer calories than expected. There is some reason to believe that this situation is the result of a metabolic derangement due to the effects of dieting. Therefore if one diets and loses weight—and then gains it back—it is much more difficult to lose it the next time. This phenomenon is seen in normal individuals as well, as demonstrated by a student volunteer who was isolated in a room for a year and fed a controlled diet. Once having dieted, his body responded to the next diet episode by conserving energy. The student was then induced to become fat, and it was found that he needed more calories than normal just to maintain that weight. He was burning up calories at a furious rate, particularly just after meals. Hence when the body loses weight it uses relatively few calories to consume food—just the opposite of when the body is obese.

What about "cellulite," or "depot fat," that people claim they cannot lose on

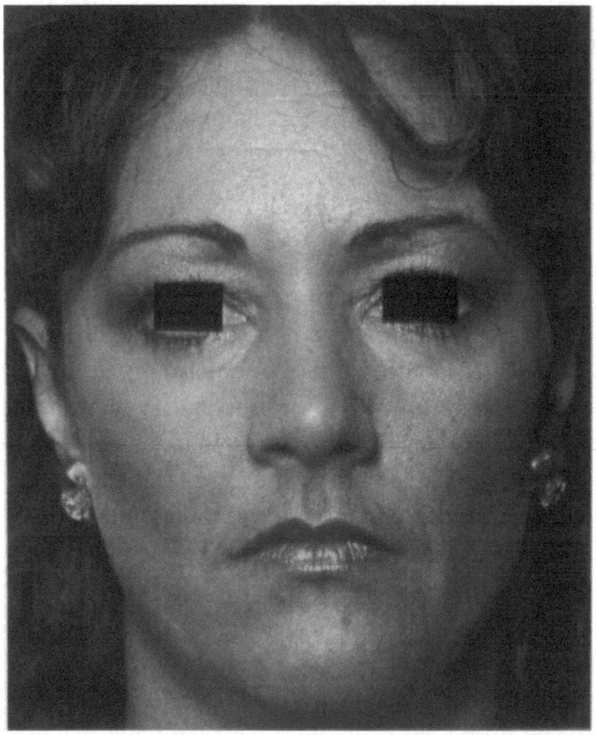

A

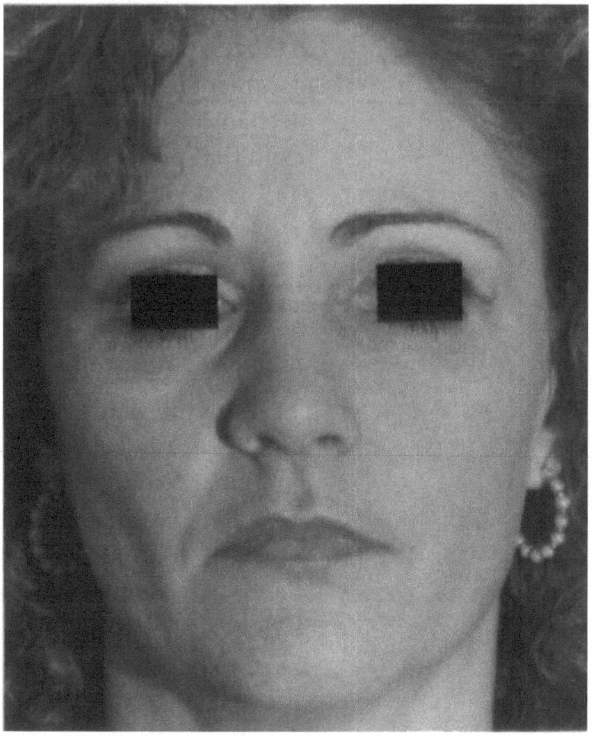

B

C

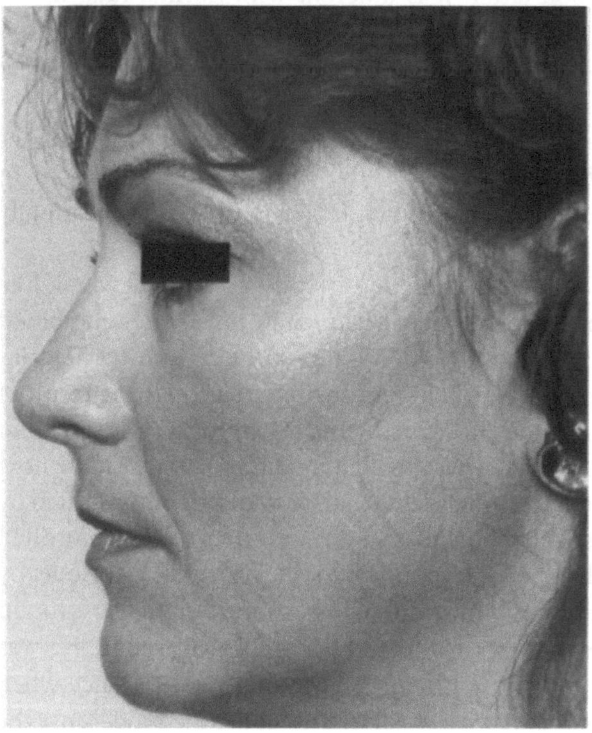

Figure 2-10. This 39-year-old woman would have benefited from a midface lift but chose to have only fat grafting and a blepharoplasty. **(A,C,E)** Her eyelids are the "hooded" type, for which one must taper the muscle excision so it is wider laterally than medially. The eyelid fat was used in the glabella and nasolabial areas, and she began a series of skin care protocols that have markedly improved the condition of her skin as noted in the postoperative photographs **(B,D,F)**. Photographs at 1

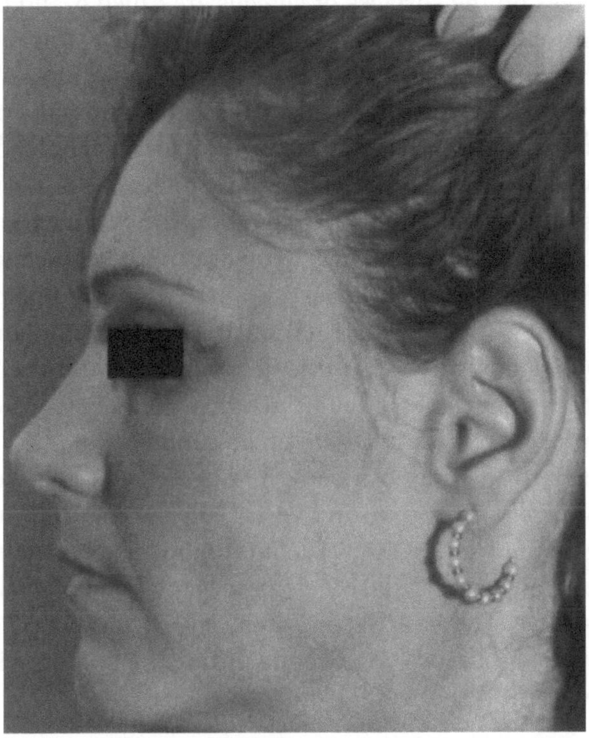

D

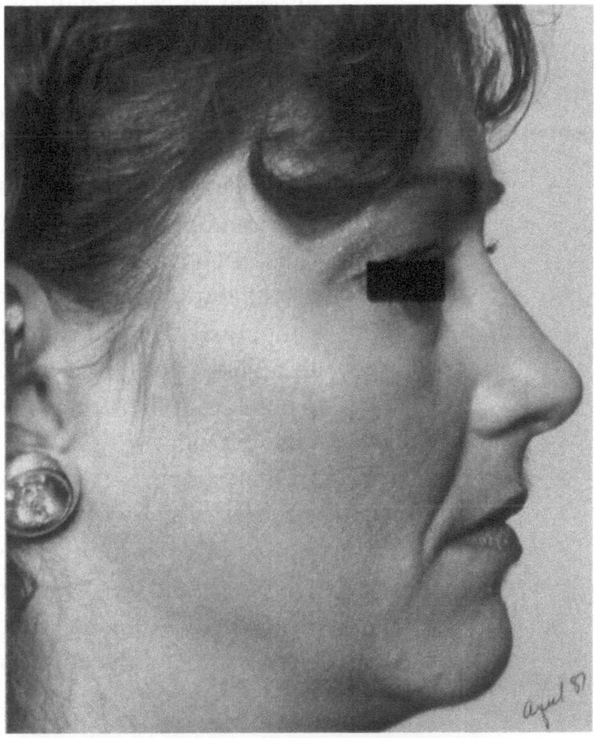

E

year after the fat grafting showed an excellent result. At 5 years she is just beginning to show lines in the forehead. Lateral views show that although the lines have been improved the patient would benefit from lifting the skin. Manually lifting the skin during her examination, as we would do with a "half face lift," completely eliminated the nasolabial lines. Without the fat grafting 5 years previously, a half face lift would be ineffective.

F

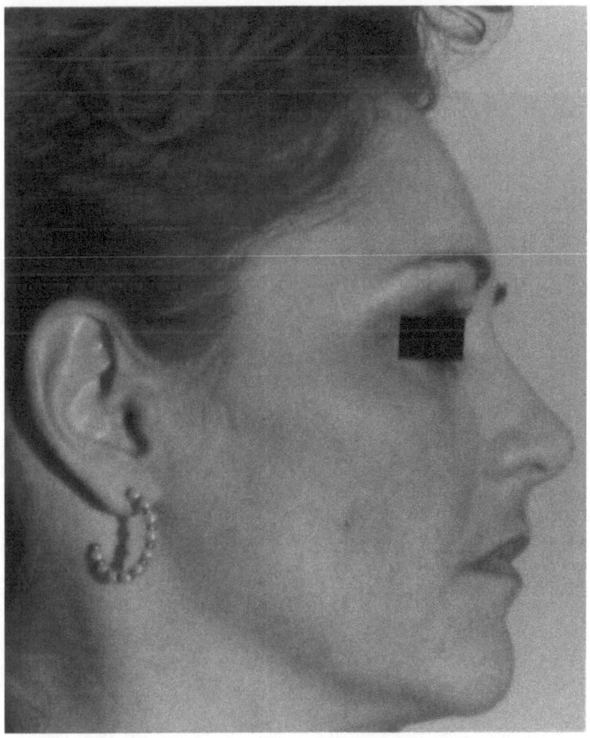

their hips, thighs, "love handles," and other areas? It is indeed composed of a different fat cell. Small molecules on the surfaces of fat cells are called α and β receptors. The α receptors control fat accumulation, and the β receptors control fat breakdown and release. Every cell in the body has its own peculiar ratio of these receptors. In the "depot" areas, the fat cells have predominantly α receptors, which means they tend to accumulate the fat more rapidly and hold it. This phenomenon explains why patients are able to maintain their figures after abdominoplasty or suction-assisted lipectomy. Once you eliminate this mass of cells that get first choice on your "hamburger calories," you do not have the same accumulation factor. When the abdomen has been resurfaced with upper abdominal skin and fat, the weight gain is more normal and does not accumulate in a "preferred" area. It also explains why it is difficult for men to lose their paunches. When they diet they tend to lose fat from other areas first: The abdominal fat with its α receptors is reluctant to give up its contents.

An important question regards dieting: Is it better to not diet at all than to diet periodically? Perhaps. When rats are put on "yo-yo" diets—resulting in gains and losses followed by gains and losses—they become highly food efficient. On the second diet, where they were forced to lose weight, they lost it at only half the rate they did on the first diet. The conclusion, then, is that the fat cells themselves are the culprits. It is not because you overate during the holidays; it is because the fat cells did not want to cooperate.

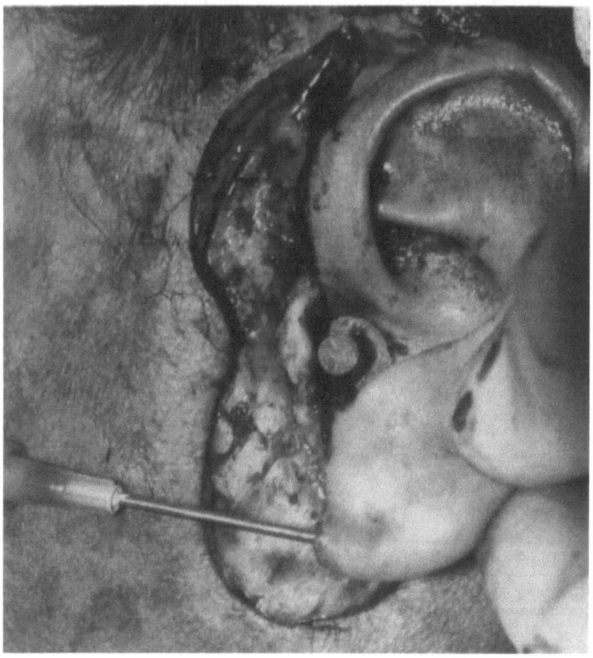

Figure 2-11. Patients do ask for help with wrinkled earlobes! We have pleased these older people by the simple technique of creating multiple tunnels in the earlobe with a 16 gauge needle and filling them with concentrated body fat as the needle is withdrawn.

Collagen Injections

There are serious questions about the safety of collagen injections. A number of collagen-injection patients in the United States, greater in number than the known incidence of disease, have developed the collagen disease polymyositis and dermatomyositis. These crippling and often fatal diseases seem to be related to their prior collagen injections that took place over a period of time.

To date, we know that patients can develop collagen antibodies. We also know that in collagen-injected patients with new cases of dermatomyositis there was a common factor: Each patient had had multiple collagen injections in the past. With the disease onset, both test sites and treatment sites became inflamed. Until the issue is resolved, our office has decided to discontinue collagen injections.

The efficacy and longevity of injectable collagen were debated at one ASPRS meeting, with little or no new information emerging. The plastic surgeons said little and were content to raise mild objections to Collagen Corporation claims. Some of the discussion did bring out some interesting facts, however.

Is the incidence of dermatomyositis greater in collagen-injected patients than in the general population? The Collagen Corporation says it is not, and yet there are studies that disagree. The Corporation says that it has never involved physicians in lawsuits, yet Dr. Jean Cukier was named by the company after he reported a dermatomyositis case. He was later dropped from the suit, but the damage had been done. The Collagen Corporation runs advertisements in women's magazines, and many of us have had the unpleasant experience of patients brandishing these photographs and demanding to know why they did not get the same wonderful result with their collagen injections. It becomes tiresome explaining to patients that collagen's effect is temporary at best, and in many patients it does not seem to be worth the time or cost.

Beef allergy is another controversial subject. There is now a disclaimer on the collagen package insert about preexisting beef allergies, yet our correspondents tell us that they reported similar problems to the company for several years and were "put on hold." The bottom line is still unclear. There seem to be some more cases than expected of dermatomyositis, and they are linked to beef allergy and collagen injections. Our patients must be adequately warned about potential dangers.

It is agreed that collagen injections can cause skin sloughs. When Zyplast was introduced we were told how good it was for deep injections. Then we were told it should be injected only into the upper dermis. The thicker Zyplast collagen does diffuse well in the upper dermis and did seem to last longer than Zyderm, but there were problems with both.

The company recently stated that localized sloughing followed "interruption of blood flow," such as through blood vessel laceration or occlusion, and

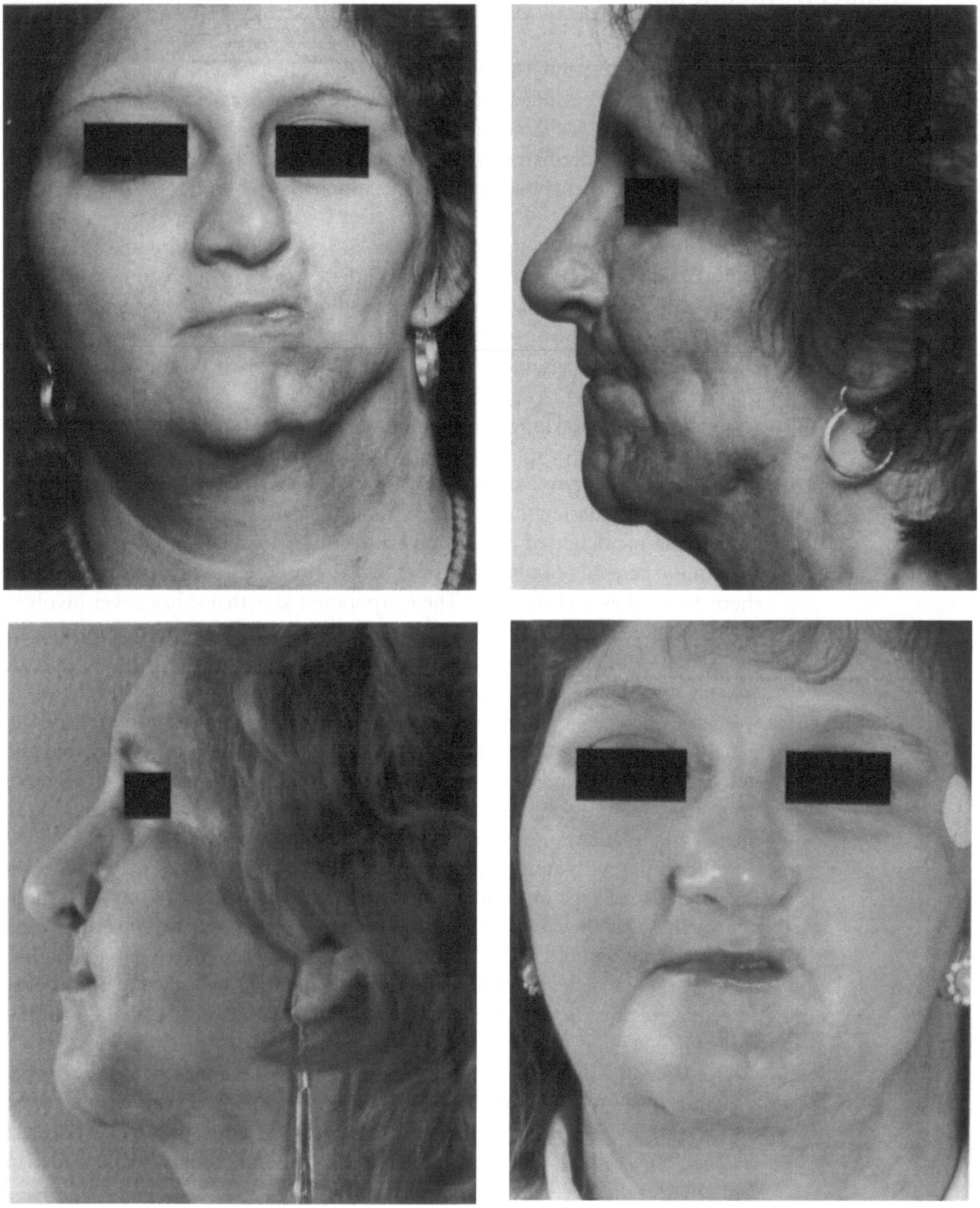

A B C D

occurred more frequently in the glabellar region than in other areas. The problem is not blood vessels; it is the fact that we pack the dermal tissues with collagen, squeezing closed the capillaries. I have seen this scenario with acne scars. More seriously, it is known that blindness is a complication of glabellar collagen injections; a skin slough may not be as devastating, but the plastic surgeon whose patients have suffered a slough are not happy with him or his work.

Paris Lips: Legal or Illegal?

According to the Food and Drug Administration (FDA) Public Affairs Notice 4169758840 dated February 22, 1990, the Collagen Corporation's promotion of their products for lip augmentation is *not* legal. "The approval of Zyderm is for soft tissue contour deformities not for augmentation of a portion of the body. Collagen's promotion of their products for lip augmentation is therefore not legal, and the company has informed FDA that they are no longer promoting the product for this purpose."

One cannot argue with a young woman's desire to have a temporary lip enhancement for a less-than-life-threatening problem, such as being selected for a modeling job. No one, however, has addressed the danger of injecting materials into a highly vascular area such as the lip. Will we encounter a rash of embolic phenomena, or is this fear unreasonable? The Collagen Corporation now says one should only inject *above* the white line—but how can one obtain lip fullness as shown in their ads without filling the vermilion? Clarification of this issue is needed by a dispassionate party. In the meantime, fat grafts *do* work and give good 5-year fullness in more than 90% of cases.

Figure 2-12. Romberg's disease. Progressive hemifacial atrophy (Romberg's disease) is difficult to treat. We have used dermal fat-free grafts, malar and manidibular RTV, Silastic implants, and other techniques with some success; in all cases, one must restore soft tissue. Before the advent of concentrated fat grafts, we had little to offer these individuals. Liquid silicone was used in the initial studies, but the late results were not good. Following the lead of Chajchir and many others, we have used fat grafts in Romberg's disease patients, and they have responded well although multiple grafting sessions are required.

Because large volumes of fat are needed, a fat trap is helpful. For the patient shown here, we used the disposable Berkeley trap because she was somewhat obese and the best donor area was a wide zone of the abdomen. The first procedure was performed under general anesthesia in the hospital. Subsequent grafts were performed with the Tulip system and local anesthesia in our clinic. **(A&B)** In 1986, before the first fat grafts and before a chin prosthesis was implanted. **(C&D)** In 1990, after the second procedure. Further graftings are planned when it suits her timetable.

Other Injectable Substances

Auto Collagen

Ever since the French went to the press about their "new and wonderful" injectable substance, auto collagen, we have been deluged by questions from patients about it. Adequate response has been difficult because the scientific data are incomplete. Apparently, individuals donate their fat or dermis which is treated so the fatty tissue is removed; the remaining cellular structures, auto collagen, are then injected back into the patient's face to fill wrinkles. The basic process, as we understand it, involves adding distilled water to the fat and then separating the collagen between a layer of saline and fat. In this country no one will add fibrin glue to the collagen to "stop the migration." Another process, preparing a fine mixture of collagen from a patient's own skin shows some promise. Is it worth the additional cost for minimal improvement? Is there a good choice between the risk of AIDS from fibrin glue preparations and the risk of autoimmune disease from blood products? Moreover, it is highly suspicious when investigators report their finding to the press before allowing colleagues to see the materials in question, thereby allowing other surgeons to independently assess a new treatment.

Liquid Silicone Injections

Despite the overwhelming evidence that liquid silicone injections cause problems, even when administered via the "micro-drop" technique, some few American physicians have continued to use them, even for such potentially hazardous areas as the vermilion of the lip. It has been illegal for years to transport liquid silicone across the state lines, which means that unless you are living next door to the Dow Corning plant you would have to use industrial grade silicone. The FDA has finally stepped in, bowing to publicity and congressional subcommittees. Reading the subcommittee reports, one stumbles across testimony that the FDA actually stormed into a dermatology office in New York City with guns drawn (a rumor perhaps?) and confiscated their silicone for analysis. Despite the doctors' claims that the silicone was legal because they manufactured their own, analysis of the fluid revealed the same impurities found in industrial silicone. At any rate, we are thankful that the FDA has become adamant: Liquid silicone cannot be used for cosmetic surgery procedures. Yet we still hear from surgeons who are actively promoting silicone injections for lip enhancement, the worst place to put silicone.

At least it is now easier to respond to patients who have had silicone injections and have come to us with glowing reports of its safety and efficacy—despite the fact that we have seen late cases of sagging, bagging, dense fibrosis in the cheeks with artificial jowl formation; hard, rocky distorted lips; and other equally terrible results. Even the late follow-up reports on the ill-fated university studies of Romberg's disease showed that late migration of liquid silicone ultimately destroyed the initially promising aesthetic result. The only good news: None of these patients exhibit the signs of auto-immune disease.

Fibrel

There seem to be several problems associated with Fibrel, for which its developers claimed "improvement" for their patients. First, it is expensive. Second, it must be mixed even after you purchase the kit. Third, if you read the fine print, a second injection must be given later with the same amount. Fourth, the published results do not clearly show such "improvement." Lastly, Fibrel cannot be an alternative to other injectables because it causes allergic reactions.

At this point one can say only that this compound is expensive, its results are erratic and disappointing, and it certainly seems to be more of a problem to the surgeon than a blessing. We would be interested to see an evaluation of Fibrel performed by a disinterested group of plastic surgeons.

Fat Injection in Hands

My first experience with fat injection of the hands involved a young woman who had been to Paris to see Fournier and had had a malar fat augmentation. Surprisingly, he showed her in a presentation a year or so later with an outstanding result. By the time I saw her she had lost most of the augmentation despite being informed that she would have to have three more injections to *maintain the correction.*

This situation would certainly not occur today. Concentrating the fat and placing the material at multiple levels in the chin, cheek, and lips is producing more consistent results, although results in the malar area are not as favorable. The patient reported above casually mentioned that she had had injections in the back of her hands to "hide her veins," but I could see little improvement. Today, I do not hesitate to use leftover fat for concentrated fat grafts to the back of the hands in my older patients. They see more improvement than I do.

There are other methods to improve the appearance of the hands of older patients. They involve stripping the prominent veins, applying TCA peels followed by a period of tretinoin (Retin-A) application. Overfill with concentrated fat grafts is one of several factors that appear to thicken the subdermal tissue. The method is not perfect, but it does help.

There is a simple way to strip veins in the elderly patient's hand that can be done easily with local anesthesia with or without ketamine-diazepam (Valium) dissociation. With a sterile paper clip make a tiny incision at the origin of the vein just beyond the wrist and pop the vein out with a hemostat. Ligate the proximal end and then make a small opening for the paper clip. Create a loop in the back end of the paper clip so when you pass it downward, there is something that acts as a stripper. Carefully thread the paper clip until you can see it inside the vein underneath the skin in the finger webs. Make a second small incision, divide the vein, and then pull it through, completing the stripping. This procedure may also be performed at the same time as a TCA peel if the hand has been prepared with Retin-A.

Comments and Commentary

1. Many of the points emphasized by the "20/20" television series on the Collagen Corporation remain unresolved. The company denied bullying and threatening plastic surgeons, which we know to be untrue. I have seen the correspondence and spoken to the plastic surgeons involved and, in fact, was threatened myself by the Corporation because of articles I published questioning their safety practices. (My questions were based on one of their internal memoranda in which a group of in-house doctors reviewed a large number of patients with symptoms of scleroderma or dermatomyositis. Two-thirds of their reports were cavalierly dismissed because the symptoms did not meet the criteria the group had established, leading to the conclusion that there was no greater incidence of dermatomyositis in collagen-injected patients.)

The Committee on Government Operations (House Report 102-1064) issued a report to the 102nd Congress of the United States in November 1992 that was highly critical of the company as well. We learned that the Corporation "fixed the books" to inflate the number of individuals who had received collagen. According to the Committee's report, it worked this way: If a patient was given six collagen injections, which was fairly common because the material disappeared so quickly, the Corporation treated the data as if they had come from six patients. This finagling inflated the number of individuals who had received treatment, thus reducing the percentage for those who developed dermatomyositis and myositis. In fact, it reduced it so much that the company was able to claim that there was no increased incidence.

The report also was highly critical of the Corporation's policy of teaching doctors the Paris lip procedure even though the FDA had told them in no uncertain terms to cease and desist. Despite the repeated warnings, in October 1990 The Collagen Corporation launched the Paris lip at a fashion show in France, claiming again that the injections would give the lush, full vermilion pictured in the photographs. This claim set off angry retorts from plastic surgeons. In addition, an epidemiologist at the Texas Department of Health testified that the Collagen Corporation had reported only 54 adverse reactions for more than 6000 consumer complaints received. The Texas Department of Health concluded that more than 800 systemic reactions, as well as other serious problems, were not reported to the FDA. Many of the problems (e.g., abscesses

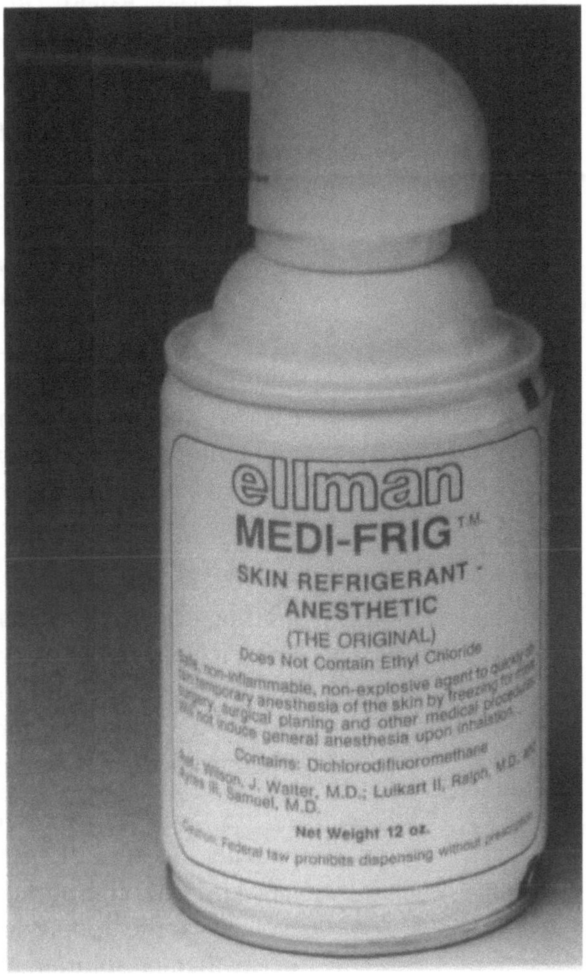

Figure 2-13. There are two ways to make injections easier. The first is the blue "Cryoglobe" shown in the Color Insert, which is held against the skin during minor operating room cases simply to diminish the pain of the local blocks. Another suggestion is the use of Medifrige sprayed on a Q-tip and lightly applied to the skin at the point where the needle will be inserted. Both techniques are effective. The Medifrige is of course more costly as it is nonrenewable. However, we have been using a single can, which has lasted 6 months and is still not empty.

and scars) were considered "not serious enough" to report, and lupus was not reported because the surgeon involved did not suggest that the lupus was caused by the "collagen," largely because the Corporation had informed doctors that their product could not possibly be the cause.

As often is stated by reputable plastic surgeons, no one can find fault with a minor procedure that brings pleasure to a patient, even though the results may be transitory. One would hesitate to perform it, however, if there were evidence that the procedure is dangerous to a significant number of individuals. It is most disturbing that the Collagen Corporation has chosen to muddy the waters by withholding information and then attacking physicians who questioned the safety of their product. It would be far better if they engaged in public education and no longer passively approved the use of their material for plumping the lip vermilion. Glossy, direct approach advertisements and the sponsorship of doctors' in-house publications that glorify collagen injections are among the practices that are most criticized and should be changed.

1. Dr. Chajchir (Buenos Aires) shows fairly good results with fat grafts in patients with Romberg syndrome at 5 years. Ubinas, Taylor, and Salyer (Dallas) use an almost identical technique and have reported the following:

> In patients with hemifacial atrophy or Romberg's disease, we have used a reverse technique of liposuction, whereby we have taken fat from the abnormal side to augment the soft tissue contour. The early results of this technique appear promising, as patients treated in this manner demonstrate less reabsorption of the lipo-injected fat than with conventional dermal fat grafts. We are in the process of documenting and quantitating the survival of such free fat transfers through lip injection.

Little else works in Romberg syndrome patients. In my longest-followed case, we had lost the dermal fat graft to infection. The patient had much body fat, and bulk fat grafts after undermining does work. It took four sessions, but the surgery was easy, thanks to disposable traps. No fuss/no mess equals a quick case and low risk. The results: A face that was far more attractive than I had hoped.

2. Sidney Coleman (New York) has had good long-term results with fat grafting. "If we talk percentage, however, we are trying to be scientists. We don't know if fat lives, but we certainly know that it lasts." Even if much of the injected fat dies, oil microcysts form and are gradually replaced with fibrous tissue, which is why we are seeing more improvement over the long term. It matters not whether the final material is fat, oil, or scar.

3. Satisfactory corrections after fat injection are less frequent in elderly patients. Because of the bulk factor fat injection has no effect on superficial wrinkles, although surface abrasion with a No. 15 blade can help. The solutions we have are temporary at best, but as one wag said, " a temporary solution is better than no solution at all."

4. Shel Rosenthal (Encino) stated, regarding his experience using fat injections:

> It has basically been associated with post-traumatic defects on the lower extremities, thighs, and anterior tibial areas, as well as some defects in the forearm and, of course, facial defects of both iatrogenic and idiopathic etiologies. I feel that it has a definite place in our armamentarium but I do not think we should elevate our hopes to expect this to be a panacea, but rather an addition to our treatment for the filling of deeper defects, always keeping in mind that there will be a loss of bulk of anywhere from 30% to 60% and that repeated injections will be required. I think the most important area is in adequately informing the patient so that they do not have unrealistic expectations but always keeping them mindful of the fact that the tissue being injected is theirs rather than a foreign material. Of course we plastic surgeons are never fully satisfied with results and are always looking for that little bit extra that will bring us closer to the perfection that we compulsively seek but are never able to attain.

3 *Submental Triangle*

WHEN THE MANDIBULOCERVICAL ANGLE IS LOST AND THE AREA underneath the jaw is no longer taut, the youthful look is gone. This area, which can be corrected by platsymorrhaphy and fat removal, (the submental tuck) may be an isolated problem in a younger patient or part of the general pattern of facial descent in a patient of older years. Cheek "slide" is a separate age phenomenon. The patient's actual age means little; general descent is seen even in patients as young as 30 to 35.

My first exposure to platysmal surgery came during the late 1970s, following the lead of Jose Guerro-Santos, Bruce Connell, and Rex Peterson. Initially, I performed submental surgery only in patients with obvious deformities. Now the submental tuck (SMT) is performed in almost 90% of our rhytidectomy candidates and frequently as an "isolated" procedures in younger patients.

These procedures are performed in the clinic under ketamine-diazepam (Valium) "dissociation," or twilight, anesthesia. Since the mid-1970s the only change in our regimen has been to substitute butorphanol (Stadol) 2 mg IV for its narcotic effect and to reduce the initial diazepam intravenous dosage to 2.5 mg. For shorter procedures, such as an isolated SMT, 2.5 of midazolam (Versed) is sufficient. These drugs allow a small dose of ketamine to give us the window of opportunity for pain-free local infiltration with 0.25% lidocaine (Xylocaine) with epinephrine. Lidocaine 1% is used for the regional nerve blocks, which are repeated at the end of the procedure using 1% bupivacaine (Marcaine) with epinephrine.

In the young patient the natural elasticity of the skin and subcutaneous tissue plus the change in the angle allow the excess skin to drape easily into the new contour, and platysmal anterior plication is sufficient. In the older patient a better sling is obtained by tightening the lax platysma posteriorly as well, which means that a face lift is in order. These individuals have too much skin anyway, and a satisfactory result is unobtainable with SMT alone.

Submental Tuck

Restoring the youthful, flat jaw and attaining a clean mandibular line are two of the goals of aesthetic surgery. Liposuction plays a role of course, but in most cases it is now confined primarily to the jowls and the nasolabial fold. At one time liposuctioning was performed indiscriminately. Too often patients are referred with prominent platysma bands and without a clean mandibular line simply because the original surgeon neglected the platysma. During the 1970s patients could not be assured that the results of plication and division would be long-lasting. As shown in the illustrations of this chapter, we should have used platysmorrhaphy in more of those patients. Today those patients are returning with droopy skin and prominent neck bands. Those fortunate enough to have had the platysmal resection plication and removal of the deep fat and superficial fatpads still have good jaw lines up to 15+ years later and require only minor skin resection and jowl liposuction. There are certain important points to note when correcting defects in this important zone.

1. Keep the incision short and high in the submental fold. Some surgeons make the scar lower on the neck, but it shows there and the patient is often displeased. Hide the scar!
2. Perform superficial liposuction as soon as the skin is incised, but do not attempt to suction the subplatysmal fat at this point. It is easier to remove it under direct vision.
3. Clear one side at a time and pack the side with iced saline, making it easier to control the bleeding.
4. Pull the platysma toward the midline and use a flat-bladed scissors to trim off the remaining fat. (It is surprising how much fat remains even after suctioning thoroughly.)
5. Divide the platysma as low as possible in the neck. Start plication of the divided muscle at the hyoid.

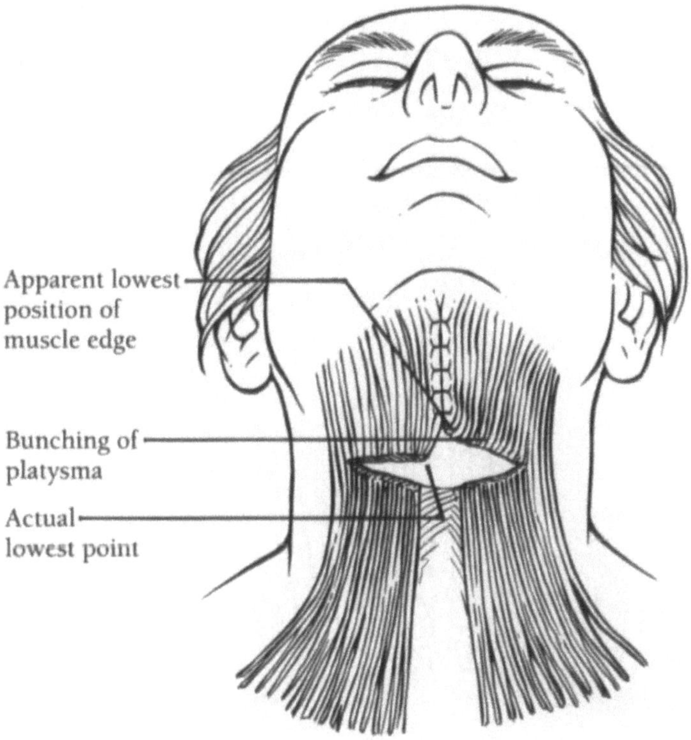

Figure 3-1. When repairing the platysma after a low division, it is important that the entire platysma be plicated in the midline. Always take a second look. As shown here, the platysma can retract. It is vital to identify this retracted area, stretch it downward, and anchor it into place. When the figure-of-eight stitch is placed, be sure to catch some of the deep tissue underneath the platysma to hold the muscle repair at a low position. In fact, it is helpful to take deep bites at intervals during the upper part of the figure-of-eight repair as well.

6. Even though it is fashionable today to talk about full neck "corset" repair, which was the procedure we used as far back as 1971, the technique is still a good one. *Caution:* If the division and repair are performed high, a "Dick Tracy" cutoff silhouette results, which is not good.
7. Always leave a little fat at the base of the dissection. It can be removed later or left in place to make the thyroid area transition zone more natural.
8. Resection of the central platysma is almost always indicated. This step provides access to the deep pad submental fat as well as an adequate muscle edge on which to sew to later.

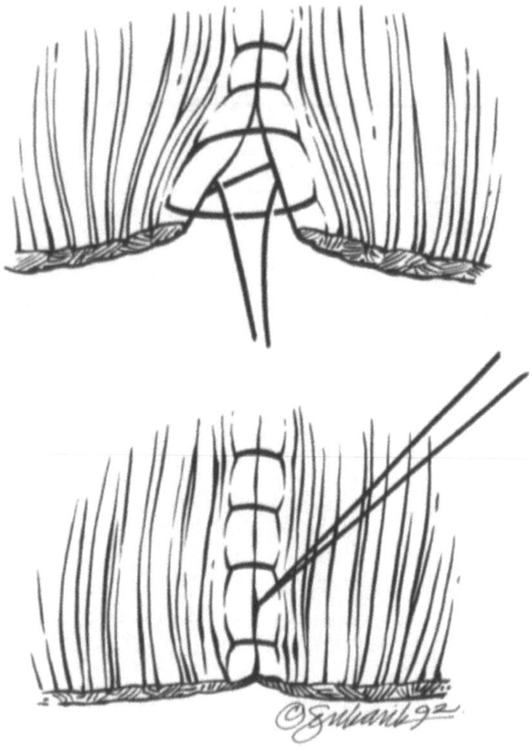

Figure 3-2. The figure-of-eight suture allows good bites of some rather fragile tissue. It is possible that many of the individuals who have separation of the platysma after several years actually had a disruption during the first few weeks after surgery but it became apparent only when the muscle bands strengthened. It is important to obtain tight closure first and then later look for fat that may have been hidden from view before the muscle was tightened into position.

9. Use figure-of-eight sutures to sew the platysma edges together, mixing absorbable with nonabsorbable sutures. Mersilene and Neurolon last longer, but all of the braided sutures have a disturbing tendency to come untied occasionally. That is not true of Dexon and Vicryl.
10. After completing the midline plication, look for fat that has not been trimmed. Put a finger on the edge of the mandible and push downward; this maneuver reveals a bulge that could easily cause a visible puff postoperatively.
11. Always drain this area.
12. At the end of the procedure reblock the regional nerves with bupivocaine (Mareaine) with epinephrine.
13. If there is chin overhang, which is common in older patients, make the first incision subcutaneously and upward, removing a wedge of fibrofatty tissue.
14. Position the chin implant first and leave the area open in case any blood accumulates. Always recheck the implant position prior to closing, as implants have been known to shift.
15. Put a hook on the mandible and exert some tension during the lateral dissection in the subcutaneous plane. Without this maneuver it is easy to inadvertently get under the muscle. Use a lot of lidocaine with

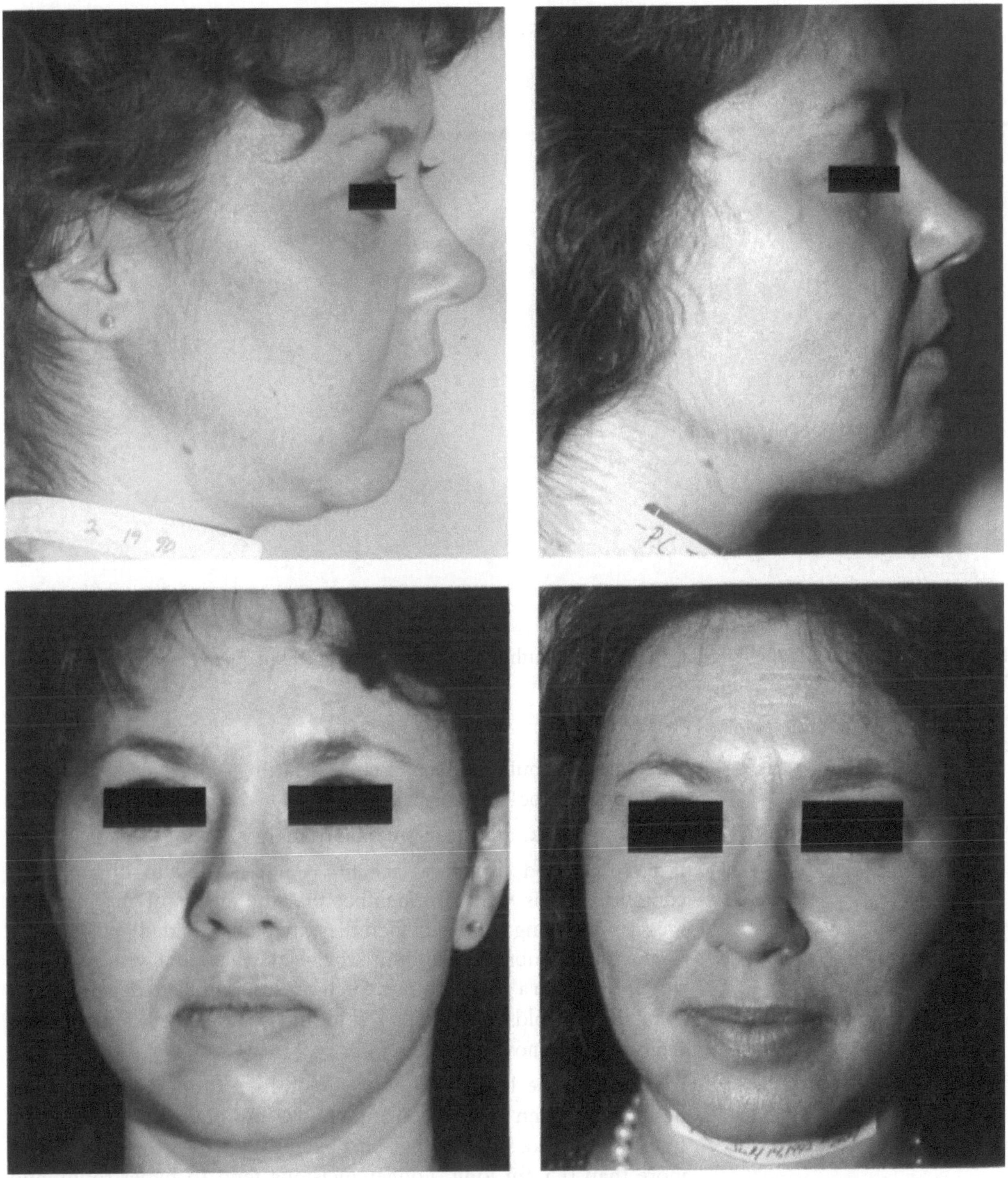

Figure 3-3. Insertion of an extended-type chin implant plus cheek and jowl liposuction to the malar eminence can make a chubby face appear hollow. This patient is shown 2 years after SMT, chin augmentation, and liposuction.

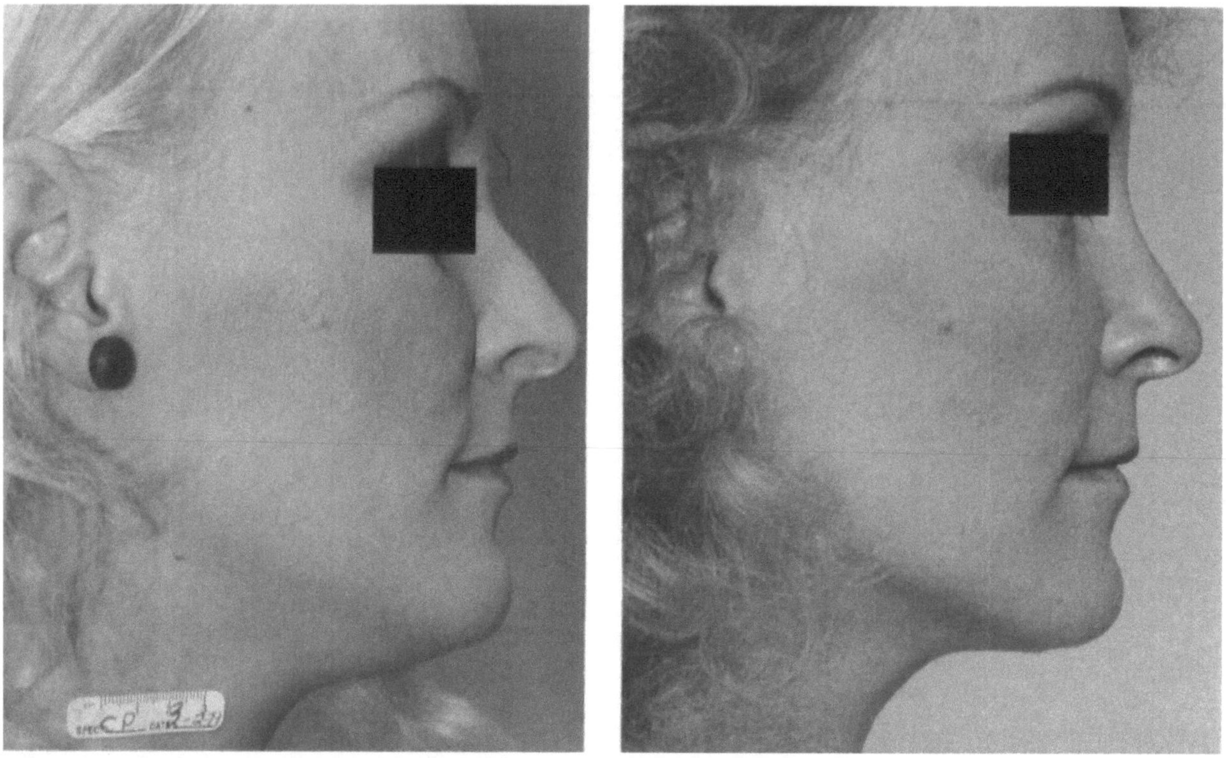

Figure 3-4. This SMT patient has maintained her youthful jawline for 13 years. Skin quality is maintained by the Retin-A and α-hydroxy acid skin care regimen.

epinephrine to puff out the tissues, so defatting is not excessive and the resulting skin looks abnormal.

16. Curetting the skin in the submental triangle is a poor idea.
17. If there is good turgor, a face lift is not needed to obtain good contouring. It is well to remember that the angles of the platysma muscles are being changed when they are being divided and sutured. Removing the submental and superficial fat in a patient with good skin turgor results in a good contour. Such a result is not age-dependent, as some 30-year-olds have floppy skin and some 45-year-olds do not require skin removal at all.
18. If there is some loose skin 3 to 4 months postoperatively, do not hesitate to reopen the incision and remove a triangle of skin, leaving a tiny T scar. Make sure the limb that extends downward on the T is no more than 0.5 cm long. Longer incisions tend to hypertrophy and cause more trouble than they are worth.
19. Some patients reaccumulate fat in the submental area. If this situation

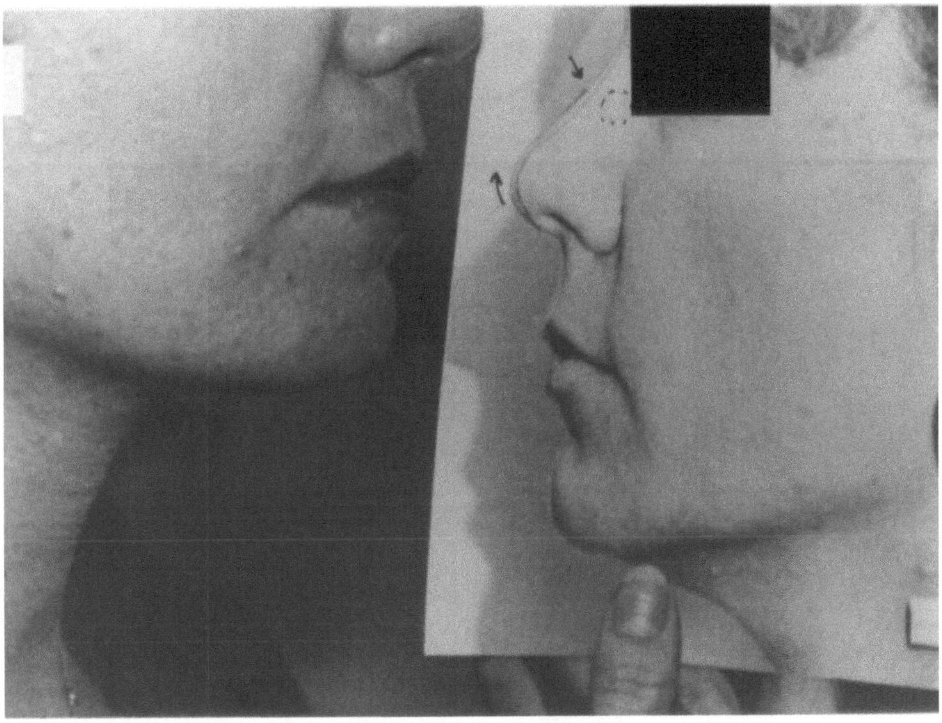

Figure 3-5. In an older patient, the submental tuck procedure is best combined with posterior repositioning and rhytidectomy. Note the effect on the nasolabial crease by subcutaneous musculoaponeurotic system (SMAS) plication and skin redraping.

occurs, reopen the incision and trim this new fat, perhaps placing another stitch or two in the platysma.

20. Platysmal bands may recur even though the platysma has been divided under direct vision. If that situation arises, reopen the incision, reach in, and excise the band.
21. Do not hesitate to suction along the jaw line, above the jaw line, or even into the cheek if conditions warrant. A cleaner jaw line results and the patient is more satisfied with the restoration.
22. For hospitalized patients, intravenous hydrocortisone (Solu-Cortef) 100 mg can be used to decrease edema. For patients on "twilight" medication, start methylprednisolone (Medrol Dosepak) the morning of the operation. It significantly lessens the swelling.
23. Instead of purchasing an expensive silicone bulb and drain system, cut the end off a butterfly intravenous set, and cut a few side holes in it; place this tubing deep in the incision, and bring it out again through the same incision. Use a vacutainer blood collection bottle taped to the

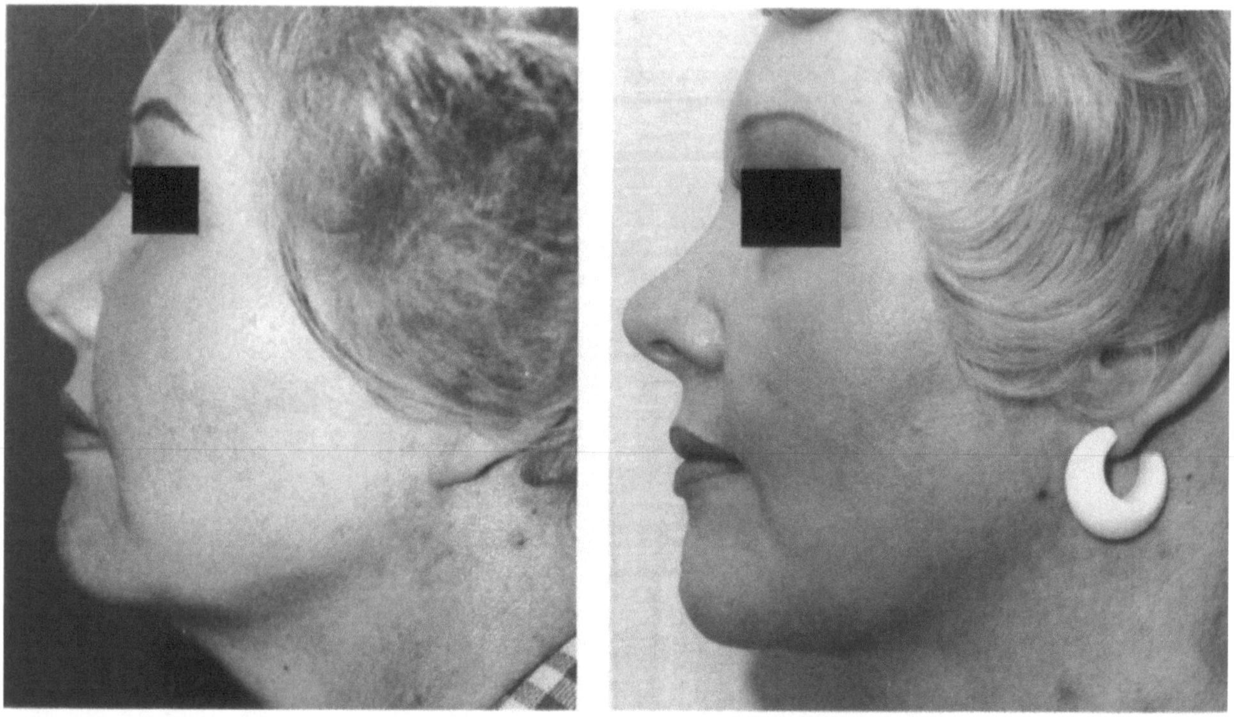

Figure 3-6. Submental fat removal and platysma resection/plication in young adults gives a cleaner, longer-lasting restoration than liposuction.

bandage of the reservoir. At the conclusion of the operation simply plunge the butterfly needle into the reservoir, creating instant suction. This method is inexpensive and effective, and the apparatus can be easily removed the next morning.

24. Choose the simplest way of closing the incision. The three-suture technique is a good one, leaving only one end suture to clip off a week later.
25. Gentle pressure massage and intermittent use of a facial support after the first week effectively maintains the contour. Always have the patient use some type of lubricating cream, not only for skin comfort but to make the massaging more pleasant.
26. Male patients are instructed not to shave up and down with a razor. Electric shavers may be used, but the patient must be wary of exerting pressure over a chin implant. It is wise to have the office staff shave the patient on the third or fourth day, allowing the patient to resume shaving himself when full sensation returns. We have had patients cut off their sutures when shaving, resulting in a gaping area at the end of the incision, even though we thought we had the stitches adequately covered with collodion and tape.

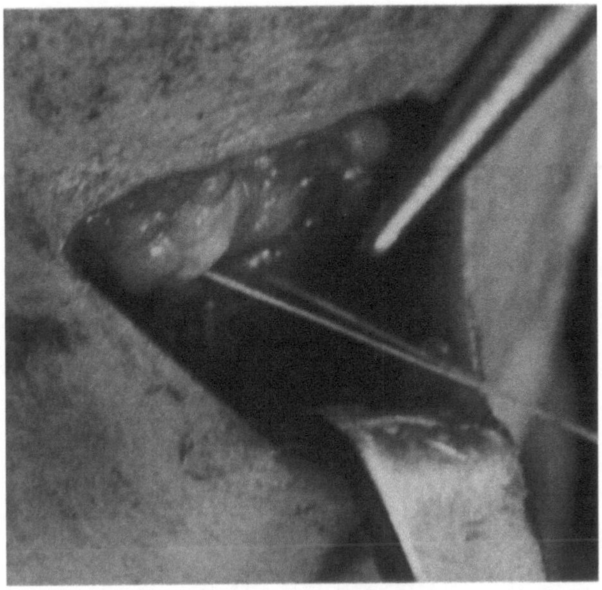

Figure 3-7. When the uppermost figure-of-eight Mersilene suture in the platysma is tightened, a small amount of unseen fat surfaces for easy removal.

Comments and Commentary

Submental Triangle

Anthony Wolff and others have stated that many surgeons regret jumping on the liposuction bandwagon. I agree, and we are now seeing many patients whose defects were not completely corrected because the muscle bands are still there. Undoubtedly, some patients are satisfied with only a moderate reduction in the bulk of the neck, but most of my referred patients obtain a clean mandibular line and flat submental triangle only by fat removal *and* platysmal surgery, which includes the deep fat. Why perform liposuction under the platysma if the platysma is open? Direct excision is precise. As well as trimming the two fat areas, do not ignore the digastrics. In some patients the digastric can create a large bulge; and if it is not flattened, cauterized, or cross-sutured, there will be ballooning in the center of the triangle even though the platysma is tightly sutured.

Almost everyone agrees that the prominent platysmal bands in the center should be resected. Plicating them one on top of the other may provide some theoretic advantage in that it prevents separation. However, if one divides these bands low in the neck and uses a series of figure-of-eight sutures from the incision line at the mandible down to the larynx, separation is unlikely. If they are not divided at least 4 to 5 cm laterally, prominent bands result that become a source of distress to the patient.

Removing the central band also provides the opportunity to lift up the platysma and remove the fat in the center. If it is extensive, it may be pushed up by a digastric muscle on either side. Therefore plicate the digastrics. By moving

A
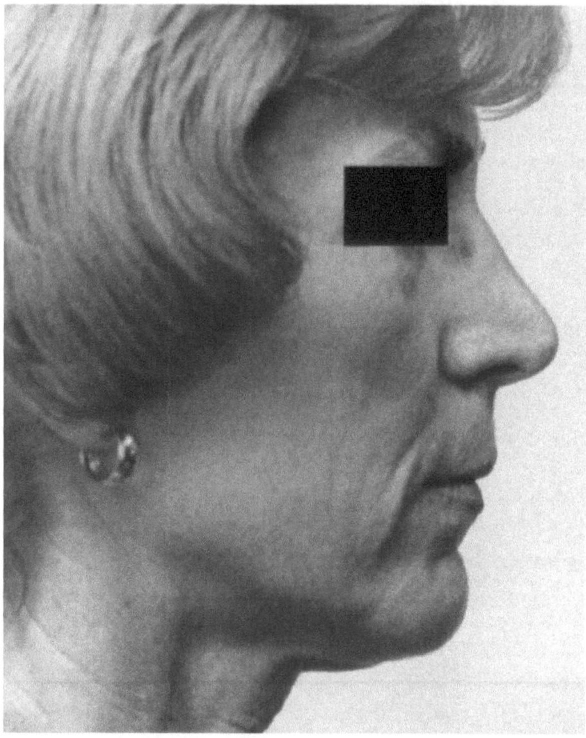

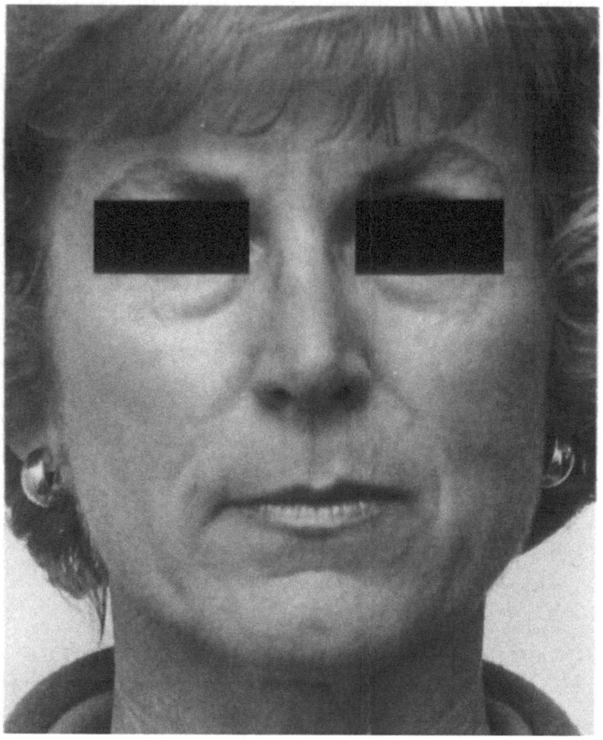
B

C
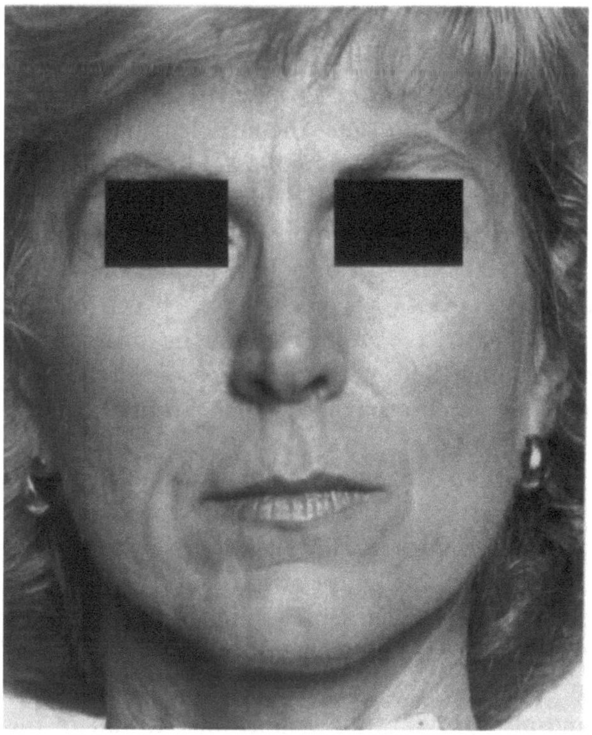

Figure 3-8. In 1982 the submental tuck (SMT) was thought to be unnecessary in patients such as this woman (**A&B**). The neck skin was taut in her 1983 photographs (**C**), but the effect was short-lived. Patients who had a complete SMT in 1983 do not show the banding and descent this patient has in her 1992 photographs (**D&E**).

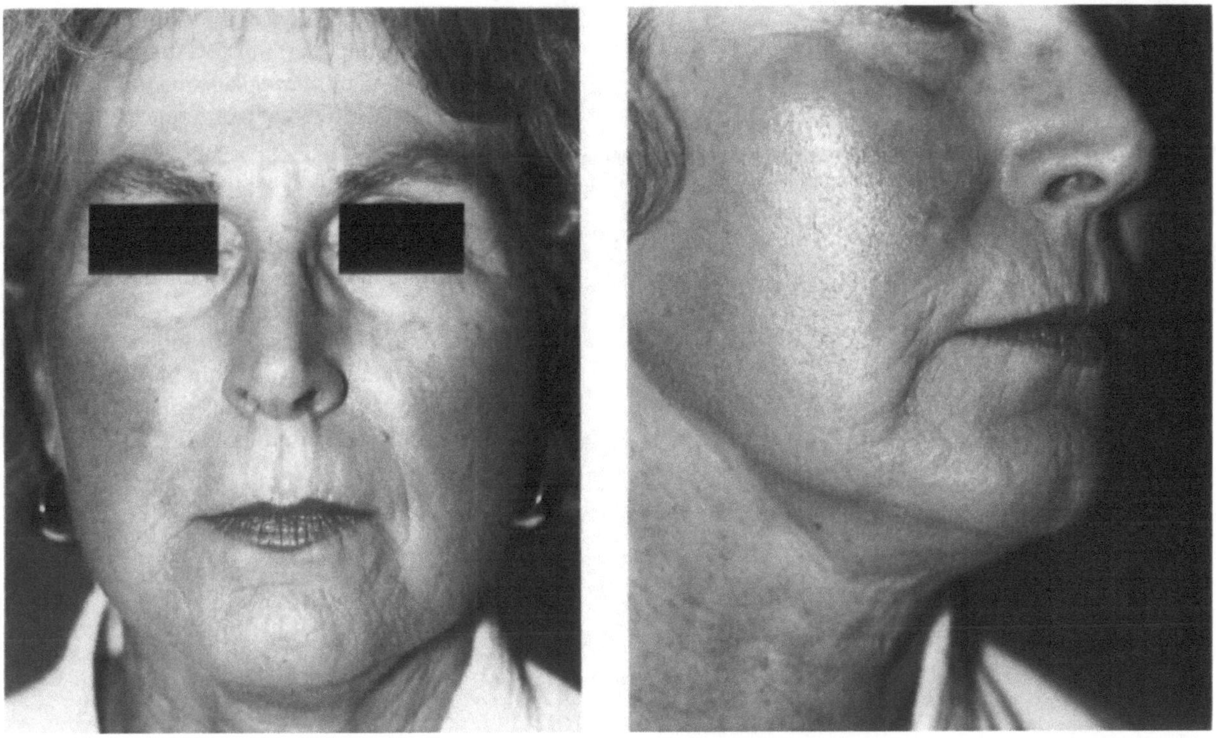

D E

the retractor from side to side, you can see everything you need to for 5 to 6 cm on either side of the midline; this view allows direct removal of the excess fat still attached to the platysma. Remember to push down at the jowl area to balloon out the fat that may have retracted upward. (If it is not trimmed now, it will certainly show later.) Liposuction may be performed in the lateral areas, opening up the planes more easily. *Caution:* Stay at a superficial level. Use a blunt tip and take care not to be so vigorous that you remove skin attached to the platysma. It is difficult to replace fat after too much has been removed. And do *not* curette fat from the undersurface of the skin!

Three-Suture Technique for Closing Incisions in the Submental Crease

Incisions in the submental crease should be closed by the simplest, quickest method, making sure the deep tissues, as well as the skin, are approximated. The technique I use precludes the need for sutures to be removed.

First, place an inverted suture using 4-0 Vicryl that catches only the deep dermis and subcutaneous fat at the lateral third of the incision and another in the center. These knots drop underneath the surface and so do not interfere with the

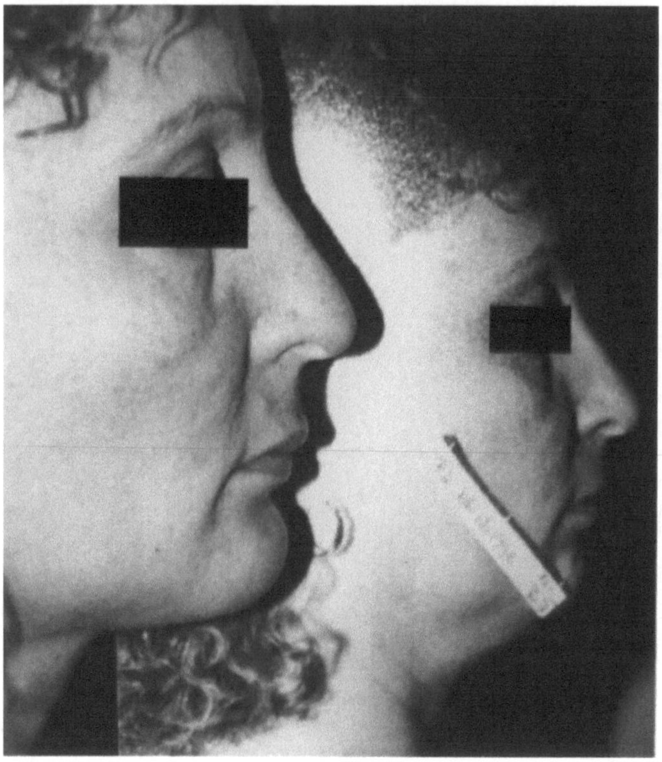

Figure 3-9. Simple liposuction cannot accomplish this result. Note in the photograph being held by the patient that the jowl descent is accompanied by descent of the platysma. Adding a chin prosthesis is helpful, but we are able to redrape the face in these young patients only if muscle suturing and deep fat removal accompany superficial liposuction. In young patients with good skin tone, freeing the skin above the mandible and to the sternum mastoid provides the best chance for successful contouring, whereas in older patients skin resection is necessary. In individuals of this age, however, addition of a chin implant and wide undermining plus reshaping the anterior neck makes skin resection unnecessary.

rest of the closure. Place the next suture at the farthest third of the incision but do not cut the long end. Use that end to close the wound subcuticularly, first to the right and then backtracking across the entire distance of the incision. When you reach the end closest to you, pass the suture through the skin and tie a loop knot. Cover it with Steri-Strips with no tension on the loop knot. The incision closes well once the butterfly drain suction is removed. Do not bury the distal knot. More often than is desirable it reappears at some time over the next few months.

REFERENCES

Wilkinson TS: The submental tuck. In JR Lewis (ed), The Art of Aesthetic Plastic Surgery. Little, Brown, Boston, 1989, p. 111.

Wilkinson TS, Swartz BE: Extended applications of platysma surgery. Clin Plast Surg 10:573, 1983.

4 Cheek

FOR MANY YEARS THE MIDFACE WAS IGNORED, WHICH IS DIFFICULT to understand, as high cheek prominence is such an important component of beauty. You cannot look at a fashion magazine today without seeing models with beautiful cheeks and sculptured jawlines.

Malar Augmentation

Malar implant surgery has encountered difficulty with the design of the implant, and whether it should be placed in the "classic" position or somewhere else. My experience with malar implants began when we had only one choice, the silastic Hinderer button.[1] This device was disliked because it created an artificial single high point. Mario Gonzalez-Ulloa, who demonstrated malar implants in 1971, anchored a ceramic prosthesis with wire sutures through the skin.

It became obvious that softer materials and "contoured" shapes were required, and I became interested in room-temperature vulcanizing silicone (RTV). We experimented with making our own prosthetic devices for the forehead and jawline. Making malar implants with RTV was messy and time-consuming; and the implants did not stay in place. I then designed an oval type (now featured by many manufacturers) and we reported our experience with it.[2] We made the still valid point that the *position of the malar prominence is the personal choice of the patient.* If you examine the models' faces from *Vogue* and *Cosmopolitan,* you can see that in some of the models the prominence occurs far laterally along the zygomatic ridge; in others it is in the classic midposition. Still others exhibit an "apple cheek," which is best achieved with the Terino shell prosthesis.[3] This malar design was an improvement on my own. Now I use a number of designs and shapes, providing a wide variety of choices. Some guidelines may be helpful.

1. Ensure that the patient wants malar prominence. If you use a silastic implant you can always remove it. A certain number of patients do change their minds, and it is difficult to remove Porex, cartilage, or other type of malar prosthesis.
2. Make the surgery as simple and as easy as possible. Obtaining cartilage from the ear and folding fascia around it is not a good idea because (1) a deformity is created; (2) the procedure is overly complicated; and (3) you have eliminated the other available choices for aesthetic insertion by creating scar tissue.
3. Terino implants (and others that are similar) are available in different heights, diameters, and curvatures. It is well to have several implants on hand so you can match them to the patient. The curvature acts like a suction cup so it is rarely necessary to use fixation sutures.

Do implants ever move? The old ones certainly did because we placed them subcutaneously, as we did chin implants. In the chin such movement makes little difference. In the cheek, however, it makes a difference. If there is insufficient periosteal cover and a few perforations, the implant will be "ballotted" or be movable under the skin. Even the best-placed implant can migrate. In one such case, the implant had obviously crept up above the orbital rim. To correct this problem we simply reopened the blepharoplasty incision, trimmed the implant, and repositioned it. Thus even though it is probably not essential that a percutaneous fixation suture be used, it is important to close the fascia if a blepharoplasty approach is used.

Submalar Augmentation

The submalar implant was touted as a logical extension of face lifting, and it was certainly overused during its development phase. Some older people are not comfortable with the loss of midface fat. Fat grafting is not as effective at that site as it is in the dense tissue of the chin, the nasolabial area, or the glabellar frown lines. Placing an implant just off the malar prominence is satisfactory to some patients but not to others. In fact, we removed such an implant because the patient thought it made her "look like a squirrel." Fortunately, it had been placed through the face lift incision, and the patient was an older woman whose skin had stretched enough to call for secondary tightening in front of the ear as well as removal of the prosthesis. The two procedures were done at the same time.

Insertion Choices

There are three ways to place implants, each with advantages and disadvantages. The simplest method is to place the implant through a short subciliary blepharoplasty incision, and the most complex is to place it during a full face lift. The intraoral approach is questionable because (1) infections have occurred and (2) it is difficult to confirm that you are under the periosteum.

What are the drawbacks of a malar implant? First infections can occur, even when one is meticulous. The main problem with blepharoplasty incisions is that some people develop a droopy lid, particularly if there has been prior surgery. For example, two women were referred to us who had undergone unsatisfactory surgeries elsewhere. The implants were upside down, too high, and in one case of different sizes and shapes. We had barely avoided an ectropion in similar cases, so we told each patient that the repair could not be done through the tight, scarred lower lid. This surgery also provided the opportunity to hide (with an intratragal incision) prominent scars in front of the ears. We also corrected the down-pulled "pixie" ears and straight-line visible scar in front of the tragus.

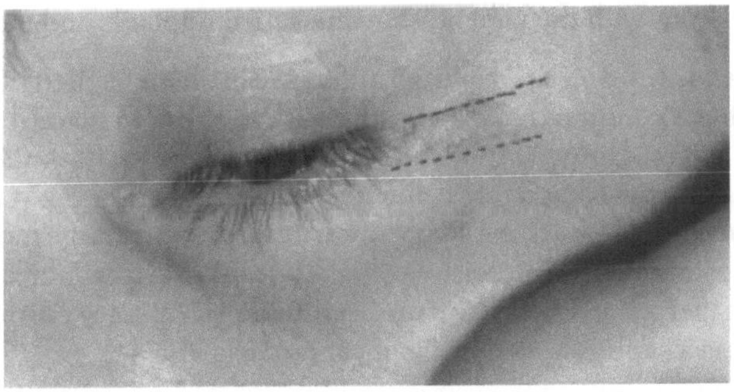

Figure 4-1. Between the dotted lines is an excessively long zigzag low incision. This length is useful if you are going to replace a malar implant, but it is not good practice to place an incision this far laterally for an ordinary blepharoplasty. The solution was to undermine widely down to the cheek and then move the normal skin below the bottom dotted line upward to the upper line, creating a single line rather than a zigzag of scars. Deep 6-0 Vicryl sutures are used to remove the tension, and the surface is simply taped or a few interrupted tacking stitches are placed.

The only good thing about this case is that replacing the malar implant became easy. Normally, this much exposure is not needed to place a malar implant. Even a short blepharoplasty-type incision provides a much easier approach to exposing the periosteum than when approaching from within the mouth.

Technique

The technical points involved in placement include the following.

1. Keep the blepharoplasty incision short unless you are already planning a classic blepharoplasty. Terino prefers the submuscular plane, but I believe that with that approach we perhaps stretch the muscle when positioning the implant. Therefore I use the standard subcutaneous approach more often.
2. Using minimal retraction, locate the orbital rim and incise it with the scalpel. Use any type of flat dissector with which you are comfortable. Stay just lateral to the infraorbital nerve and work backward.
3. If planning off-malar positioning for a low placement or use of a wider, flatter "shell" prothesis, push away from the lower edge of the malar prominence, which means that some of the implant is not covered by periosteum.

Figures 4-2 to 4-5. In certain cases consider overcorrecting everything. It may mean that a larger malar prosthesis is used to overcome the differences between the left and right sides of the face. (We use the same process for asymmetry during breast augmentation because a larger breast implant can hide the differences between left and right and can minimize the differences in nipple/areolar positioning.) A large Terino "shell" prosthesis or a higher-projection, more narrowly based "contoured" malar implant may fit the needs of one person better than another. One should discuss the possibilities with the patient, showing actual implants and molds.

Figures 4-2, 4-3, 4-4. Note the difference in diameter, height, and projection of the two "medium" contoured malar prostheses. We chose to place the prosthesis partly on the malar bone to provide some projection as well as to fill in the submalar zone. I do not place implants completely below the malar eminence; there must be an overlap. Most patients benefit by at least some upward and outward projection. Note the positioning of the prostheses. The one with the higher projection is trimmed and used in the side with the smaller natural bone structure. A different shape is used on the opposite side because it covers a slightly wider area and yet projects less.

Figure 4-5. This photograph was obtained 10 days after rhinoplasty, chin augmentation, fat grafting, rhytidectomy, blepharoplasty, and malar augmentation. Note the slight swelling of the dorsum of the nose and in the areas along the nasolabial zone where fat grafts have been placed. Although she no longer has the hollowed-out midface, there is an appropriate curvature on both sides—illustrating what we mean by subtle differences.

If a number of implants are available and you have a good idea of the shape you wish to achieve, it may be more matter of trial and error in the operating room than preoperative planning. Occasionally, it is best to stand back and take a good look. You may want to exchange one implant for another from a different manufacturer to obtain a subtle difference in projection or size. The same applies to the selection of chin prostheses.

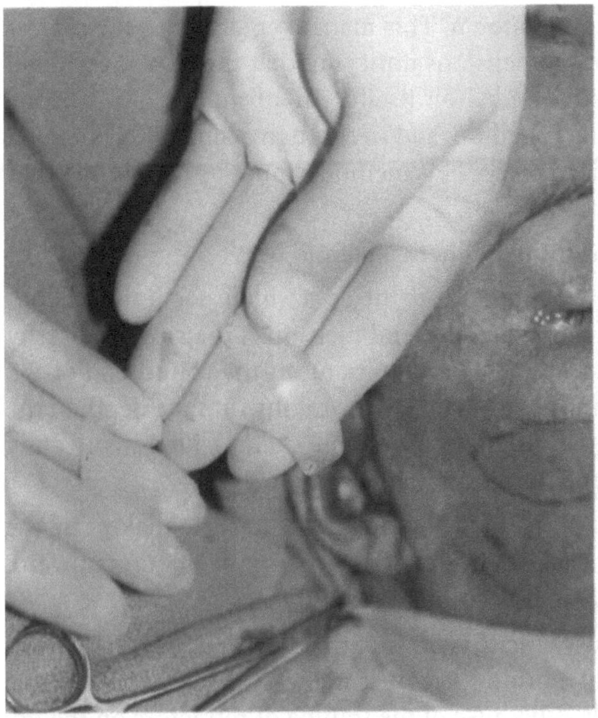

Figure 4-2

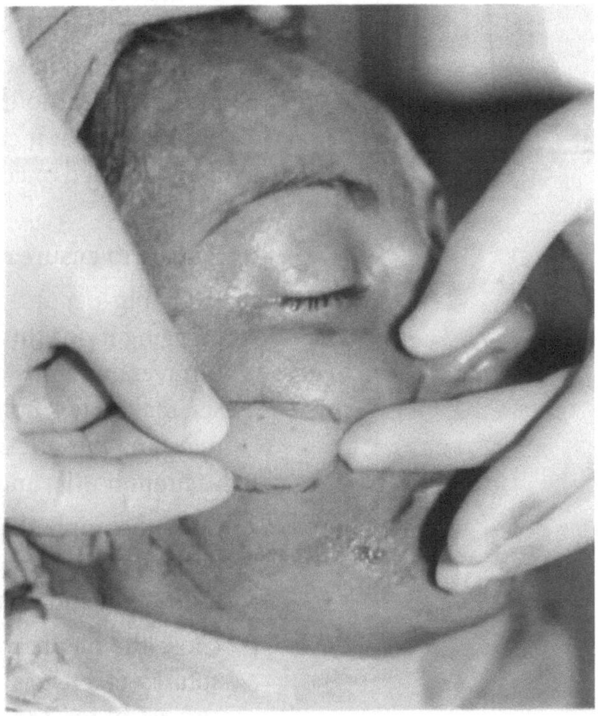

Figure 4-3

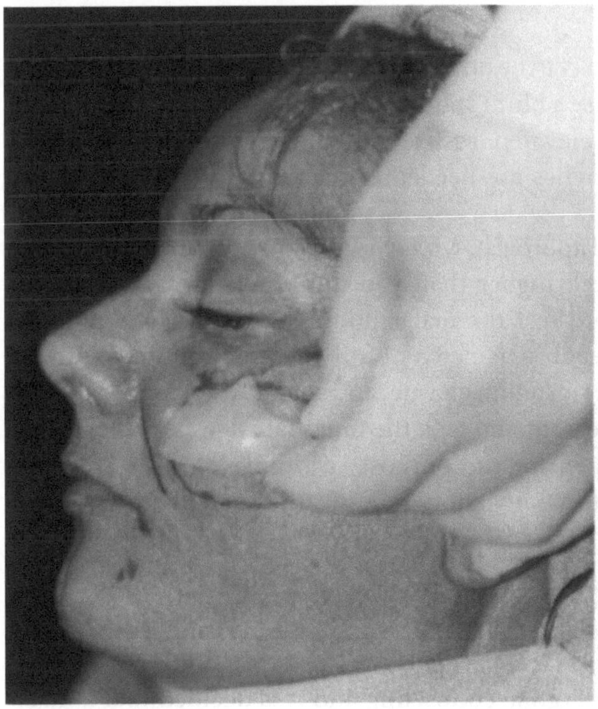

Figure 4-4

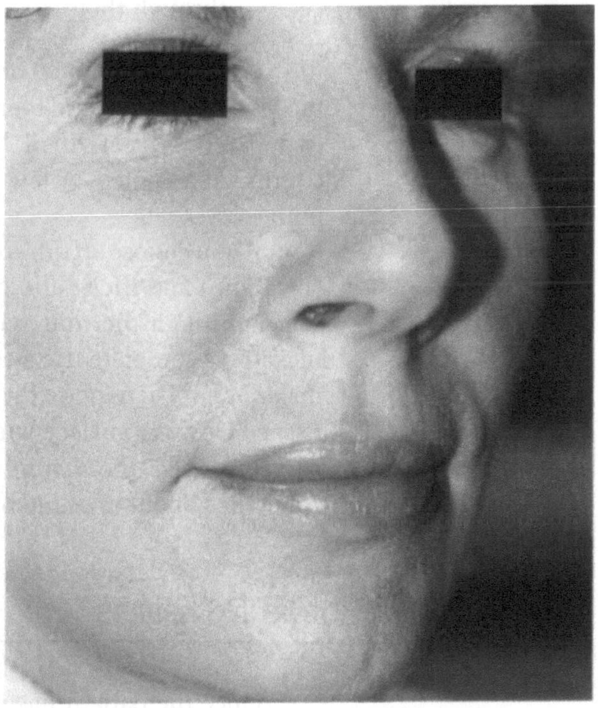

Figure 4-5

4. To ensure correct positioning, slide scissors into the pocket, turn the scissors sideways, and open them. This maneuver stretches the periosteum. Stretch in several dimensions until sure that the implant will fall into place without being folded on itself. (An advantage of a silicone implant is that it can be rolled up, slid in through a small incision, and then unrolled once it is in place. This method cannot be used with other materials.)
5. Palpate to ensure everything is where it should be.
6. If oozing occurs, do not hesitate to place a small suction catheter, bringing it out through the lateral eyelid incision. Try using a butterfly intravenous infusion set for suctioning. (Cut off the round end of the set, make a few holes in the side, and lay the tubing into the depth of the incision. Put the needle point into a small suction blood-collecting vacuum bottle, and tape it to the patient's temple.)
7. Once the implant is in place, use a few tacking stitches to make sure the periosteum is closed. (If a patient should then push the implant upward, it does not slide into a high position as easily.)
8. Close the blepharoplasty incision, as described earlier, with *suspension sutures* to ensure that nothing becomes "stuck." I leave these Frost sutures in for 3 to 4 days because of the trauma of retractors on the lid. It is a preventive measure to keep the eyelid undersurface from sticking to the orbital rim. (Remember, people lie in bed and watch television through their toes.)

If the malar augmentation is to be done during a face lift, it is easy to palpate the distal malar rim and then use a blunt splitting dissection until the periosteum is apparent. It can then be elevated easily and safely, with the procedure continued as noted. A few stitches are needed in the fascia to cover the entry point.

If you choose an intraoral approach, wipe the interior with povidone-iodine (Betadine) and incise the cheek higher than you think is necessary. Put your finger through the mucosa and feel the malar imminence. Once the mucosal incision is complete use a spreading maneuver until you are in contact with the malar bone. Then incise the periosteum, elevate, and so on. Always close the soft tissue below the surface with catgut and tack the mucosal edges together. Some surgeons leave the wound open for the purpose of drainage, but I am more concerned about possible bacterial infection underneath the implant.

Size and Shape Decisions

Once the patient has undergone counseling and it is decided that a malar implant is wanted, how do you decide on the size and shape? It is well to have a

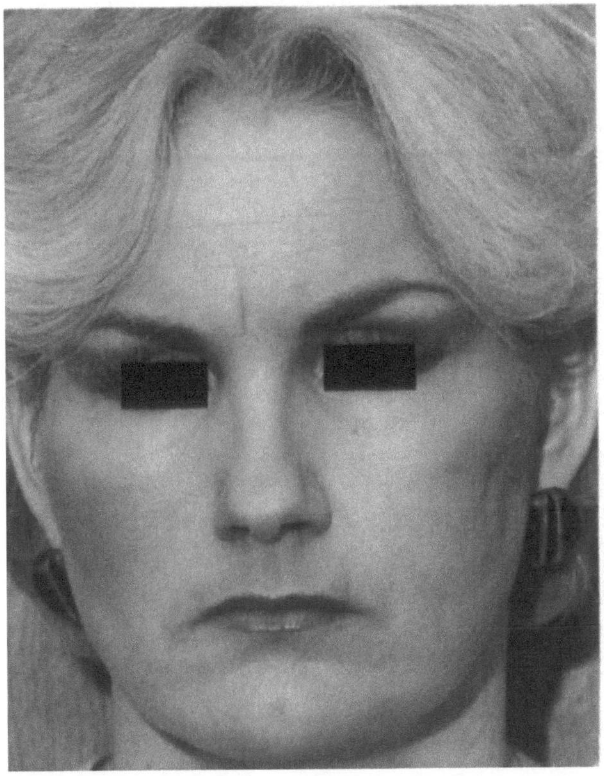

4-6

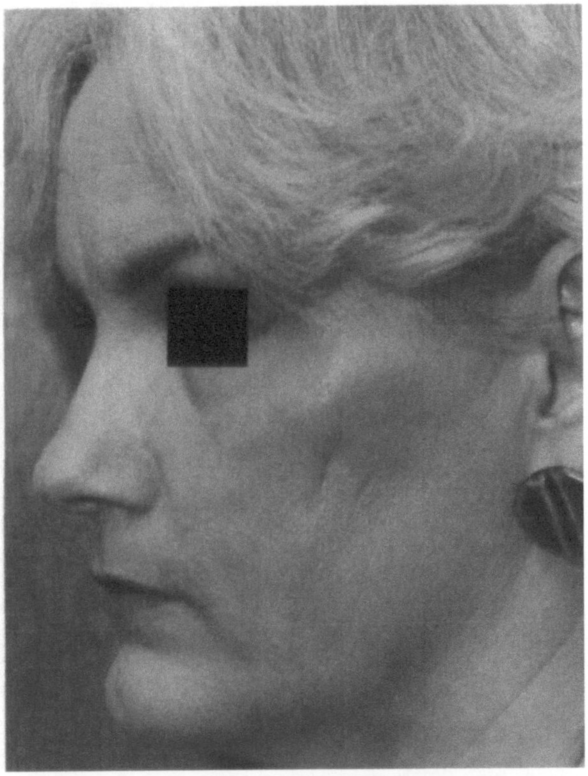

4-7

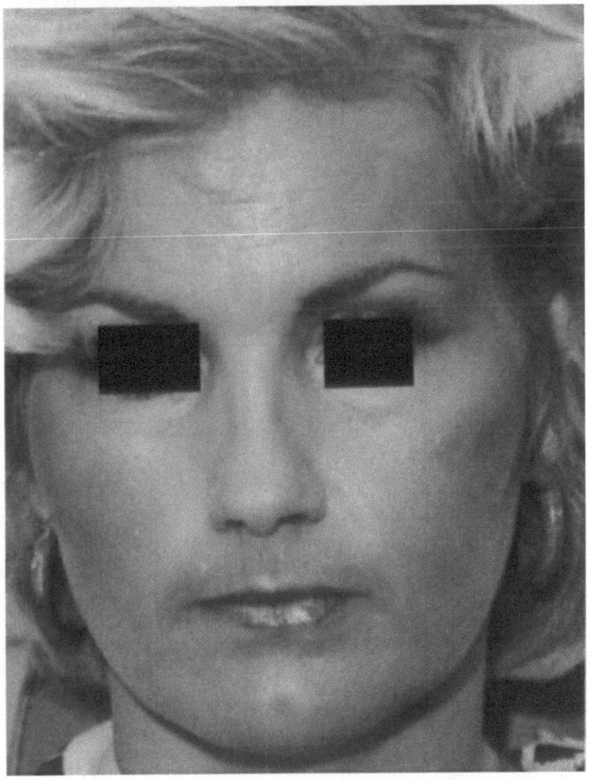

4-8

Figures 4-6, 4-7, 4-8. In 1982 a woman presented who had had a severe soft tissue injury just below the malar zone with bone resorption, scarring, and soft tissue loss (**Figs. 4-6, 4-7**). This situation is one of the few for which the malar zone can be approached directly, with a scar revision being done at the same time. Simple deepithelialization of the scar bed and then using this bed as an anchor for the deep stitches can prevent scar widening. In 1982 we used softer gel-type implants with Dacron fixation patches. They were sufficient for soft tissue repair but not for bone replacement. Although the long-term result with this woman was good (**Fig. 4-8**), one of the problems was displacement of the soft gel-filled implants. One implant rolled up into a ball 3 months after we had inserted it.

Our first malar implants were home-made, and they worked. Before 1976 we saw few complications with these RTV silicone implants, but we also used them in a limited number of patients. Today we can categorize complications as preventable or nonpreventable. With the wider, contoured-type implants, displacement or failure to fill a specific zone is rare.

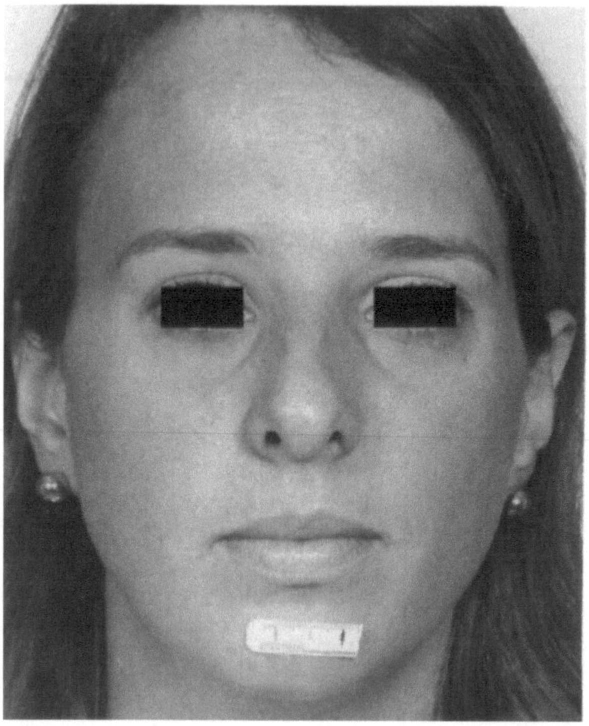

Figure 4-9

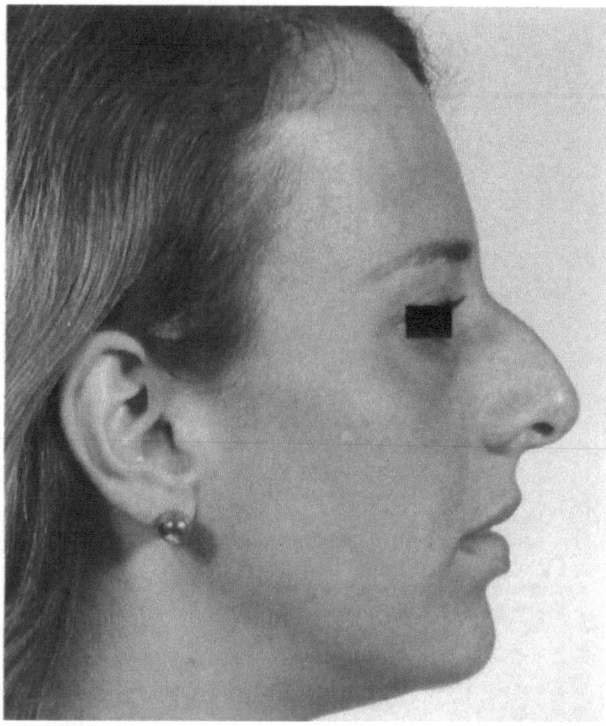

Figure 4-10

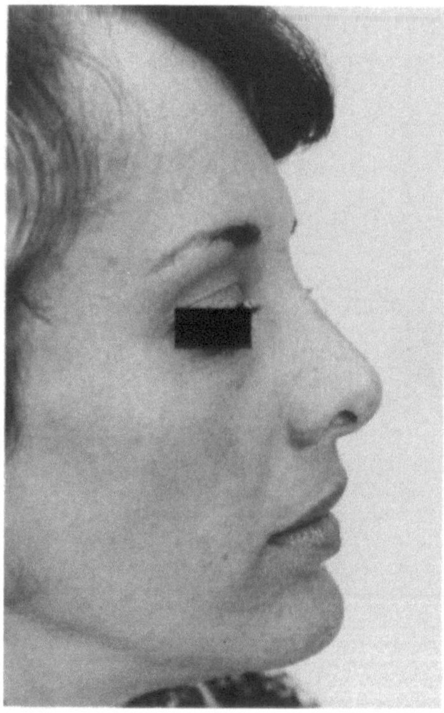

Figure 4-11

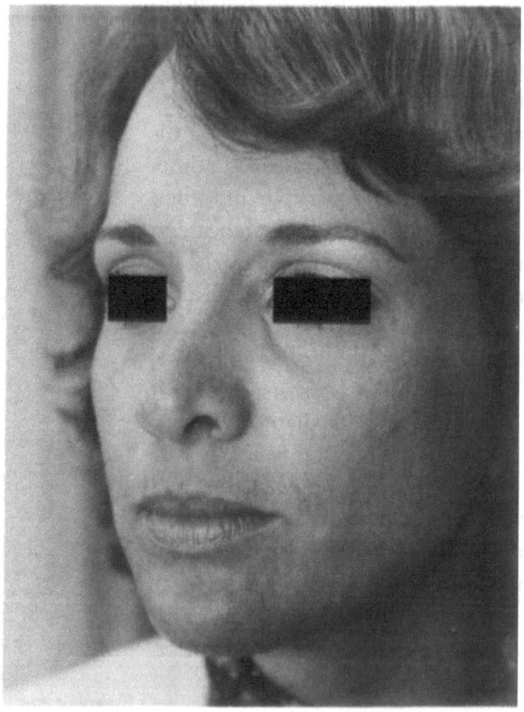

Figure 4-12

number of manufacturers' products on hand. As can be seen from the illustrations in this chapter, the implants vary by diameter and height, and each provides a distinctly different appearance. For example, if the patient already has fullness on either side of the nose, an extension that crosses under the intraorbital nerve is not needed. If the face is flat, a higher profile is needed. If the patient desires that the lateral zygoma zone be accented, choose a smaller, flatter implant.

The next step is to sketch the proposed changes on a facial diagram. Then outline it on the patient's face with a washable red pen. The choices become clearer to the patient using this method, and the two of you can then make the appropriate decisions. This time is well spent, as it is easier to erase red pen marks than to reposition a malar implant. Make it clear to the patient no one's face is symmetric. (The reversing mirror introduced by Mark Gorney is valuable for this purpose and is used during all of our preoperative facial consultations.) A different shape or design may be needed so the left side matches what has been chosen for the right side because of the difference in the amount of soft tissue or bony prominence.

When analyzing facial contours considered beautiful in Western culture, there are few fixed points of reference. Facial bone structure varies so much in individuals it is impossible to use one formula. The only guideline I recommend

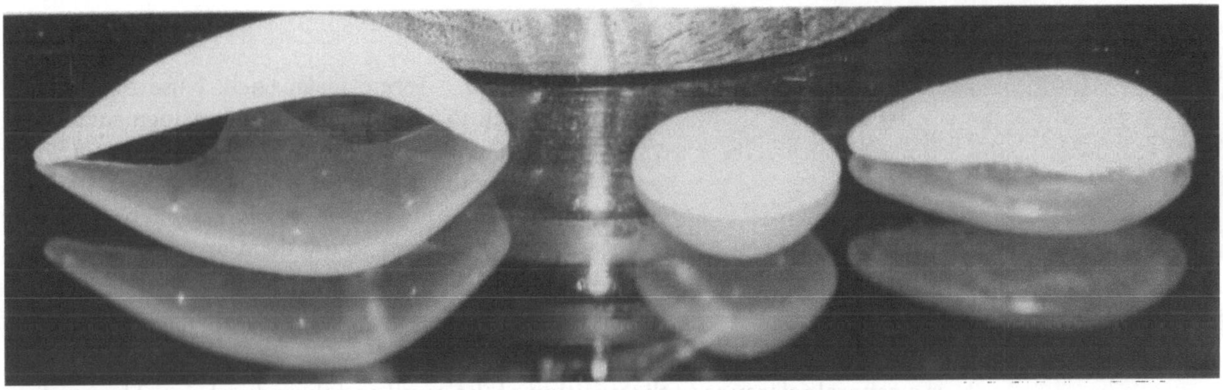

Figure 4-13

Figures 4-9 to 4-13. Oval malar implants. During the early 1980s this woman underwent malar implant (**Figs. 4-9 to 4-12**). The prosthesis was placed in the "classic" position with more fullness posterolaterally. We achieved a reasonably good match with the oval implant of my design. (There is still a place for this implant, in certain patients.) Note in the preoperative frontal view that she has good fullness in the anterior zone just below the orbit. Many patients do not and so require an "extended," or contoured, prosthesis to fit beyond the vertical line from the pupil.

Fat grafting can be used to fill out the area around the edge of the implants; and in fact a good degree of correction can be obtained with fat grafting alone. I have never thought that fat grafting is effective or predictable in the malar area, even with a second or third regrafting in superficial and deep layers. If a patient does not have this central fullness, it is far wiser to choose one of the contoured implants (**Fig. 4-13**). Contrast the original "button" type implant designed by Hinderer with my original oval shape beside it. The button does not correspond to any natural malar variation. We use many more of the various contoured designs.

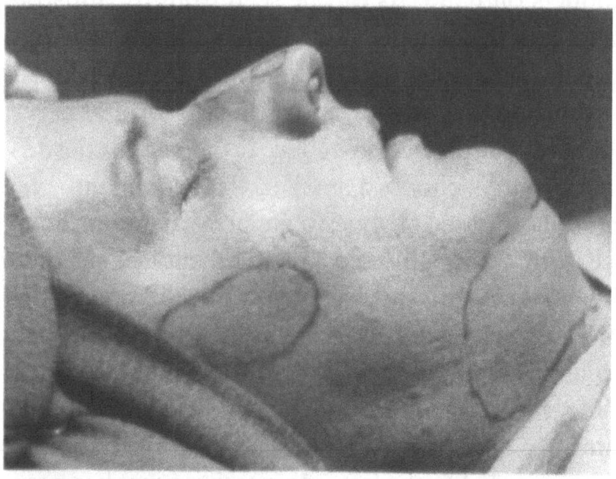

Figure 4-14. Classic versus lateral prominence. Note the posterolateral placement in this patient. The entire prominence is located posterior to a line dropped from the corner of the eyebrow. Surprisingly, many of my patients desire this correction rather than the classic high anterior or apple cheek types. Also note the markings for simultaneous submental fat removal, platysmal plication, and rhinoplasty. The patient was offered chin augmentation as well but declined. Simply reducing the bulk of the nose, freeing the upper lip so it can drop to a more natural position, and widening the face by this far lateral placement can minimize the chin deficiency. It was his choice (not mine), but we were both pleased by the final result.

Complications can occur, as in patients whose implants move about laterally with smiling. Such implants had been placed subcutaneously or off-center, or they may be floating in an overlarge pocket. Hematomas and infection occur infrequently. They are largely preventable by inserting drains and giving preoperative antibiotics.

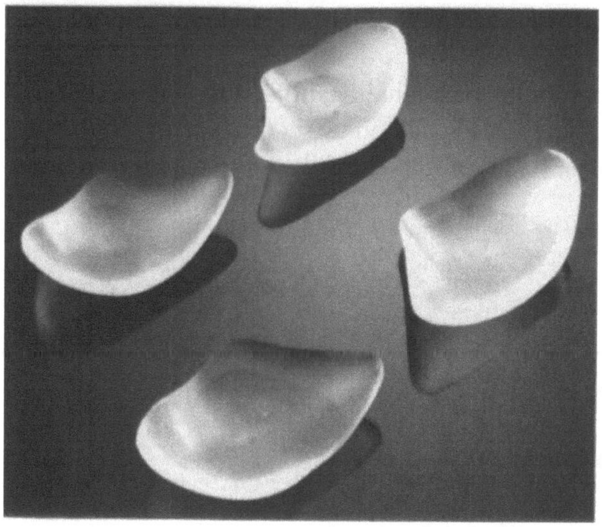

Figure 4-15. Terino malar shell. I use this implant more often than any other for malar augmentation. It gives an "apple cheek" look because it covers a wider area but without as great a projection as a standard implant. These implants may be wider, but because they are thinner it is easy to roll them up and slide them in through a small opening.

is a general reference to the position of the pupil and the orbital rim. The implant can be placed just at the rim or in the "apple cheek" area, bringing the leading edge directly in line with the pupil; or the entire prosthesis can be made to sit over the lateral malar fullness.

Finally, be prepared to remove the implant from a number of patients. All of our work and counseling may be overturned by one look in the mirror. After all, it is the patient's face and he or she certainly has a right to choose how it is restructured.

In two cases young men requested that the lower portion of the cheek be filled out. One man was dismayed because he had a "Mick Jagger" look. The solution was a Terino shell malar implant, which extends downward in the cheek but does not produce a dramatic change in contour. We added to this new look by fat-grafting the lower cheek both subcutaneously and in the facial musculature. It was done with concentrated fat grafts. In fact, it is good practice to take any fat left over during a face lift and inject it along the malar rim, producing submalar fullness without adding to the facial swelling. True malar augmentation also fills the submalar zone. This step causes the height of submalar implants to fade a bit.

Technical point: Be particularly careful with posterior dissections if a long implant is being used. The periosteum becomes tenuous posteriorly, and it is easy to cause bleeding by tearing tissues. If you are unsure about the positioning, remove the sharp elevator and use blunt, curved scissors. Then continuously press and spread until there is the required space plus slightly extra.

Avoiding Problems

If the dissection is clean with no bleeding and a Frost suspension suture is left in place for a few days, patients are less likely to develop an ectropion or lower lid retraction problem. This unfortunate result may occur, however, especially if the surgery is being done to reposition an implant in someone who already has the problem. It is then best to use one of the other two incisions.

A temporary ectropion is not rare. Massage, heat, suspension, or even a temporary tarsorrhaphy may be required. We leave the Frost sutures in place for 48 hours and then begin gentle massaging when the patient changes from cold packs to hot packs. For the most part, however, if the exact pocket needed has been created and filled with a rolled up silicone prosthesis that is then unrolled and positioned, there is not likely to be migration or movement.

A good subperiosteal pocket is essential. It has always been a problem when the intraoral approach is used. It is difficult to identify the periosteum and to verify that the implant is in correct position. Moreover, there is a risk of infection, especially a massive infection that can easily spread to vital structures. In such cases remove the implant and plan to replace it within a few months. Do not give in to patients' urgings to replace the implant as quickly as possible; it is essential that you wait until the infection has completely cleared.

Technical point: Once the periosteal dissector has passed across the created pocket, use it as a lever to stretch the periosteum. This maneuver provides more space in which to work superiorally, laterally, and medially. Another suggestion (from Steve Hoefflin) is to notch the edges of the malar implant; the notches keep the implant from moving because soft tissue grows across it, thereby implementing fixation from the through-and-through holes.

My technique for the uncomplicated case is as follows. If there is no indication for a lower lid blepharoplasty, the incision is made from the midportion of the lower lid and only slightly longer laterally. (Do not make it as

(Text continued on page 97)

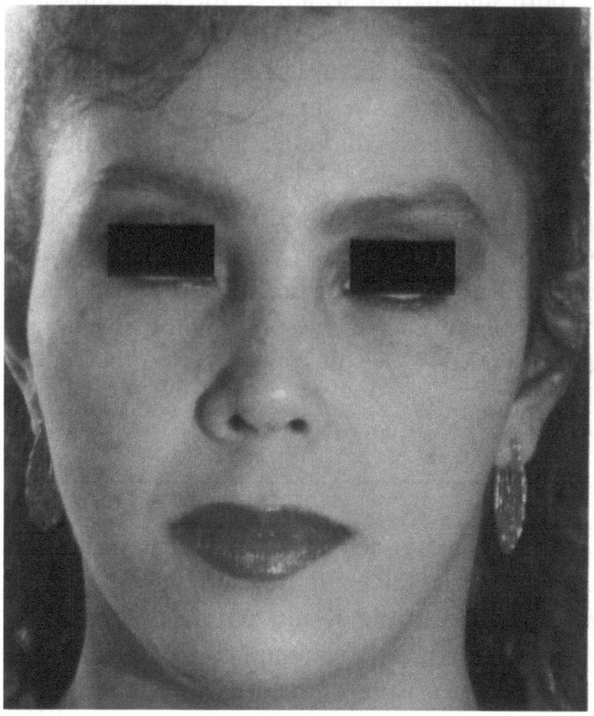

Figure 4-16A

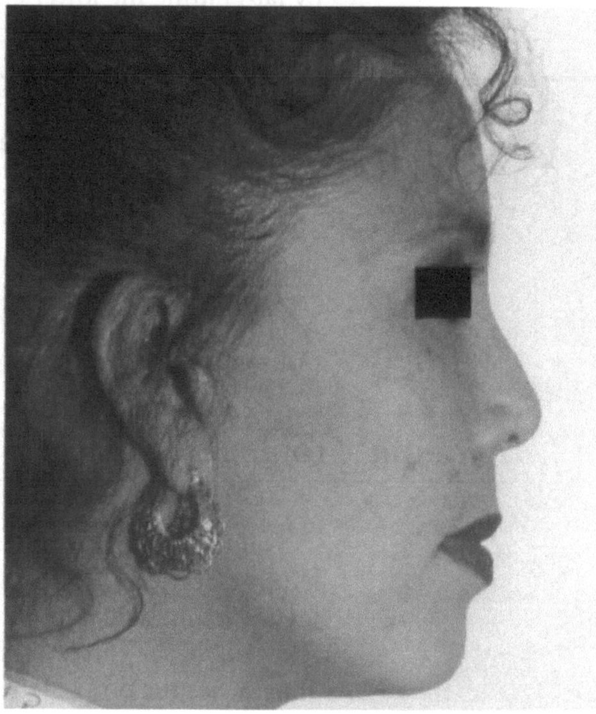

Figure 4-16B

Figures 4-16 to 4-19. This patient provided a learning experience in handling ectropions. She had undergone a blepharoplasty elsewhere, and Silastic contoured malar implants had been inserted. Even after two adjustments the asymmetry was obvious (**Fig. 4-16A–C**), although the ectropions had resolved. I tried to avoid repairing this area again, despite the success we had had with her submental tuck, lip rolls, chin implant, and fat grafts (**Fig. 4-17A–C**; see also color section). However, we decided to explore the malar area, and it was a mistake. There was scar tissue everywhere. Two dissimilar malar implants were found and replaced (March 1991). Two days later she had an "accident" with eyelid trauma, and later suspension sutures were broken. Bizarre bilateral ectropions occurred and recurred. Kuhnt-Symonowski procedures did not help. Finally, in April 1991, we did skin grafts (**Fig. 4-18A–C**). Although the malar area looked good, we replaced the right one with a larger shell at her request—but only when she agreed to a preauricular approach (June 1992). We were able to hide the scars from her original surgery with placement inside the tragus. She requested that the skin grafts under each lid be removed at the same time, and because more than a year had passed since their placement I agreed. The final resolution came with the tarsal tuck procedure and lateral tarsorrhaphies (July 1992). Note the following details in the final closeup (**Fig. 4-19A–C**): The nasolabial lines and lips are full (2.5 years after fat grafts and lip rolls). The ear lobes are full, and the preauricular scar is hidden (1.5 years after revision). The chin line is full and natural, and a youthful submental contour is evident (2.5 years after submental platysmorrhapy, liposuction, and an "extended" Silastic chin implant). The full apple cheek malar augmentation has restored left and right malar balance.

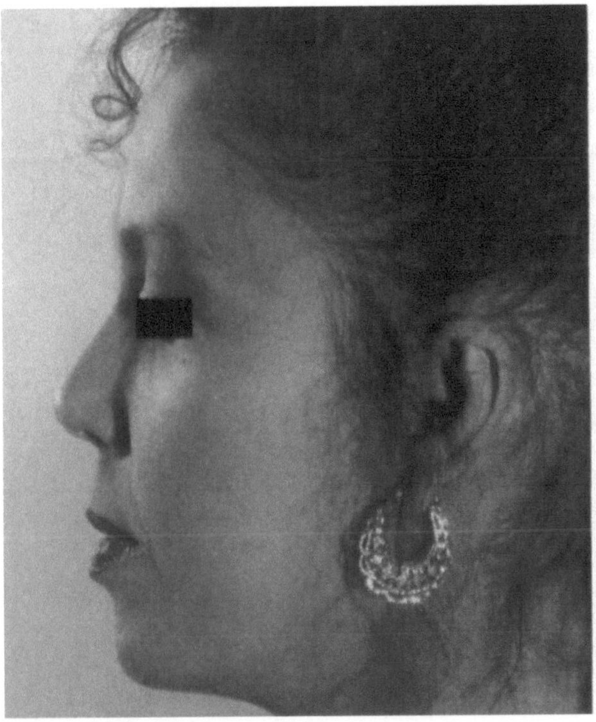

Figure 4-16C

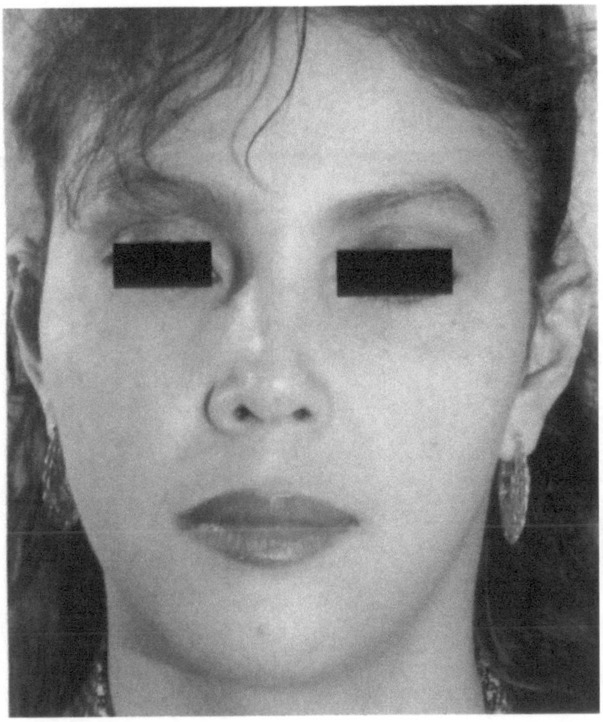

Figure 4-17A

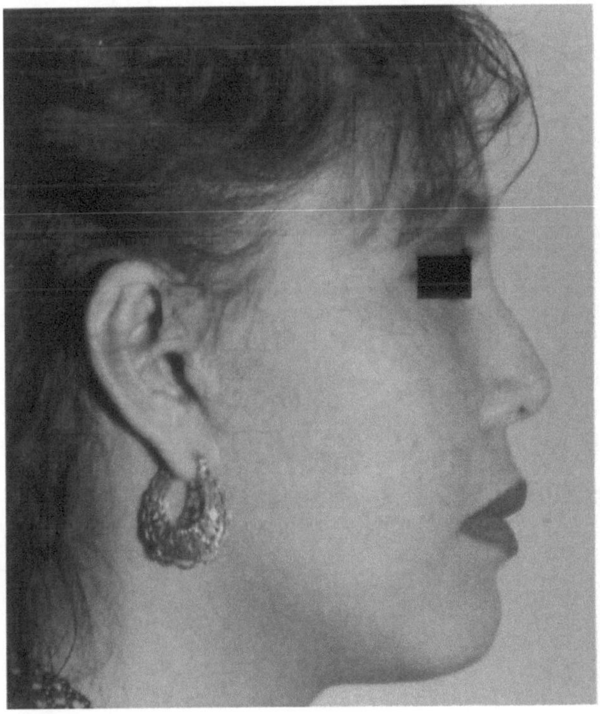

Figure 4-17B

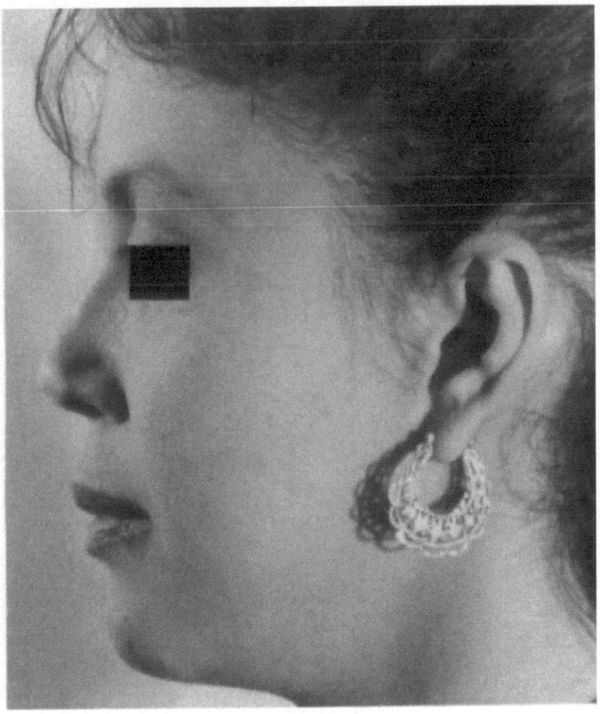

Figure 4-17C

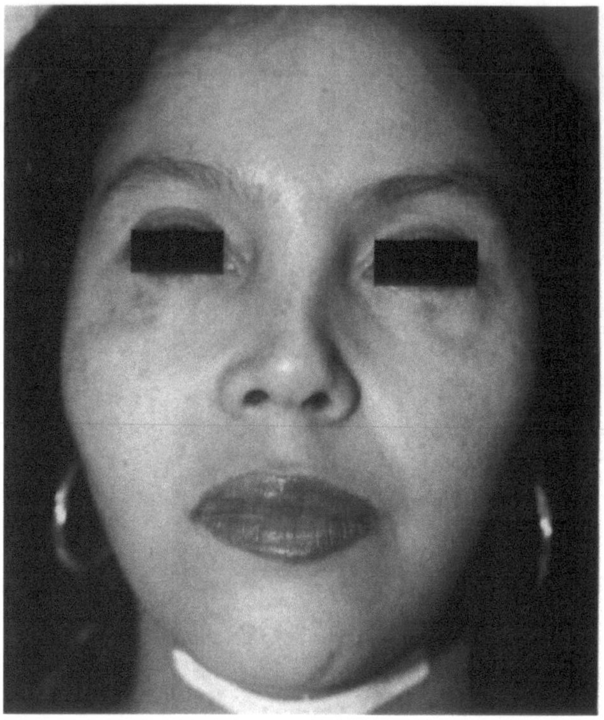

Figure 4-18A

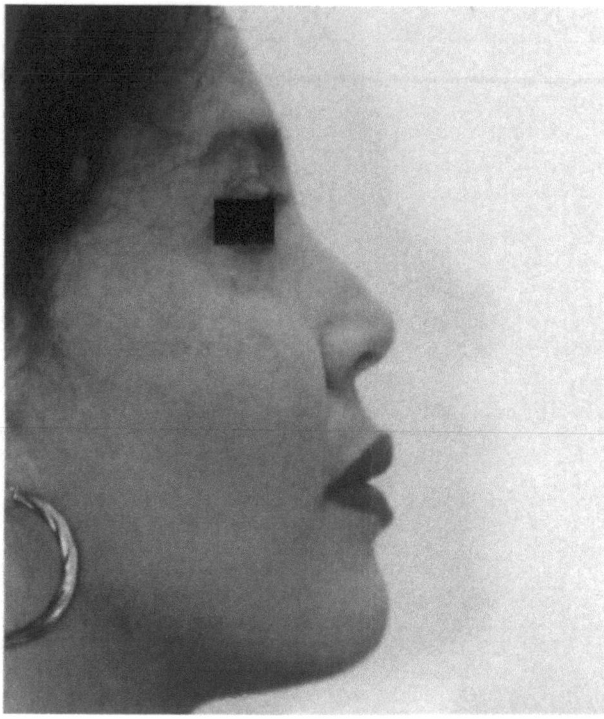

Figure 4-18B

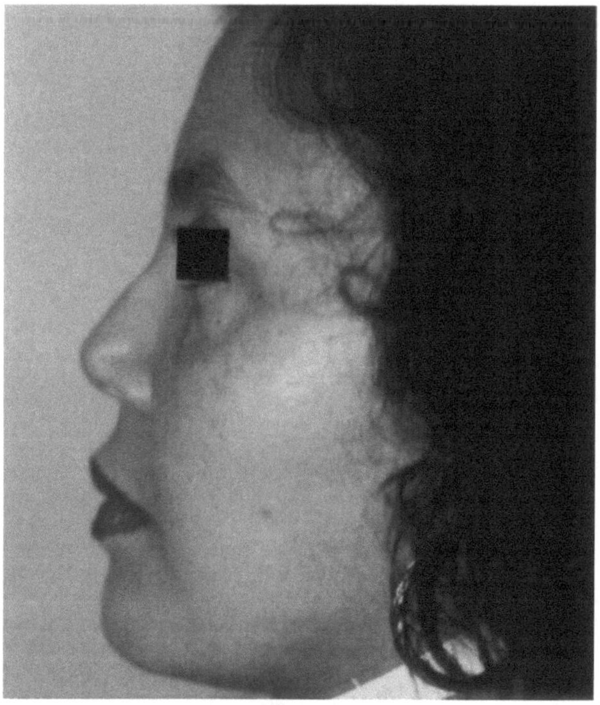

Figure 4-18C

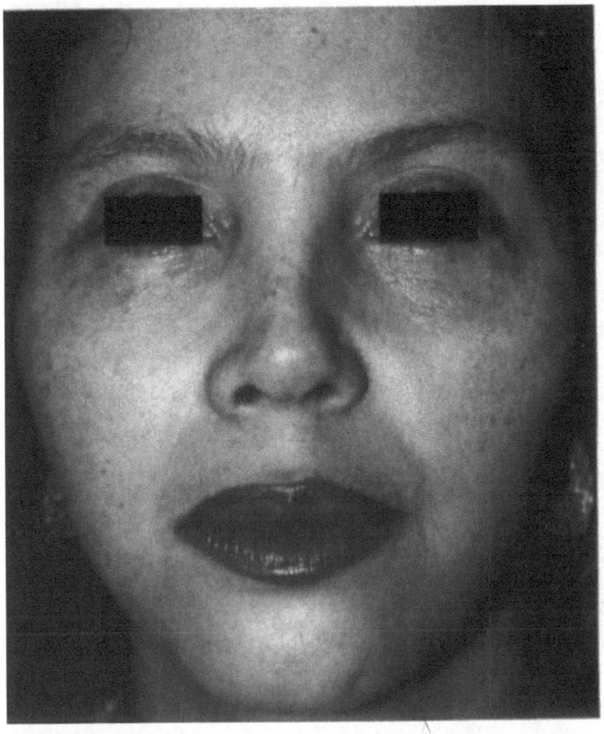

Figure 4-19A

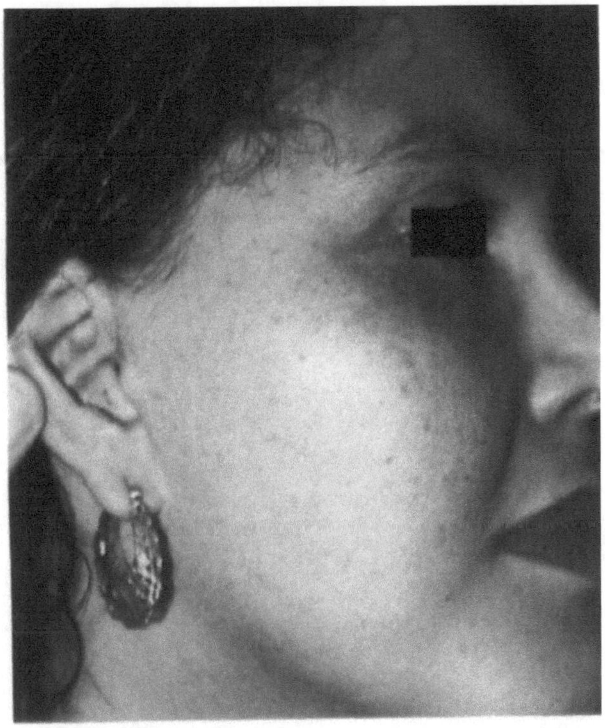

Figure 4-19B

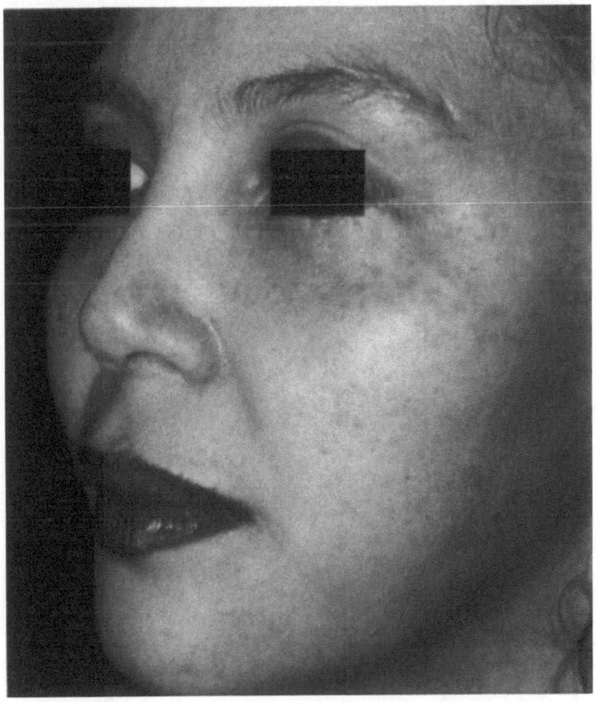

Figure 4-19C

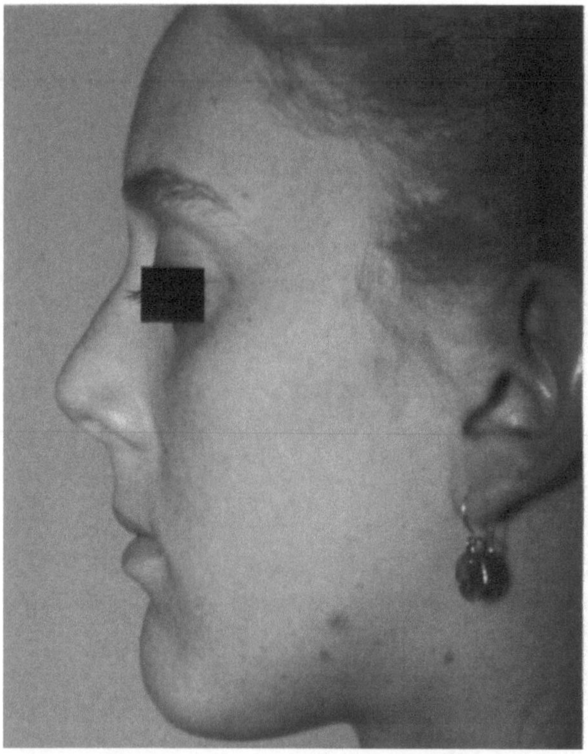
A

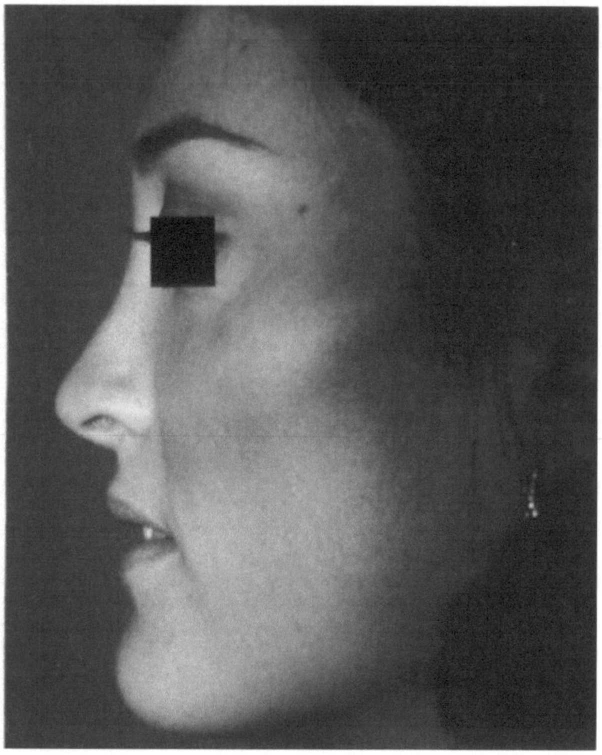
B

C
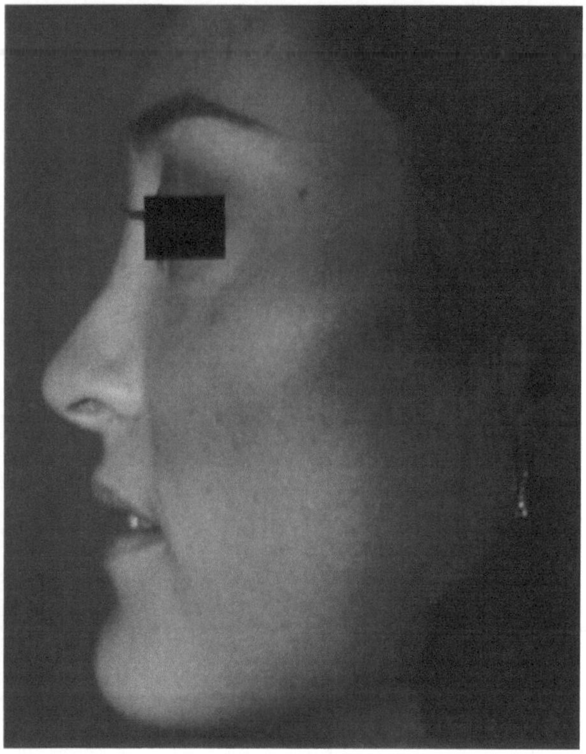

Figure 4-20. Classic malar augmentation. When making selections for facial contour, one choice is to use an oval prosthesis in the classic posterior position. In the preoperative photograph **(A)** this patient has fullness in the anterior face lateral to the nose. Her concept of "high fashion" was a far lateral placement, as shown in the postoperative photographs **(B&C)**. Reducing the length of the mandible shortens the distance between the lower lip and the chin line, giving better balance to the midface. A lip roll procedure for fullness of the upper lip, a reduction rhinoplasty, and a Silastic moderate projection chin prosthesis of the wraparound type completed this facial balancing.

long as the incision in Figure 4-3. This patient had had two parallel incisions, and the revision was a struggle.) The opening is made directly under the orbicularis and continued as far as the orbital rim, as for an orbital floor fracture. Extra fat in the area can be cauterized to keep it from puffing out forward. Use the scalpel to incise the entire length of the orbital rim and then carefully dissect the periosteum, with your fingers in place above the desired space. Taking note of the position of the intraorbital nerve, slide the periosteal elevator back and forth and up and down and lever it until an adequate space has been created. (By now the shape, size, and contour of the implant have been determined, so the dimensions of the space required should be clear).

Fat Sculpture

Some patients request a reduction in the bulk of facial fat in order to accent flat facial planes, whereas others associate this look with being old. With the exception of Oriental patients, it is probably a waste of time to dissect the fatpad of Bichat. This fatpad is approached from within the mouth and is carefully teased away from the nearby facial nerves. I believe, however, that this maneuver leaves a dimpling effect in an unnatural position, rather than accomplishing true facial planing in most cases.

The combination of malar augmentation and liposuction, or fat grafting, of the triangle below the malar prominence may be effective. The best word to describe malar augmentation is "enhancement." We begin with the natural beauty of a face and finely tune it. We create a look that is pleasing to that person and, as with rhinoplasty, provide a subtle yet distinct and visible change. Particularly in young patients, a dramatic change in facial appearance is effected by this maneuver when combined with the submental incision for exploration and control of submental zone bulging.

Placement Decisions

When I designed the "extended" silicone malar prosthesis,[5] the procedure was not often requested, as it is today. Problems such as extended recovery time, floating implants, and infection have largely been eliminated by changes in the choice of materials and technical maneuvers. Correspondence and discussion with other surgeons in the field of aesthetic plastic surgery, however, reveal several trends. Few surgeons choose autologous material or Proplast.

In the real world of aesthetic surgery, the use of ear cartilage is an academic exercise. Patients must be able to return to normal activities in a short time without percutaneous sutures, visible scars, or other indications of cosmetic surgery. The employment of contouring silicone malar prostheses allows one to

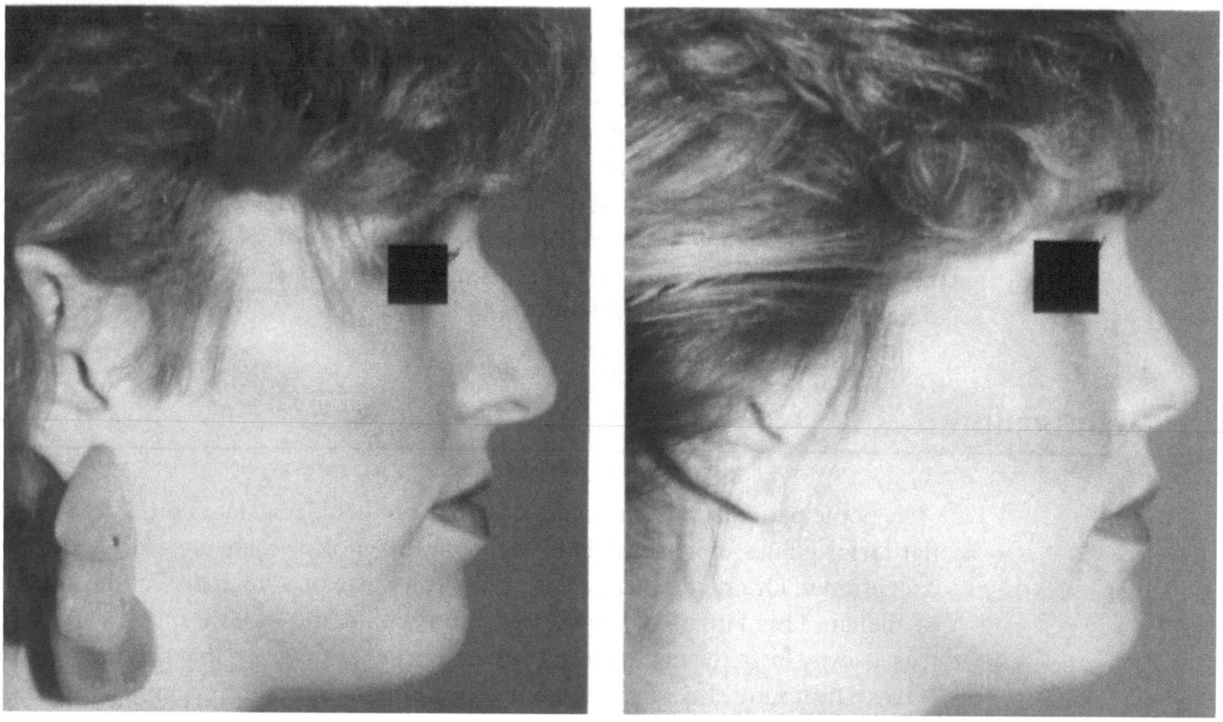

A B

Figure 4-21. Patient choices for facial rejuvenation. The primary concern of this patient was the height of the nose. Our preliminary drawings showed a preference for a high tip and a straight dorsum. A malar augmentation was selected as well. Note that the nasal spine has been addressed, so the lip can fall into a more normal position. The lip roll procedure gave more fullness to the upper lip, and the malar implant of the extended type developed fullness below the original malar highlight. Addressing the lip deficiency as well as the nasal contour results in more pleasing facial balancing.

reach this goal. If the patient should decide on a change or removal of the prosthesis, such procedures too can be accomplished easily without a residual defect. For this reason alone, autogenous materials are not recommended. In certain instances one may use temporalis fascia. I have placed fascia over silicone prostheses with good results. Temporalis fascia is harvested through an incision hidden within the hairline, thereby satisfying one of the requirements for aesthetic surgery.

An advantage of preformed silicone malar prostheses is that they can be folded and inserted easily through a shortened eyelid incision. Both the "extended" and the "anatomic" silicone prostheses have been satisfactory for aesthetic appearance, rapid recovery after surgery, and immobility of the prosthesis. My patients return to normal activity within 36 hours and require little more than the services of a cosmetologist trained in postoperative makeup application.

For chin augmentation, supraperiosteal placement of a silicone prosthesis seems to work as well as subperiosteal placement. Exposure of the subperiosteal space for accurate positioning is a definite requirement with prosthetic materials in the malar area, however. For this reason, the trend is to avoid intraoral incisions. The shortened lower lid blepharoplasty incision allows rapid, accurate subperiosteal dissection and implant placement. I have encountered several patients with movable supraperiosteal malar prostheses whose defects were corrected by subperiosteal placement through the eyelid. It may be significant that the only infections I have encountered were after transoral placement.

Malar augmentation should be reversible without morbidity or deformity. Harvesting ear cartilage leaves a permanent reminder of an experience that may later be viewed as unpleasant. A number of my patients with malar augmentation grew to dislike their appearance. The major "complication" was dissatisfaction with the projection or positioning of the high point of the prosthesis. Proplast, autogenous cartilage or bone, and Dacron-backed prostheses are not easily removed or repositioned.[6] The various contoured prostheses have this advantage plus a unique suction effect that prevents motion even if the desired placement position extends beyond the periosteum.

There are several measurement formulas to determine placement of the high point of the prosthesis.[7] Use these measurements only as a reference point, not for a final determination of position. A rapid perusal of models in fashion publications reveals wide variation of positioning of the natural high point of the malar prominence. Individuals have their own ideas of natural beauty and may choose role models that vary from the standard. I use facial photographs of different placement sites and compare them with drawings on the patient's photograph before we (the patient and I) jointly determine the choice of projection, extension, and high-point positioning. It should be noted, however, that despite this careful preoperative counseling and analysis, a number of patients return for repositioning of the prosthesis, sometimes as little as .1 cm elevation.

Several colleagues have reported achieving good resolution of infections around malar implants by simply draining the area through the mouth and using antibiotics. With Dacron backed implants, of course, the implant must be removed because the infection does not clear otherwise. The more modern solid implants do not present the displacement problems encountered with the earlier implants, or at least not to the same degree.

Errors of placement are generally overcome by ensuring the patient's cooperation during the preoperative planning. We sketch the proposed changes on the patient's face with a red washable felt-tip pen at the first consultation and then transfer this diagram to a preprinted facial form and to a photocopy of facial films. Because there are so many possible variations, it is essential that each patient bring in magazine photographs that illustrate the placement they desire.

Comments and Commentary

1. True malar augmentation also fills the submalar zone. One must confess, however, that there are individuals with high cheek bones who do not have fullness in that central facial plane and desire it. One way to correct this situation is to use a smaller version of the "anatomic" malar prosthesis and place it a bit lower. The other is to make a separate pocket just off the malar fullness for true submalar positioning. Each of these prostheses is placed in the subperiosteal space. Note that the periosteum begins to fade away and becomes tenuous posteriorly.

2. Technical point: If a long implant is being placed, be particularly careful during the posterior blunt dissection so as not to tear a muscle or cause excess bleeding.

3. Suggestion for pain control: Because pain is not likely to be great now that we are using postsurgical bupivacaine (Marcaine) instillation or nerve blocks—and knowing that it takes only one-fourth the dosage of any analgesic to *prevent* pain that would be required to *relieve* pain—try using acetaminophen or aspirin every 4 hours (not "as needed" but around the clock) for the first few days. Synthetic drugs such as hydrocodone (Vicodin), which is more powerful but has fewer side effects than codeine, may also be used.

4. The early malar implants were crude by today's standards. In 1971 Spatafora presented a case using polyethylene, placed using a preauricular oblique approach. Hinderer reported cases in 1972 and 1973 and used the intraoral approach. Gonzalez-Ulloa followed in 1974 with the rhytidectomy incision. Ceramic implants were replaced by perforated silicone rubber implants in three sizes. None of these efforts compare to the elegance and naturalness of modern surgery, primarily due to our selection of materials, contours, and appreciation of male and feminine beauty.

5. Our Oriental colleagues often ignore a microgenia or a flat malar eminence but jump at a chance to reduce a prominent angle of the mandible. These differences in approach to a problem can be attributed to perceptions of beauty by the various cultures.

6. Most complications associated with malar implants are due to secondary procedures. It would not be as simple if one used alloplastic material or bone (repositioning the malar bone by cross-cutting and grafting the open wedge). Another advantage of silicone malar implants is that one can easily choose a different size implant for the two sides of the face. Sixty percent of patients require different sized implants for the two cheeks in order to achieve better symmetry. These onlay techniques are far simpler than transection of the zygomatic arch or the onlay of alloplastic bone.

7. The Binder II implant design is an improvement on the original submalar design for face lift patients who had too much hollowing of the cheek. The long tail end of the Binder I was mobile, and a number of these implants worked through into the mouth simply because the distal end lies free of the bone and can be rubbed by chewing. Although the Binder II implant is wider, I prefer an implant that covers more of the lower edge of the bony prominence.

8. What do you do with the thick tissues that overlie the malar eminence, the notorious cheek pads? You have probably tried cutting them out (they come back), injecting them with steroids (they either do not go away, or you end up with an atrophic spot), or ignoring them. The consensus now is to use a 3-mm suction cannula, approaching from a distance, to remove the deep underlying tissue. We have had consistently good results with that approach, but the patient must be warned that results are often unpredictable.

9. The manufacturers of Proplast are combining their product with hydroxyapatite to make a firmer material that they suggest will become fixed bone. Proplast is a black, crumby material that was a problem when it was extruded. The new Proplast HA may be an improvement because it is heavier and firmer.

10. Fixation or no fixation? Usually fixation is not used. If you choose to use a temporary percutaneous stitch, it can easily be placed using a sheathed needle. Instead of a suction tip, Steve Hoefflin uses a tuberculin syringe to sheath the needlepoint. Either way, the needle can be passed to the exact point where you want it within the pocket; it can then be punched through the skin.

11. Another unsubstantiated statement was made by someone who favors buccal fat pad excisions: "Large malar implants cause unnatural results." There is a place for Bichat pad removal, particularly in Oriental patients, but removal is more often associated with "unnatural results" than are malar implants.

12. Bob Flowers (Honolulu) has noted the use of new implants he found useful. One fits below the rim of the orbit for those individuals who have depressions, and another fits in the area below the nasolabial fold as part of an extended malar implant.

REFERENCES

1. Hinderer VT: Malar implants for improvement of the facial appearance. Plast Reconstr Surg 56:157, 1975.
2. Wilkinson T: Room temperature vulcanizing Silastic in facial contour reconstruction. J Trauma 15:449, 1975.
3. Terino E: Alloplastic facial contouring: surgery of the fourth plane. Aesth Plast Surg 16:195, 1992.

4. Wilkinson T: Discussion: malar augmentation using autologous composite conchal cartilage and temporalis fascia. Plast Reconstr Surg 83:401, 1988.
5. Wilkinson T: Complications in aesthetic malar augmentation. Plast Reconstr Surg 71:643, 1983.
6. Whitaker L: Aesthetic augmentation of the malar-midface structures. Plast Reconstr Surg 80:337, 1987.
7. Powell NB, Riley RW, Laub DR: A new approach to evaluation and surgery of the malar complex. Ann Plast Surg 20:206, 1988.

5 Chin

THE SMOOTH CONTOURS OF THE CHIN ON EACH IDEALIZED FACE represent one of the goals in plastic surgery; that is, we want not just to restore beauty but to create it. Facial balance is a major goal. In western society the chin is a symbol of masculinity for men. In women, the chin accents the sensuous lip. A full chin line is rarely accompanied by submental muscle descent, which spoils our quest for a youthful "clean" jawline.

Implanting a chin prosthesis and applying liposuction can create the same jawline in the young patient that submental tuck creates in older patients. Eventually, aging changes and redeposition of fat above and below the platysma require intervention, but in the meantime a chin prosthesis can suffice. Even with occlusal problems, patients choose simplicity (chin prosthesis) over perfection (sliding genioplasty).

Keep it simple. Choose lesser fullness with centrality for women, and overfill for men with heavy features or large noses. Forget the soft gels with Dacron backing; there are better, less problem-plagued designs. These implants are not problem-free, of course, but they have technical advantages that matter.

Proper Placement

"Extended" chin implants can be too prominent and hence objectionable to the recipient. It is essential that the extended implants be placed in a small subperiosteal pocket just along the edge of the mandible. Because they are tapered, it is easier to place them posteriorly. There are two types of Silastic extended implant. One extends to the edge of the jowl area and is a soft material; others are longer and are composed of a firmer material. We prefer the firmer material because it can be easily placed in the pocket and gives a prominent contour.

Aesthetic results have been satisfactory in patients in whom we removed the prominence of the chin (using an electric drill bevel) and then placed a small soft, contoured, extended implant above the bone edge. In our experience, use of an extended chin prosthesis is a rapid, less traumatic way to achieve a smooth, rounded chin without lateral depressions. Grafting fat into the lateral area is effective, but the best result is seen when the grafts are combined with subperiosteal prosthesis implantation.

Augmentation or Genioplasty?

Arthur Ship (New York) advocates the use of genioplasty, citing cases in which the distal end of an extended chin prosthesis was palpable. (We have had such a case as well, although correcting the problem was simple. The incision was reopened, and the palpable end of the prosthesis was removed, trimmed, and reinserted—all in about 20 minutes and as an outpatient procedure.) Ship has virtually abandoned alloplastic chin prostheses, despite the fact that he had extensive experience with prostheses of his own design. He tried a variety of extensions, wings, and materials but considered them insufficient. He eliminated the need for wiring the bone segments during genioplasty by appropriate placement of a "miniplate." As he stated, "The contour of a reconstructed chin preserves the integrity of the original soft tissue anatomy."

We differ regarding this concept in that the original tissue may not be the size or shape desired. In older patients there is a crumpling effect due to atrophy. No matter how skilled the surgeon, genioplasty is a complex procedure; and miniplates, wires, and cephalograms are not inexpensive.

I prefer not to use the sliding genioplasty, a procedure that many plastic surgeons find too complex for most patients. We do agree, though, that patients should be offered the alternatives and be presented with the advantages and disadvantages of each.

Design Problems with Chin Augmentation Prostheses

At a 1985 symposium several surgeons discussed their preference for contoured chin augmentation prostheses. They correctly pointed out that standard Silastic prostheses fill only the anterior chin. In older persons there may be soft tissue atrophy lateral to this area in a triangle almost directly underneath the oral commissure. "Extended" prostheses help to fill that area. Technical point: Ensure that the prosthesis extends into a subperiosteal pocket and that it lies along the margin of the mandible (not across the mental nerve). Some extended prostheses simply do not look good in some people, however.

After examining the usual gel chin prostheses and some of the contoured prostheses, the difference becomes obvious. The gels are wider in their central dimension and do not project as far. It is impossible, though, to produce a gel implant that can be placed in a small pocket far posteriorly; a compromise is reached by choosing a harder silicone. Some hard silicone prostheses are round, causing abnormal projection, even in patients with adequate soft tissue.

The solution to this dilemma is to keep many implants available in the

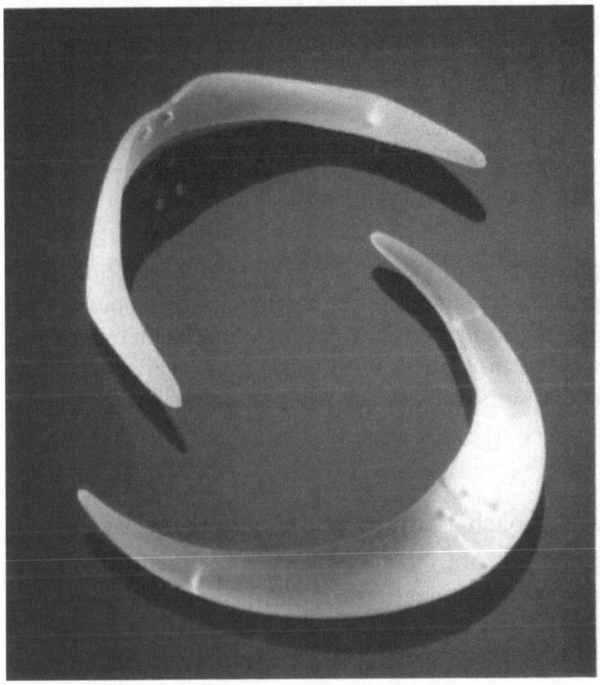

Figure 5-1. Chin implants of radically different design. The upper one ("pre-jowl" Mittelman type) is designed for the patient with good chin projection but no lateral fullness. To date, however, we have found that it is far better to fill these areas with autologous fat grafts. The lower design is typical of the extended chin implants in use today. One chooses the amount of projection according to the requirements and to the person's preferences. I would not choose this much projection unless the patient is male, has a large face, and has practically no chin.

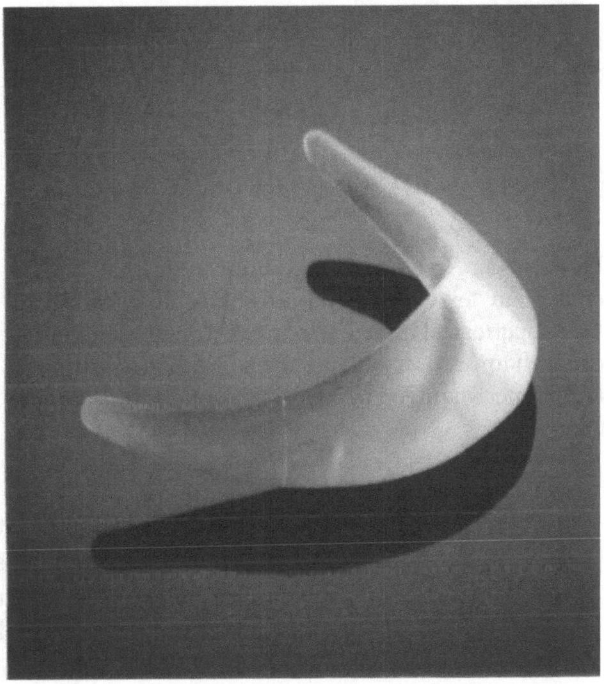

Figure 5-2. Flowers' mandibular glove chin augmentation device. It is designed to fit over the mandible, not just above it, giving some forward and downward projection. This device would be appropriate in someone who does not have a normal distance between the mandible tip and the lip. All other chin prostheses fit directly above the mandible and are covered with periosteum. Total periosteal coverage of a chin implant is not as important as it seems to be for malar augmentation.

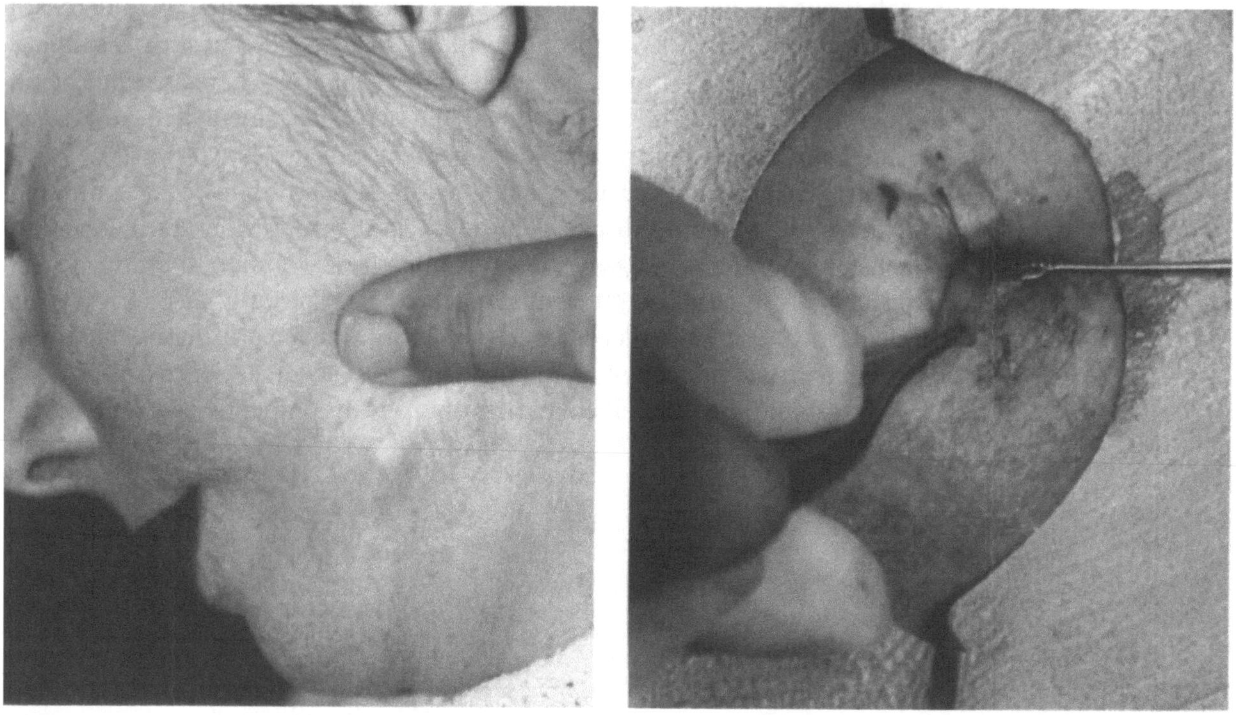

Figure 5-3. Even when you are certain that the far ends of an "extended" chin prosthesis are lying flat in the subperiosteal tunnel, the tip can turn up. The center can drift upward as well, despite tapes, internal sutures, and properly applied facial elastic support. If this complication occurs, simply fix it. Reopen the incision. If the problem is simply an annoying tip-up, apply a local anesthetic, make a tiny incision on the undercurve, and clip the prosthesis. With a spreading maneuver of the iris scissors, the silicone will pop up easily.

operating room. Whether the approach is through the mouth or, as Adrian Aiache prefers, through the submental zone "to avoid infection," the implant can be chosen on the basis of the preoperative evaluation and how it looks once in position. A long extension looks best in some people and a short extension in others. If there is adequate soft tissue, the defect can be corrected with a standard gel prosthesis.

Antibiotic coverage is universally recommended. It is well to remind the patient that infection can occur; and if it does it is almost always invariable that the implant must be removed. Fortunately, it does not always have to be replaced. If the patient receives a sufficient injury to dislodge the chin prosthesis or if it becomes infected, usually enough soft tissue thickening develops to give the appearance of the presence of an implant. This situation has occurred in four of our patients over a decade and in each case the patient's appearance was almost the same after implant removal as immediately after implant insertion. Furthermore, none has asked to have the implant replaced.

Chin Reduction

Any evaluation of the face should be based on the concept of equal distances in the central, upper, and lower thirds of the face, as proposed by Mario Gonzalez-Ulloa. More often than not, I have been consulted by patients who have had satisfactory rhinoplasties but were vaguely dissatisfied with their overall facial appearance. A simple analysis of the remaining portion of the face indicated that adding malar implants or reducing the length of the chin would have been a valuable adjunct. Several of these patients are shown in the color section.

The technical approach to this problem is as follows. It is not important whether the redundant bone and soft tissue is approached from the submental crease incision (so long as the entry is high enough) or intraorally. The latter approach is somewhat easier.

For the intraoral approach we use ketamine-diazepam (Valium) "twilight" anesthesia to establish regional blocks. We then flood the soft tissues with 0.25% lidocaine (Xylocaine) with epinephrine. After placing two sterile sponges to collect any run-off in the lateral gutters just outside the teeth, an incision is made

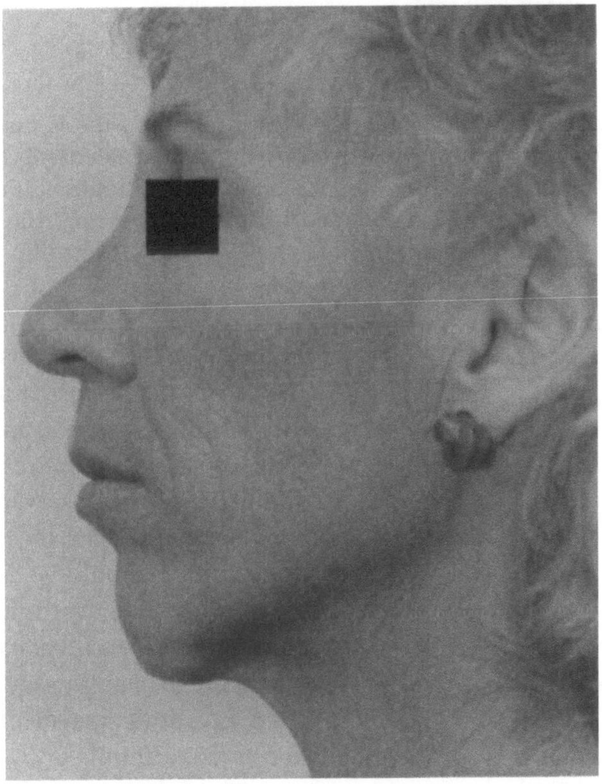

Figure 5-4. Note the position of the chin implant—below the mandible and floating freely in the subcutaneous tissue. The patient's frustration was compounded by the fact that the illustrated problem occurred after the *third* repositioning. We found no evidence of prior dissection in the proper area and easily repaired this defect to the patient's satisfaction with a chin prosthesis in the correct position just above the edge of the mandible. We also repaired her polly-beak nose.

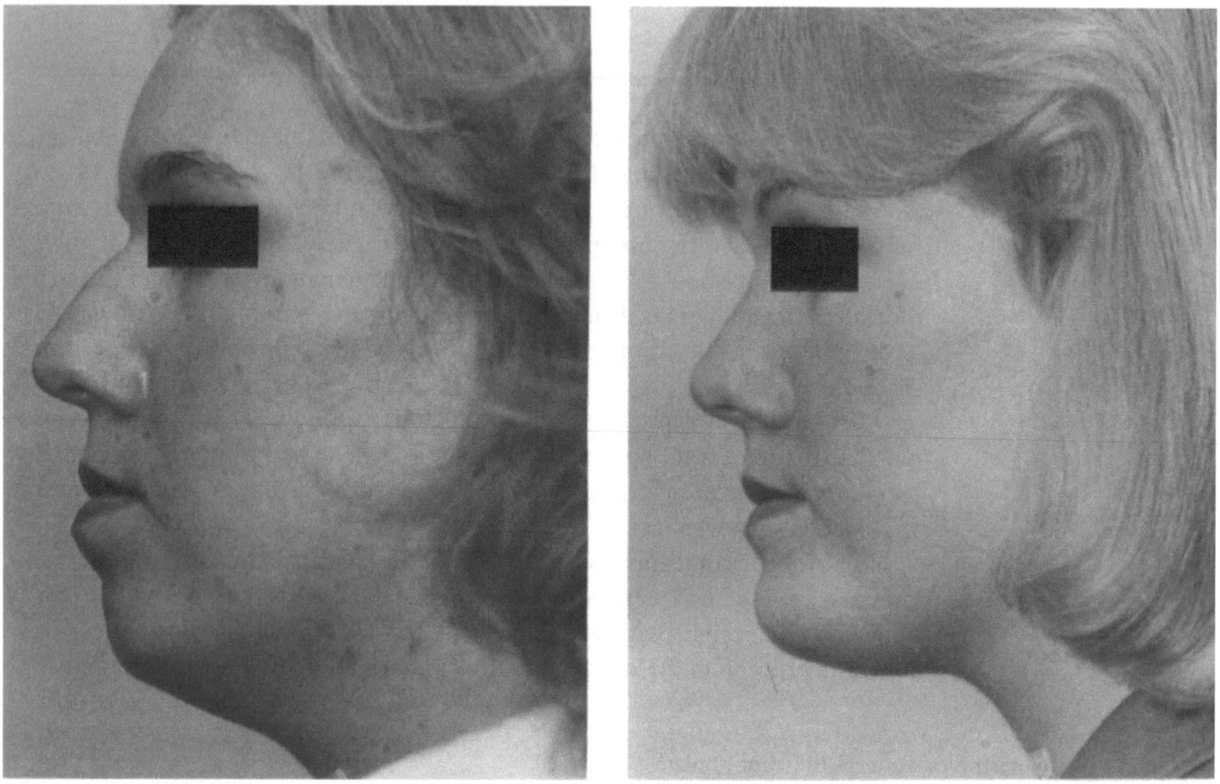

Figure 5-5. A properly selected chin prosthesis can correct many apparent cases of "submental droop." Some cases require an incision in the fold underneath the chin with defatting and anastomosis of the partially divided platysma. In other cases, such as the one illustrated, simply changing the angle of skin pull with the prosthesis can erase the problem. In this individual the repair from the nose down was infinitely more important to her overall appearance than the rhinoplasty.

4 mm above the sulcus inside the lower lip. The muscles are carefully dissected away from the periosteum. It helps to perform the final periosteum dissection with cutting cautery, as many tiny blood vessels come through this area. Using good retractors, the area can thus be cleared safely, almost to the area of the nerve origin. It is not necessary to go that far, however, because the plan is to reduce the bony section only 2 to 3 cm back from the center. During the preoperative evaluation, it should be determined if it is necessary to remove a wedge of soft tissue. This maneuver is easy to accomplish. Many female patients have only a bony point, a masculine habitus that is neither soft nor feminine; whereas others have a bulge of soft tissue where the chin rounds. Approach this bulge directly after separating the mentalis muscle. Removal can be accomplished with a liposuction cannula or by direct excision.

The anterior part or visible part of the bone has now been cleared. At this point, use electric cautery to go around the edge, separating the muscle

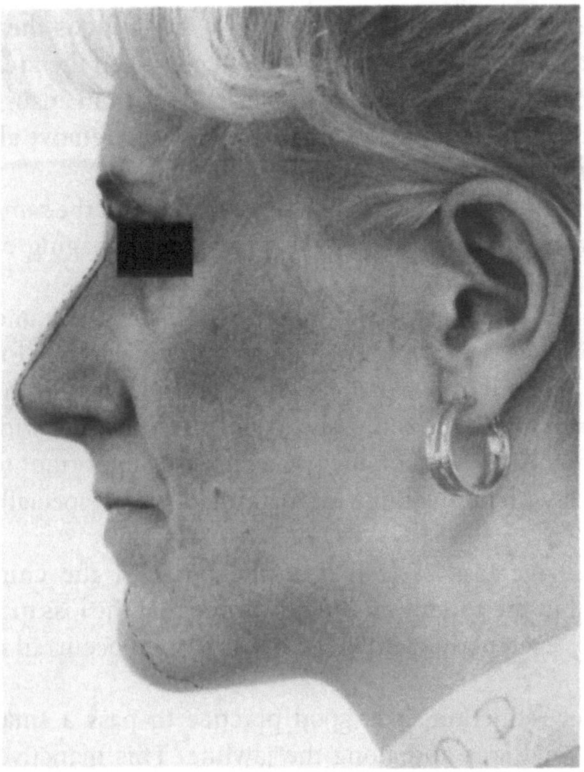

A

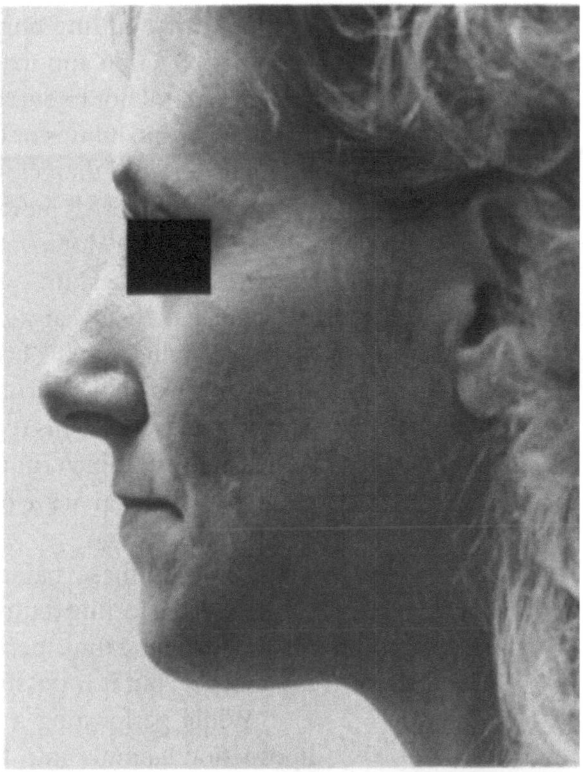

B

C

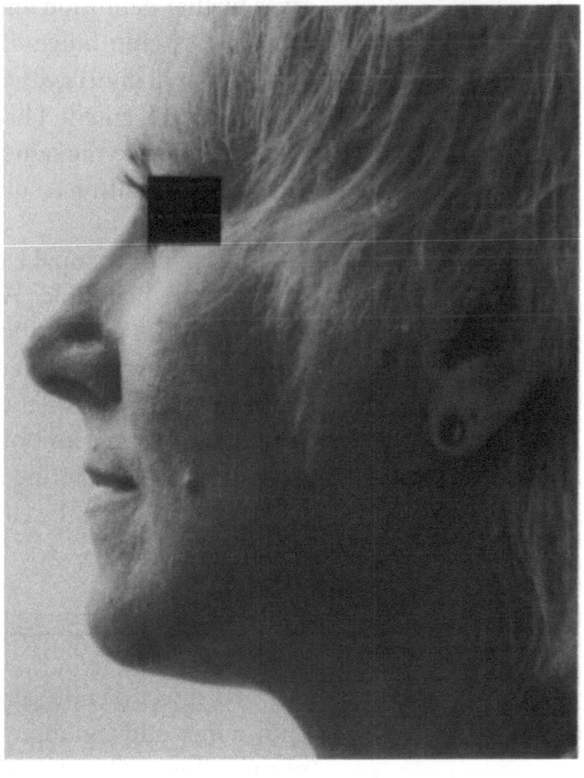

Figure 5-6. Chin reduction. This young woman has successfully pursued a public entertainment career since her original surgery in 1981. Her rhinoplasty was not difficult. Removing the bony point of the chin protrusion made a major difference. Note that it has been reduced in anterior projection as well as in length **(B&C)**. A too large "lower third" of the face violates Gonzalez-Ulloa's rules of facial symmetry. In these individuals, reduction of the nose is as important as reduction of the chin and shortening the vertical distance. **(C)** This 1992 photograph shows that the facial symmetry is retained.

attachments until all the bone to be removed is exposed. We use the "hand-engine" with a cutting burr, as it is safer than using chisels. The bone is then smoothed. Suction and irrigation are ongoing during this step to keep the area cool. Be careful not to overcorrect. Once the bone is reduced about 1 cm ensure that there are no bumps or lumps laterally. Finally, irrigate the area to remove all the bone dust and then close the wound without a drain.

The procedure is more difficult using the submental approach, but the same principles apply. Moreover, with good assistance you can avoid damaging or overstretching the skin.

Our patients wear a protective compression dressing for 5 days, day and night, removing it only once or twice a day. After that, they wear the dressing for an hour or two in the morning, an hour or two in the evening, and all night for the next several weeks. This regimen forces the soft tissue to shrink to position with less chance of visible crumpling. At the end of *any* procedure it is important to establish a regional nerve block with bupivacaine (Marcaine), but it is especially helpful in this area.

Some of these patients have loss of feeling at the point of the chin. Generally, the feeling returns, but the patient should be warned that the loss may remain for a long time, perhaps even permanently. Such loss has not occurred in my practice, but it is possible.

While performing a chin reduction, it is good practice to pass a small liposuction cannula into the jowl area and along the jawline. This maneuver gives further definition and breaks up the skin adherence in this area.

Just as chin bulge can be successfully reduced by liposuction, it can be enhanced by a multilayered fat grafting technique, which is described in Chapter 6 for lip enhancement. I have had only a few such patients, but their chin fullness is intact almost to the same degree that could be achieved using a chin prosthesis. The good fat grafting results have persisted in these patients for almost 7 years at this writing.

I have no personal experience with the implants that are being used at the angle of the mandible. Adrien Aiache has reported good results with these prostheses. It is interesting to think that certain Asians want these wide angles of the mandible resected because they think it makes them too ethnic, whereas most Americans consider that Maria Shriver look as very attractive. According to Aiache, using an intraoral incision, sharp subperiosteal dissection of the masseter, and implanting a preformed prosthesis over the end of the mandible, like a cap, has been the easiest way to accent this zone of the face.

Witch's Chin

To resect or not to resect, that is the question. Treatment of the hanging chin, commonly but discourteously called the "witch's chin," involves a number of procedures. One may operate from within the oral cavity, resecting fat and advancing the soft tissue upward with a series of anchoring sutures. That procedure corrects part of the overhang but does not fill the depression in the submental fold, nor does it correct the commonly seen "crumpling" of skin across the chin. Ewaldo de Souza Pinto prefers a direct incision in the chin area. He advocates a hat-shaped removal of tissue despite the resultant scar, which is in a visible area. My choice and that of many other surgeons is to open the submental triangle and turn down a flap of subcutaneous tissue after defatting. This turned-down flap allows one to fill the submental depression. In the most common case, it is better to resect the soft tissue that overhangs the mandible rather than depend on it for support.

If crumpled skin is the major problem, it is simpler to use a minor turned-down flap to fill the submental fold depression, defat the remaining overhang area, and add a wraparound silicone chin implant. The balloon effect stretches the soft tissue so the Retin-A program and light chemical peels can finish off the crumples. The advantage is that there is a single incision hidden in the submental fold, which allows correction of other defects if they are present.

The turned-up flap of soft tissue can be used to give fullness to the chin. One patient refused chin augmentation because she did not want anterior projection. The witch's chin that resulted from shortening the pointed mandible was partly a result of tissue edema and partly the result of lack of anterior support. Our choices in this case were sliding genioplasty or removal of the pointed downward projection of the mandible and the simpler addition of a chin implant. The patient refused all of the above. During surgery, I rotated the soft tissue of the hanging part of the chin upward into an anterior position.

The technical points of correcting a witch's chin are as follows: First, reopen the submental incision that was used for the platysmal repair during the face lift. (Do not try to do an up-turned flap procedure through the mouth; it is almost impossible.) Once you open the submental area, dissect the skin away, leaving a small flap of fatty tissue. This maneuver easily exposes the extra soft tissue. Create a space just above the periosteum in which the tissue can lie. Pass percutaneous sutures through the skin at the point where the new chin fold is to be created and then through the leading edges of the flap; pull the flap into position underneath the skin. The front side of the subcutaneous flap is thus turned upward so it lies in contact with the periosteum and is now posterior. Tie the sutures loosely to create the fold. Instead of the flat chin with a hanging witch's chin protrusion, there is now a smoother jawline and an anterior projection.

Fat Grafts and Soft Tissue Flaps

There are other ways to augment the chin. As discussed in Chapter 2, fat grafting has proved useful in the marionette zone and for enhancing the lip. We speculated that if we could create a thick, fat lip by crisscrossing multiple tunnels filled with concentrated autologous fat, perhaps we could do it in the thick fibrous tissue of the chin.

Why, you may ask, would you do that instead of a chin implant? The answer lies in the fact that some patients fear the use of silicone despite our reassurances and the scientific studies of Silastic, which has been used in medical devices since the mid-1950s. Other patients do not want a "foreign material" in their face. Hence we must look for alternative solutions. One alternative is to use a turned-flap of soft tissue, particularly for a witch's chin. A second is to use our experience with lip fat grafting to create a fuller chin using the multiple tunnel technique.

The patient shown in Figure 5-7A was counseled regarding his neck deformity and was offered a chin implant. He declined. A chin implant would have tightened the skin and given a better angle to the jaw, but we acceded to his wishes and instead asked him if he would agree to be one of our early patients with multilevel fat grafting. He agreed, and as can be seen from the photographs

A B

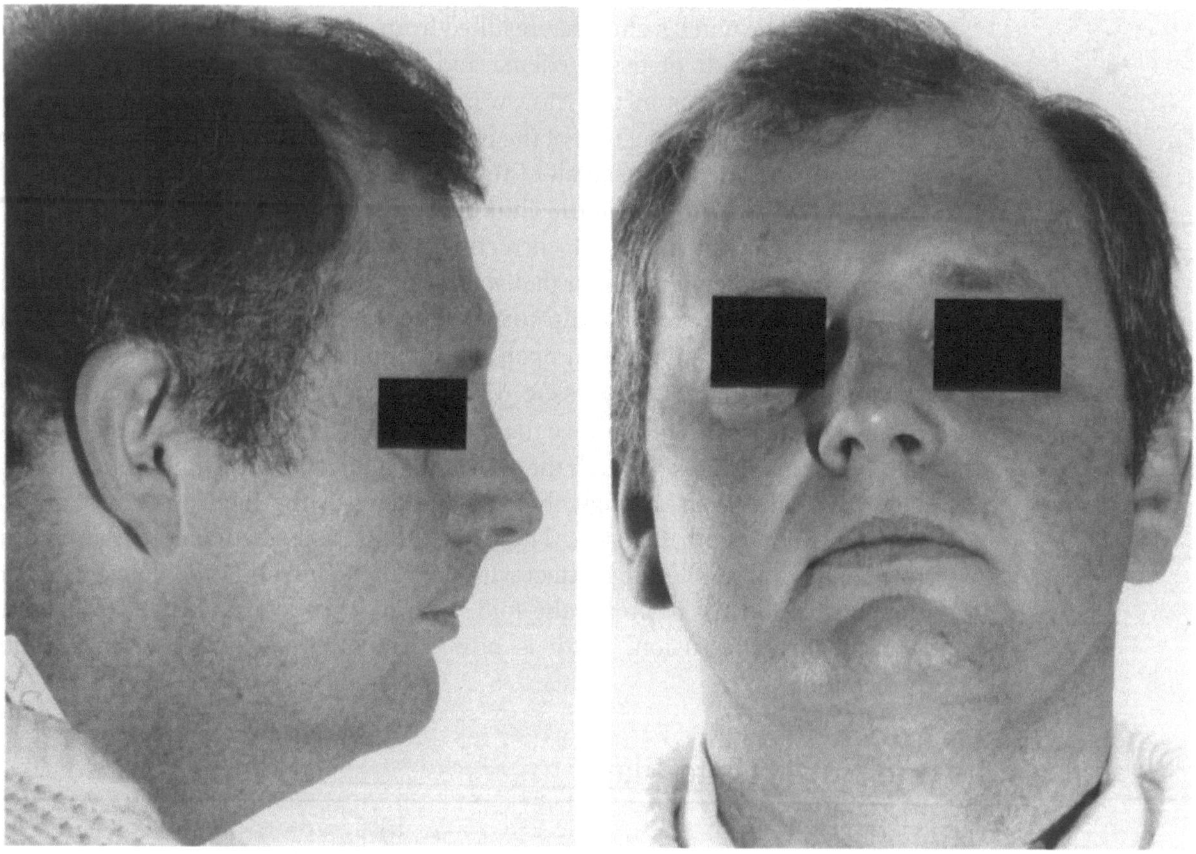

Figure 5-7. See text for description.

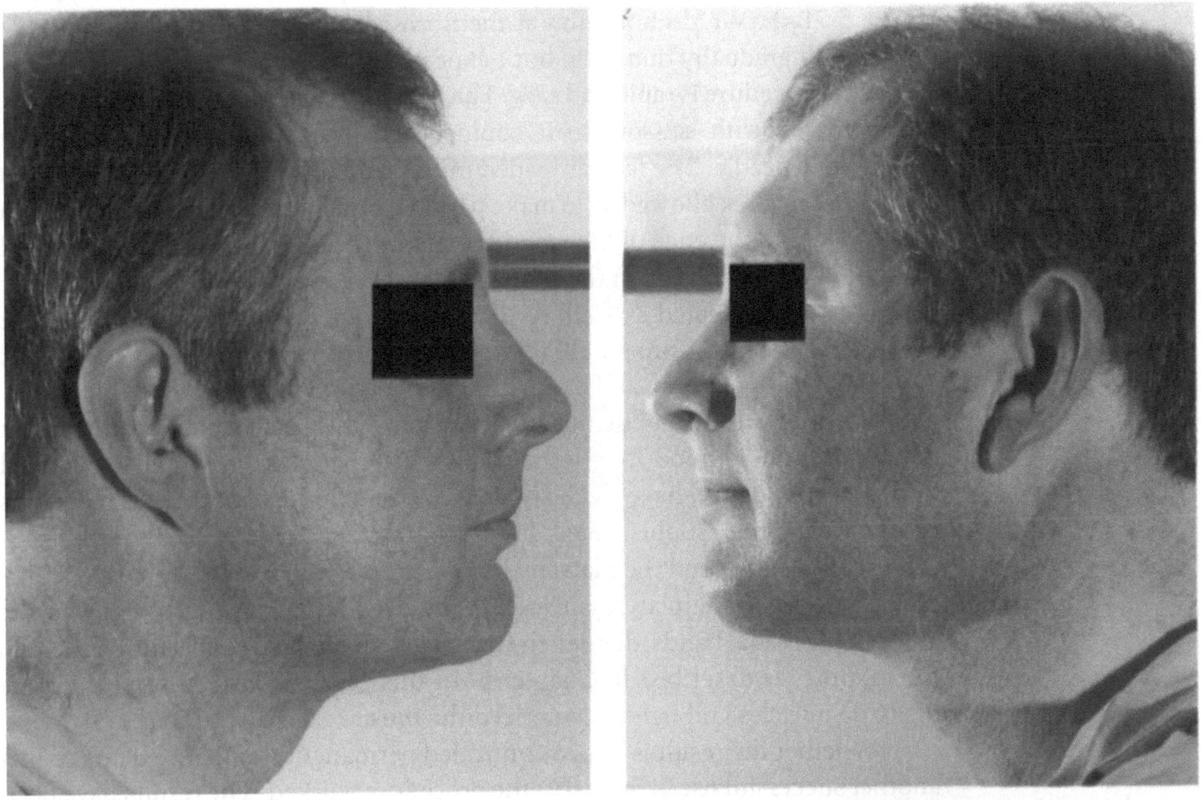

C

D

Figure 5-7. Continued

E

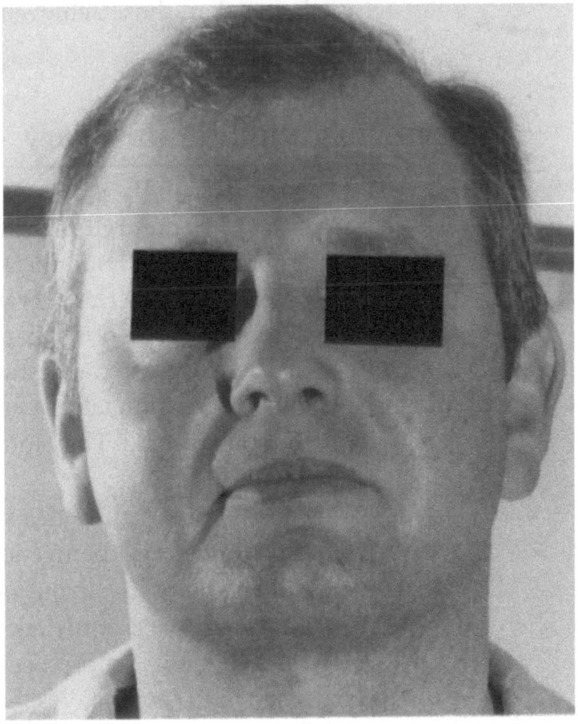

good chin enhancement has been achieved. The patient is shown at 1 year in Figure 5-7B–E. We do not know if the fibrosis that is created in the multiple tunnels will gradually diminish, but I expect not.

The procedure is rapid and easy. The fat, which was obtained from his neck, was prepared with scissors so it could be passed through a long 16-gauge hypodermic needle. The fat was loaded into a "fat gun" for precise placement. A percutaneous stick allowed us to make parallel tunnels underneath the skin from the chin fold to the edge of the mandible. As the needle was withdrawn, a small amount of fat was placed in the tunnels. A second and third layer in the deeper soft tissue were created as well. At 1 year, we expected to see a clean jawline because men's skin shrinks well. (Unfortunately, women's skin does not shrink as well in this age group, and one frequently must perform a lower face lift.)

We know from submental tuck patients that platysmal repair and fat removal produces good long-term results. The patients on whom I operated during the 1970s still have clean jawlines. Liposuction, of course, has made this procedure far more sophisticated. For the patient in Figure 5-7, we prophylactically suctioned beyond the platysmal center above and below the mandible line and then opened the platysma to resect the deep fatpad. We also removed the anterior platysmal bands, divided the bands low in the neck, and sutured them in the midline, as described in Chapter 3. In this case, we also sutured the large digastric muscles and lightly cauterized the muscles to flatten them.

Whether the result is due to controlled permanent traumatic edema or just another successful use of fat grafts, the procedure worked. The results have been better than those achieved with turned-up flaps.

Comments and Commentary

1. In the argument about oral surgeons versus plastic surgeons and why we ignore the "really important" aspects of the patient's case came a short, cutting comment from Hans Freihofer (The Netherlands): "Because you have good occlusion does not mean there are good aesthetics." This well-taken point implies that it is the aesthetics that interest the patient. A millimeter or two in dental occlusion takes a far distant second in terms of importance. "People want to look normal." They tolerated minor tooth offsets, but not a "wimp" receding jawline.

Pursuing this idea, Ian Munro (Toronto) reviewed the importance of cephalometrics, roentgenographic dental models, and so on and concluded that *examination of the living face* is by far the most important. The facial appearance after surgery certainly takes priority over dental aspects.

"Patients ignore occlusion problems. They simply want a good cosmetic result." Ed Terino (West Lake Village Calif.) was discussing patients' preferences for simple chin augmentation versus the more complex jaw suctioning with advancement. Our oral surgery colleagues are greatly in favor of the latter procedure for predictable reasons. Patients, however, are willing to overlook minor occlusive problems for a simpler solution to what they perceive is the problem.

2. A rotating chin prosthesis may be a problem. For example, a young woman presented 5 years after insertion of a smooth, firm contour chin prosthesis that had been inserted during a routine chin augmentation. To the amazement of the patient and the surgeon, the prosthesis had abruptly rotated 180 degrees. This bizarre appearance occurred over a period of several days without prior trauma or signs of infection. Needless to say, it was promptly replaced, with successful restoration of the contour.

3. Part of the aging process, according to McGhan Medical's instruction data, is a reduction in the size of the bony mandible with absorption of the alveolar processes. When soft tissue atrophy continues and the jowl pads increase in size, this "marionette" groove becomes visible. Although the defects can be filled with repeated fat injection grafts and suctioning of the jowl, an extended prosthesis provides an advantage. With the models that are available, one can choose the degree of anterior projection as well as the degree to which the lateral groove or marionette zone is filled.

4. There are few if any patients who do not require *some* anterior projection as well as lateral filling. Most of the marionette defect is closer to the lip, and the Mittelman design does not help there. Fat grafts and standard extended implants should be used in these cases.

5. Ed Baccari (Omaha) mixes 4 ml of lidocaine with adrenaline and 1 ml of sodium bicarbonate to reduce the pain of injections. Bicarbonate neutralizes the acidity of the lidocaine but does not interfere with its effectiveness. Baccari uses this combination particularly in children. It could also be used to advantage in the emergency room (ER). Another suggestion applicable to children is to have the nurse mix equal parts of 4% cocaine with lidocaine and apply it topically to the cut with a sterile 2 × 2 gauze on arrival. By the time the ER physician examines the child there is sufficient topical anesthesia to make injections less painful.

6. Ed Terino irrigates chin implant pockets with antibiotic solutions, 50,000 units of Bacitracin and saline. Irrigation is performed under pressure with a 25-gauge needle and syringe to clear out blood clots and other debris. Incidentally, Ed agrees with me that intraoral incisions for malar augmentation have more problems and complications than blepharoplasty or rhytidectomy approaches.

7. It is unlikely that hydroxyapatite will replace silicone chin implants the way contoured extended chin implants are replacing Proplast.

6 Lip Enhancement

MOST INDIVIDUALS HAVE PERSONAL IDEALS OF LIP SIZE AND shape. Perhaps it has something to do with our culture and ethnicity. One solution to the aesthetic surgeons dilemma with these choices is to have patients bring in photographs and compare them with an office file of photographs from magazines and actual patients. The surgeon and patient must be certain before surgery about the size and shape desired as well as the presence of asymmetry.

For lip enhancement, the most common technique is multilevel fat grafting. The degree of fullness of the vermilion depends first on the number of tunnels and second on the amount of the fat graft placed in each tunnel. Those patients who show no vermilion require a lip roll procedure of either the advancement or the V-Y type.

There is a difference between male and female changes. Some men want to resemble the full-lipped models in magazines, whereas others believe that these lips look too feminine. There is also the unusual situation that we call the double lip. Such individuals have a division from an inner and outer lip. One woman who presented for a secondary face lift was as concerned with her lower lip protrusion as she was with her pixie-like earlobes. A simple examination revealed that she had a second lip roll fold, a congenital type. This double lip made her upper lip seem to protrude. Simple excision with a wavy line scar was the answer.

In 1971 I began a series of lip enhancements based on a vague recollection of a type of undermining that I had seen in a paper by a Swiss surgeon. I believed that the edema I would create in the advanced vermilion was more important than the amount of tissue that was advanced. I later described this procedure as "lip roll." These patients have continued contact with our clinic, and their lips are soft and natural to this day.

I strongly advise against the proposed operation that requires skin excision above the white roll to give a "lift." As described in my letter to the editor of *Plastic and Reconstructive Surgery* that will be published this year, excision is not a "safe procedure." Scars are highly visible and unpredictable in size or tendency to hypertrophy. This has created a medico-legal nightmare for several good surgeons. Similarly, use of non-FDA approved materials such as "Gore-Tex" are associated with extrusions that nullify the advantages of simplicity. Overall it is best to enhance the lip by an internal maneuver, such as grafting or mucosal advancement, because it gives the illusion of the white roll area having been lifted as well. I have seen more individuals with abnormal length between the nostril and the vermilion. The operation appropriate for them is "lip lengthening." In others this area has elongated too much with age, and so a "lip shortening" is worth considering, particularly for older face lift patients who are aware of deformity.

The principal lip enhancement procedures are as follows.

1. *Lip enhancement by transverse mucosal advancement.* This proved technique (lip roll) involves an incision just above the frenulum at the labial sulcus and undermining of the dry and wet mucosa. Advancement and fixation in a forward position leaves an uncovered area of muscle, but fullness and an increase in vermilion height and projection are obtained. The size of the vermilion can be controlled by the degree of advancement and undermining (Figs. 6-1 to 6-4). Disadvantages include an occasional case of prolonged edema in the upper lip just below the nares (Fig. 6-5).
2. *Lip enhancement by excision of the white roll.* This technique, which was used to make the lips "full," has largely been abandoned because of the incidence of hypertrophic scarring as well as the obliteration of the natural white roll (Fig. 6-6). It is better to simulate an increase in the height of the lip by internal advancement. In older patients, it may be advantageous to remove an ellipse of skin below the nostril, which shortens a long upper lip (Fig. 6-7). Disadvantages include visible scarring across the columellar base.
3. *Lip lengthening.* In many individuals lip enhancement techniques involve not only mucosal expansion but lengthening the distance between the nares and the white roll. Our internal technique has produced excellent long-term results with few complications (Fig. 6-8). The labial

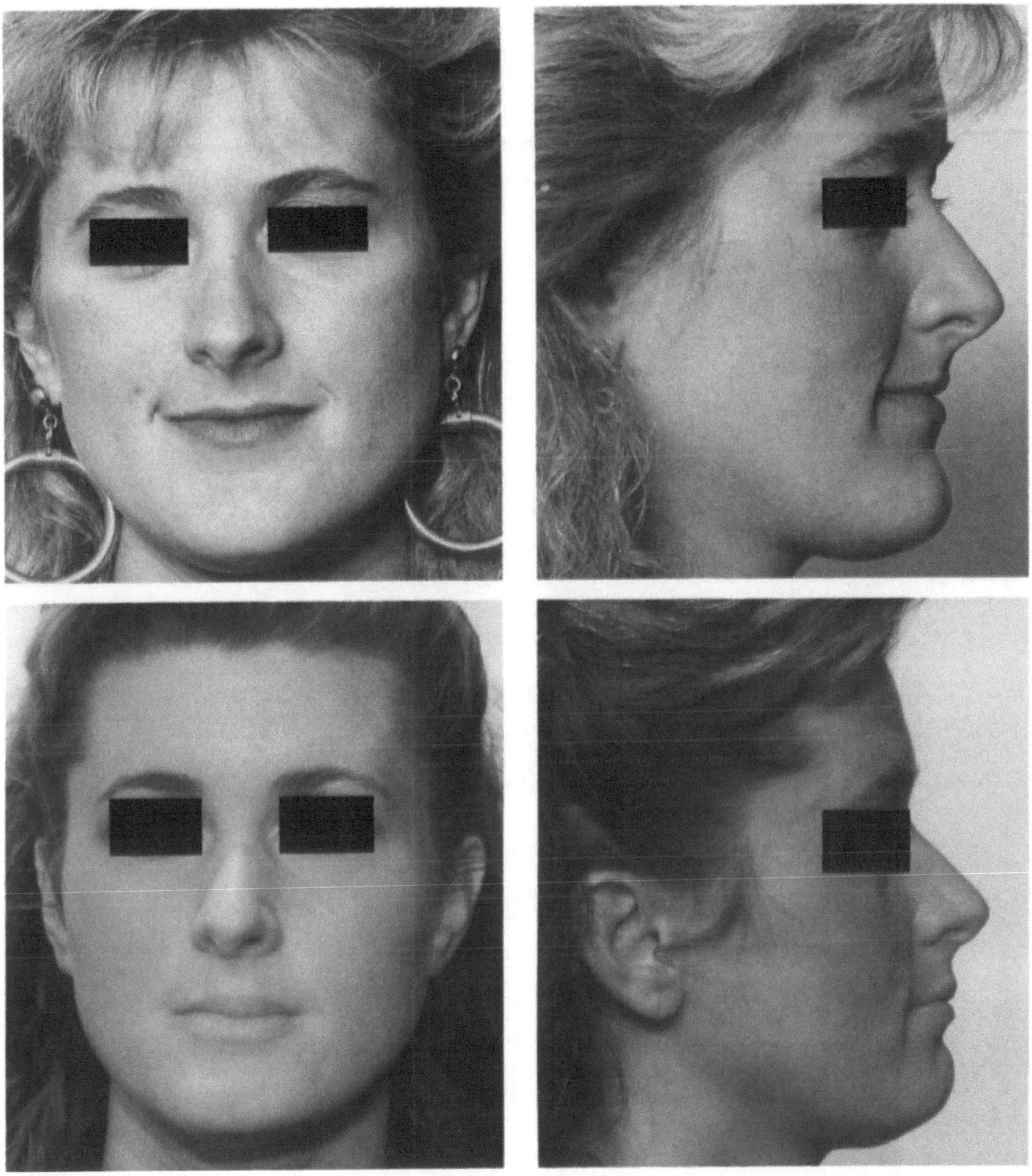

A B C D

Figure 6-1. **(A&B)** Balancing the lower third of the face may include lip enhancement. A flat malar zone and a large chin often accompany thin lips. Reducing the chin (intraoral approach, bony reduction with a hand-held engine and bone cutter tip) helps, but the added effect of an upper and lower lip roll both soften and balance the face and adds a sensuous element. Note the "apple cheek" position in which the contoured Silastic malar implants were placed. **(C&D)** One year after surgery.

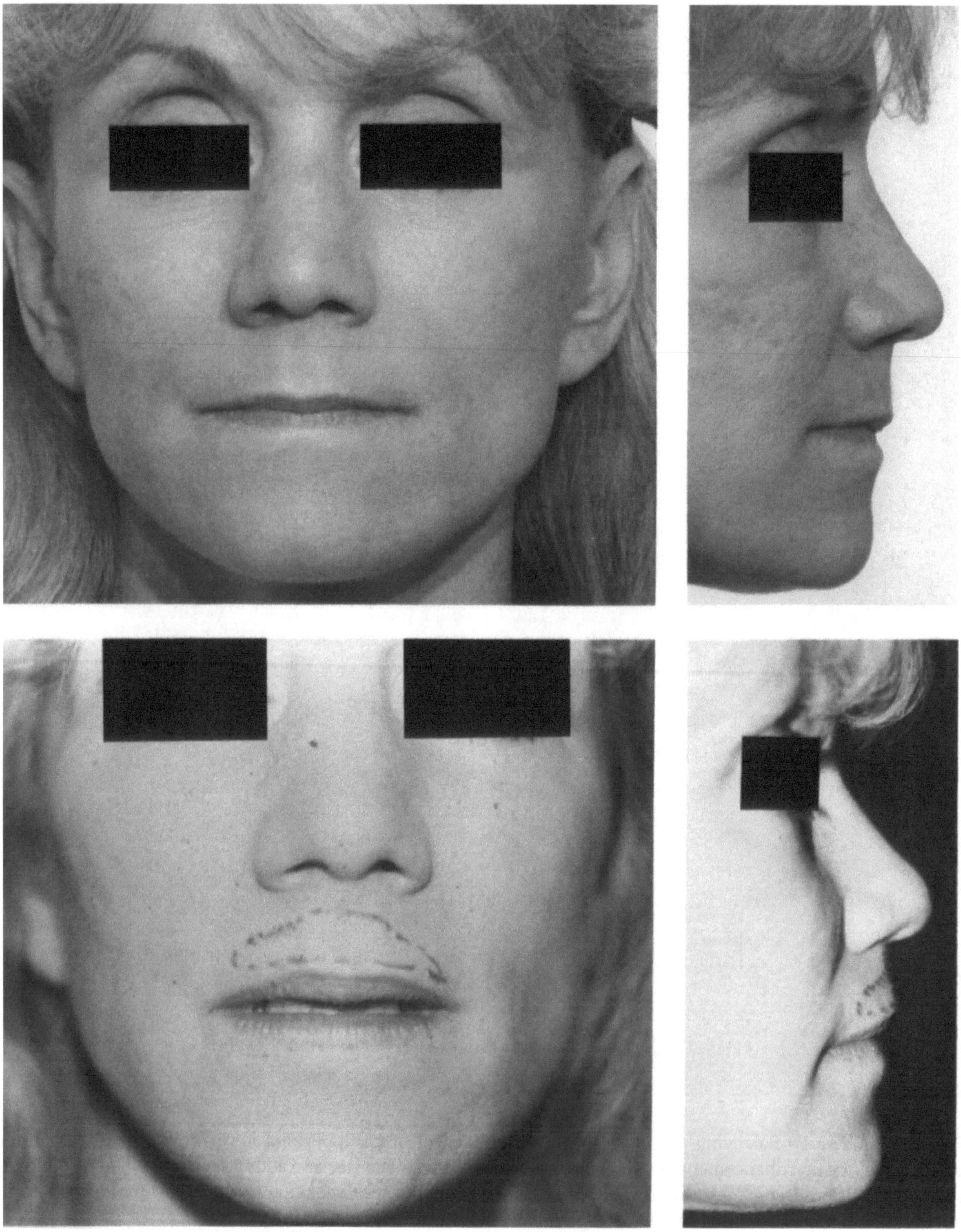

A B C D

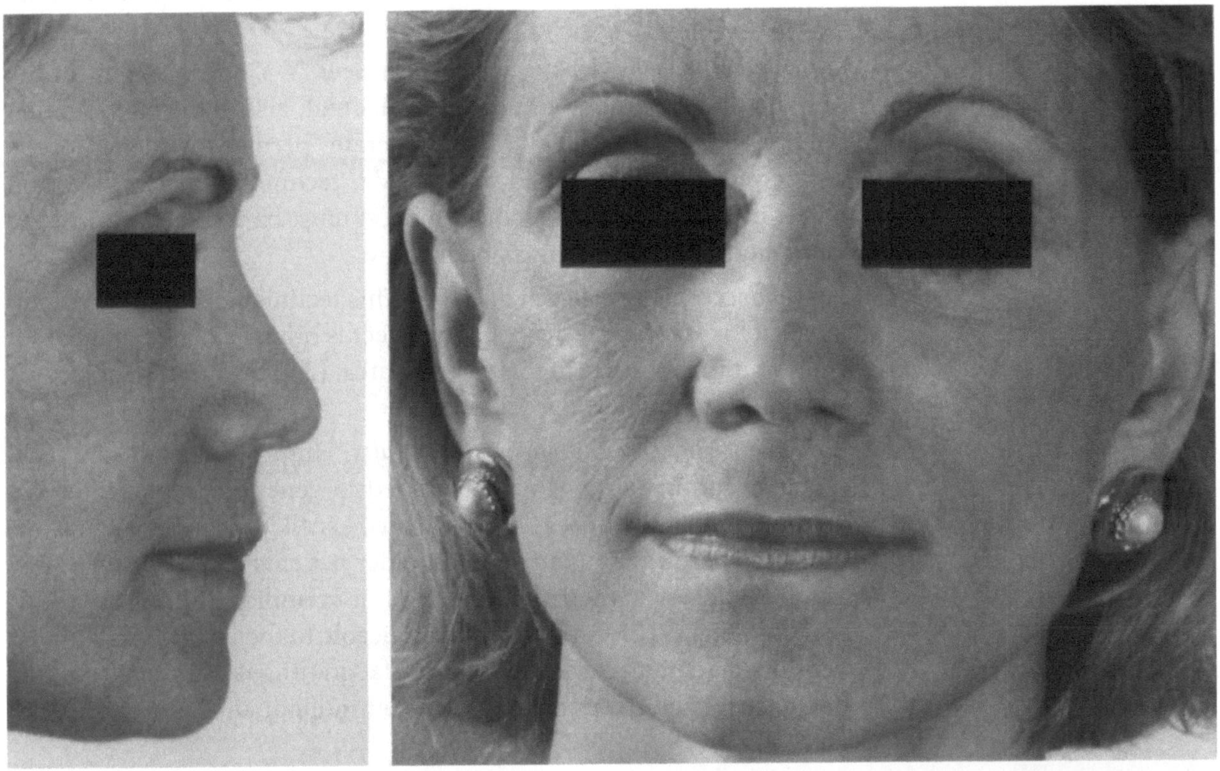

F F

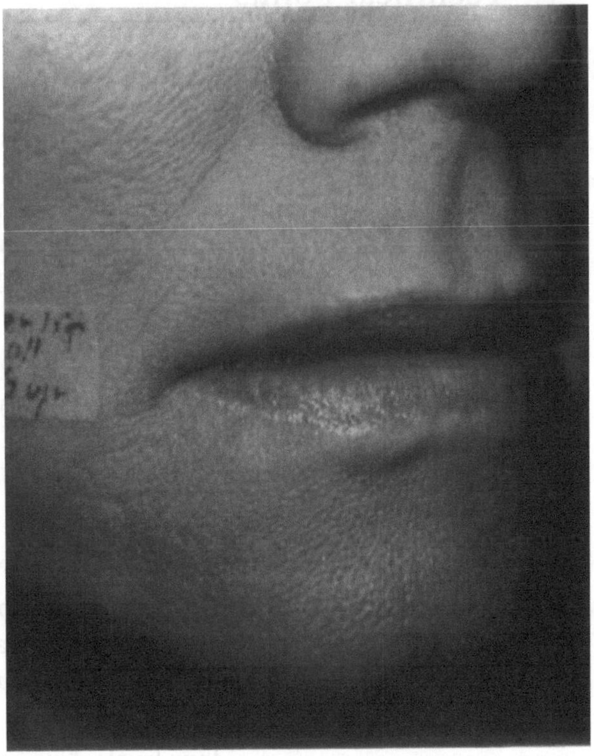

G

Figure 6-2. Complications of minor lip roll. It may have been a tip-off that this patient had a fairly prominent soft tissue development just below the angle of her nose, but I was unprepared for the prolonged swelling after a relatively minor lip roll procedure. **(A&B)** Preoperative state. **(C&D)** Six months postoperatively, she still had too much fullness just below the nostrils, which can be controlled by pressure (a thin tennis headband looped behind the neck and brought across the upper lip for several hours each day) or by a series of dilute triamcinolone (Aristospan) injections. We chose the latter method, and the thickness resolved to a more acceptable fullness than noted in her preoperative photographs. **(E&F)** At 21 months after surgery. **(G)** At 2.5 years she has continued to show the same fullness of the upper and lower lip.

sulcus is repositioned, with division of the orbicularis oris at the nasal spine and laterally.

4. *Lip enhancement by double V-Y enhancement.* V-Y advancement of the wet and dry vermilion, vertical or horizontal, also achieves vermilion fullness (Figs. 6-9 to 6-11). More moderate "permanent edema" of the visible vermilion is obtained with the V-Y technique than with lip roll procedures. A shortened recovery period must be weighed against the more modest fullness that is obtained.
5. *Lip enhancement by collagen injection.* This technique cannot be recommended for several reasons: (1) The effect is brief. (2) The potential for embolization is greater in this vascular area. (3) The question of local or systemic reaction is not yet resolved.
6. *Lip enhancement by autologous fat "grafts."* Improvement in the technique of grafting autologous fat has led to general acceptance of this method for lip fullness. We have obtained excellent enhancement of the crumpled vermilion in our series of older patients followed since 1987 and have achieved moderate increases in vermilion fullness in young patients (Fig. 6-12). Although not applicable to the congenitally underdeveloped lip, multilevel concentrated fat grafting is now the procedure of choice for the atrophic lip of the older individual.

Technical Points

Fat Graft Enhancement

For patients who desire a fuller, "pouty" lip contour and have *adequate vermilion,* fat tunnel grafting is a valuable procedure. If there is insufficient vermilion, one must use the internal mucosal advancement V-Y or lip roll technique, more complicated procedures. Fat grafting is a cost-free addition for older face lift patients. They usually have sufficient vermilion, but their lips are atrophic.

1. Obtain concentrated fat from a convenient source (we prefer the periumbilical area). We use either the inline filter (M.D. Engineering) or a Tulip system.
2. Mark the areas to be corrected. One side may require more than the other (Fig. 6-13). Plan to overcorrect each by 30% to 40%. Remove a small amount of extra fat for the nasolabial groove.
3. Do not use the spatula-type "Rhytid dissector" under the vermilion, although it is a great help in freeing vertical lines above the white roll for grafting and of course in the nasolabial area.
4. With lateral entry points, pass a 1½" 16-gauge disposable needle into four levels, "injecting" fat only during withdrawal (Fig. 6-14). Do not

"inject" using pressure. One level is directly under the vermilion. For more fullness, make another series deeper in subcutaneous tissue. Each tunnel is parallel to the next and is filled with concentrated fat. For the fullest vermilions, add one more level just above the orbicularis oris. If the patient has shown you a photograph of a "mega-lip," favored by some fashion models, lay in a few fat-filled tunnels in the muscle itself (Fig. 6-15).

5. Postoperatively, instruct the patient to apply iced saline compresses. Avoid the pressure of ice packs. Crushing or extruding the fat defeats the purpose of the procedure.
6. After 2 weeks, any areas that are too full or too prominent may be adjusted by fingertip squeezes—the crushed fat then dissipates.

Lip Roll Technique

Lip enhancement means filling the vermilion to create greater puffiness and roundness; it is also used to restore youthful fullness in the older patient. A number of patients have an upper lip that simply did not develop; when this defect is combined with overdevelopment of the lower lip, the appearance is bizarre.

The lip roll technique, often combined with lower lip reduction or fat grafting, solves the problem of facial balance (Fig. 6-16A–E). My 1976 presentation of a series of lip rolls was based on a single European report. Today, this procedure is the one most commonly asked about in my lecture series and requested by patients. With the lip roll one can create a uniform fullness of the entire upper or lower lip, and the incision is hidden in the sulcus (Fig. 6-16F–H). The undermining makes a gradual increase in the bulk of the newly exposed vermilion, which I attribute to a "permanent edema" (Fig. 6-16I–L). The one disadvantage is that the area that is left bare can stay swollen for a longer time than one would like. Most of the edema in the visible area starts to disappear by 10 days. If not, edema persists below the nose. To avoid this problem, the patient can wear a thin tennis headband hooked behind the nape of the neck and across the upper lip or lower lip. The pressure it exerts speeds resolution. Night taping also helps. If swelling is still visible after the third week, plan a few dilute triamcinolone (Aristospan) injections at weekly intervals; this method is always effective.

The area left open on the posterior aspect, just below the sulcus, becomes completely reepithelialized within 3 to 4 weeks. The vermilion that was rotated outward has now become thicker owing to the dependent effect of the undermining and repositioning.

Do not use long-lasting fixation stitches such as Dexon or Vicryl: They remain in place too long. Use 4-0 chromic suture material to anchor the mucosa.

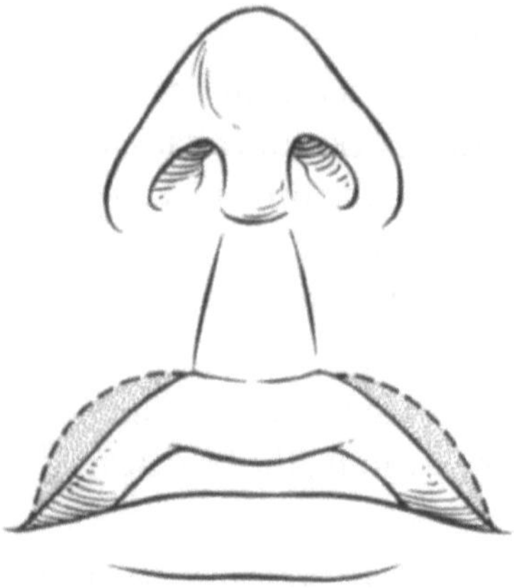

Figure 6-3. Austin lip lift.

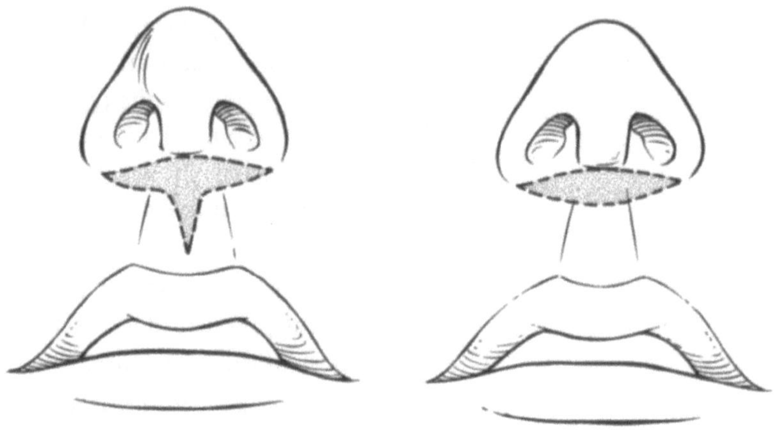

Figure 6-4. Reduction of long upper lip.

Excision Above the White Roll of the Upper Lip

Excision of lateral skin just above the white roll has been reported by Harvey Austen to produce a higher prominence only in that zone.

He places a dot exactly at the commissure and extends the line medially from the dot along the skin–vermilion junction for 12 to 16 mm. Next, he extends the line from that dot toward the top of the ear, stopping just short of the nasolabial crease and creating an angle of about 120 degrees. When this line is connected, the suture incision is extended beyond the normal commissure and the triangle that extends only about one-third of the way toward the nose is outlined. Excising this triangle with a curved incision that goes just above the white roll and slightly laterally lifts the edge of the lip. If one considers this technique as only a "corner lift," one would expect fewer complications than with an excision across the entire length.

Lip Reduction

We have discussed the various techniques of lip enhancement but have only briefly reviewed the time-proved techniques for lip reduction. It is primarily a lower lip procedure in Caucasians and an upper and lower lip procedure in African Americans and Latinos (Fig. 6-17). The patient's desire to fit the norm is the most important factor when planning the operation. Steve Hoefflin asks his patients to bring in photographs from magazines, a good idea for both enhancement and reduction patients. A quick look through *Vogue* or *Cosmopolitan* reveals the large variation in the "acceptable" size of the upper or lower lip. It is valuable to put together a reference book for your office that shows all of the characteristics desirable in faces and lips. Our patients are more comfortable discussing a model's appearance than they are their own.

First ask the patient to judge the amount of lip that should be reduced. One-half? One-third? Have them physically hold the lip in its new position with an underfolding to give you a good idea of how much to remove and how much to leave. The surgical excision is on the posterior inner aspect of the mucosa. It is rarely necessary to remove muscle to achieve the desired reduction. Make a wavy line rather than a straight one (Fig. 6-17C). Some surgeons advocate placing an occasional Z-plasty or W-plasty in the center, but it is not necessary. The length and width of the incision depends on how much reduction is desired. For some people it is only the central half of the upper lip or central two-thirds of the lower lip that requires reduction. For others, the reduction extends from commissure to commissure. Technical point: After excising mucosa, use a tacking suture that will dissolve in a reasonable length of time. It is a difficult task to go back later to remove a buried Vicryl knot. 4-0 Chromic sutures are a good choice. We routinely follow the procedure with compression, ice packs, and head elevation. Steve Hoefflin prefers intravenous dexamethasone (Decadron) and diphenhydramine HCl (Benadryl) 50 mg IV to reduce swelling. We have been satisfied with methylprednisolone (Medrol Dosepak) and local measures.

Collagen Injections

My main objection to the collagen-enhanced "Paris lips" is that they are painful and transient, and they give an artificial appearance. The only good thing you can say about the technique is that the collagen eventually disappears.

Bioplastique was introduced by Robert Ersek. He has reported good results as well as real problems. In theory, the tiny clusters of solid silicone that are implanted are just large enough not to migrate and small enough to be injected easily through a tiny needle. The body surrounds them with scar fibers, which creates a firmer enhancement than one could obtain with fat grafts or with normal edema. As Ersek would be the first to admit, there are difficulties associated with using this material. He claims, however, that he has made all the mistakes for us. Bioplastique is in use in Europe today but probably will not be approved in our lifetimes in the United States because of problems with the liquid silicone injectables. In both cases, one cannot remove the material once implanted. The FDA now prohibits liquid silicone usage.

A number of unscrupulous surgeons are still using silicone injections in lips and at various other sites with disastrous results. I have seen patients with such injections in the lip as well as the cheeks. The news media provide us with graphic reports of silicone migration into the orbit and other undesirable places accompanied by subsequent fibrosis and distortion. By contrast, fat grafts generally stay in place. If the fat has not moved to a new position by 2 weeks, it is highly unlikely that it would move from the implantation site. The other advantage (discussed in Chapter 2) is that fat grafts can be purposefully crushed during the first 10 days. The body then simply removes the liberated oil, resulting in the original or a reduced fullness.

The Collagen Corporation has down-scaled their claims dramatically. They now describe the Paris lip as being created by collagen injections into fine rhytids and the white roll, not the vermilion. (The U.S. Food and Drug Administration had ordered them to stop advocating injections into the vermilion itself).

I worried also about the tendency of collagen to travel through the bloodstream. Cases of blindness following glabellar injection have been reported, indicating that the collagen material had moved directly through the tiny needle used for the injection into a blood vessel and then lodged in the retina. Bioplastique could easily follow the same route, no matter how careful the operator. It is therefore incumbent upon us to stay with the safe, tried and true methods of lip enhancement.

Bob Harvey (San Francisco) gave a completely negative report on the use of collagen injections for lip enhancement. More than 50% of the collagen they injected into willing individuals' lips had dissipated within 4 weeks, and the rest of the patients who were followed for more than 4 weeks eventually reverted to their original condition.

Lip Lengthening

We have developed a series of maneuvers designed to lengthen the upper lip and permanently reattach it at a lower gingival level so the lip covers the upper portion of the incisor teeth. This method differs from previously reported transoral approaches in that the incision is not opened to the contaminated oral cavity, and complete release of the orbicularis muscle of the mouth is obtained transnasally.

The patient is prepared for surgery with oral, intramuscular, and intravenous sedation. When a satisfactory level of analgesia has been obtained, the infraorbital nerves are blocked.

If the base of the nose is flared, lip lengthening is carried out through a Weir-type incision, which curves around the alar rim. A wedge of tissue is then removed from the nostril floor. If the nose is not flared, a unilateral incision is made at the mucocutaneous junction by the columellar base. A bilateral subcutaneous tunnel is created, paralleling the curve of the upper lip; it extends from the nasal spine (which is freed or resected, if necessary) to within 0.5 cm of the commissure. A parallel tunnel is made above the maxillary periosteum. Blunt-tipped scissors are then introduced, one blade in each tunnel, and the orbicular muscle of the mouth is divided atraumatically (Fig. 6-18). In the nasal

(Text continued on page 138)

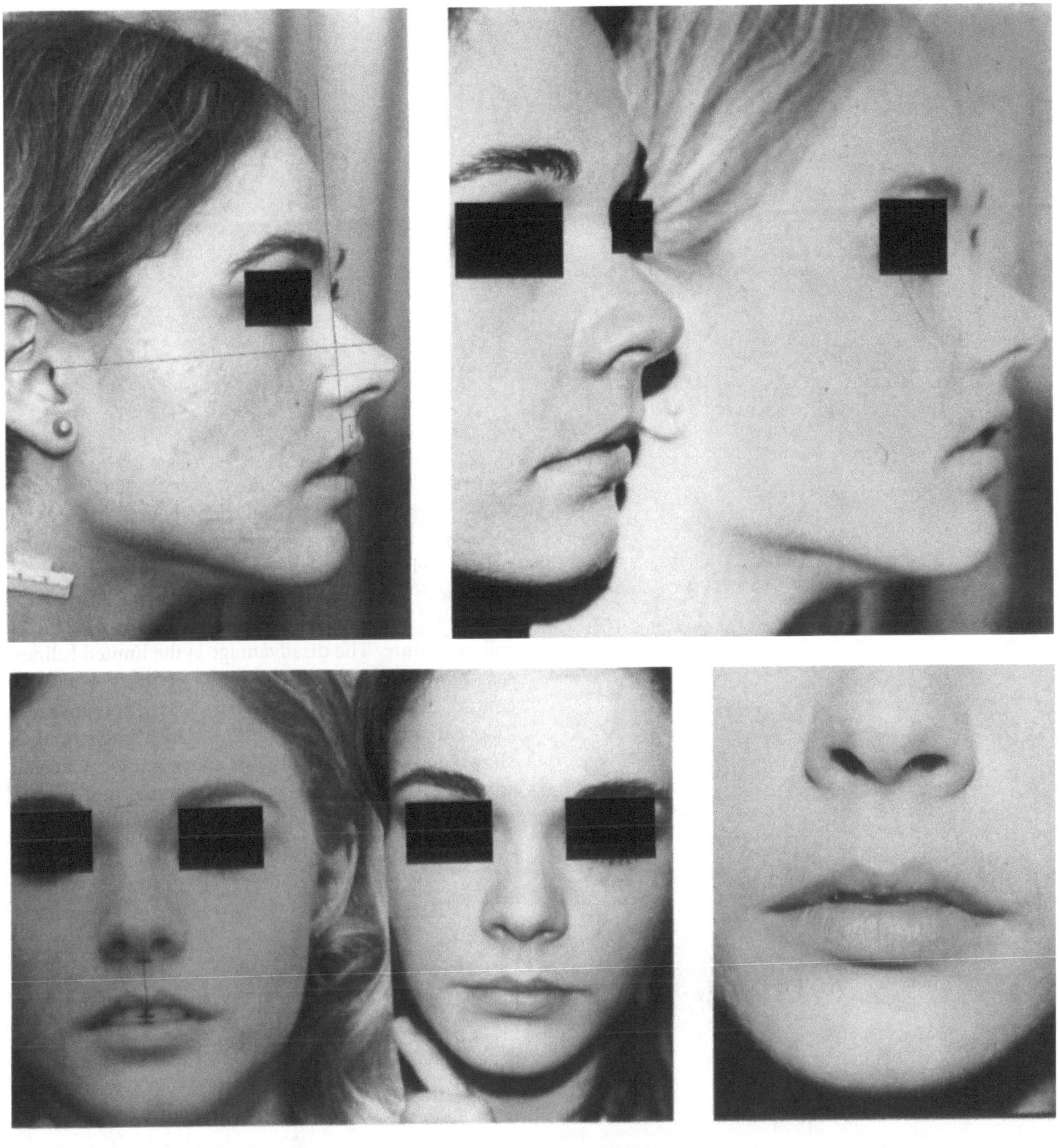

A B C D

Figure 6-5. Lip lengthening. Simply freeing the attachments of the upper lip to the nasal spine does not achieve the degree of lengthening that has been obtained in this patient. **(A)** Note in the preoperative photograph that the gum in the normal resting position, but it is obscured postoperatively. The lip is taped in an exaggerated lengthened position after freeing of the tissues and unfurling of the mucosa from the upper labial sulcus. Using an intranasal approach, the muscle is divided as well. **(B–D)** Patient's appearance 12 years later. The lip position is still excellent. At this point, we would offer her the option of a lip roll to further enhance the fullness of the upper lip itself. Interestingly, several of our long-term lip-lengthening patients have retained this fullness of the upper lip, presumably due to permanent edema from the surgery performed years before.

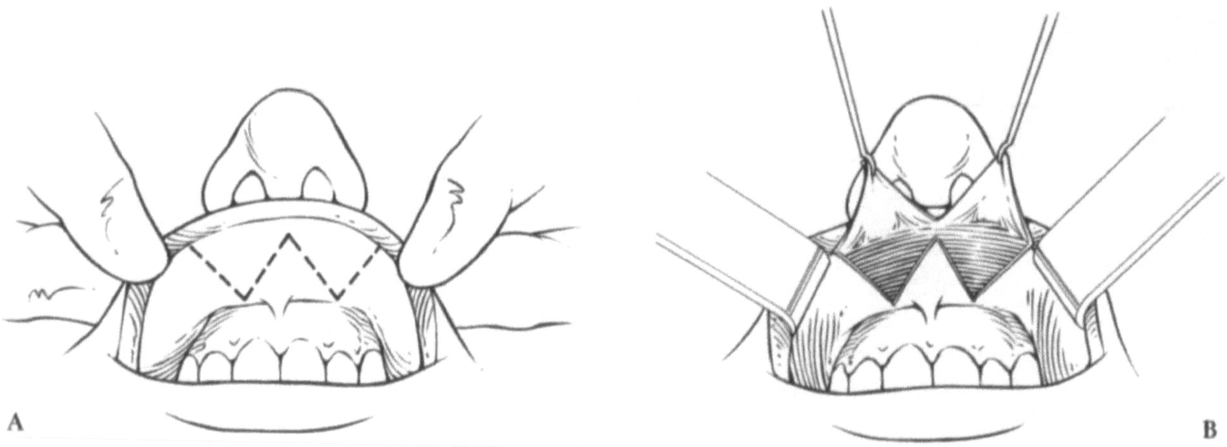

A

B

C

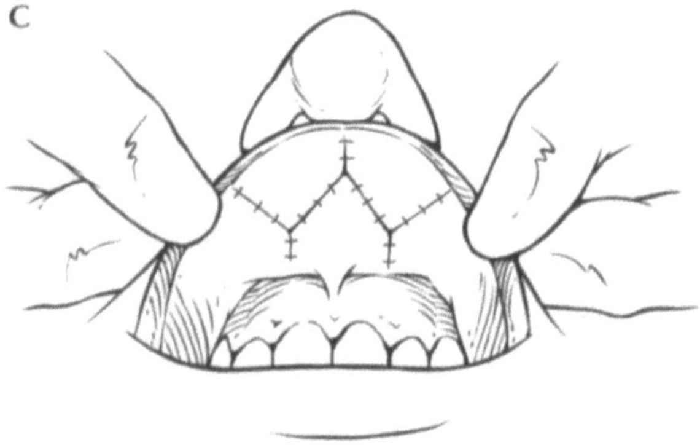

Figure 6-6. Lip enhancement by the Aiache double V-Y procedure provides excellent lateral and central fullness and is the procedure of choice for young patients who do not have severe lack of development. The major advantage is that there is not an exposed muscle zone that must be reepithelialized as with the lip roll procedure. The disadvantage is the limited fullness that may be obtained. The limbs of the V-Y may be central, as shown, or extended toward the commissures. Take care not to injure the V tips. Use a single hook as shown and dissent sharply just above muscle. Chromic sutures ensure the repositioning, converting each V to a Y.

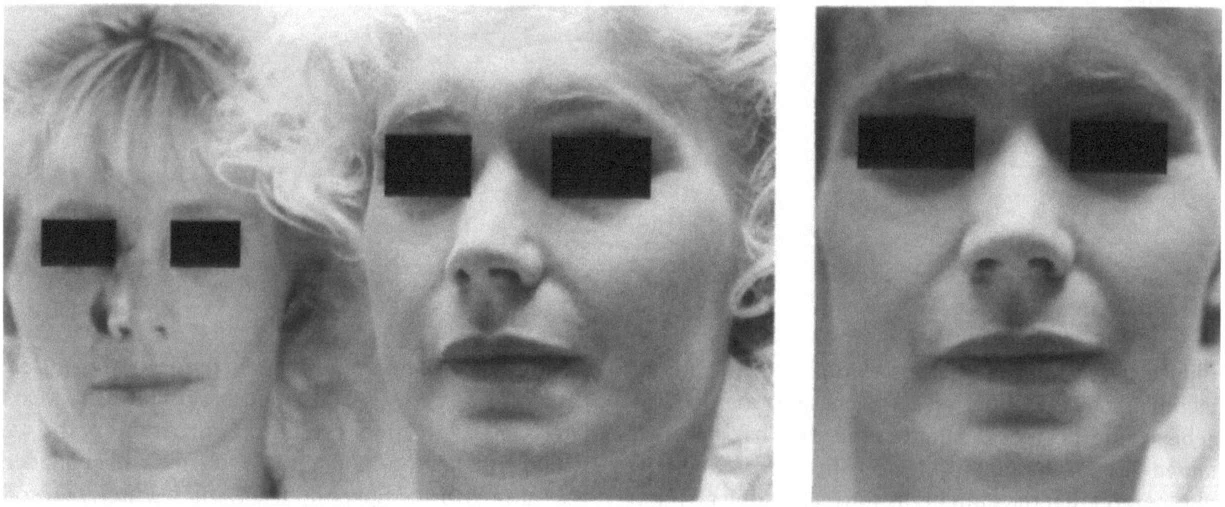

Figure 6-7. Lip enhancement by double V-Y. In many patients the thin upper lip requires enhancement only in the central zone, and the relatively full lower lip can be filled with fat grafts alone. In this patient, fat grafting was also used to build up the mandibular angle area. She thought that recent dental surgery had caused the

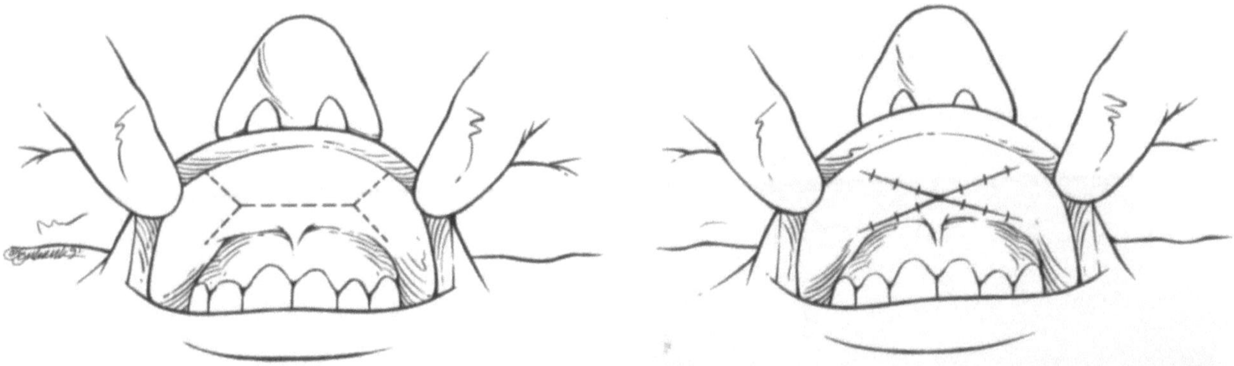

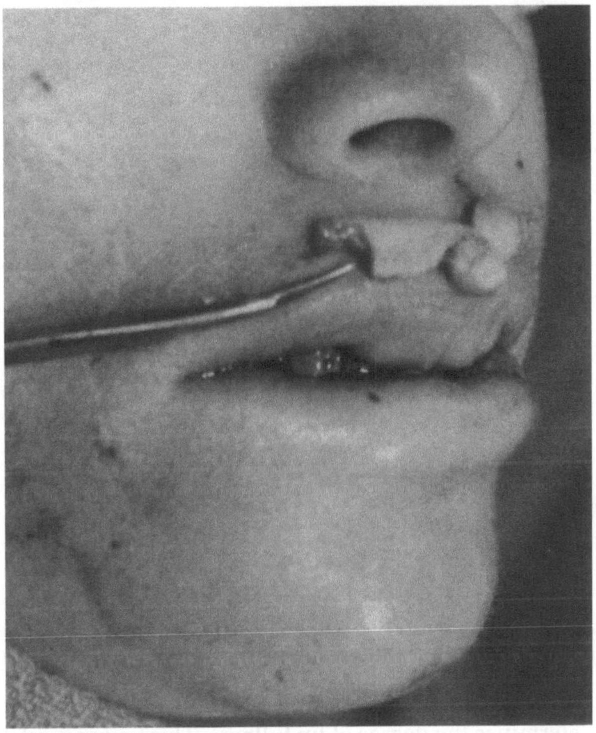

Figure 6-8. **(A&B)** The Lassus V-Y technique entails a horizontal rather than a vertical incision and may be used to create modest mid-lip fullness. Claude Lassus reported a series of patients in whom this horizontal V-Y was employed alone or with a buried graft of dermis. I prefer to use tissue other than dermis, which often absorbs completely or may give rise to dermal cysts. It is simpler and more effective to add fat grafting at the same time as a lip roll or V-Y enhancement. For unusual problems, such as a cleft lip enhancement, one often has exposed the mastoid fascia, facial subcutaneous musculoaponeurotic system (SMAS), or temporalis fascia during the combined procedures of facial repair. Rather than harvest fat, I use fascia for added fullness. Suturing the fascia **(C)** creates the shape required for augmentation of specific areas of the lip.

infolding and atrophy of the soft tissue, which is evident in the preoperative photograph that she is holding. The nasolabial areas were filled as well and have maintained this fullness. With the double V-Y procedure, there is less likelihood of edema below the nostrils from the healing advancement site, but a lesser degree of fullness is obtained.

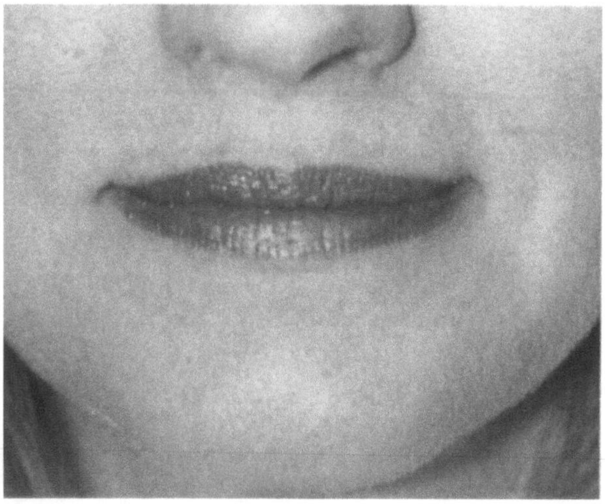

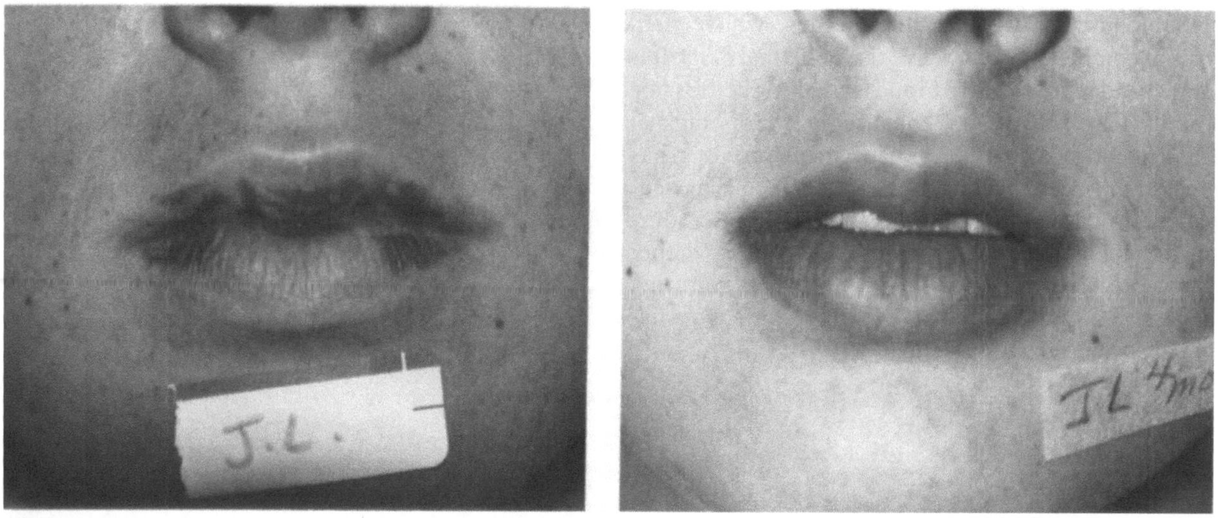

Figure 6-10. Degree of lip enhancement. The patient determines the degree of lip fullness. This young model wished only a small amount of lateral fullness and a buildup in the center of the lower lip. In addition, she requested a slight increase in the fullness of the upper lip, the areas marked preoperatively (**A**). In these cases, only a small amount of fat is placed in each of the tunnels, and the tunnels are limited to those areas to be increased. Had this patient desired a much fuller lip, I would have recommended a lip roll or a more aggressive fat grafting program to fit with her plans for a photography engagement, which was carried out successfully 3 weeks after the lip fat grafting. She has maintained the correction shown in her 4-month photograph (**B**) for more than 12 months now.

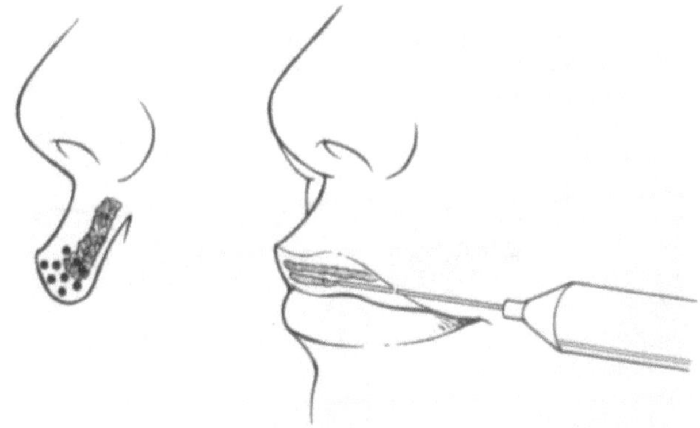

Figure 6-11. Fat graft enhancement.

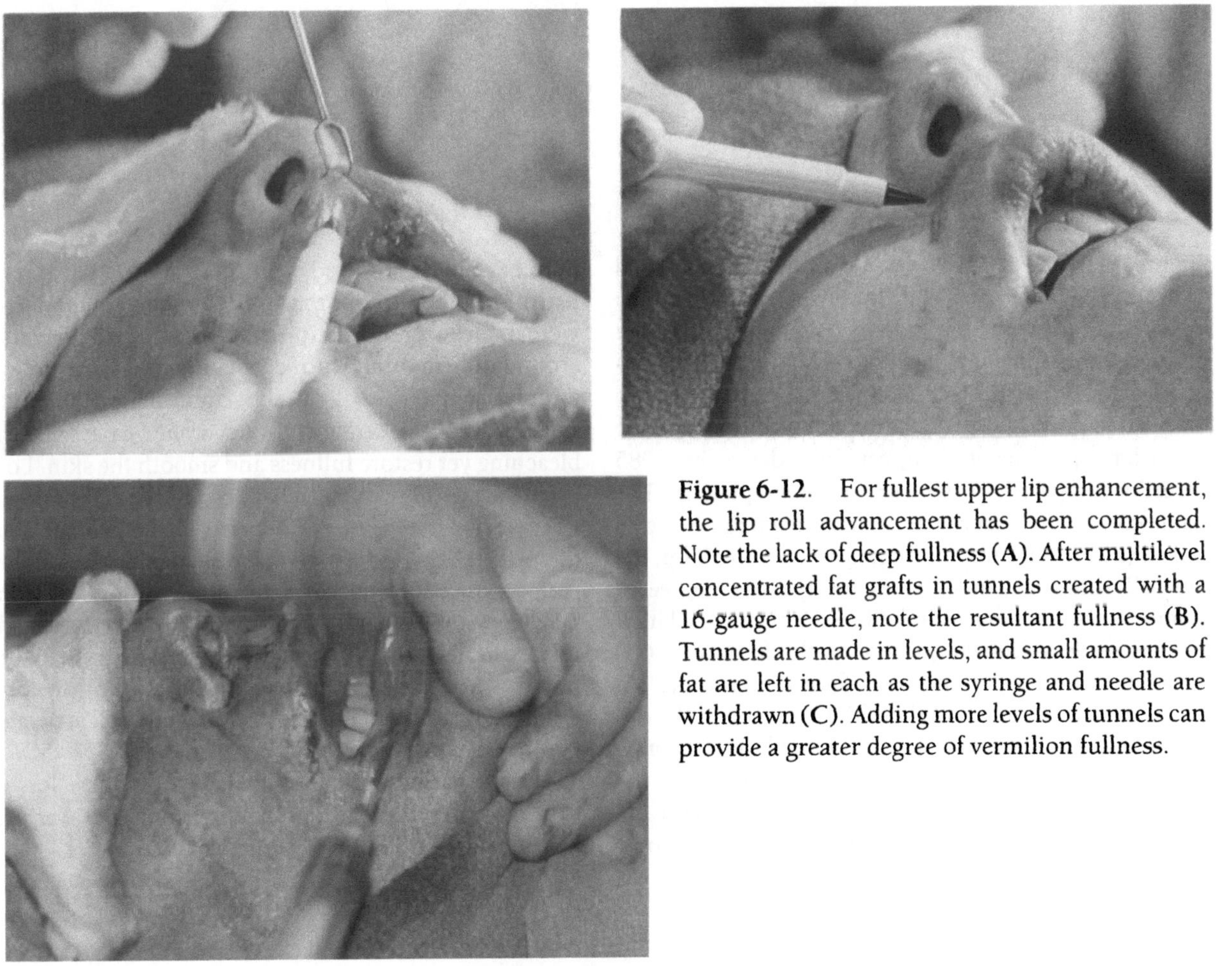

A B C

Figure 6-12. For fullest upper lip enhancement, the lip roll advancement has been completed. Note the lack of deep fullness (**A**). After multilevel concentrated fat grafts in tunnels created with a 16-gauge needle, note the resultant fullness (**B**). Tunnels are made in levels, and small amounts of fat are left in each as the syringe and needle are withdrawn (**C**). Adding more levels of tunnels can provide a greater degree of vermilion fullness.

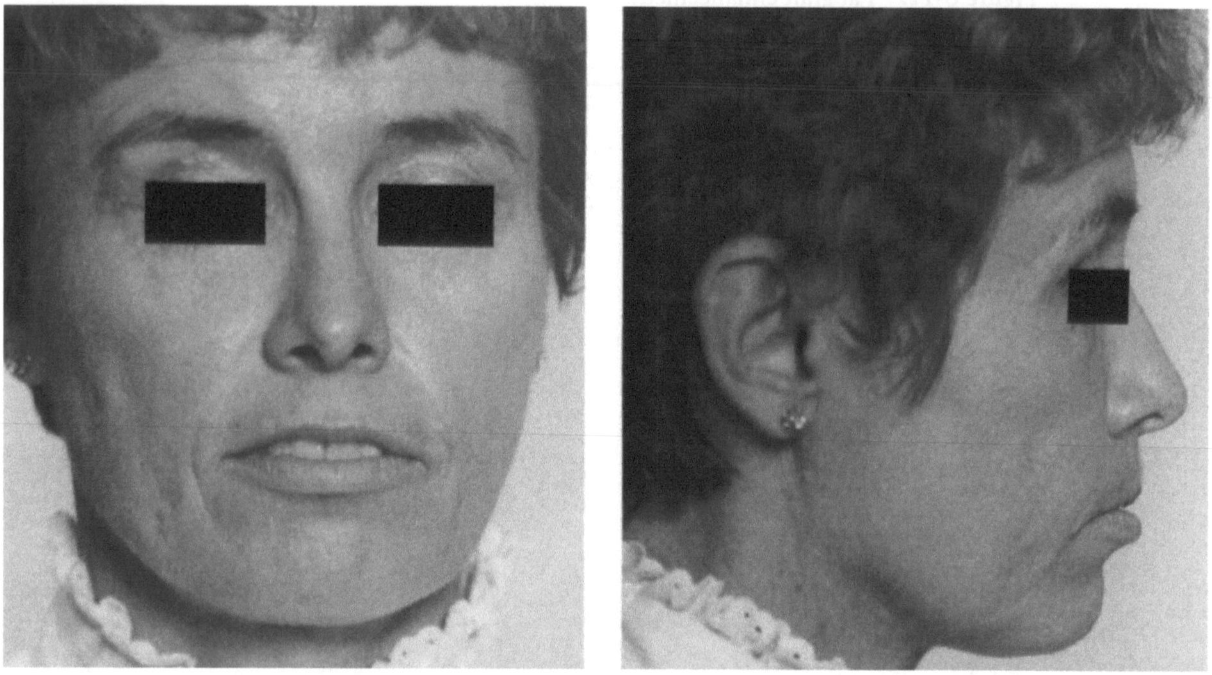

A

B

Figure 6-13. For this facial type, an upper lip roll procedure is combined with lower lip reduction. The occurrence of upper lip underdevelopment and lower lip over-development is not unusual. **(A&B)** After upper lid and lower lid blepharoplasty. The patient then decided to proceed with lip correction (1985). Note the persistent postoperative upper lip edema in 1985 **(C&D)** compared to the 1986 photograph **(E)**. The same correction balance has been maintained now for 8 years. **(F)** For the atrophic or congenitally small lip, the lip roll enhancement provides the greatest degree of commissure-to-commissure fullness. The mucosal incision is made as shown, preserving the frenulum. **(G)** Dissection just above the orbicularis oris muscle extends from the incision to the white roll beyond the dry vermilion. The mucosa is then positioned. **(H)** Chromic sutures secure the advanced mucosa. Much of the subsequent edema of the dry and wet vermilion becomes permanent fullness. Patients having this procedure have been followed since 1976. **(I–M)** Lip roll as part of a combined approach. A common complaint of women over age 30 is premature aging in the area around the mouth, with deepening lines, vermilion atrophy, and vertical lines above and below the white roll. As with the senile lip, one wishes to avoid skin bleaching yet restore fullness and smooth the skin. Low eyebrow position, eyelid changes, and the prominent chin **(I&J)** were primary concerns of this woman, but the perioral changes **(K–M)** complemented the rejuvenation. Procedures performed were as follows: (1) upper and lower lid blepharoplasty; (2) coronal (forehead) lift; (3) transoral chin reduction (bone and soft tissue removal); (4) fat grafts to vertical lines, root of nose, forehead lines, nasolabial lines, and white roll area; and (5) light chemical peel of the oral triangle (35% TCA). The rejuvenation was accomplished without the loss of skin coloration, and the upper lip vermilion was enhanced with a lip roll procedure.

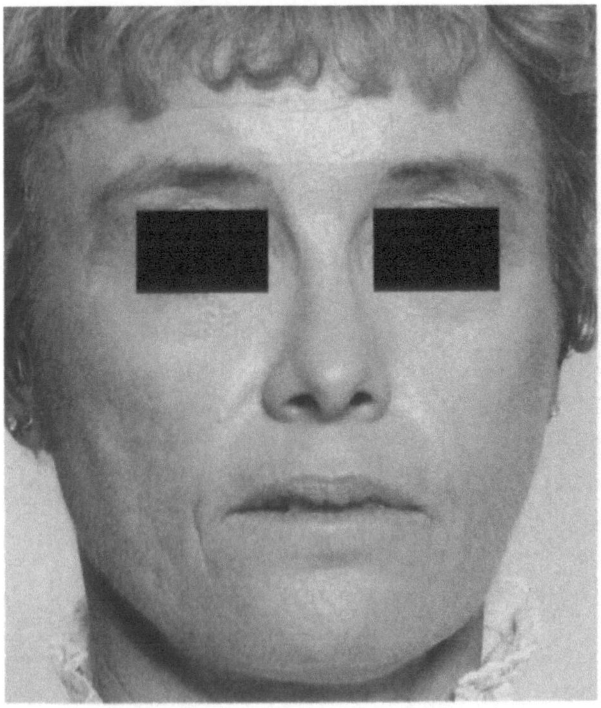

C

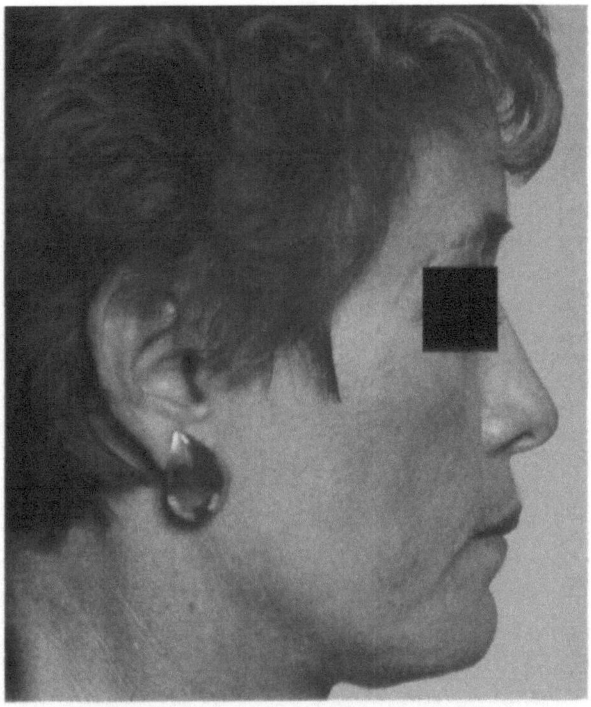

D

E

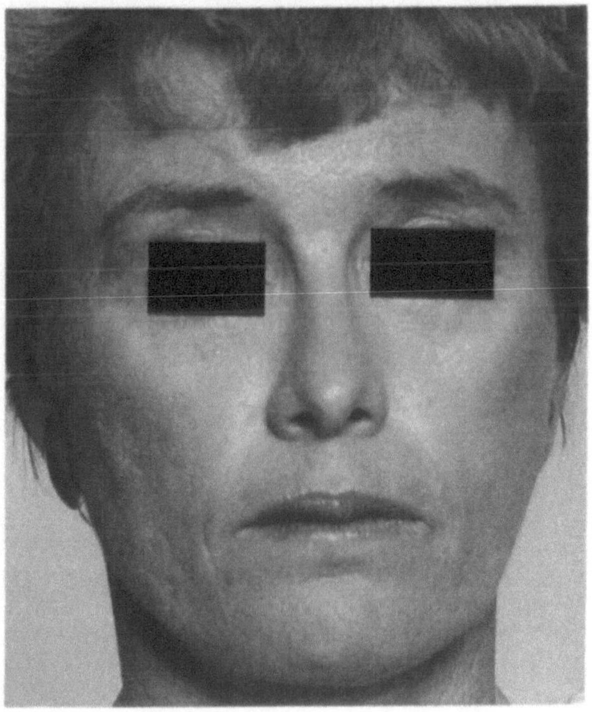

F

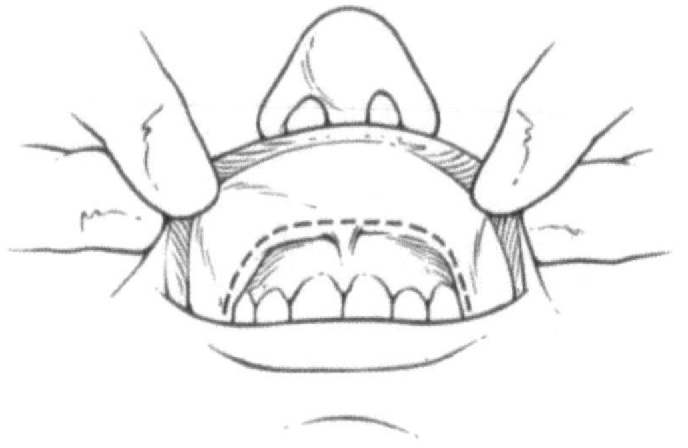

G

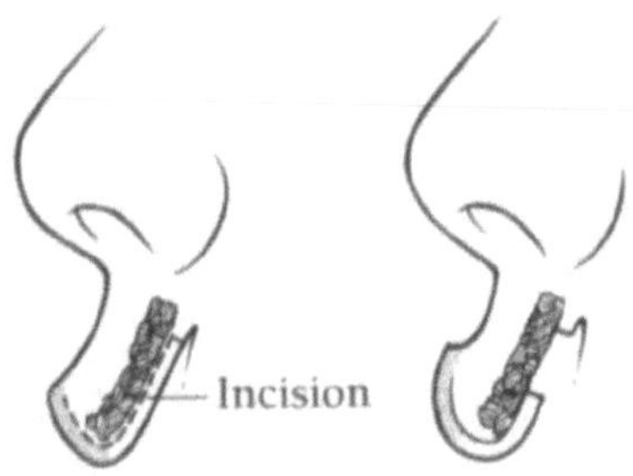

H

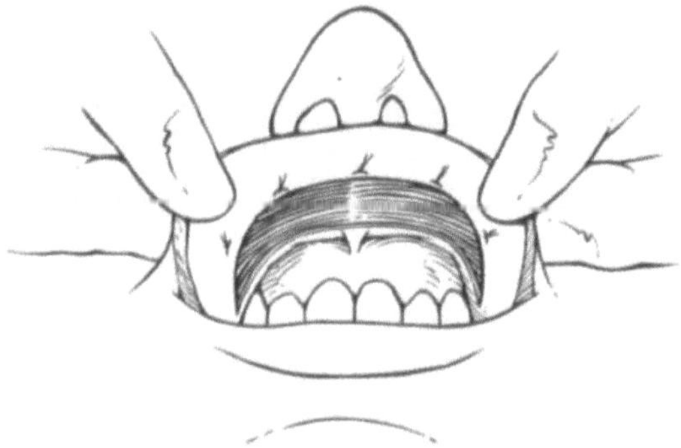

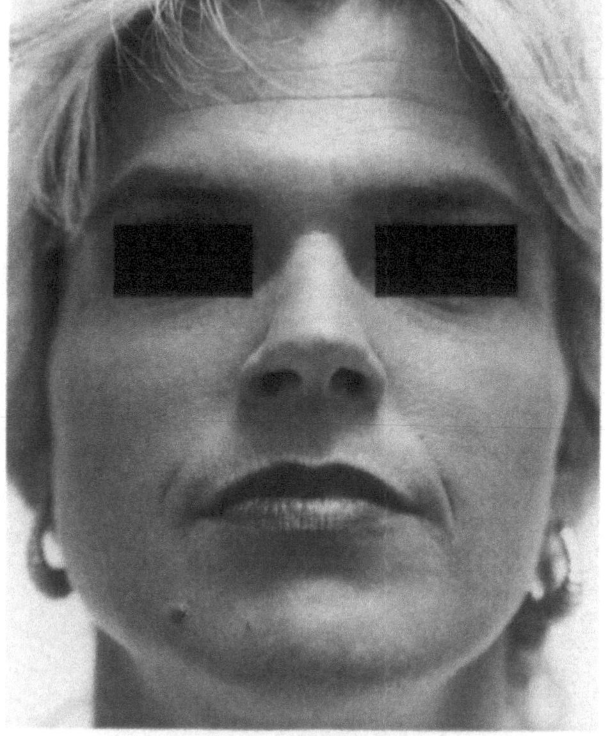

I

J

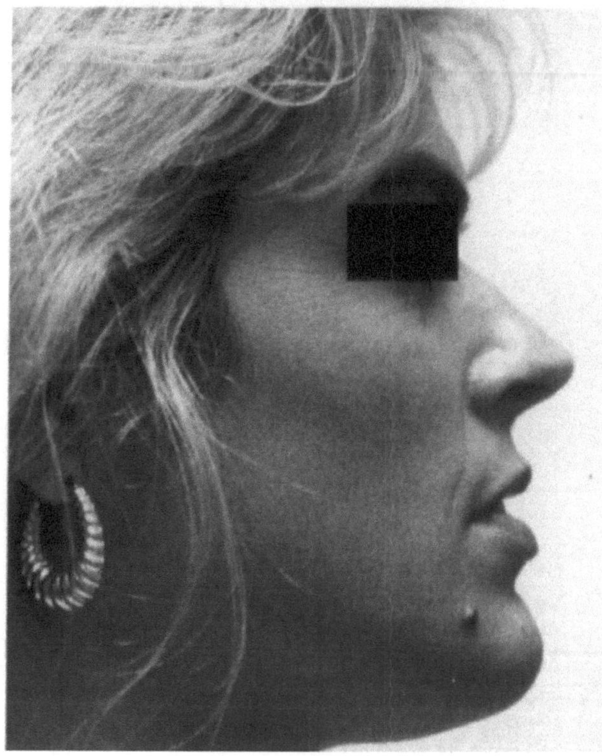

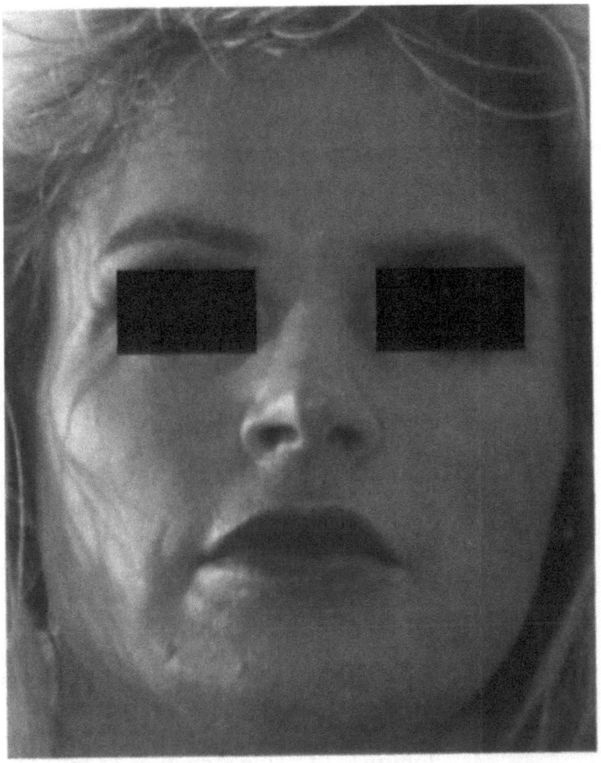

K

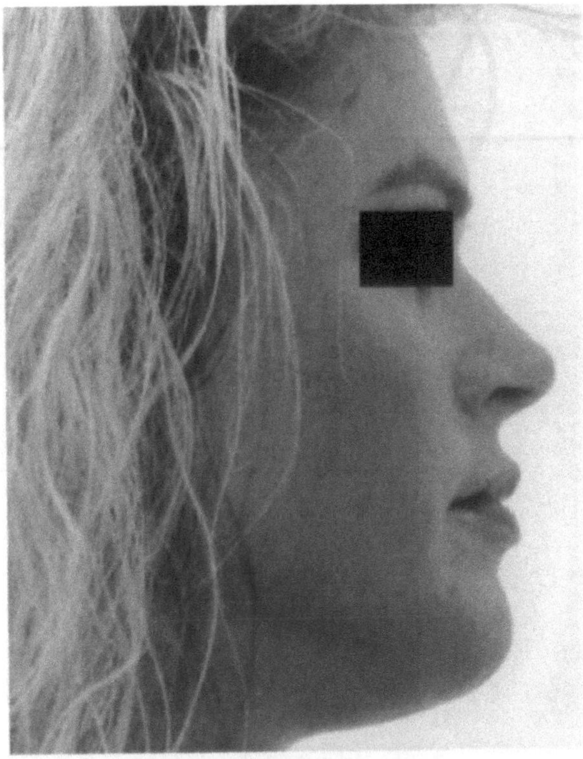

L

M

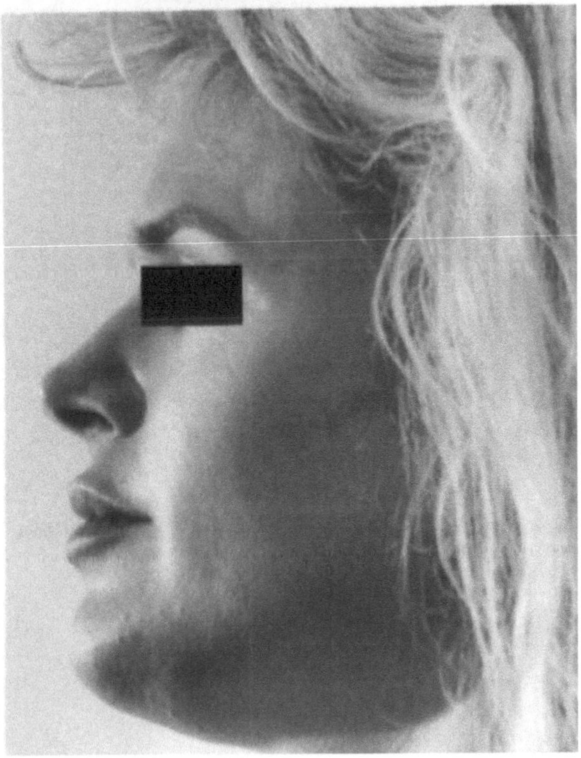

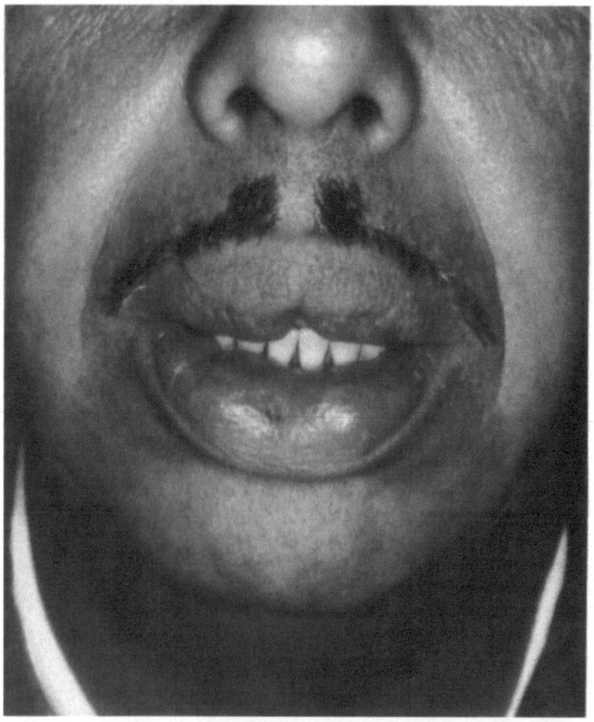

A

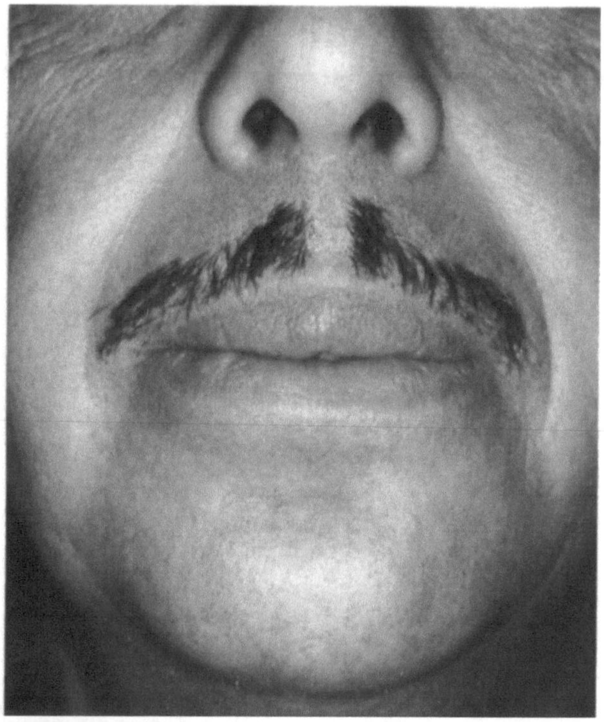

B

C

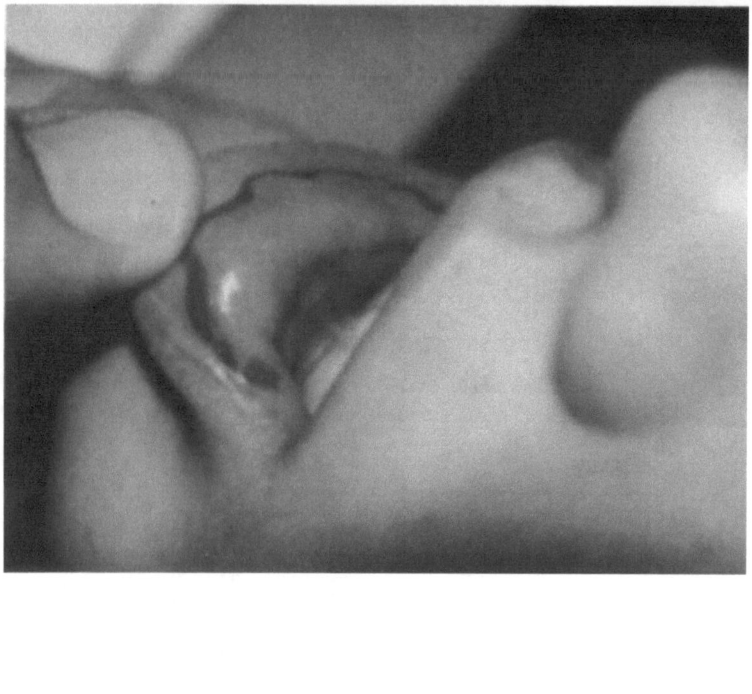

Figure 6-14. Lip reduction. **(A&B)** The first type of lip reduction is for simple hypertrophy. It is important to determine preoperatively exactly how much reduction is desired and what type of balancing should be obtained. In this patient the upper lip was left relatively full and the lower lip reduced to a greater degree. (The feminine lip is often the opposite with a greater degree of fullness in the lower lip.) **(C)** The "double lip" is a ridge of tissue that develops on the inner surface. When the lip is everted, as shown, there appear to be two major vermilion prominences. Simple excision and closure are in order.

Figure 6-15. Lip lengthening. When one wishes to make the lip hang at a lower position, it is necessary to separate the fibrous attachments between the orbicularis oris and the base of the nose. It can be easily accomplished through an intranasal incision. The idea is to separate the muscle and reflect the gingival mucosa down to the teeth. This raw area then seals when the lip is taped in its new lower position and prevents the lip from riding upward. Always overcorrect with the taping so there is a maximum amount of contact with the subdermal tissue of the lip and the bare periosteum of the upper maxilla.

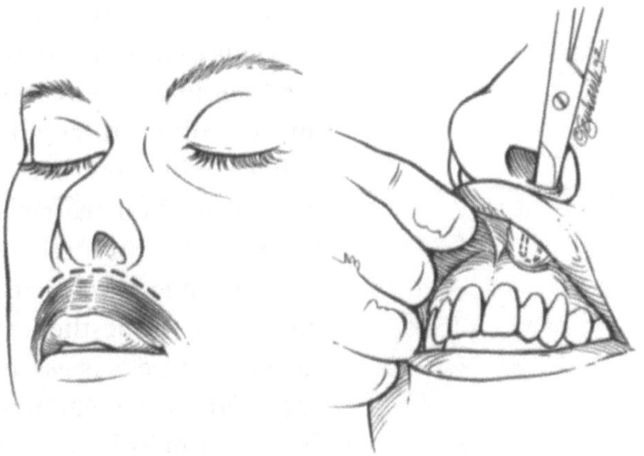

A

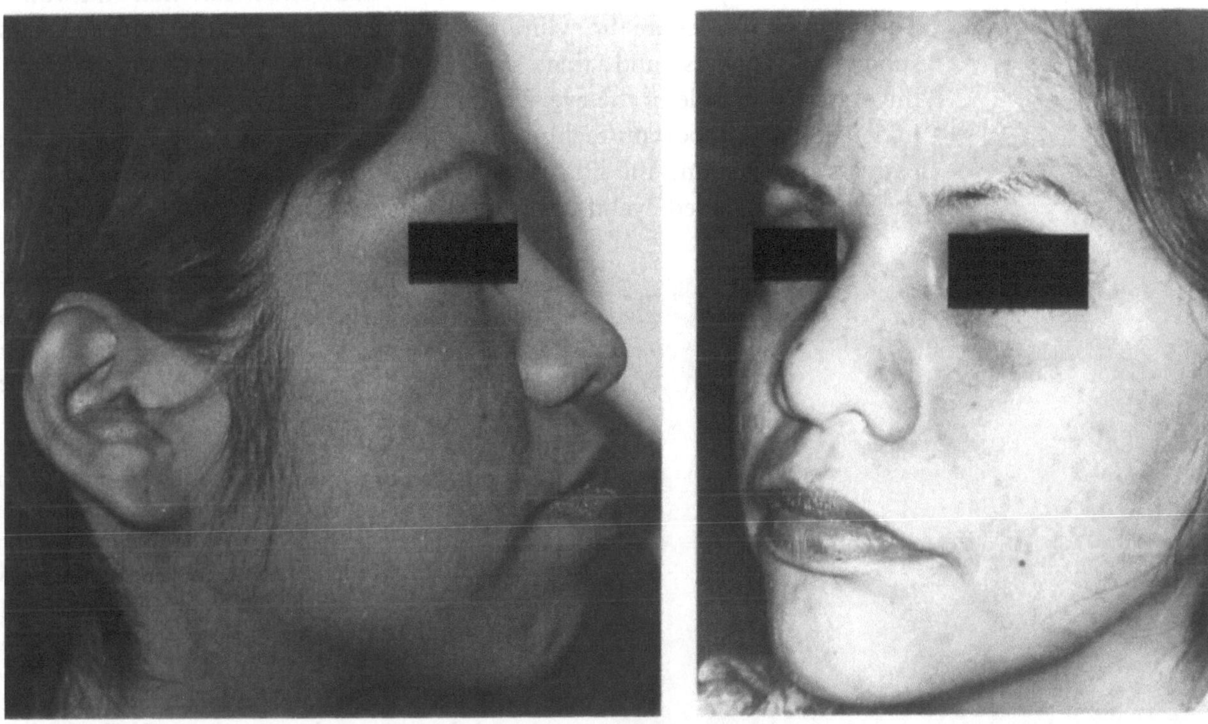

B

Figure 6-16. This patient is typical of the short upper lip/hooded eyelid group. She is shown before **(A)** and after **(B)** lip lengthening, chin augmentation, and blepharoplasty. Over the ensuing years, the upper lip has not only maintained its length, but there has been an increase in vermilion fullness.

spine area, a periosteal elevator or the same blunt scissors are introduced to reflect the entire width of the oral mucosa from the gingiva to below the level of the frenulum. After completion of the facial incision, the upper lip is taped into an overcorrected lengthened position so the raw undersurface of the lip is in contact with now bare upper gingiva. In effect, the upper sulcus has been repositioned for reattachment 1 cm or more downward. Eliminating the open "fish-mouth" or "rabbit-mouth" appearance by upper lip lengthening via repositioning the sulcus and division of the orbicular muscle of the mouth completes the aesthetic restructuring. Maintaining overcorrection with elastic tape for 2 weeks is essential in these patients. Fixation continues separation of the divided orbicular muscle and allows an adhesion to form that keeps the upper lip sulcus in its new lower position.

The syndrome of short upper lip and heavy-lidded eyes or hooded upper eyelids was the subject of a 1980 paper of mine (*Aesthetic Plastic Surgery* 4:73, 1980). The heavy eyelid occurs commonly in Latin American men and women. The major anomalies are the cylindrical role of orbital fat, rather than the classic subdivided "pockets," and a thick fatty areolar tissue layer on the undersurface of the orbicular muscle of the eye. There may be total absence of a developed lip fold. The most important technical maneuver during blepharoplasty for these patients is deepening the lid fold by a modified supratarsal fixation. In most patients with hooded eyelids, removal of a strip of redundant upper orbicular

A

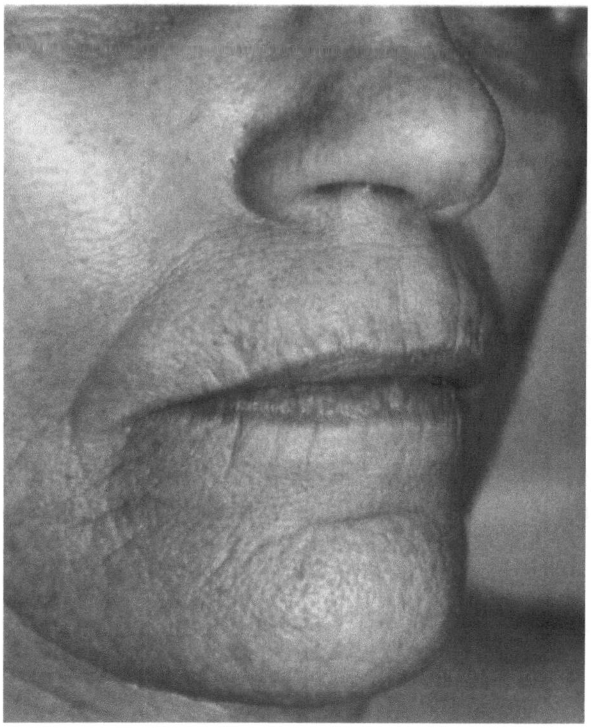

Figure 6-17. The goal of correcting the wrinkling and discoloration of the upper lip is to achieve a reasonable degree of smoothness without whitening. Undermining the central vertical rhytids and placing fat grafts underneath them is a major component of the procedure **(A&B)**. First, each line is outlined prior to injection of local anesthesia under the ketamine/diazepam (Valium) "window of painlessness." **(C)** Note that provision has been made to fill the marionette zone below the commissures. During the face lift procedure, a scalpel is used to lightly abrade the rough areas along each rhytid and along the lip edge. **(B)** It leaves these results, and we are now preparing to apply 35% TCA. Note the fullness of the lips from the fat grafting and the improvement that is evident at this point in the procedure. **(D)** The final step is application of TCA to the entire triangle and then Baker formula phenol, using the latter only along the white roll line, where the deepest rhytids were seen in the preoperative photograph. Final touch-ups with 35% TCA may be required after 6 weeks, as some of the deeper rhytids do not respond as completely as others. These patients maintain lip color, and the fullness is restored.

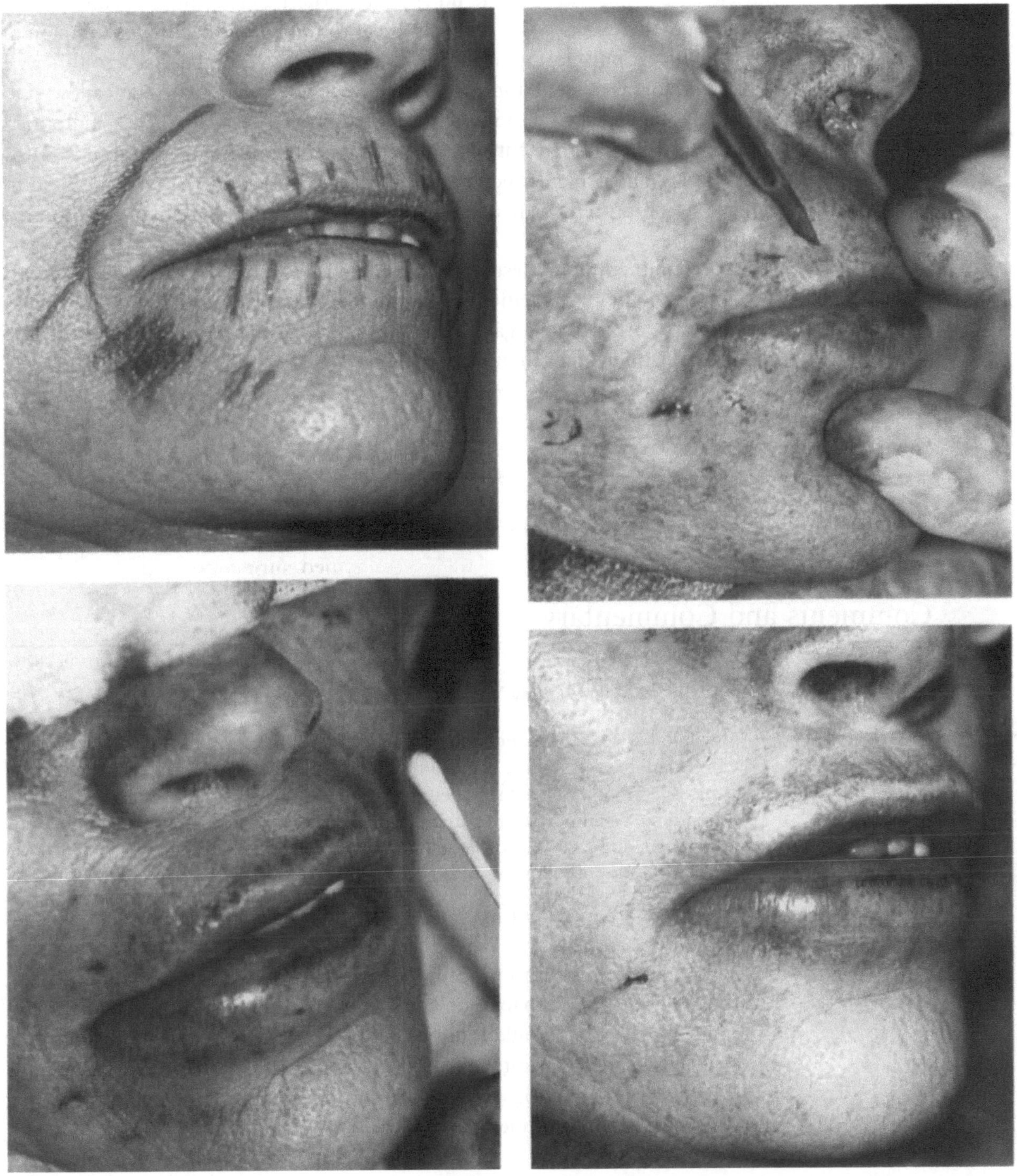

B D C E

muscle across the width of the lid is as important as the suture fixation. This excision completely exposes the cylindrical roll of fat and facilitates eversion of the orbicularis muscle for trimming thickened fatty areolar tissues. If a well defined lid fold is present, the edges of the resected orbicular strip are allowed to fall freely into place without suture fixation. Otherwise, I use simplified supratarsal fixation that consists in percutaneously joining the skin, levator aponeurosis, and orbicular edge. This technique is usually all that is required to achieve a sculptured, well defined upper lid in most patients with hooded eyelids.

Lip lengthening in these patients is then performed by internal repositioning. Interestingly, in the patient in Figure 6-19, late thickening of the upper lip vermilion occurred, which gave a pleasing fullness not present originally. These changes are still evident in our original patients at 10 and 12 years.

Senile Lip

See Figure 6-17 for discussion of the senile lip.

Comments and Commentary

1. James Norris (New York) on lip reduction:

> I would like to caution individuals who perform lip reductions that it is extremely important to consider the occlusion of their patients. An overzealously performed lip reduction may leave the patient with failure of lip seal. This can be a disastrous situation. It is important in patients with bimaxillary protrusion that orthodontic treatment and possible orthognathic surgery be first completed, then the lip reduction should follow.

2. There are excellent methods for thickening the lower lip that leave no evidence of the procedure. Why, then, do colleagues insist on excising skin above the lip? Claims that a procedure leaves "insignificant scars" do not stand up to close scrutiny. Perhaps one could make a case for such excisions in an extremely long lip, but would it not be better to excise the extra tissue *under the columella* rather than disrupt the natural white roll reflection? No surgical scar is as normal to the casual observer as an untouched lip. An incision above the cupid's bow is not a good idea, no matter how much one might prefer to have a higher lip roll.

3. At a recent dinner, I observed several European women who had obviously undergone poorly performed lip enhancement. The upper lips were taut, full, and totally immobile. More than likely they had undergone liquid

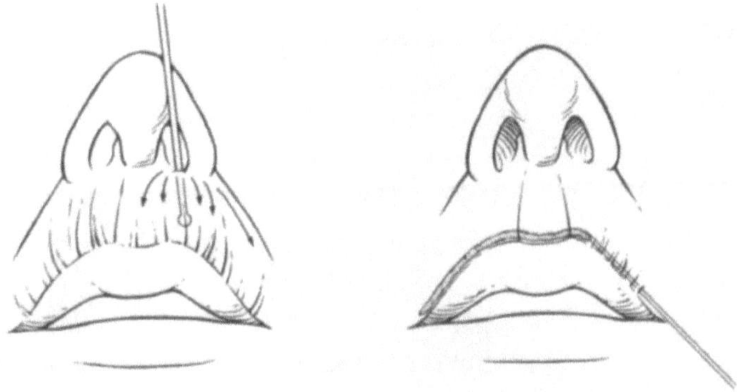

Figure 6-18. (A) Adding fat grafts under rhytids that have been elevated with a transnasal dissector fills the "valleys" of the senile lip. (B) For the severely wrinkled lip, I undermine the white roll as well and then graft this area. Concentrated autologous fat is deposited in the space created by passing a 16-gauge needle under the white roll. Light surface abrasion of the ridges flattens the "hills." Light chemical peel application is the final touch.

A

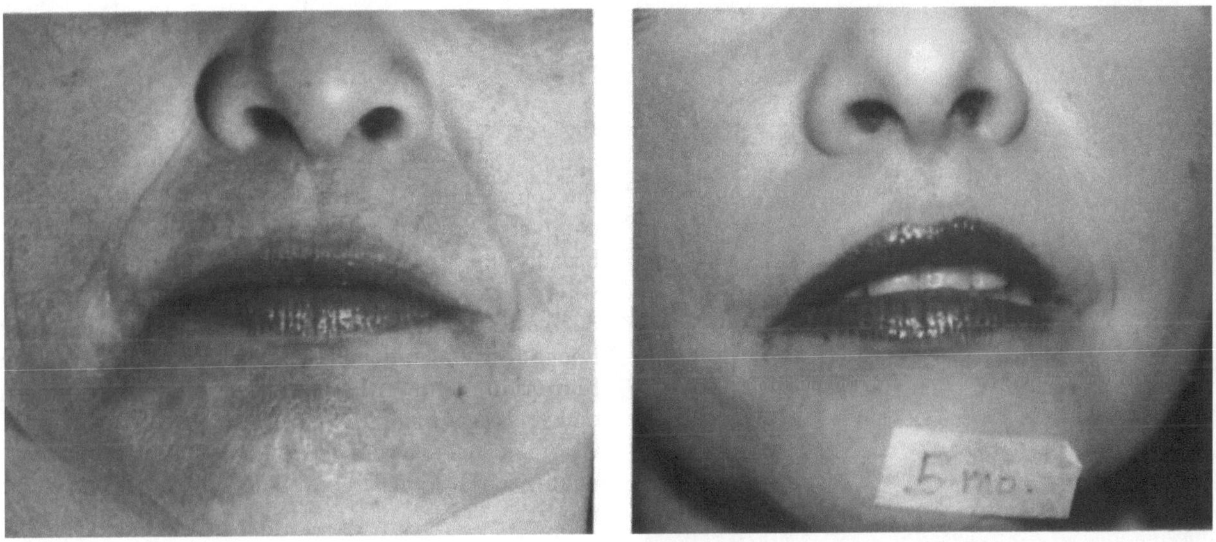

B

Figure 6-19. Lip rejuvenation in the middle-aged patient. (A) Pigmentation and fine lines mar the appearance of the lip in this patient, yet the wish for rejuvenation did not include whitening of the lip. In a Hispanic population especially, rejuvenation includes a slow regimen of Retin-A and α-hydroxy acids with iodoquin, and then facial fat grafting. We did not use a light peel in this case. (B) Note the fullness of her lips from the fat grafting into the subvermilion area. There is no demarcation line between the cheeks and the lip; yet the only correction was blepharoplasty, fat grafting to the nasolabial fold and vermilion, and topical creams and bleaches.

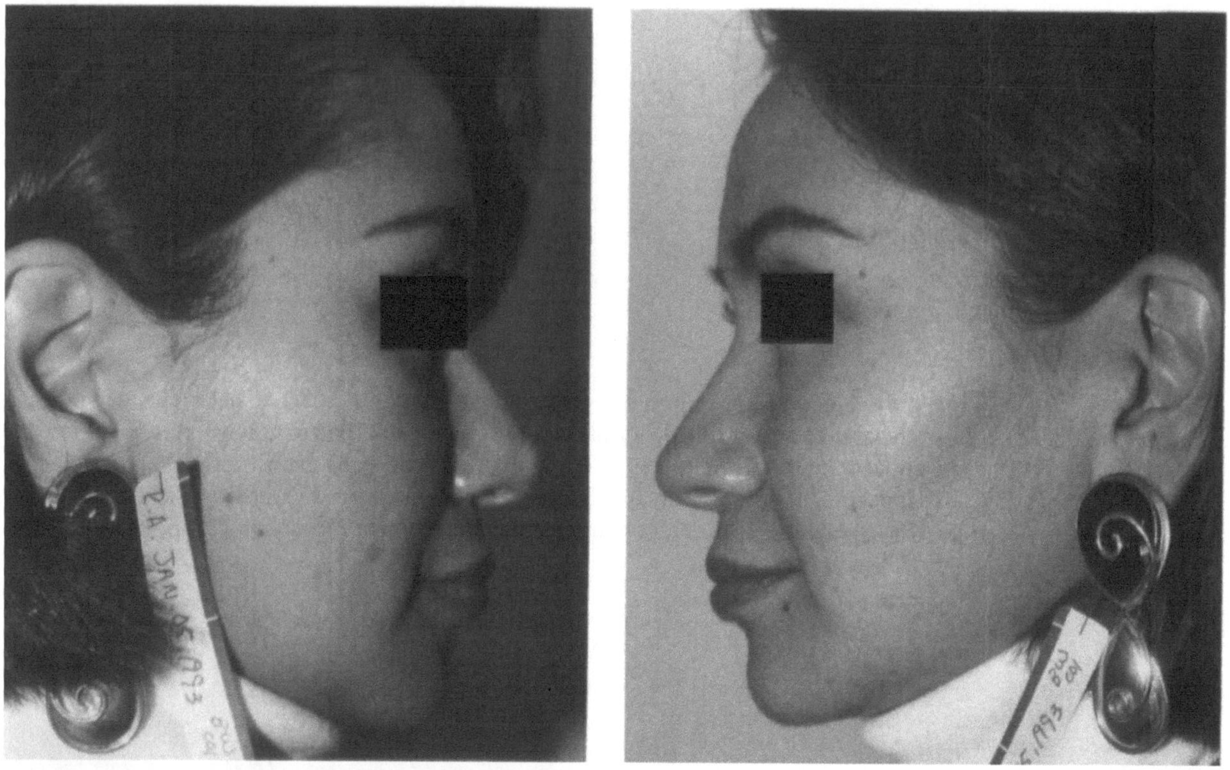

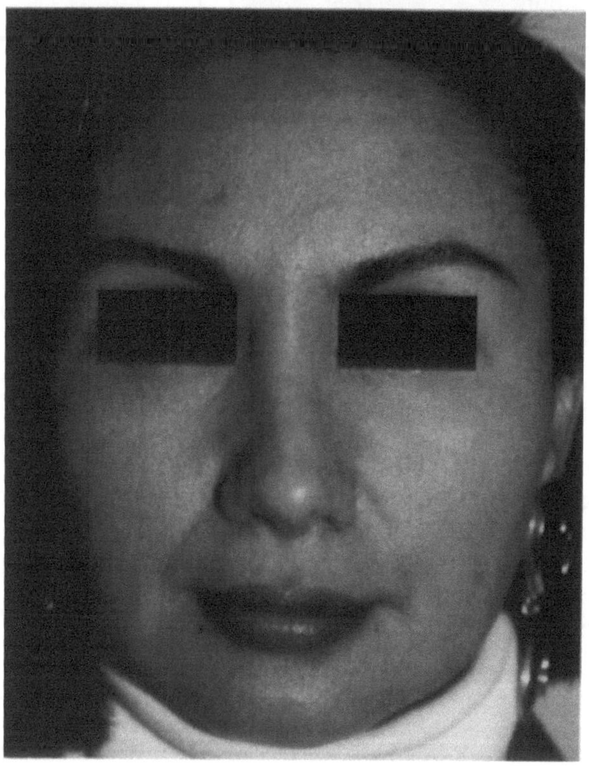

Figure 6-20. Lip enhancement 4 years after lipografts and lip roll procedure. This patient is also depicted in the color section showing a complication of less-than-complete lipografting. When this patient smiled broadly, the upper inner portion of the lip flattened, whereas the visible portion did not, and this situation distressed her. It was corrected by an additional minor lipograft to the undersurface. She also requested more fullness to the lower lip. Patients are counseled preoperatively regarding the choice of the size of the lip, yet it is not unusual to have a patient request further enhancement even after what I would consider an excellent result.

silicone injections into the rhytids and suffered the consequences of dense fibrosis. There was also evidence of phenol peeling with permanent whitening that even their makeup could not cover. This result is not necessary. You can restore the aging lip with fat grafting, rhytid elevation, trichloroacetic acid (TCA) peels, and good skin care.

That type of complication is almost uncorrectable. Liposuction in an area of liquid silicone injection may help some, but it creates as much scarring as the original silicone. It is effective only if there are specific areas of fibrosis and liquid silicone deposits. The edema and swelling of the upper lip following lip roll surgery corrects with time and does not require surgery.

One plastic surgeon consulted me because a patient/friend was upset with him. He had performed a lip roll and had created an attractive vermilion, but the upper lip was still stiff. There are two ways to approach this problem. The first is to instruct the patient to wear a thin tennis headband hooked behind the neck and across the upper lip, wearing it at night and occasionally during the daytime. Supplement this treatment with digital pressure. Eventually this rare form of upper lip edema resolves, and the vermilion remains in the full state intended. If this regimen is not effective within a short time, follow the advice I offered the other surgeon. Use of series of dilute triamcinolone (Aristospan) injections into the deep tissues. Be careful not to overdo it and make the injections deep so there is no surface change. This measure speeds resolution.

4. I strongly agree with Gene Courtiss, who discussed a lip enhancement technique presented in the December 1992 issue of *Plastic and Reconstructive Surgery*. Earlier presentations by French surgeons touted the convenience and efficacy of threading strips of Gortex under nasolabial areas and described placing this material within the lip. My comment at the time was that the material is firm and palpable; hence the lips would not look natural. Furthermore, there is a concern about eventual extrusion of the material. As healing occurs, fibroblasts and collagen penetrate the polytetrafluoroethylene. Why would it not contract thereafter, and how would one treat such contraction? The submucosal area of the lip is subject to trauma and is located next to an area that is contaminated with some of the most potent bacteria we know.

Lastly, a 13% complication rate is far too great for the type of individual who seeks lip enhancement. The worst complication with the multilevel fat grafting technique is that the lips do not retain the fullness achieved during the first two postoperative weeks. In our experience, however, some 75% of patients report that fullness noted at 2 weeks is still present at 4 to 5 years. It is a simple thing to add more fat for greater fullness. After 3 months, the lingering decrease in sensitivity allows this procedure to be rapid and relatively problem-free.

REFERENCES

Countiss EH, Glicksman CA: Discussion. Plast Reconstr Surg 90:1091, 1992.
Kesselring VK: Rejuvenation of the lips. Ann Plast Surg 16:480, 1986.
Wilkinson T: Augmenting the upper lip. Techn Forum 9:10, 1986.
Wilkinson TS: Correction of the congenital short upper lip and heavy-lidded eyes. Aesth Plast Surg 4:73, 1980.
Wilkinson T: Lip enhancement. Techn Forum 13:4, 1990.
Wilkinson T: Lip lengthening and lip roll combination.
Wilkinson TS: Upper lip lengthening. In J Lewis (ed), The Art of Aesthetic Plastic Surgery. Little, Brown, Boston, 1989, p. 503.

7 Blepharoplasty

YOU WOULD THINK THAT AN UPPER AND LOWER LID BLEPHAROplasty is a straightforward procedure. Wrong. Some of the problems with this operation date back to the early days of plastic surgery, and some are recent ideas that just are not acceptable. For instance Howard Gordon has made the point that the surgeon should "stay off the nose." It is difficult to believe, but sometimes incisions are made onto the nasal skin as well as into the upper lid lateral zone, a highly visible area. The blepharoplasty scar should follow the natural curvature of the lid fold and then stop. Do not carry the incision high and lateral in an ill-advised attempt to raise the corner of the eyelid. Another mistake is to remove too much skin and muscle so the eyes look skeletal and not natural. Leave a little fat, and limit the muscle resection.

At one time we were advised not to resect orbicularis muscle but to touch it with electrocautery. The worst ectropion that developed in my practice occurred during the early 1970s after using that technique. Conversely, do not overuse cautery for bleeders; ice packs can control most of them. In fact, do not overdo *anything* when performing blepharoplasty. In women it's perfectly alright to create "the deep sculptured eyelid". In men, leave it alone. Don't take as wide a muscle strip, don't take as much fat and leave the crow's feet alone. A male has to look masculine. We cowboys like a little Clint Eastwood around the eyes.

Blepharoplasty is a procedure with little margin for error. Small technical errors can ruin a perfectly good result or spoil what should be a rapid recovery. When done well, the operation does not need "fixing."

Some surgeons who use lasers to dissect the upper lid skin make extravagant claims, such as that when a laser is used as the cutting instrument there is no edema; yet we know that most bleeding comes from subcutaneous tissue or when fat is removed for regrafting. If the fat is cut with a laser, valuable fat is lost. Other bleeding derives from the muscle edge, not from skin. Bleeding should not be a problem if you puff up the area with local anesthetic with epinephrine, keep the patient lightly sedated, and pack the area with iced saline during and after the procedure.

We offer each of our patients the option of reusing the fat to fill the nasolabial areas or to plump up the lip. If you can do that without additional cost, or even for a minor surgical fee, you have an advantage. It is a better marketing tool than making extravagant claims for laser surgery; moreover, it is not necessary to go back and excise the skin edges that were burned by laser.

The other media-touted "innovation" is transconjunctival removal of lower lid fatpads. There are two sides to this issue. Those who advocate the procedure justifiably claim that it is quick and easy, and that there is less bruising. Those who oppose this technique wonder why the patients still have skin wrinkling. There are two solutions to the latter problem. One proposal is performing transconjunctival fat removal and then later removing the skin. (Why operate on the patient twice?) I remove skin with a simple maneuver, after which the fat can be trimmed, saved, or cauterized. In other words, *the original transcutaneous operation works*. The only theoretic advantage of the transconjunctival method is that in certain individuals a trichloroacetic acid (TCA) peel on the skin removes all the lines. Entry into the fatpads using this approach is from behind skin and muscle, sometimes a risky procedure.

We now use peels with our submuscular flap fat and skin removal. The submuscular route is safer and adding a TCA peel on the skin is not risky. No type of peel should be used on the extremely wrinkled lower lid. These patients benefit most from the standard blepharoplasty, which is a *subcutaneous*—not a submuscular—dissection. Going subcutaneously allows me to unravel the crumply skin to a greater degree.

Technique

Blepharoplasty is the most common operation performed by private practitioners. A few guidelines may be helpful.

1. Always remove less skin than you think you need, particularly from the lower lid. To create a full sculptured eyelid in women, remove a strip of muscle wider than the skin you excise on the upper lid. Remove more muscle laterally in women than in men.

2. Unless there is severe skin wrinkling and damage, use a submuscular approach for the lower lid. Lifting the skin muscle flap eliminates lesser degrees of skin wrinkling.
3. Transconjunctival fat removal on the lower lid is not a benign procedure. Most patients have extra skin as well, and you do them no service by leaving it in place. Removing the fat transconjunctivally is said to allow the skin to "shrink and contour to the new shape," but in most instances visible wrinkling results, which is disturbing to patients.
4. For the upper lid, angle the ends of the incisions slightly upward but stay clear of the visible zone laterally and medially.
5. If you must use a lower lid extension because there is more loose skin laterally, keep it short. The visible scars are the ones 2 to 3 mm beyond the lid.
6. Upward fingertip massage of the lower lids and Frost sutures to reduce the risk of temporary ectropion.

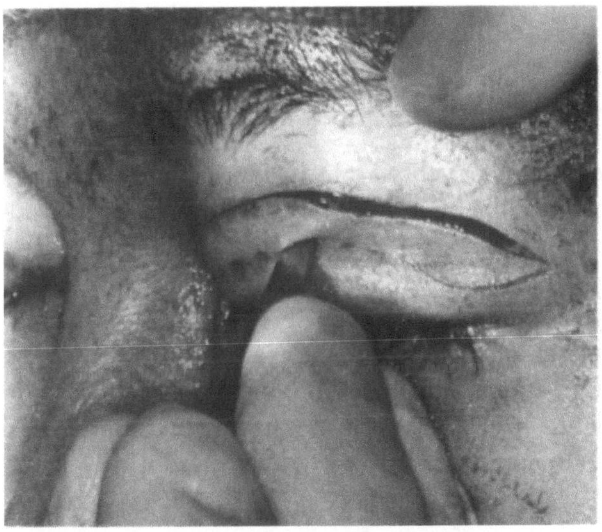

Figure 7-1. Blepharoplasty. For the upper lid, curving the lower incision upward just beyond the natural lid fold maintains the elevation of the lateral corner, and the lid remains well within its natural lines. It is a major mistake to extend an incision laterally or above the point shown here because these areas are visible and scars may be unpredictable.

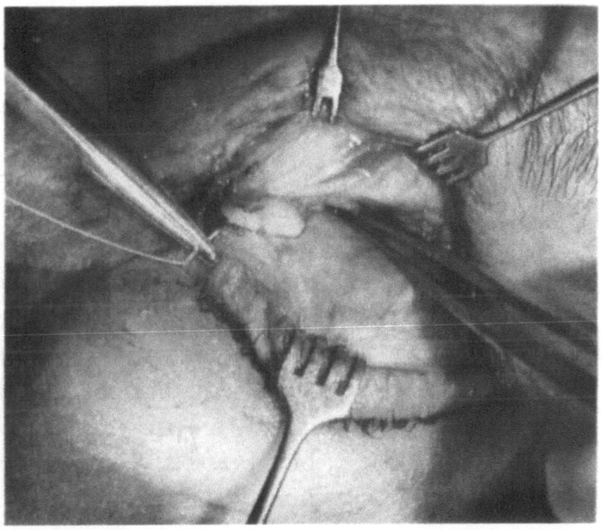

Figure 7-2. Blepharoplasty. Do not forget the lacrimal gland. In patients who have lateral fullness, look for the gland so as not to damage it. It is easy to find after local anesthesia has infiltrated the area. The simplest way to correct lacrimal gland ptosis is to pass a Vicryl or Dexon suture through the gland and then expose the undersurface of the orbital rim. Pass the needle next throughout the periosteum on the undersurface of the orbital rim. Usually one suture suffices to tuck the gland out of sight so it is not damaged.

7. Close eyelid incisions the easiest way. Remember how painful suture removal is, so use fast-dissolving catgut on the lower lid. Do not trust it laterally or in the upper lid, however, as it may dissolve too quickly.
8. Once fat removal is complete, tuck an iced saline pad in the defect. Leave it in place as long as possible. If a face lift is the next procedure, close the eyelids only after they have been ice-packed for 10 to 15 minutes while you do something else. Take one last look to see if there is a persistent bleeder, as occasionally you do find one.
9. Use a single Frost suspension stitch in the center for most people. For elderly patients, use one on either side of the pupil. Do not tie the stitch; jut loop it through the skin and tape it to the forehead. In older patients, leave it in place 3 to 4 days.
10. If the older patient shows signs of early ectropion before surgery (lid rebound test), use some type of suspension reefing of the orbicularis or even nail the tarsal plate to the periosteum. Give the patient Steri-Strips to tape the lower eyelids at night. Some older patients develop a full-blown ectropion 3 to 4 days postoperatively. It usually responds to hot and cold packs, night taping, a night eye cover to keep allergens out of the eyelids, and gentle massage.

Eyebrows

A common mistake is to overlook eyebrow ptosis. Is it better to raise the eyebrow first and then perform the blepharoplasty, or should you finish the blepharoplasty and then perform the rest of the face lift? I prefer the latter method. If care is taken with the preoperative skin excision lines, a short eyelid does not result. Raising the eyebrow is part of practically every face lift. Even in those who require a full coronal lift and resetting of the eyebrow, it is acceptable to work on the upper lids first. Close the skin later, after using iced saline. If the cavities are packed with iced saline, you save time by not having to cauterize tiny blood vessels. Ninety percent of these tiny bleeders will have disappeared by the time of closure.

Upper Eyelid

Repairing the upper eyelid is basic. Numerous diagrams can be drawn, but they all boil down to a few simple rules. For the most part, follow the curve of the lid where it breaks in a natural groove. For those with hollow recessed eyelids and little fat, make the incision as high as possible. For normal eyelids choose the

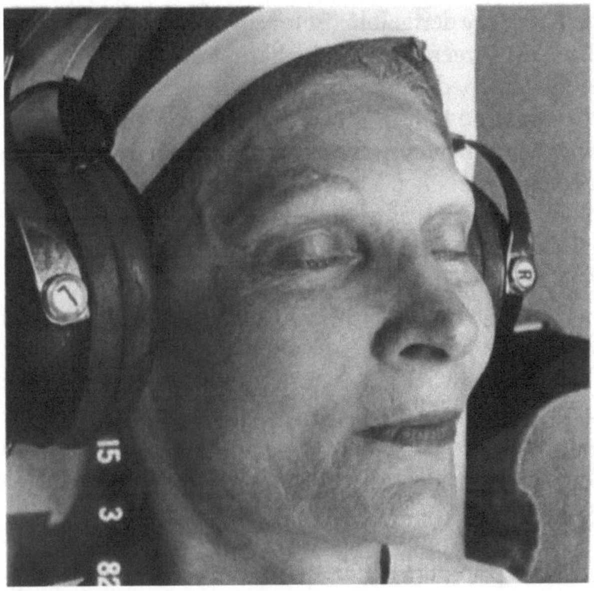

A

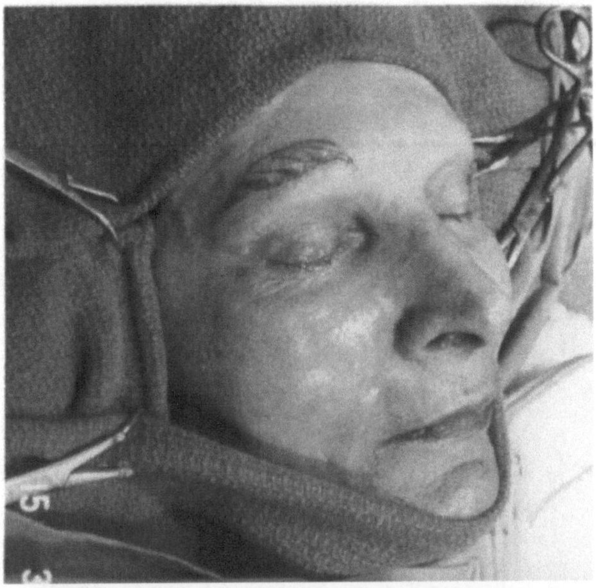

B

C

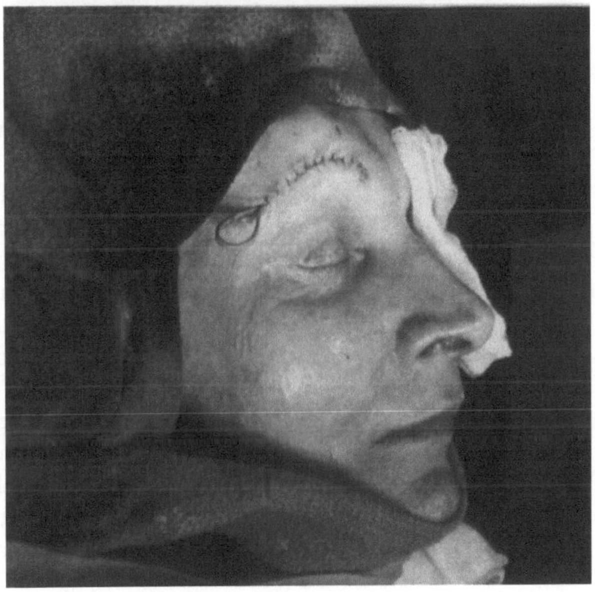

Figure 7-3. Direct excisions to lift the eyebrows are favorites of some ophthalmologists. The scar is obvious, however, no matter how well closed. In many older people unconcerned about aesthetics, visual obstruction is due partly to excess upper lid skin and partly to brow descent. Direct excision is quicker and easier than a coronal brow lift. One of my unhappy male patients had what he called a "gash" in the midforehead, performed for these reasons. We were able to minimize the scar with a turn-under suspension flap; but we restored some of his sensory loss only by carefully lysing scar tissue.

(A–C) This ptotic brow resulted from an old injury. We reepithelialized the scar and undermined upward. The edge of the scar tissue was then attached to galea and the skin edges back-cut so the next layer of sutures everted them. A few tacking 6-0 Nylon sutures were placed and a drain inserted. The brow was suspended by the deep flap, not the skin. Good balance was achieved with only a minimally visible scar.

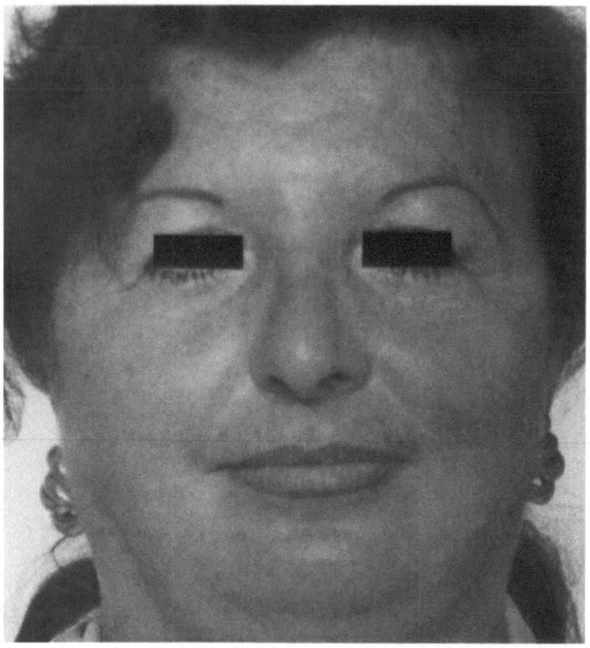

Figure 7-4. Dermatology blepharoplasty. This patient had been to a dermatologist for correction of her defects. The first surgery was a "blepharoplasty," which apparently consisted only of removing some skin just above the upper lid lashes. When the patient predictably was upset that her eyelids had not improved much, the dermatologist then excised skin at the lid fold. It is obvious that his procedure in no way resembled what trained surgeons consider an upper lid blepharoplasty. At surgery we found considerable scar tissue above the muscle. The difficulty was to identify the levator and then clear the extra muscle and scar on either side of the incision. In such cases remove no skin. Creation of the upper lid fold takes up any excess. We undermined the skin with a scalpel superiorly but left skin attached in the tarsal area. It was then easy to identify the orbicularis and the untouched volumes of fat.

The technical maneuvers associated with surgery for such patients include speculating whether the original surgeon was totally untrained or partly trained. The latter would be far worse. In this case, he had attempted to divide the orbicularis and put extra scar tissue in the fat (it would have been more difficult to isolate and individually remove the lobules of fat). Scar tissue around the muscle is also a problem. The desired result is an attachment to the levator area laterally with blunt spreading dissection. Once you identify the levator—and in this patient it was not difficult because no attempt had been made to resect muscle—you can clear a path and carefully trim the muscle. This patient's problem was obvious. There has been no removal of muscle, no attempt to create a fold, and no attempt to remove the ordinary upper lid fat and the fat that attaches on the undersurfaces of the orbicularis laterally. When sculpturing an upper lid in a female patient, it is important to evert the orbicularis and manually trim the fat with scissors. Limit this dissection to the outer third (for details see the drawings in my articles on heavy lidded eyes in *Aesthetic Plastic Surgery* 4:73, 1980). Cautiously proceed until all the anatomy can be viewed. Then perform the trimming and make the appropriate attachments. In this case, we preferred the Baker technique of surface-anchoring sutures using 6-0 silk. This suture passes from skin to levator edge and back to skin. Sometimes placing one or two of these stitches shows that you have not removed enough muscle on the upper edge.

break point and remove somewhat less skin than you think you will need. Medially, angle the incision slightly upward and do the same laterally in more of a curve. Whether this maneuver is responsible for reducing the thickness of the scar or just makes the extra skin in the upper inner canthus disappear, it is a helpful modification of the standard technique.

For women, remove a wide muscle strip (wider than the skin strip). If the muscle is pinched with forceps, it can be removed with a single passage of the scissors—essential for creating the sculptured look. Always lift the lateral muscle above the incision and take a look underneath. Many patients have extra fibrofatty tissue under that muscle. If it is trimmed in the outer third, a sculptured contour results. At this point the fat is visible. Do not be shy about removing the lateral fat as well as the "white fat" medially. Pass the scissors tip deeply and open the scissors. Exert a little pressure on the globe, causing the fat to come out. After trimming the yellowish fat, another push usually results in a fairly large glob of white fat to come into view. It usually has no blood vessels, so it is safe to cut it away. Should you miss this fat, the patient will likely appear 5 years later with a fat bulge at the inner canthus.

For treating the Oriental eyelid to remove the epicanthal fold, you can use the Mustarde or other elaborate diagrams, or you can utilize a simple procedure: A small ***Z-plasty*** (not a giant one) in the ascending limb can be performed that allows the skin to lie down. No incisions are needed on the nasal skin with this technique.

Suturing the upper lid is the next step. Some surgeons promote the use of subcuticular closures, others use interrupted sutures, and still others prefer deep tacking sutures as are used for the Oriental eyelid. There is a simple suture procedure: To ensure that the new lid folds at the right place, place two 6-0 silk sutures at intervals. Catch the skin and muscle on the lower part as well as a bit of levator (do not catch it too high or the patient will not be able to raise the eyelid). Bypass the muscle on the upper part and come out through the skin. Tie these sutures loosely and remove them in 4 to 5 days. The sutures also help line up the skin so there is no mismatch.

The simplest way to close the rest of the skin is to use a continuous over-and-over running Prolene stitch. It makes no difference whether it is done subcuticularly or on the surface, so do it the easiest way. We do not tie the central part—just place a Steri-Strip and leave the Prolene taped across the bridge of the nose. On the outer aspect there is usually some tension and some movement, so it helps to make a loop knot and then tape it down. Use Prolene so it can slide out easily.

Lower Eyelid

For the lower lids, the only decision is whether you should approach via the usual subcutaneous plane or deep to the orbicularis (skin-muscle flap). We had husband and wife patients who had these repairs. The wife came back to us angry because she had a bruise on the fifth day, and her husband was doing fine with no bruise. The difference was that her skin damage extended to the midcheek because we had performed a standard subcutaneous dissection to the midcheek, and then simply split through the muscle to reach the fat. For most patients there is muscle folding and skin folding but little skin excess. Use of a skin-muscle flap is easy, fast, and effective; and it hides any blood accumulation so no bruises are seen.

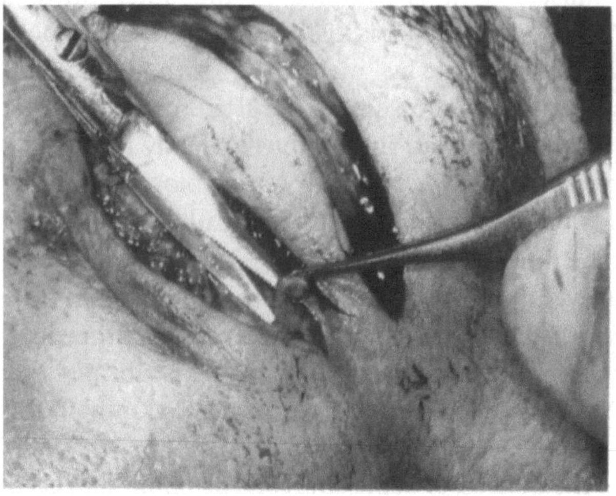

Figure 7-5. When skin is dissected away from muscle (particularly in the wrinkled lower lid skin syndrome) the orbicularis muscle is elevated when the skin is tailored into the outline of the incision. In this figure, note that the lateral extension of the incision is only 2 to 3 mm. This figure represents a plea for shorter incisions. Incision need not extend 4 to 6 mm to obtain lateral lift except in the elderly patient in whom you are planning a Kuhnt-Symonowsky lid repair at the same time. In this photograph the forceps is holding a resected portion of orbicularis muscle taken just below the outer canthus. When you lift the skin into position, you will note buckling in this area. First make sure there is not an aberrant fatpad, which would be located toward the globe and not nearly as deep as the usual pads. You should be able to detect it preoperatively (except in lids that have massive fat deposits). To avoid this buckling of muscle, simple elliptical excision can be done directly through the full thickness of the muscle in this area. This maneuver also helps the skin flap lie in position and avoids the unsightly "trap door effect" that can occur in the corner. As an added note, one should always check the skin flap to make sure that extra muscle or dermis has not been left on the skin flap just inside this corner. Trim it to the same thickness as the rest of the eyelid skin before placing the corner sutures.

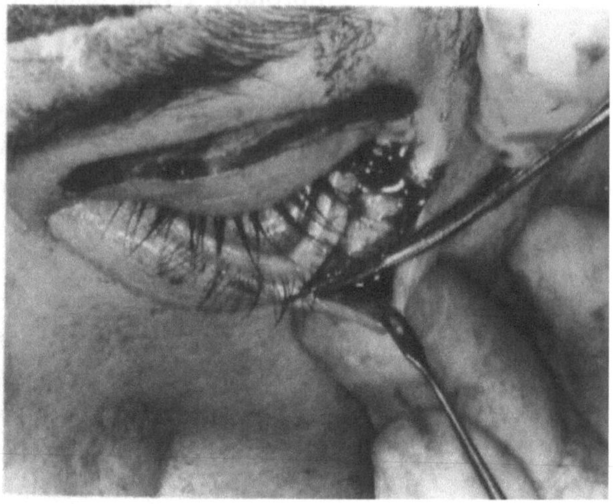

Figure 7-6. Have you ever looked back at a lower lid blepharoplasty incision and found that there was an irregular line that dipped too far below the lash line? Here are a couple of technical points that not only can speed up the surgery but can prevent those irritating minor problems. First, note in the figure that the scissors is curved toward the lid, that is, with its curvature paralleling the curvature of the incision and the lid curve. Turning the scissors over would just make it more difficult to cut a curved line. Second, how do you keep from cutting the lashes when you are placing an incision in this preferred close-in position? Use a serrated edge scissors such as the Kaye blepharoplasty scissors. Once you are in the groove, be it subcutaneously, or if between the orbicularis and the skin for a skin-muscle flap dissection, just push. The serrated edges turn the lashes away, and the extra tension exerted by the hook allows you to separate the incision line smoothly with little effort.

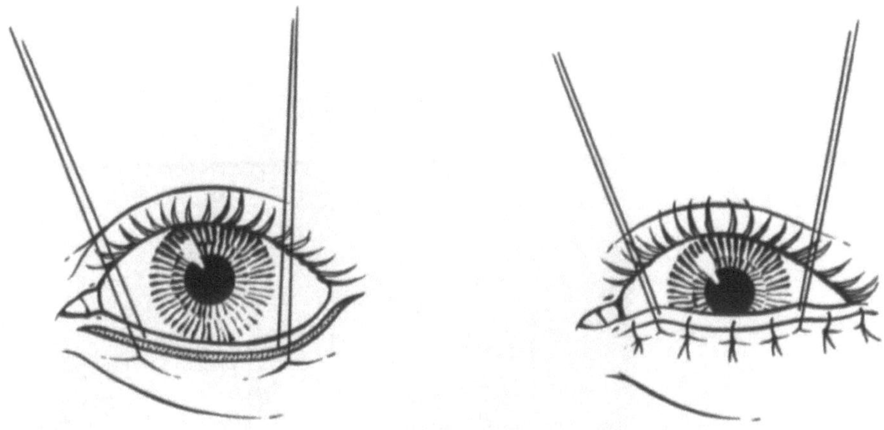

Figure 7-7. The basic idea is to hold the lower lid in an overcorrected position so the orbicularis muscle does not drop into the cavity formed by the fat removal and become entrapped by the serum clot. Lying in bed and watching television over one's feet can cause this complication. We use the Frost suture routinely for all blepharoplasties but leave it in place for only 24 hours in normal lids. If a lid is half-way between normal tone and a tone for which you would use Tom Rees' wedge excision (as a modified Kuhnt-Symonowsky procedure), leave the Frost suture in for 3 to 4 days. There is no discomfort if it is taped to the forehead without overvigorous suspension. Patients appear to tolerate these sutures quite well.

Note one modification: The Frost suture is not knotted on the lower lid, thereby eliminating digging around with pointed scissors to try to cut a silk suture. Loop the Frost suture through and lift it up, tie it in a knot, pass a Steri-Strip through it, and tape it into position after eye ointment is instilled at the completion of the blepharoplasty. Removing it is simple if there is no knot.

Another advantage of using the Frost suture is that when your assistant lifts on either suture, the two edges come into direct apposition, making it easy to add 6-0 catgut. It also is a means of protecting the cornea, as you pull the lid up and over during closure.

Note that the lower lid is "tacked" with only a few sutures. Fast-dissolving 6-0 plain catgut holds long enough and falls out rapidly.

When the upper lid incision has been outlined with the scalpel, the lower lid lateral cuts can be undertaken—always in a skinfold and never at less than a 30-degree angle. When these cuts are complete, place blunt scissors through the incision and dissect either subcutaneously or submuscularly. I prefer Bernie Kaye's scissors because the serrated edge makes it easy to perform the next maneuver. Turn the scissors on their side and push along the eyelash margin. You do not cut eyelashes using this method, but you stay close enough to them so you need not return to remove 1 mm of skin. If you drift down 1 to 2 mm, the scar will be visible. (Another common mistake is to suture lower lid skin edge to skin edge after the resection. The muscle then retracts, leaving a noticeable depression.)

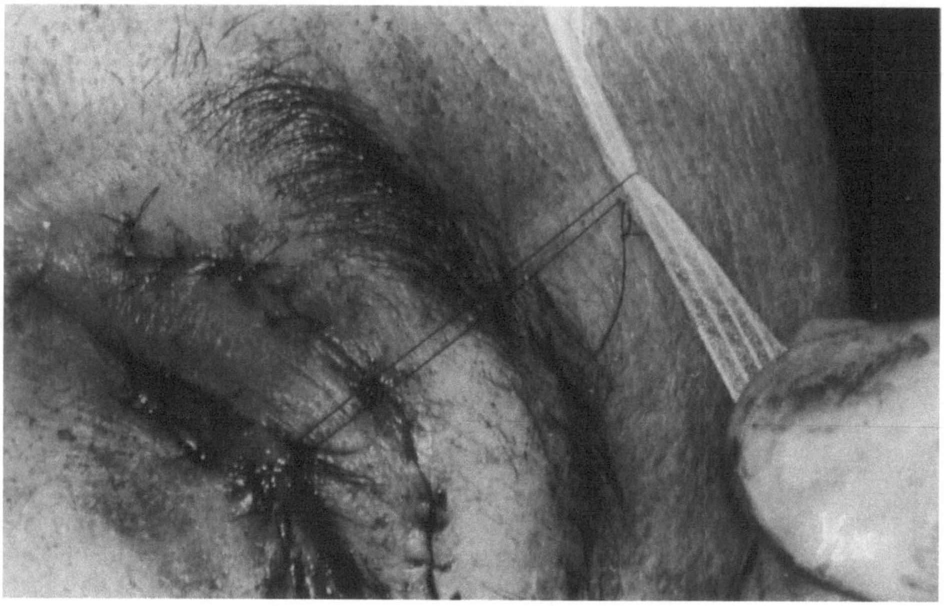

Figure 7-8. Routine use of a suspension suture for the first 24 to 48 hours after lower lid blepharoplasty has several advantages. Not only is the lower lid elevated and protected from incidental trauma or corneal exposure, but the orbicularis oculi is stretched to prevent its entrapment. This point is particularly applicable to the standard blepharoplasty in which one dissects underneath skin and then enters the fat compartments directly. The cut edge of the muscle can easily become entrapped and give a temporary or permanent downward slant to the lower lid. With skin-muscle flaps, the suspension suture makes certain that the muscle is in full contact with the incision edge and cannot retract and form a visible fold.

Note in the figure that traction on the suspension suture can speed up closure. We prefer this type of running suture because of its ease of removal and low incidence of skin markings. With skin-muscle flap lower lid blepharoplasty, the suspension suture pulls the muscle edge (which it includes) upward and makes it easier to catch it with running sutures.

A hint on anchoring the suture so its removal is relatively pain-free: We do not tie this suture at the lid edge. We simply loop it through the lash line, muscle, and skin and then tie it in a long loop for suspension. If you pass the instrument through the loop first as shown and grab the half-length Steri-Strip, it is easy to pull it through. Use the Steri-Strip to anchor the suture loop. Lift up so there is moderate tension on the lower lid, and apply tape directly to the forehead. Be sure to reinforce this tape with several other Steri-Strips because it is easy to dislodge a single strip. Patients do perspire and sometimes wet dressings can loosen the Steri-Strips.

With three rakes, hold the area open so you can see all the fatpads. I like Gonzalez-Ulloa's idea of splitting the whole area open so you can see what is there and what is not. If the fat is not needed for grafting and it is not excessive, cauterize it; otherwise, lift it up, clip it, cauterize any obvious bleeding vessels and then lightly cauterize whatever is left after the fat has been harvested for grafting. Scar tissue seals the rest in place. During the muscle trimming, be conservative, and be sure to take a little extra muscle in the outer third. Once the skin is aligned, apply fingertip pressure to ensure that no muscle remains. If the extra muscle is not removed, an extra bulge appears in the lateral curve. Although this step does cause bleeding, and cauterization will probably be necessary, a smoother eyelid results. Closure becomes easier if silk tacking stitches are placed laterally followed by a Frost suspension suture (do not tie it, just loop it). Holding the suture makes it easy to place a series of interrupted sutures because the skin edges are thus pulled together.

Interrupted stitches are placed in the lower lid because they do not require removal. A few years ago we took a suggestion from Byron Green and changed to fast-dissolving 6-0 catgut. The plain gut sutures dissolve quickly when the patient performs lower eyelid massage with oils. The upward massage is to make sure that nothing becomes stuck in the cavity left by fat removal (serving the same purpose as the Frost stitch). I close the lower lids with fewer tacking stitches today, and the catgut goes through skin and orbicularis and then back through the edge of orbicularis and up to the skin.

Leave a small strip of orbicularis right below the lash margin to be sure there is no depressed scar. The normal youthful eyelid has some fullness just below the lower lashes.

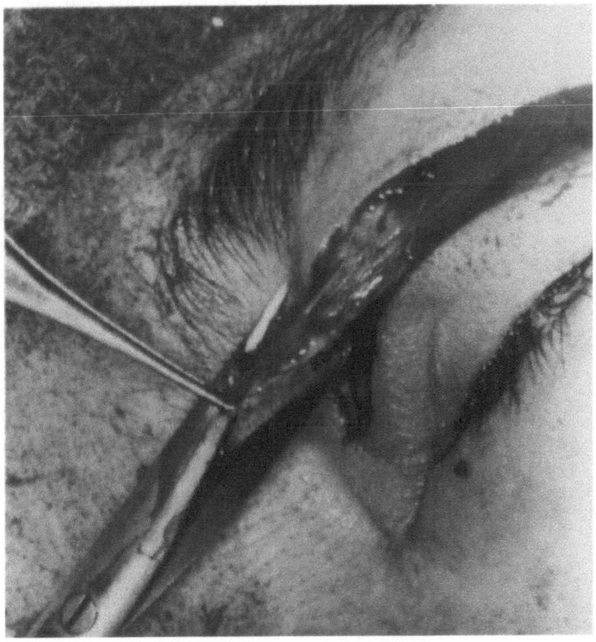

Figure 7-9. Process of lifting the lax orbicularis away from the underlying fibrofatty tissue and aponeurosis of the levator. The worst mistake you can make during this procedure is to cut completely through or damage the tarsal plate. First, apply the forceps carefully, lifting the lax tissue away. You may eventually want to remove more muscle, but it can be done easily after fat removal during the final phase of sculpturing the upper lid. Do not forget the lateral fullness, and look underneath the orbicularis for the thick fibrofatty layer on the periosteum. Most of it is removed when converting a hooded eyelid to an elegant sculptured one.

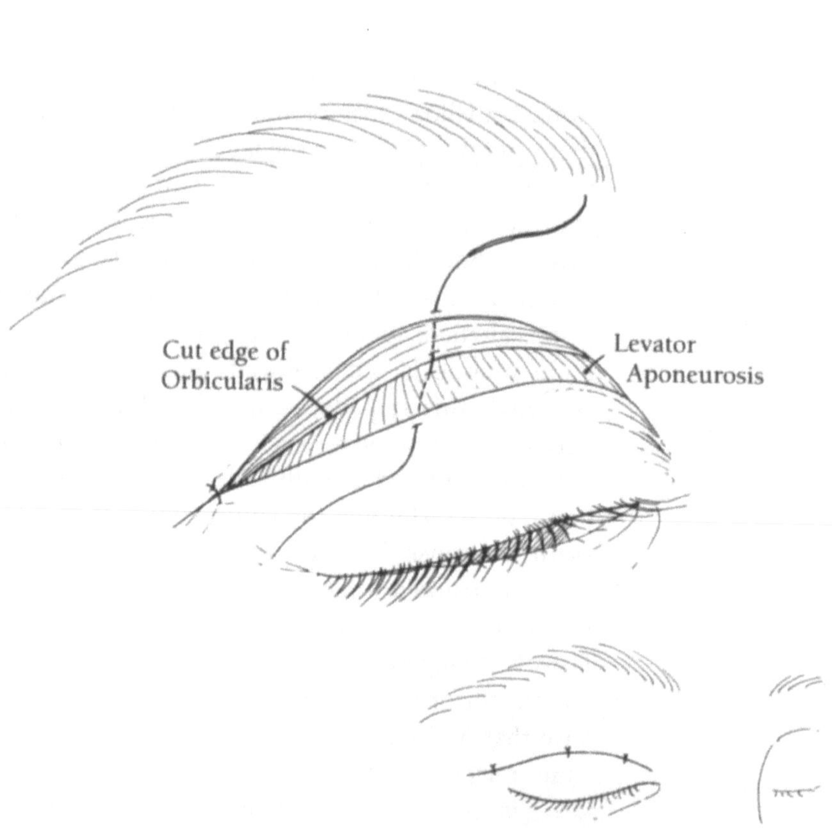

Figure 7-10. Surgeons disenchanted with the complexity of the anchor blepharoplasty, the multiple buried silk sutures that were advocated for the eyelid of the Oriental patient, or the "nonbreaking" type of sutures would be advised to try this simplification. When the eyelid does not have a definite fold on opening, we use these techniques to establish contact and fixation of the lower skin with the upper edge of the tarsal plate and levator. Thus when the eye opens, the skin fold is tucked backward, hiding the inelastic upper lid skin. Rather than spend the amount of time necessary to suture individually, we recommend this technique.

Three tacking sutures are used to establish contact between the cut edge of the resected orbicularis and the levator aponeurosis. To ensure that the upper muscle does not retract and that the two skin edges meet at this exact plane, the suture is first placed through the skin, then dipped through the line at the levator aponeurosis, up through the cut edge of the orbicularis, and out through the skin. Once these three tacking sutures are in place, a continuous subcuticular or running nylon suture is used to join these edges together at their fixation points. Failure to fix the cut edge of the orbicularis can lead to a "double break" appearance on opening the eye. These three tacking stitches take only a few minutes to put in. They have the advantage of helping adjust the skin edges as well, so there are no "dog ears" on either end.

Terino Lateral Lower Lid Support Procedure

For the elderly patient who shows early signs of ectropion, one must give added support to the lower eyelid. The tarsal tuck (see below) and overfolding of the orbicularis are two approaches to the problem. Another excellent idea is the lateral support described by Ed Terino.

Once the incisions have been completed and the skin has been trimmed, tunnel from the upper lid incision under the lateral raphe to the lower pocket and slip through this area two 4-0 Vicryl sutures and then anchor them. The first suture goes through the lateral raphe and the canthal tendon. The second goes through the skin muscle flap. Before passing the sutures through the periosteum, pull them up until the right amount of suspension is created. Then pass both sutures to the orbital rim periosteum 5 mm above the horizontal of the eyelid. Proceed then with the routine blepharoplasty closure. This suspension remains effective for several weeks after surgery.

Aftercare

During the aftercare phase, it is best to use iced compresses for at least 3 to 4 days. We have added another component. Medical Cosmetic Services composed an oil for us that is aloe-vera-based and contains vitamin E and a number of other ingredients. Called Extremely Effective, it is similar to the night cream oils from major cosmetic companies but with a difference. We can put this oil directly on sutures. Our face lift and blepharoplasty patients apply the oil on the stitches starting the day after surgery. Contrary to what I would have once thought, there is no resulting oil granuloma or irritation. The crusts come off easily, and the incisions stay soft and smooth. The patient puts a droplet on a fingertip and presses it into the lateral part of the blepharoplasty incision and lower lids, for upward massage. The oil must not get into the eyes. The patient places a fingertip at the orbital rim and pushes gently upward two or three times a day, a maneuver that also seems to remove some of the edema. Needless to say, other stitches should be removed early enough to avoid stitch marks and late enough so the patient cannot inadvertently open the incision. A small amount of collodion on the lateral incision and a drop or two along the upper lid after suture removal helps keep the incision intact.

We supply patients with see-through eye masks and cold witch hazel compresses for use at home. These items should be kept in the refrigerator and applied several times a day. The eye pads soak up tears, and the witch hazel is soothing. When the patient wants to be up and about, they can remove the see-through blue ice mask from the refrigerator (not the freezer) and wear it to read the paper or walk around the house.

After the third or fourth day it is time to apply hot packs. The same blue masks can be placed in hot water and worn three or four times a day starting at breakfast time. Our skin care and makeup team takes over on the fourth or fifth day, when it is safe to cover the incisions with hypoallergenic makeup and eyeshadow.

Even though one tries to avoid ectropion with conservative resections and Frost sutures, some older patients develop a "pseudoectropion." If one occurs, prescribe topical steroid eyedrops and tape the lower lid in an overcorrected position. Make sure the patient is massaging the eye. Replace the tape every 2 to 3 days so skin irritation does not result. This regimen stops the process in most cases. For others, (patients who ignore your instructions) plan a Kuhnt-Symonowski (K-S) procedure at the time of the initial blepharoplasty or do one after 6 weeks.

If an older patient has a preoperative ectropion with minor lid pressure, do not hesitate to correct it during the initial surgery. The two choices are tarsal tuck and K-S wedge resection. The K-S procedure is complex, but it is easy to run a 4-0 Vicryl through the lateral edge of the tarsus and into the periosteum as a support. Jim Smith (New York) suggested plicating the orbicularis muscle in these older patients with a couple of catgut sutures. This helps in my experience.

Tarsal Tuck Procedure

An early report described tacking the lower lid tarsal plate to the lateral periosteum in patients with lax lower lids. Experienced surgeons find a few problems with this procedure. First, the cosmetic results are not good. A large amount of lax skin remains, along with lines that are unacceptable in an aesthetic surgeon. Perhaps the clue to resolving this problem is that the authors of the original article stated that they *always* used a submuscular approach. I believe that there are times when you should dissect underneath the skin simply to elevate that extra folding of skin. Those authors also reported a patient who had only fat prolapse that was corrected with transconjunctival fat removal. In my experience, such patients are rare. Removing the fat accentuates the wrinkling of the skin and muscle in most eye lift candidates.

Several procedures are helpful for correcting the "round eye." The simplest is plication of the orbicularis muscle to the lateral canthal area to support the lid. Carefully done, it results in no extra bulge under the skin when performed during a subcutaneous dissection of the lower lid.

Lastly, one should consider the Faivre fixation technique to reduce the weight pulling on the skin of the lower lid. Jacques Faivre (Paris) presented a subcutaneous dissection down into the midcheek at the level of the infraorbital nerve foramen, then elevation and fixation of the cheek's soft tissue to the periosteum of the orbital rim. This technique has been useful to us in several cases. One then would dissect the skin freely so the eyelid, which returns to its original position, can be draped without tension. The use of Frost suspension sutures to provide a tissue expander effect for several days is helpful as well. Pass these loop sutures through the skin and the rim of the lid and then tape them to the forehead. Use at least two of these sutures.

One must employ techniques in addition to some form of fixation when a severe ectropion occurs. The K-S wedge resection technique has long been effective. Properly done, it does not create notching of the lid, and one is left with firm tissue on both sides of the suture.

One more point: Do not use 7-0 silk sutures that you have to remove! Fast-dissolving catgut stays in place long enough and disappears on its own, particularly if the patient begins lower lid massage with a drop of oil on the fingertip for lubrication. The oil then creeps upward and saturates the sutures, allowing them to dissolve without pain or discomfort.

Putting It Together with the Patient

Putting it all together for a patient involves much dialogue. For example, one of my patients is an over-35 Latin American woman who has a budding career on the stage. She went to a plastic surgeon and had an upper and lower blepharoplasty and a partial face lift done with less than gratifying results. The right eye was far too deep. Questions that arose during our consultation: Does she want to keep it that way and match it with the left, or should we add fat grafts? Can we move the high blepharoplasty incisions down to a hidden spot because they certainly show as a white line on her darker skin?

It is easy to perform a submental tuck and add a chin implant to shape her neck. Her original face lift left bald spots above the ear that can easily be removed. Her new rhytidectomy incisions can be placed inside the tragus. The defatting technique can make a more normal tragal appearance and hide the fact that she had a face lift. Malar implants can provide more balance to her face.

She chose a moderate projection with more classic placement and the skin care program with light peels on the lower lids. We can add some phenol touches to the dark spots scattered throughout the upper face and then let the Retin-A and α-hydroxy acid regimen blend these spots with the rest of her skin. Six months later we can discuss a TCA peel for further refinement.

It is not unusual to see these early signs of aging in young women. They do not have to live with them, though, and they do not have to look "plastic" when we are finished.

Unusual Cases

Just when you begin to believe eyelid surgery is easy, an unusual case presents. Earlier you read about measures used to prevent ectropion in older patients: leaving the frost suspension sutures in place for 3 to 4 days, using Jim Smith's suggestion of tacking the orbicularis of the lower lid into the fascia of the orbital rim, taping the lower lid, and so on. We followed this procedure in a 70-year-old woman, and the eyelids were level the next day. Five days later, however, *severe* ectropion occurred on the left and less so on the right.

In such cases, before considering more surgery (i.e., a K-S procedure or temporary tarsorrhaphy), try topical steroid drops and have the patient retape the eye once or twice a day. This regimen alleviates some of the pressure and relieves the irritation. Emphasize the importance of wearing a sleeping mask. Many patients show sclera when they are sound asleep, and those who have undergone blepharoplasty may do so to a greater degree. Those who react to household dusts or pollens or who sleep with the window open may experience irritation of that open eyelid. Applying Lacri-Lube at night helps, and steroid drops do the rest. In the case of our 70-year-old patient, this conservative treatment was effective.

What about the patient with minimal ptosis? The goal here is to make the patient appear slightly more bright-eyed. I place two tacking stitches between the lower incision and the levator in the upper lid skin. This method is certainly simpler than the complete row of stitches suggested by others. The two tacking stitches simply reestablish a deeper fold. If you want to raise the eyelid just a bit more, place three stitches to plicate the levator to the tarsus.

For the "hooded" eyelid, do not neglect the fat that sits on top of the orbital rim bony prominence. Adrien Aiache, Malcolm Paul, and Thomas Biggs have emphasized this point. In an early publication, I described patients with hooded upper eyelids and short upper lips that required lengthening. Everting the orbicularis to expose this fat and fibrous tissue is still a good idea, so long as you do not "skeletonize" the upper lid. Once the strip of muscle is removed and the usual fatpads trimmed, a skin hook is placed under the muscle and the muscle lifted. A thick layer of fibrofatty tissue becomes apparent on the bone edge and slightly below it. Trim this tissue, but conservatively. Then trim the fibrofatty material on the undersurface of the orbicularis. It is at this point that tacking stitches can be inserted to hold the eyebrow at a higher position (if desired) because the whole area is exposed. These maneuvers should result in smoother contour and a more feminine eyelid. Do not do this procedure in men, as it does make the eye appear somewhat feminine.

Eyebrow Lift

The best technique for eyebrow lifting is the temporal face lift: an incision back in the hairline, dissection along the bone level, freeing the soft tissue along the orbital rim with blunt and sharp dissection, and pulling the entire flap upward. I favor Bruce Connell's technique for preventing hair loss along the incision. Use one of the scalp advancement clamps to push the posterior scalp downward so there is no rebound relaxation. Pull the skin upward and bite in, which indicates the amount of scalp that needs to be removed. Split the temple hair up to that point and place a strong 2-0 nylon anchoring stitch. Should you continue this procedure all along the line, hair is lost. Bruce's idea was to leave an extra 2 mm of scalp on the advanced flap between two of these fixation sutures, so the areas between those two tacking stitches touch without any tension; then one or two extra stitches can be added to keep them in place. That procedure is called the temporal lift and is usually done with our standard face lift.

If the patient refuses the temple lift, try eyebrow tacking from below. I have tried several ways to make this work with inconsistent results. The direct approach is to anchor subcutaneous tissue at two lateral points from underneath the flap. Do not give in to the temptation to excise skin above the eyebrow. Scars in that area are highly visible regardless of your technical skill. Use this excision only as a last resort.

An occasional young patient has lateral eyebrow ptosis. In combination with their excess eyelid hooding the ptosis gives them a sad "hound dog" appearance. Simply working with the eyelids is not enough. One should also offer eyebrow elevation.

Try tacking the eyebrow's undersurface to the orbital fascia at a higher position. If only slight elevation is needed, the procedure is done as follows.

Once you have removed the muscle strip from the upper lid, simply dissect upward underneath the remaining muscle until you can easily identify the orbital rim. A bone-cutting burr can be used to remove part of this rim, although I have not done so often. Free up the soft tissue with blunt dissection for at least 1 to 2 cm above the orbital rim. This step helps the skin fall into position more easily.

There are two ways to attach the eyebrow. I use Vicryl or Dexon sutures from periosteum to subcutaneous tissue. Place three or four, and overcorrect slightly. A surface suture may be added to hold the eyebrow in exact position. I then pass a large nylon suture through the center of the brow, look at the undersurface, and pass the suture through the periosteum and then back out through the eyebrow. I tie it loosely so it does not kill any of the hairs. The two suturing techniques together produce a good result.

Malcolm Paul reported anchoring the undersurface of the eyebrow directly to the fascia of the upper orbital rim instead of using a coronal lift to keep the eyebrows up. It is not a bad method, although it does not hold well. John Lewis had reported undermining the forehead skin so a skin redrape might help hold the eyebrow. My way is the third approach. One variation of combining an undersurface set of sutures with a skin surface suture is to use a buried suture placed through a tiny stab wound in the eyebrow. In several cases I passed a Vicryl suture through the stab wound, into the fascia, up through the skin, back through the same hole, and then subcutaneously to reach the stab wound. I tie the knot and then cut off the Vicryl suture and let it fall below the surface.

If you are planning to raise the eyebrow while doing a forehead lift, remember to incise the periosteum and free it completely from the orbital rim. The eyebrow then floats upward when you tighten the forehead lift.

Matt Gleason has noted that the frontalis fat can slide over the supraorbital rim and drop into the upper lid. He has agreed that simply removing a wide muscle strip and lateral fatpad is not sufficient in these "hooded" cases. Gleason sutures the edge of the orbicularis to the orbital rim to create a skin–muscle flap with fixation and relieve the effect of the eyebrow ptosis. Having little experience with this method, I can only emphasize the importance of not overdoing any type of eyebrow lifting, particularly in men, as well as not overdoing fat removal.

Avoiding Problems

At one time, joining the upper and lower lid incisions just beyond the lateral canthus to the left of the eye was considered aesthetic. Unfortunately, the scars that resulted ruined the effect, as these scars are in a highly visible area. Everyone who has tried this approach has abandoned it. The same applies to the "fishtail" incision, which also creates scars in "no man's land." Revising these scars with tiny, delicate subcuticular sutures to relieve tension and applying surface Steri-Strips makes a bad situation only slightly better. Keep the incisions short, and keep them away from each other.

There is a place for the Bob Flowers canthoplasty in conjunction with a lower lid blepharoplasty. Flowers does not advocate the medial to lateral tilt of the eye in most cases but, rather, uses canthoplasty to restore a normal, youthful contour with a slight, upward tilt. Although it is not readily visible when an eyelid ages, the lateral canthal tendon begins to stretch and the lower lid falls to a slightly lower position. This "Sophia Loren" effect can also be attained by superficially undermining from the temple to the outer canthal area. It is not always necessary to divide the orbicularis as Sherrell Aston and others have discussed.

Upper lid incisions tend to migrate superiorally with time. Howard Gordon seconds the recommendation to make the upslants short and at the end of the incisions. There is no disagreement between Howard Gordon and Tom Baker that removing the muscle strip accomplishes the same fold fixation as the elaborate suturing techniques described in the literature for "westernizing" the Oriental eyelid.

Do not try to cut a curved line with a straight scissor. The Kaye scissors can be used to push the lower lid at the ciliary margin. Dissect a subcutaneous groove first, then place the scissors, with the curve matching the curve of the eyelid. Continue to push, which results in a clean cut with no irregularity and little chance of losing eyelashes.

Once-hyperthyroid patients occasionally present a problem when they have unilateral proptosis. This condition is not a true proptosis; it is just that more sclera is visible in the lateral half of the eye. Correction can easily be accomplished by removing a little extra deep fat during the blepharoplasty and performing a small lateral canthoplasty. It is also helpful to perform an upper lid blepharoplasty on the opposite side with wide muscle strip removal. This technique makes the upper lid on the opposite eye open more and gives better balancing.

Do not hesitate to use two Frost sutures in older people with stretched orbicularis muscles. Loop one laterally and one medially so the patient can see between them. Leave them in place for a week or more if tolerable.

A strange syndrome of which to be aware is the oculocardiac reflex; it consists of bradycardia following manipulation of the eyelid or orbital fat. It is commonly seen in young women and occurs most often with medial fatpad removal. The bradycardia does disappear, even though one may continue removing multiple fatpads. The reflex may simply be a diminished effect of lidocaine on the trigeminal fibers.

Bernard Kaye (Jacksonville) has reported seeing the oculocardiac reflex once or twice. "It can be reduced or prevented by preoperative administration of Atropine or Robinul." My theory is that it is easy to "prevent" something that does not in reality happen. One or two instances of this syndrome in Kaye's busy practice does not convince me of its existence.

Tom Biggs (Houston) has reported seeing bradycardia following tugging on the medial fatpad. "I've always felt that it was due to ineffective infiltration of the local [anesthetic] than some kind of pain. I don't have any way of knowing what the cause of it is, however." Currently, Biggs performs few blepharoplasties under local anesthesia, as he reports being more satisfied "without fooling with any of that mess" of local anesthesia.

Robert Allan Smith (Jackson, Miss.) recalls watching McCarthy DeMere performing lower lid surgery. For some reason DeMere preferred to isolate the inferior oblique muscle. Perhaps he did it to show residents that when he tugged on it there was a prompt, sometimes profound bradycardia. Smith believes that those who discuss bradycardias may be reporting muscle-tugging bradycardia rather than fat-removal bradycardia.

Cheek Pads and Orbicularis Festoons

Those annoying thick areas just above the malar ridge and just beyond the orbital ridges have been referred to as "cheek pads." They are annoying because they are difficult to eliminate. Steroid injections may work but they may cause the undesirable side effect of a "hole" in the face. No surgeons excise directly through the cheek skin any more: Scars are too visible. Passing a suction lipectomy cannula against the malar bone and suctioning some of the deep soft tissue is a better way to solve the problem. Reaching down and directly excising through the blepharoplasty incision, in my experience, has been fraught with hemorrhages, recurrences, and failures. At times we thought it was almost better to leave them alone. Advocates of subperiosteal facelifts suture this thick fibrofatty tissue to temporal fascia. This is a lot of surgery for a little improvement.

Howard Gordon advises a wedge resection of the orbicularis with suturing to lift the redundant portion upward—during a face lift, of course. This method seems to be the best approach for the "festoons" of muscles that may lie directly underneath the redundant lower lid skin. Bruce Connell approaches the orbicularis from this face lift incision. He simply splits the orbicularis muscle and resects some of the redundancy. Sam Hamra divides the muscle and repositions it at a higher spot with a series of suspension sutures. Each approach is somewhat different from the more complex procedure proposed by Sherrell Aston several years ago.

A certain amount of the deformity can be removed during blepharoplasty with skin-muscle flaps. Aston uses larger muscle resection laterally than medially. This eyelid lift takes out some of the redundant or folded orbicularis.

Ice and Ice Bags

Cold compresses can be used to reduce initial edema, whether it is from a blepharoplasty or a sprained ankle. We have often followed the example that Peter Stokley (Miami) discussed years ago, which is to use iced saline as a continuous compress in open wounds during blepharoplasty. It also takes care of the small amounts of blood that would eventually work their way to the surface to form a visible blue or yellow mark.

The easiest way to prepare iced saline is to place a plastic jar filled with saline in the freezer 30 minutes before surgery. The saline gets cold enough but does not form enough ice to make it difficult to pour on 4 × 4 gauze pads.

Remove skin strips from both upper lids first. As soon as you have removed the skin strips for the upper lids and are ready to attack the fatpads, alternately pack these areas with iced saline. Once you have completed the lower lid, tuck the saline down deep in the incision and use it to cover both while you are working on the opposite side. Continue alternating these ice packs until you are ready to move the patient from the operating room. If you prefer to do blepharoplasty before rhytidectomy, as do most surgeons, it is easy to reduce edema by continued cooling with the iced saline pads.

It has been argued for years whether the delicate blepharoplasty procedure should be done when one is "fresh," or if raising the eyebrows during rhytidectomy would create distortion if the blepharoplasty skin excision is premarked. Long experience indicates that the latter concern is not valid, and the choice of precedence is a personal one. Most surgeons prefer performing blepharoplasty first.

Technical point: If the patient bleeds easily during the blepharoplasty (e.g., if taking aspirin or someone with labile hypertension), do not tie the final sutures—leave them open for later closure. Place a rubberband drain in the lid incisions and leave it in place for as long as 24 hours. It does not cause problems, and any remaining bloody fluid can be squeezed out later and the outside suture tied. We add Steri-Strip supports over the suture at that point. If you apply them earlier in "wet" cases, they slip free and are ineffective.

Cooling the operated area while the patient is in the recovery room is another important issue. Malcolm Paul and I once worked to improve the design of a blue gel ice pack that was commercially available. We could not, however, induce the manufacturer to accept a design for a thicker face mask cooling device that would hold cold long enough to be practical. You cannot freeze the mask because frozen it could cause a nasty skin burn; moreover, freezing a gel ice pack creates considerable difficulty in contouring it to the patient's face. Unfrozen it does not hold cold well. We finally gave up on the blue icebag face masks and switched to a more economical device, called Icebag. These devices are reusable and are practically indestructible. The Icebag is a plastic bag with a fold-over closure that is long enough to fit over the eyelids with room to spare. The thickness of the plastic allows filling the bag with crushed ice and placing it on top of wet pads, such as Tucks, which provide skin protection. We have seen no skin burns with the Icebag, and it is inexpensive.

Transconjunctival Blepharoplasty

Transconjunctival blepharoplasty is a hot topic because of the theoretic advantage of the incisionless operation. Steve Hoefflin believes it to be a good way to insert cheek implants because it provides easy access to the malar area with a periosteal elevator. He uses stabilization sutures, which is probably a good idea when working through this blind approach. Hoefflin suggests passing a tuberculin syringe through the incision and then bringing it out under the skin. A nylon suture is passed into the tuberculin syringe and withdrawn, similar to the way we once placed dermis grafts using the tip of a steel suction tip. Hoefflin passes the suture through the implant, positions it, and then passes it back out through the skin, tying it loosely over a bolster. I have not used this approach and feel constrained to warn readers against the concept of performing blepharoplasty from within the eyelid.

The first consideration is that transconjunctival approaches are not complication-free. We have always suspected that there are no surgical procedures without problems, but reports of complications went beyond simple ones such as conjunctival cysts and mild ectropions.

My objection to the transconjunctival blepharoplasty is that it simply is not a good procedure unless the patient has perfect, tight skin. Using the standard blepharoplasty, many patients have had wrinkled skin after fat removal—hence the idea of performing blepharoplasty transconjunctivally to remove fat and secondarily taking a strip of skin from under the lashes. If skin is to be removed, why not go ahead and do the operation, which provides the opportunity to hike up the muscle as well as tighten the skin? I cannot remember a single blepharoplasty patient since the 1970s who has not had some excess skin and who did not look better when that excess, no matter how small, was removed.

Critics point out only that removing fatpads left wrinkled skin (unacceptable to most patients) and did nothing for the redundant orbicularis muscle. Adding a TCA peel will help. We routinely peel our blepharoplasties now, but this only smooths tiny surface wrinkles.

Serious complications from transconjunctival blepharoplasty include bowing of the lid, lid malposition, dry eyes, and permanent diplopia—which are more serious than the minor problems of conjunctival cysts and prolonged bruising. Among five reported cases there was an injury to the inferior rectus and in three an injury to the inferior oblique. The last case was an injury to the lateral rectus. Ophthalmologic consultation and possible muscle surgery are indicated for all these patients.

Oculopharyngeal Dystrophy

Oculopharyngeal dystrophy is a strange syndrome. Matt Gleason (San Diego) reported a family with a combination of bilateral eyelid ptosis and myotonia of the esophageal muscles. Apparently this autosomal dominant disease is carried in families, appearing only after age 50 to 60. Approximately half of the members in the family he reported were affected.

Because the muscle is already weakened, Gleason advises leaving it alone and reducing the width of the tarsal plate using the Mustarde technique. With this method there is no interference with the function of an already weakened levator. He vertically pinches the tarsus up to move it away from the eyelid and then carefully cuts through it, finishing the cut with blunt scissors. Usually 8 mm can be removed. Gleason has stated that it is almost impossible to overcorrect the defect in these patients. A single-layer closure, leaving the conjunctiva in apposition, is adequate.

Use of Fish Oil and Postoperative Hematomas

An article in *Technical Forum* has warned about the antithrombotic effect of fish oil, which is being touted as a health aid. The promotion of fish oils, or marine omega-3 lipid concentrates, is based on tenuous scientific evidence of a reduced incidence of heart attack or stroke in Eskimos. Rex Peterson noted a case that demonstrated prolonged bleeding after ingestion of these compounds. The platelet reaction to fish oils is similar to that seen with ingestion of ibuprofin (Motrin, Advil, Nuprin). Peterson wrote: "I was very impressed with the ability of this material to cause prolonged surgical bleeding. My patient did not have a hematoma, but I had to work very hard to stop the bleeding from numerous minute and small bleeding points. This was much more dramatic than most people that I have operated in the past who have taken salicylates."

Although there is no strong evidence to support the claims, patients ingest fish oils because the oils are supposed to lower cholesterol and "decrease platelet activity." Query patients preoperatively about such intake because it takes 2 to 3 weeks to clear the patient's system of these oils.

Schirmer's Test

Schirmer's test, a measurement of tear flow, may be done in patients over age 40 for legal reasons, but does it make sense medically? The consensus is that this test is useless. It is more important to determine if a patient has a weak Bell's sign or infrequent blinking; these individuals are the ones who will have dry eyes or irritation problems after blepharoplasty. Should a routine tonometer test be done instead of a Schirmer's test? Perhaps if the patient is hypotensive and perhaps if there are symptoms suggesting glaucoma. The fact is that patients who reported "grittiness" or irritation of the eyes after blepharoplasty were equally divided between those who had a positive Schirmer's test and those who had negative tests.

It is useful to ask patients if they have had eye symptoms and then determine if they have a condition that limits tear duct production. Such individuals can be better evaluated by sophisticated ophthalmologic tests.

Comments and Commentary

1. "Ping-pong ptosis" is a term used to describe drooping of the opposite eyelid after a unilateral ptosis repair. The reason for the condition is probably reduced stimulus to the levators, which accents a mild ptosis that was not appreciated preoperatively.

2. It is not unusual to have to reoperate ptosis patients. Jim Carraway, one of the most knowledgeable ptosis surgeons, has said that it is not unusual to operate at least three times on the same patient. In fact, about 10% of his cases require reoperation. Seventy-five percent of surgeons favor levator shortening for this problem.

3. Few surgeons continue to use the French lateral extension procedure for upper lid blepharoplasty. Some plastic surgeons had become accustomed to seeing anguished patients with an upper lid incision that crossed the visible zone between the lid fold and the eyebrow. Apparently, someone had decided that elevating the corner of the eye was attractive and did not consider the effect of placing a highly visible scar on a suntanned area.

4. Among U.S. aesthetic surgery patients, who are discriminating and perhaps even overinformed, there are no acceptable "inconspicuous" scar areas.

5. If a favored blepharoplasty incision leaves "dog ears," you are doing something wrong.

6. When do you treat an ectropion after blepharoplasty? Tom Rees suggests waiting at least 6 months. His reasoning is based on the desirability of waiting for softening of tissue and the fact that many ectropions resolve with massage and compression.

7. Normal brow projection is 8 to 10 mm beyond the cornea. Do you care? This fact is important to Douglas Ousterhout, who designs acrylic onlays to correct flat foreheads. Ousterhout's group no longer uses cranial bone grafts because of the resorption rate. Their preference today is methylmethacrylate, and they reported 75 patients with excellent results. Modifications in the technique include molding directly onto the forehead with the scalp reflected. The disadvantage, according to Ousterhout, is that the exposure must be large enough that one does not spend all day filing down the excess amount of methylmethacrylate.

8. I prefer running Prolene sutures for the upper lids because the tension can be adjusted with the edema using Steri-Strips over the ends and because these sutures are easy to remove. On the lower lids removal is not as easy, but we have had consistently good results using a fast-dissolving catgut on the lower lids. One note of caution: Use a removal silk or nylon suture at the lateral canthal area because slight edema can pull this area apart if you rely on a catgut suture.

9. Another operation has withstood the test of time. Several years ago *Technical Forum* discussed the advisability of using tacking sutures to create a new supraorbital fold in non-Caucasians (Caucasians as well) with "hooded" upper lids. It was pointed out that elaborate suturing techniques produced results identical to those obtained by removing a wide muscle strip. Howard Gordon (Miami) reviewed his lengthy experience with the latter procedure and reported that he still believes that muscle strip removal is a better operation than classic supratarsal fixation.

10. Howard Gordon reminds us that incisions tend to migrate superiorly with time. Therefore it is good practice to place an inferior curved incision lower

on the upper lid than would normally be done and make the upslants medially and laterally. Gordon also believes that fewer inclusion cysts result in the upper lid if you use a subcuticular pull-out for skin closure. Others disagree. Whether you use subcuticular or running sutures that are removed every 4 to 5 days, it is good technically to use Prolene instead of nylon. (Removing subcuticular nylon sutures from an eyelid is extremely painful.)

11. Sal Castanares was once threatened with a lawsuit charging that he had caused unilateral blindness by his blepharoplasty technique. For some reason no one had checked the patient's vision prior to surgery. Fortunately, medical records existed that described the already-present blindness. I myself have had a new employee fill out the vision test form without looking at the patient—who later was shown ophthalmoscopically to have total corneal opacity. There is a lesson to be learned by these cases. An ophthalmologist is not needed to screen blepharoplasty patients, but you do need a simple vision and reading test for each eye plus your own ophthalmoscopic examination. Insurance companies are now requesting second opinions regarding patients with true obstruction of vision due to blepharochaliasis. It is at this point that the ophthalmologist is needed.

12. Crow's feet. Sherrell Aston still likes to operate on the orbicularis, although he reemphasizes a point that is clear to all veteran aesthetic surgeons: Not all patients derive cosmetic benefit from such a procedure. Is the extra dissection using Sherrell's approach to the lateral orbit worth the time and effort? I have always thought it was more a matter of separating the muscle from the skin, but Sherrell believes that skin undermining is not the most important part—splitting the muscle ring is. We concede that this procedure can make a significant difference in individuals with exceedingly heavy folds.

13. Sudden proptosis due to (presumably) deep bleeding is rare. In my single experience I followed the advice of an ophthalmologist, and gave intravenous acetazolamide (Diamox), to which there was a rapid response, and left all incisions open for drainage. He had said, "Don't even think about opening the anterior chamber." He was right. Within a few hours the globe was back in position, and we closed the incisions the next day.

14. We must agree with the conclusion that the blepharoplasty technique itself probably has little to do with the incidence of bleeding during and after the operation, and that the most important factors are failing to detect preoperative hypocoagulation states, debilitating disease, systemic hypertension or vasculopathies. We assume, of course, that such a state indicates the presence of mild, controllable hypertension.

15. Despite the furor in the past, few aesthetic surgeons fear retrobulbar hemorrhage to the point of its affecting their judgment in individual cases. One excellent San Antonio surgeon won his court case in a blepharoplasty–blindness action involving an elderly patient by emphasizing the truth of the matter: A vascular accident can occur before, after, or during any operation and may or may not have severe consequences for the patient. It has been said that surgeons "rightly" do not mention blindness when counseling preoperatively. I certainly mention this possibility to my patients, but only to reassure them that the chance of such an eventuality is remote and that more people suffer eye injuries while riding in automobiles with windows open than suffer injuries during eyelid surgery.

16. Robert Flowers (Honolulu) on eyelids:

> The comments on my presentation of "Canthopexy with Lower Lid Blepharoplasty" were read, and enjoyed. I was, however, left with a distinct feeling that there was some misunderstanding. I am not advocating in most cases an increased medial to lateral tilt of the eye, but rather the restoration of the normal youthful contour of the lid. A slight upwards tilt from medial to lateral of the intercanthal axis is a normal feature of eyelids, and when slightly exaggerated, can make for exquisite beauty. If you think about it, that, perhaps more than anything else, is the secret of the beauty of many of our loveliest ladies—Sophia Loren, for instance. The aging of an eyelid results in attenuation of the lateral canthal tendon, and stretching of the lid margin, resulting in a lowered posture of the lower lid. A properly done lower lid blepharoplasty should address first of all the problem of reduced tonicity, restoring it to a normal position, and secondly the removal of redundant or excessive tissues. The restoration to a normal position requires an initial overcorrection to result in a normal long-term result.

17. Can we believe that fat obtained during blepharoplasty makes a better graft than other fat? The cells are smaller, the lipase activity is less, and it has different fatty acids—but are these traits important? A lower cell turnover rate in a bulk graft (which also needs a blood supply) is supposed to make a difference.

18. European surgeons allow long scars after blepharoplasty. Moreover, the scars they create curl upward and cross the visible zone between the eyebrow and the upper lid crease. U.S. patients would find these scars unacceptable.

19. Sheldon Rosenthal (Los Angeles) has reported his use of laser blepharoplasty. Theoretically, using laser should decrease edema and ecchymoses, but Rosenthal is not sure about that. First it is easy to burn tissue with laser, and second is the time involved. Most of the oozing seen during blepharoplasty derives not from skin but from muscle edges, and a quick touch with cautery stops this bleeding. Perhaps for a patient who cannot take epinephrine laser is an advantage. Patients who undergo laser blepharoplasty take longer to heal. An advantage of laser blepharoplasty is that you do not have to worry about losing the lashes on the lower lids.

20. Alberto Sanchez (San Juan, Puerto Rico) on blepharoplasty: "For the upper lid, take twice as much as you think you are going to need to remove. On the lower lid, take only half as much."

21. Anthony Sokol (Beverly Hills) has had some success with an *eyebrow suspension* in which he turns back a flap of soft tissue and imbricates it. Apparently the wider area of soft tissue (the flap is based superiorly and is a square measuring 2 to 3 mm in each dimension) provides more permanent adherence and holds the brow in its new position above the rim. He says the brow then stays there.

22. John Lewis (Atlanta) on *eyebrow elevation:* "This . . . technique that I reported . . . has worked well for me, though I find the permanent suture is necessary for many patients who raise and elevate their eyebrows a good bit or are very expressive in their faces. The absorbable sutures simply don't hold long enough to allow for good support and fixation."

23. Pain in the hand syndrome. The nurse has just started an antecubital intravenous infusion and the first dose of diazepam (Valium) is injected. The patient suddenly grabs his hand, which is turning white, and screams with pain. What happened? Probably the needle is in the artery. *Do not remove the needle.* It is in perfect position for flushing out the artery and preventing distal thrombosis. Dexamethasone (Decadron), lidocaine (Xylocaine), 1 ampul of phentolamine (Regitine), and heparin should be given directly through the intraarterial line until the spasm subsides and arterial flow is reestablished.

24. Ron Gum (El Paso) is another who has abandoned subcuticular closure on the upper lid. He was not satisfied with the approximation achieved and the fact that sutures occasionally broke during removal.

25. For loose lower lids in elderly people, make the wedge resections for the modified Kuhnt-Symonowsky (K-S) procedure laterally, not medially. Stay about 2 mm from the commissure and resect a full wedge. Tom Rees made this point and emphasized that separate closures of the conjunctiva (a là Mustarde) are no longer done. There is still a place for imbrication sutures laterally to support these lax older lids. The lateral muscle can be directly excised with the same effect.

26. Beware of microcauterization blepharoplasty. A review of blepharoplasty procedures has included the technique of multiple pinpoint cauterizations to tighten the elderly patient's orbicularis muscle. There may be a place for this procedure in some patients, but I can attribute two definite complications to the technique. If it is necessary to resect the muscle, do so—it is a clean, safe procedure. If you must elevate it and tack it, do that. Cautery may result in a difficult situation by creating a band of scar tissue in the muscle that can pull the edge of the eyelid down. A second surgery to release the orbicularis band is the embarrassing solution to the problem.

27. Ulrich Hinderer suggested a simple technical maneuver before performing blepharoplasty in elderly people. In addition to checking the "rebound"

of the lower lid, measure the length of the border of the lower lid. If it is greater than normal, plan a lateral Kuhnt-Symanowski wedge excision.

28. Matt Gleason (San Diego) added a new dimension to alleviating the heavy or "hooded" upper eyelid—skin debulking. He pointed out that frontalis fat may slide over the supraorbital rim and descend into the area of the upper lid. Simply removing a wide muscle strip and the lateral fatpad may not be sufficient. Removing these fatty areas underneath the orbicularis can be an important contribution to a high, curved aesthetic eyelid. I must warn against excessive removal in men, however, and point out that everting the orbicularis may reveal a thick fibrofatty layer, the removal of which may be sufficient. Gleason also advised suturing the edge of the orbicularis to the orbital rim, which creates a skin-muscle flap with fixation in the normal eyebrow position and relieves the effect of eyebrow ptosis.

29. What do you do about the patient with intraocular lenses after cataract resection who needs a blepharoplasty? Must you worry about dislodging the lens? With modern lenses the fixation devices are relatively secure. It would take enormous pressure on the globe to force one of them out of its fixed position. The consensus is that intraocular lenses are not a contraindication to blepharoplasty.

8 Rhinoplasty

Rhinoplasty is still one of the most difficult and challenging procedures of cosmetic surgery. Pollybeaks, scar retraction, "floppy septums," and other problems will plague us to the end of our days. Despite the problems, we are doing a better job now than we were during the 1970s. Back then we used nasal saws to cut through the bone. Now we use a chisel and simply pop the bone inward. We no longer transect the tip cartilages, and we do not see the superresected bird-beak tips that we once associated with Latin Americans. When we add grafts for tip elevation, we choose cartilage, with or without an overdrape of temporalis fascia in the tip of the nose, and know that it will stay there. The open technique has added a dimension to the difficult nose repair, although it is certainly not the procedure of choice for the average rhinoplasty. We are more aware of the turbinates and do not hesitate to cauterize and out-fracture the inferior or even the medial turbinate or resect them, as needed. We are aware that in most rhinoplasty patients only the distal part of the nasal bone flares and a complete bony transection is not necessary, a procedure that certainly caused distressing edema and ecchymoses.

Technical Overview

Most nose surgeries are safely and easily performed in an office setting under Ketamine Valium (K-V) anesthesia or some other type of sedation. We no longer use Vaseline nasal packing, as it contributes to discomfort and spreading of the nasal bones, and it creates a painful interval for the patient when it is removed. During the 1980s we took Gene Courtiss's advice and began using Gelfoam packs not only for hemostasis of the turbinates but to hold the nasal bones in place. The Gelfoam packs, K-V anesthesia, and postoperative bupivacaine (Marcaine) blocks of the infraorbital and paranasal nerves have made rhinoplasty a relatively pleasant experience.

It is helpful to use blowup photographs and have the patient sketch with you. I am not a fan of the computer imager; it makes people look too good, and the image cannot be reproduced in real life. I would rather have the patient work with me and understand the limitations. We take lifesize photographs and obtain copies on the office copier. The patient can then erase and draw with me to their heart's content.

Have a plan before you start and write it in the chart during the first interview. Add details at the second interview. A preprinted anatomic sheet is helpful. Look for the hanging columella and the alar widths. See if you can reduce the columella width or even resect soft tissue in a thick nostril. Can you smooth the dorsum with a sander, or is more needed? I have given up chiseling the dorsum because the method is not easily controlled. Have a variety of rasps on the operating table and use the rough ones first, the smoother ones next, and a "polisher" last. It is much easier to remove a little more than to build it back up because the chisel took away too much bone.

Always be ready to do a touchup at minimal cost. Turbinates sometimes swell and press the nasal bones to a wider position. At times skin refuses to shrink despite massaging, night tape pressure, and an occasional steroid injection.

Always check the airway of any rhinoplasty patient. You can almost always create more airway space by pressing toward the vomer and away from the vomer with a flat "cake knife" spatula.

Dressings are of paramount importance. In our specialty, we learn the value of proper taping and support of tissues. I paint the nose with Benzoin and then use small overlapping strips of 0.5 inch paper tape, which usually lets moisture through. Be careful to change the strips regularly, avoiding such complications as full-thickness scars. Avoid excessive edema with ice packs on the eyes and some type of oral or intravenous steroid. Choices are intravenous hydrocortisone (Solu-Cortef) or methylprednisolone (Medrol Dosepak). If bruising should occur, administer hyaluronidase (Wydase) with lidocaine (Xylocaine) injections, particularly in self-conscious patients (a Steve Hoefflin idea that works well).

Postoperatively, our patients start a nasal spray on the third day. It soaks the Gelfoam packs, keeps down some of the swelling, and eventually opens the airway more rapidly. Prescribe any good antihistamine to start on the day after surgery. I prefer 12-hour Ornade.

Other technical tips: once you have a plan for reducing the width of the

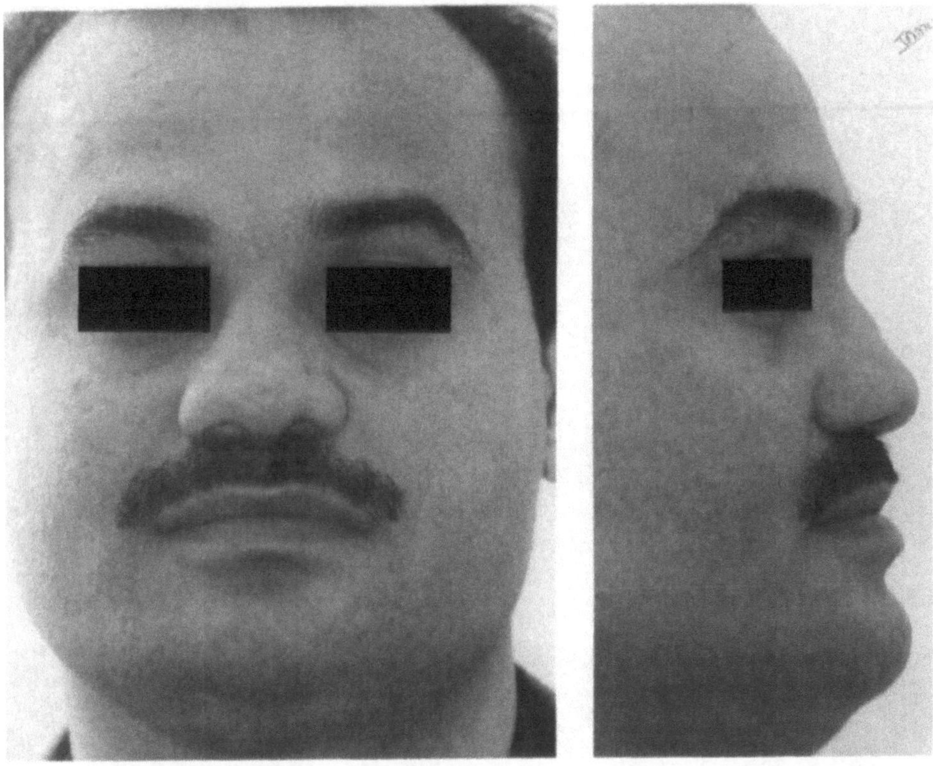

Figure 8-1. For a tough secondary rhinoplasty such as this one, the main concern is the airway. Next comes tip bulk and the splayed-out nasal bones. In this case the anterior septum had been resected, leaving this retraction. The turbinates were giant-sized. Our plan included the following.

1. Cauterize and out-fracture or resect the lower and middle turbinates.
2. If the septum is too scarred and the mucosa atrophic, try blunt repositioning rather than resection.
3. Debulk the tip with LLC excisions and direct thinning of the subdermal tissue and subcutaneous fat.
4. Remove an alar floor wedge.
5. Place a cartilage and fascial graft to the supratip depression.
6. Place a tip graft for elevation. LLCs are not separated, so the open technique with midline suturing of LLCs is not indicated.
7. Sand the maxilla adjacent to the origin of the nasal bones, then in-fracture.
8. Swing the septum back to center with chisel separation from the nasal spine back to the vomer.
9. Either graft the nasal spine area or use the "star-fighter" preformed Giunta premaxillary implant.

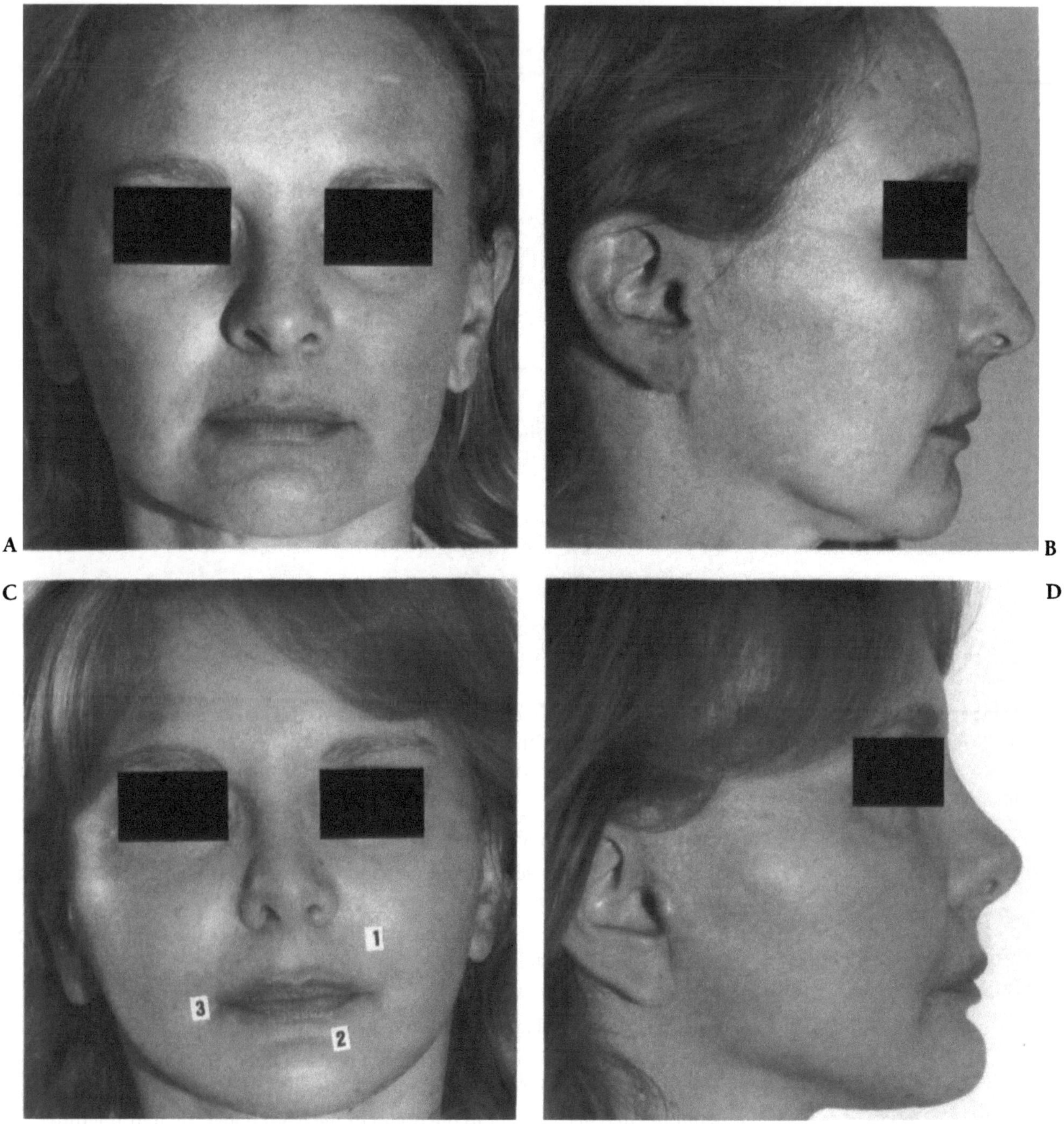

Figure 8-2. **(A&B)** The closed technique is best for this patient. Her columella "show" was corrected by partial posterior resection of the descending LLCs and suturing to the newly tilt-trimmed distal septum. The right nostril was advanced more than the left. **(C&D)** At 30 days postoperatively expect to see an almost finished nose. Note the tragal size and position, the effect of jowl liposuction, nasolabial and lip fat grafts, and the submental tuck effect combined with a rhytidectomy. The chin and malar prostheses effect is

lower lateral cartilage (LLC), consider removing some of the foot plates and cross-suturing the *base* of the columella. Simple rasping of the dorsum and some trimming of the midline upper lateral cartilage (ULC) keeps the nose flat and slender. Consider scoring the domes, particularly for a pointed nose, to allow the LLCs to fall downward. Consider resecting the distal LLC in "Pinocchio" tips. We use the closed (not open) technique. Use blunt scissors to free the nasal skin *widely* to give it its best chance of contracting to the new shape. If the nasal bridge is too wide, make a cut on either side of the septum with the saw and then in-fracture. Removing this 1 to 2 mm of bone creates a more attractive dorsum.

Helpful Hints

1. Have the patient bring magazine photographs showing the nose type he or she likes. This practice then allows you to point out facts they may not appreciate. Point out differences in the angle, bone structure, skin quality, and so forth. Emphasize the points that you wish to achieve, such as a thin tip, high points, and narrowing; point out how his or her nose will differ from those in the magazine. This exchange gives you and the patient a good basis for planning the final shape of the nose.
2. Prepare a counseling book. Show "before" and "after" pictures with good and bad results. The bad results should reflect cases in which texture of skin, healing problems, and acne played a role. Show touch-up surgeries and describe them in detail. Show the various profiles that may or may not fit the patient's face.

---

still too pronounced at this point. Patients should be forewarned that softening of the facial features may take 6 months or more. We did not ignore her flat midface and signs of aging: atrophy in the nasolabial area of the lips and the area below the commissure that we call the marionette zone. These problems can be corrected at one session. Suction in the jowl area was important too. For young patients' face lifts, it is important to place the incision *inside* the tragus because for some reason many of them form thicker scars. At 1 month postoperatively the malar implant is in place but is slightly prominent. The wrap-around low-profile extended chin prosthesis is too prominent. It is well to remember that the implants settle within a month or two. At the preoperative counseling book session, she chose a high tipped nose, and we grudgingly obliged. The patient and I sketched it in on her own 8 × 10 photograph. At 1 month, if a nose is too high, the patient can gradually smooth it down with downward fingertip massage.

This patient is a good illustration of the methods employed to make the tragus smaller when one places the face lift incision inside the ear. The deep suture of 2-0 Dexon anchored in the pretragal fascia not only relieves tension in front of the ears so the scars are as good as this one at 30 days, it makes a more natural-appearing tragus.

3. When possible perform the rhinoplasty under K-V anesthesia. Less bruising occurs with this method because the patient stays quiet and relaxed for hours.
4. Use ice packs immediately after surgery. The see-through packs should be kept in the refrigerator, not frozen.
5. At home the patient should have a package of witch hazel pads (Tucks) in the freezer. These ice-cold pads can be alternated with the see-through blue mask. The pads also soak up tears if the patient has had a blepharoplasty at the same time.
6. Use dissolving packs of Gelfoam. They create little pressure, there is no pain on removal, and the patient is comfortable with them.
7. At the end of every facial surgery, particularly rhinoplasty, block the nerves and then the whole area with 1% bupivacaine with epinephrine. Flush the solution into the dorsum under the skin that you elevated. Make the rhinoplasty a pleasant, easy procedure.
8. Do not hesitate to discuss other facial changes. Point out that, for example, a patient has no malar prominences, or has a deep, lateral groove that can be filled with a fat graft, or lacks fullness in the chin, or perhaps has a short upper lip.
9. If there is a short upper lip remove a portion of the nasal spine and free up the soft tissue subcutaneously with blunt scissors point.
10. Do not waste time carefully dissecting the periosteum away from the dorsal nasal bone. Sand it all off. Use a series of rasps of varying degrees of roughness and finish with a fine polisher after the nasal in-fracture is completed.
11. If the columella protrudes too far forward ("columella show") resect the back edge of the descending portion of the lower lateral cartilage. During mucosal closure be sure that the mucosa is tacked *directly* to the septal cartilage; otherwise it drifts down.
12. Use alar wedges for nostril width reduction in most patients. Shortening the nose always widens the base.
13. At the end of every nasal surgery, cosmetic or otherwise, use a flat blade to out-fracture the turbinates and to centralize any deviation in the vomer. One or two moments of pressure in each direction provides a better airway.
14. Do not hesitate to cauterize normal-appearing turbinates. If the patient has a history of allergies, the benefit of this measure will manifest 5 years later when their nasal passages do not become as congested. Large turbinates can enlarge during the immediate postoperative period and spread nasal bones.

(Text continued on page 183)

Figure 8-3. (A) This patient had had a chin augmentation in 1983 and an eyelid peel and facial fat grafts in 1987. **(B&C)** Preoperative photographs. **(D&E)** Note the lasting effects of the nasolabial fat grafts. Unfortunately, she has developed a complication after a rhinoplasty done elsewhere in 1990. **(D–G)** Preoperative worksheets for a secondary rhinoplasty. We chose spreader grafts, splint grafts for the septal curvature, turbinatectomy, and alar rim grafts. We also planned to remove intranasal nostril floor scar tissue and a collapsed left LLC **(G)**. **(H–K)** Results are shown at 4 months and 1 year. The transcolumellar scar is less obvious, and she has excellent airflow. The only remaining problem is the slow descent of the tip. At 4 months the tip position was good **(H&I)**, but at 1 year it was not **(J&K)**. It is not a major problem and can be corrected easily without a third open approach.

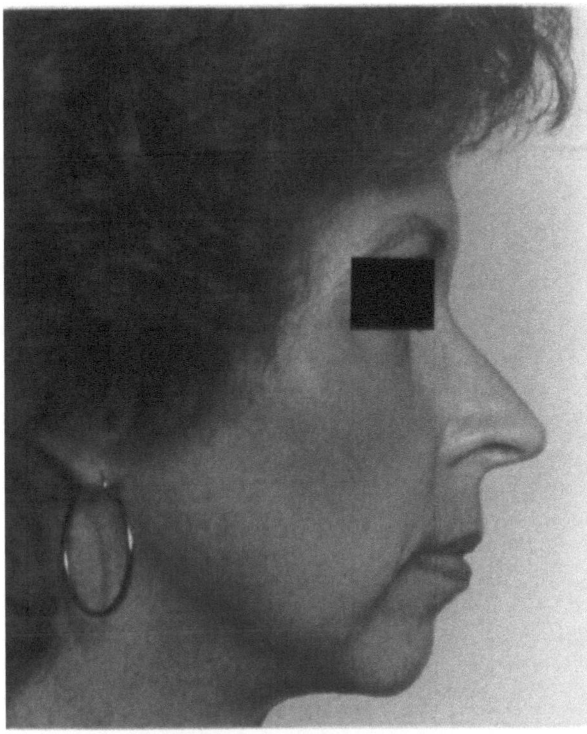

A

B

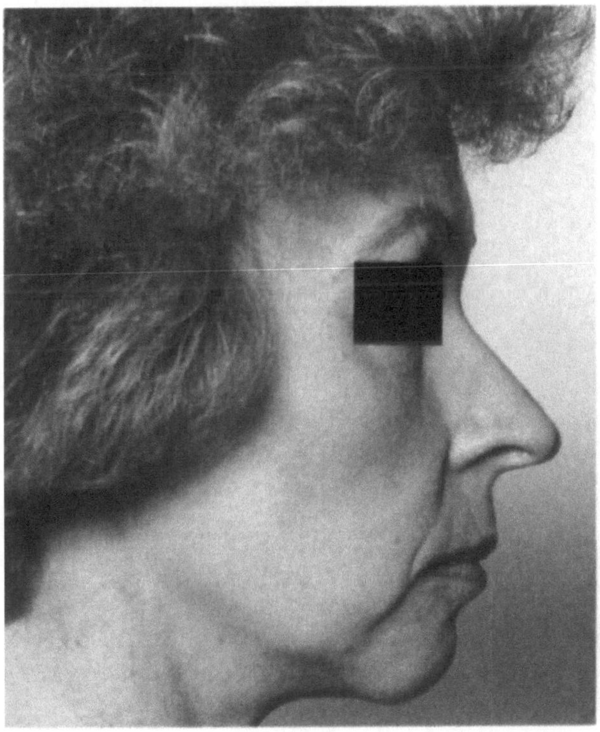

C

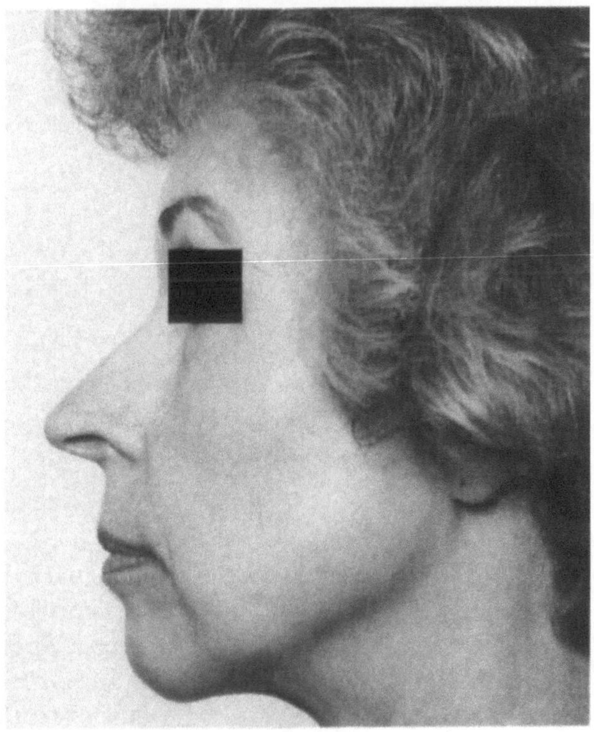

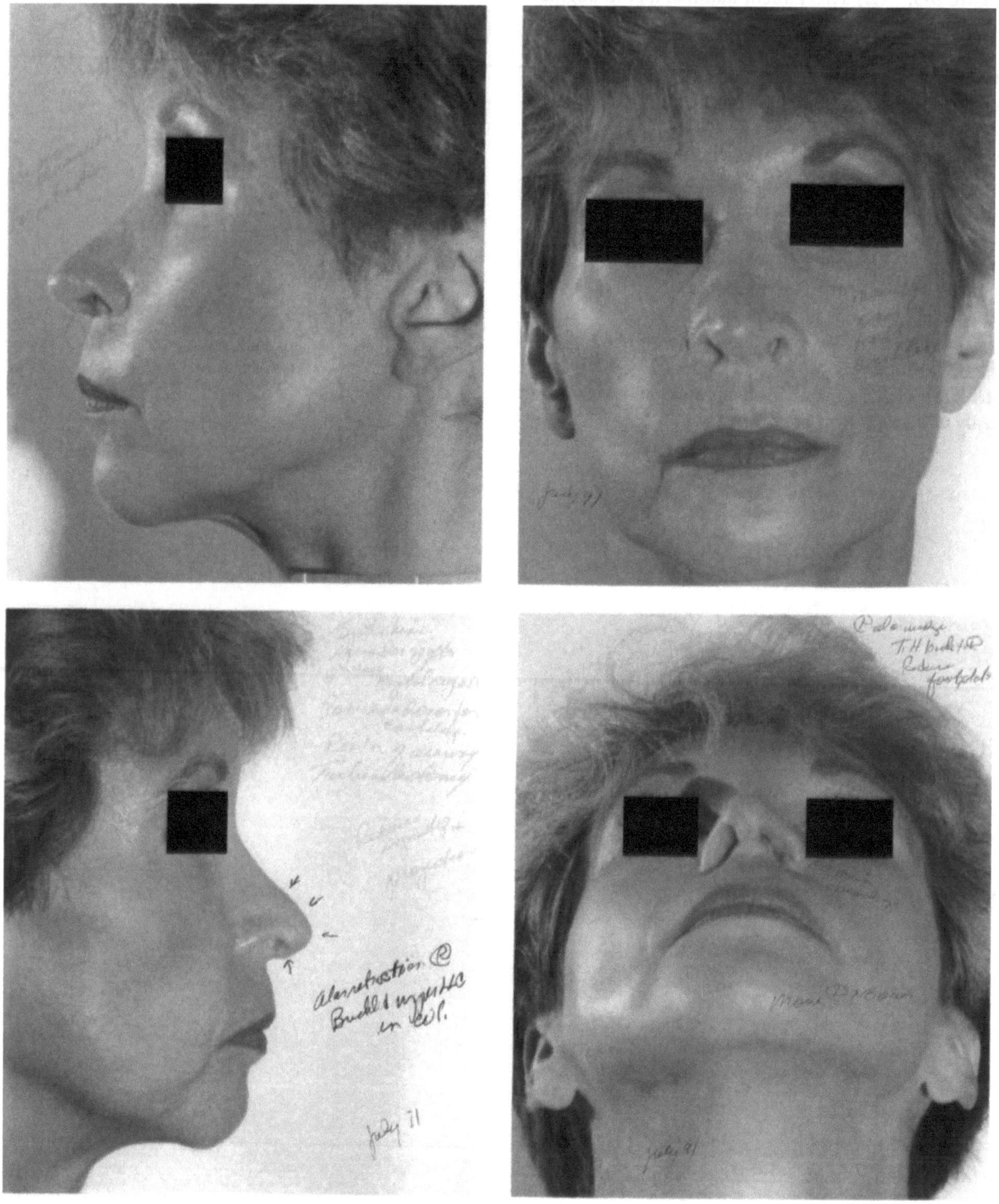

D E F G

Figure 8-3 (continued)

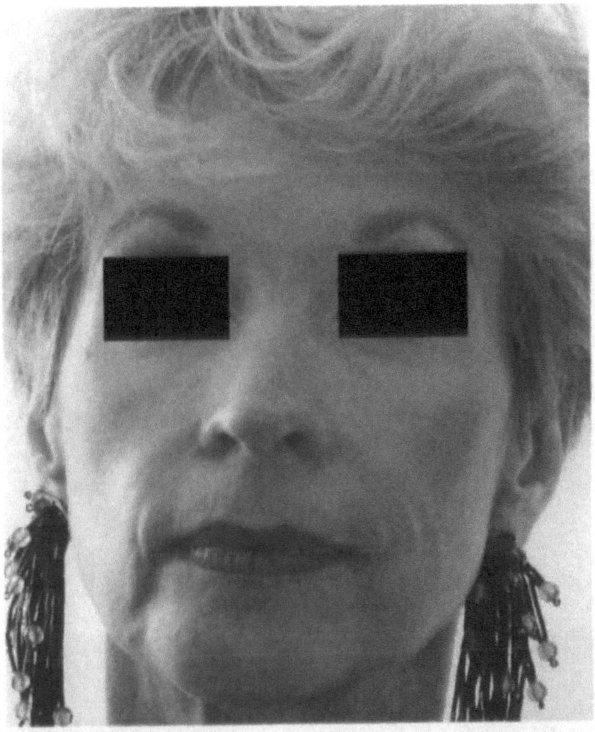

H

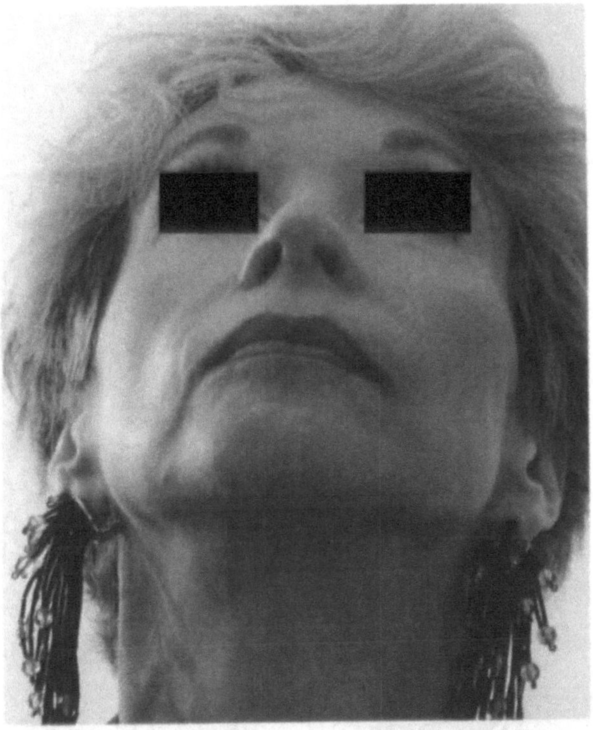

I

J

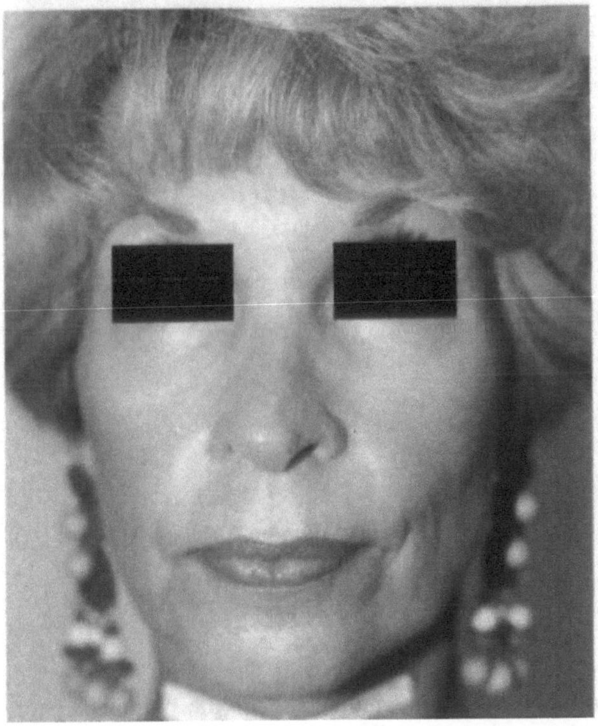

K

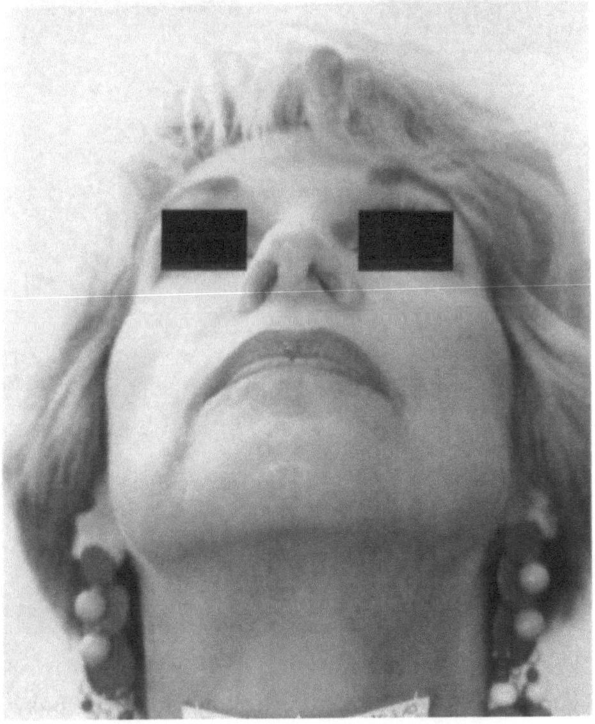

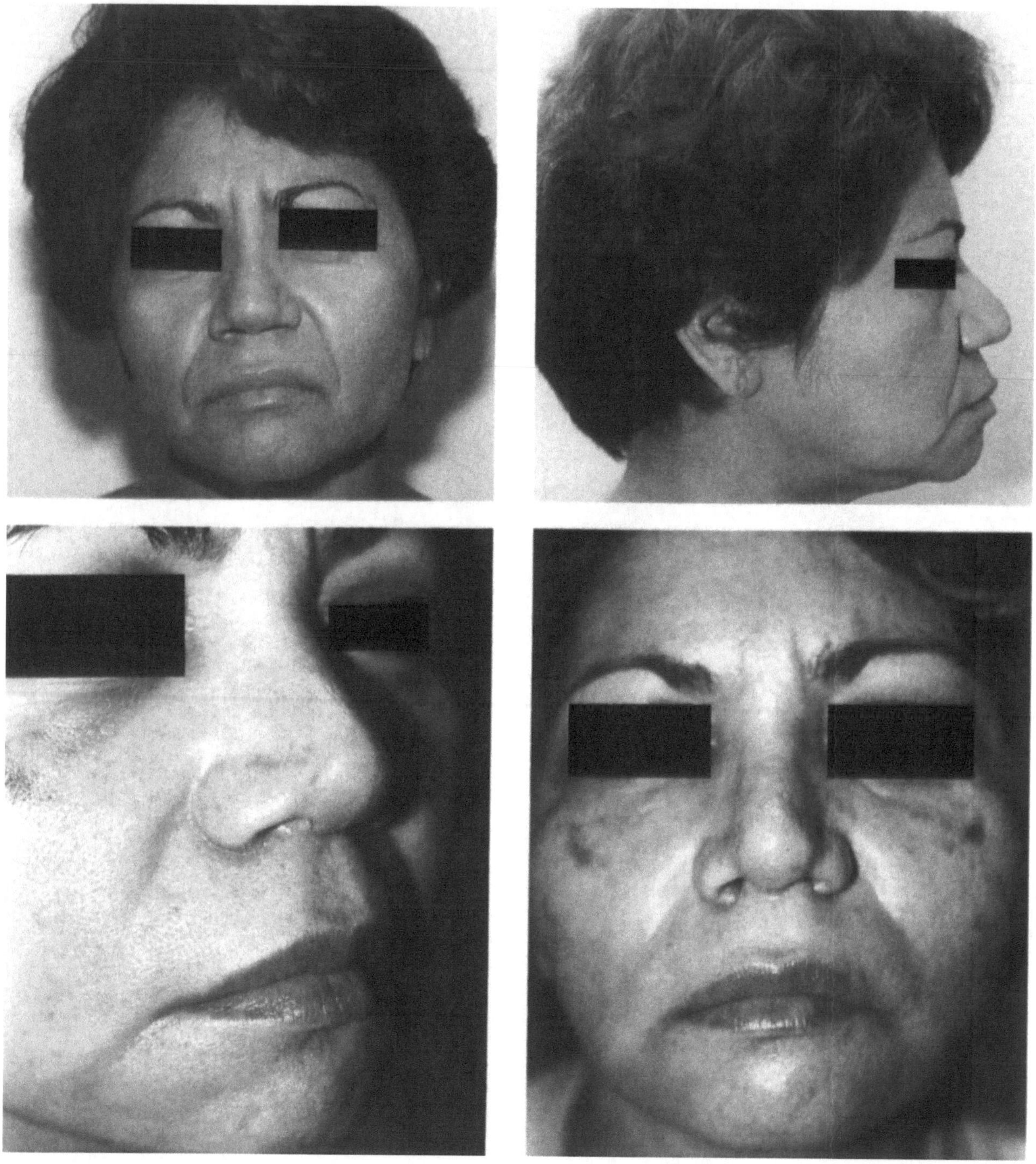

A B C D

Figure 8-4. **(A&B)** With thick skin, wide ULC, boxy tip, and a retracted columella, this patient is a good candidate for open rhinoplasty with a septal cartilage tip graft. Note the alar incision scars **(C&D)** tucked out of site. For pigmented skin, I prefer to place the open columella incision at the base of the columella, not midway. Note the effect of the midface rhytidectomy with liposuction of the nasolabial fold zones and fat grafts to the lips and nasolabial folds. The LLCs were sutured together to elevate the tip as well.

Rhinoplasty for African Americans

Steve Hoefflin (Santa Monica) has extensive experience with rhinoplasty for African Americans. The same principles apply to Mexican American noses as well, which have a similar bulky, wide appearance. Among Hoefflin's "commandments" are the following.

1. Establish realistic goals, making sure the patient understands that it is not possible to obtain a thin, tapering tip, for example.
2. He also advises staged procedures to approach the thinness gradually because of the particular anatomy. These noses have less supportive cartilage and abundant subcutaneous tissue.
3. Use every method possible to reduce edema, such as antibiotics, diphenhydramine (Benadryl) 50 mg IV (to decrease histamine release), and dexamethasone (Decadron) 10 mg IV. (Hoefflin believes the Medrol Dosepak is ineffective, whereas I found just the opposite.)
4. Do not use septal cartilage for the tip projection, as it is too firm. (Others I canvassed disagreed. Often the lower lateral remnants are not thick enough or the right size.)
5. An important technical point: Tape the patients' noses at night for about 6 weeks. Decrease salt intake, and remind the patient that edema in the tip is the last to disappear.

Hoefflin has never had a keloid develop from a Millard-type alar arch thinning excision. The incision is just inside the edge.

Technical point: When preparing the tip of the nose, be sure to free all the fibrofatty tissue and trim it as necessary. Vicryl mesh or temporalis fascia can be used over tip grafts to smooth the contour. Finally, remember that swelling in African-American noses may take 2 years to subside fully.

Difficult Rhinoplasty and Open Rhinoplasty

The nose that is difficult to repair can be fixed easily with the open rhinoplasty approach, particularly with noses that have had prior surgeries. The bumps, dips, and displaced tip grafts are in plain view using the open approach. Reaching the septum to obtain graft material is somewhat difficult, but it can be done. The advantages of the open approach are as follows.

1. One can see the LLCs and easily suture them together to decrease columellar width and to raise the tip.
2. Scoring the LLCs is easy (and necessary to make a graceful curve).

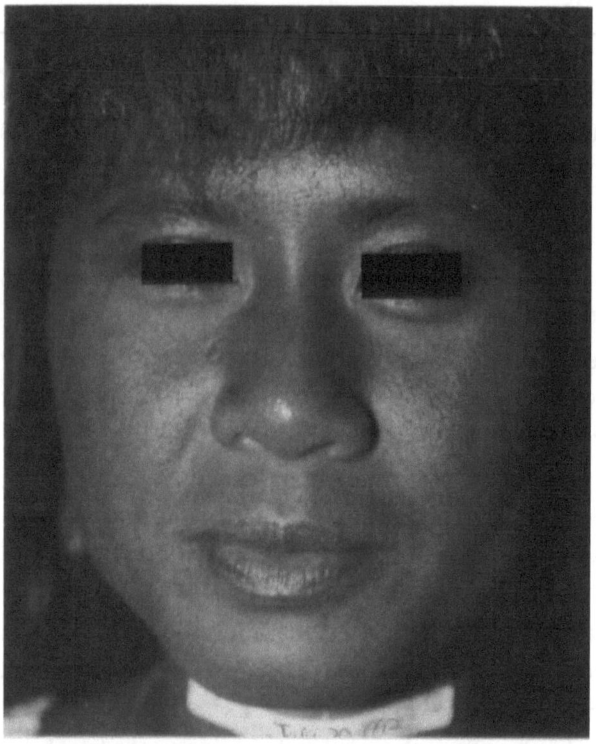

A

Figure 8-5. **(A–C)** This young woman with a mixed racial background (Asian plus African) complained that her nose dominated her face, making her look masculine, and that her Oriental eyelids were not attractive. Our task was to approach both at the same time to create a more harmonious face. A skin care program was instituted to change the texture and lighten the color of her skin. An open rhinoplasty was planned with alar wedge advancement and resection of the nostril above the nasal groove. This maneuver shortens the distance between the tip and the base of the ala. A tip graft placed by the open technique would follow resection of the excess LLC, sanding of the dorsum, and midline suturing of the mobilized remaining LLCs. For the eyelid, we chose a modified double Z-plasty along with upper lid blepharoplasty to remove the excess fat. **(D–F)** Note the

B

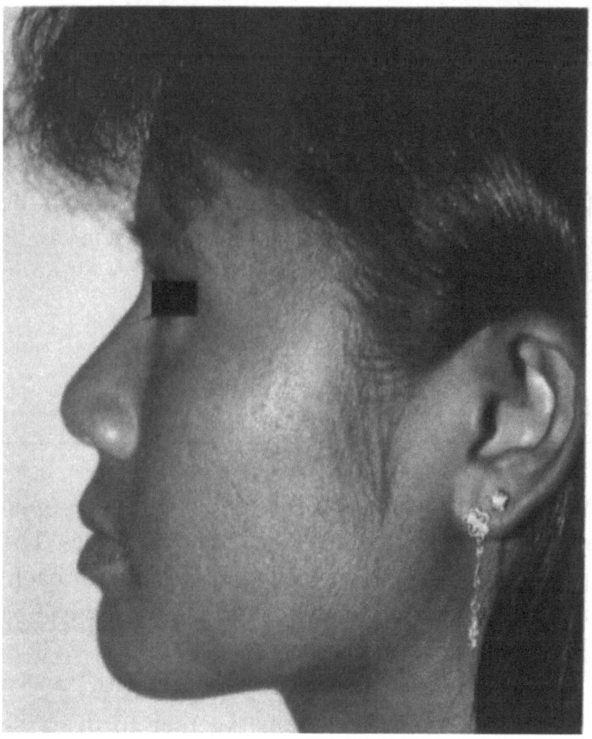

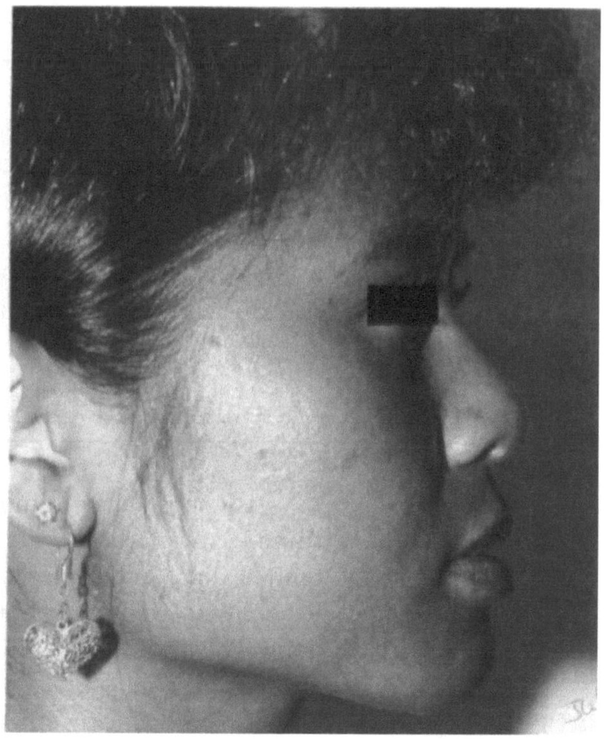

C

deepening of the eye, elevation of the tip of the nose, decrease in the width of the nose, and barely visible scars lateral to the ala. These scars must be tucked under with a deep suture of Dexon or Vicryl so they do not drift outward into the visible zone. These 3-month photographs show good resolution of the process. Defatting of the undersurface of the nasal tip, easily accomplished using the open technique; allowed more rapid contracture and decreased the bulkiness. Note the effect of good skin care and bleaches. Scar massage was started during the second or third postoperative week. Until then, protective taping was used to avoid shifting or pulling due to sudden motion. Patients sometimes move around and create problems when they are asleep. Note the change in pore size and skin texture that has resulted from the α-hydroxy acid and 0.05% Retin-A regimen.

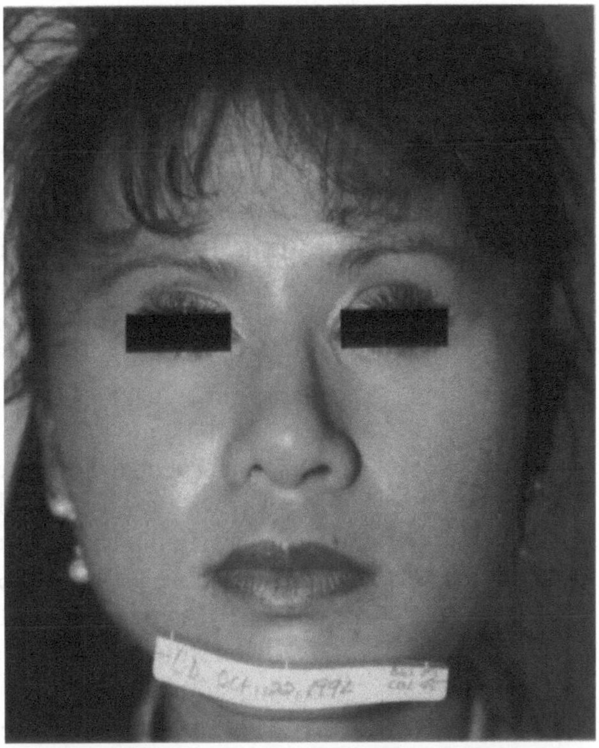

D

E

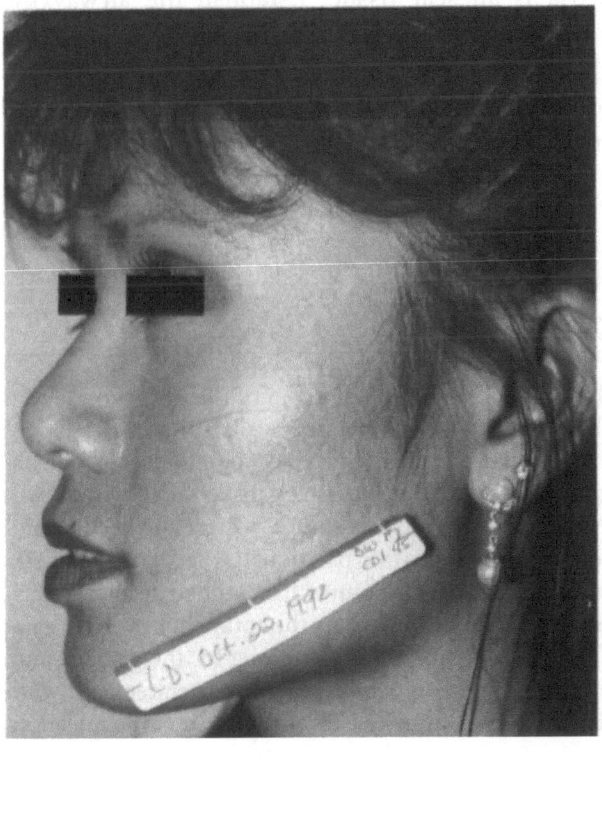

F

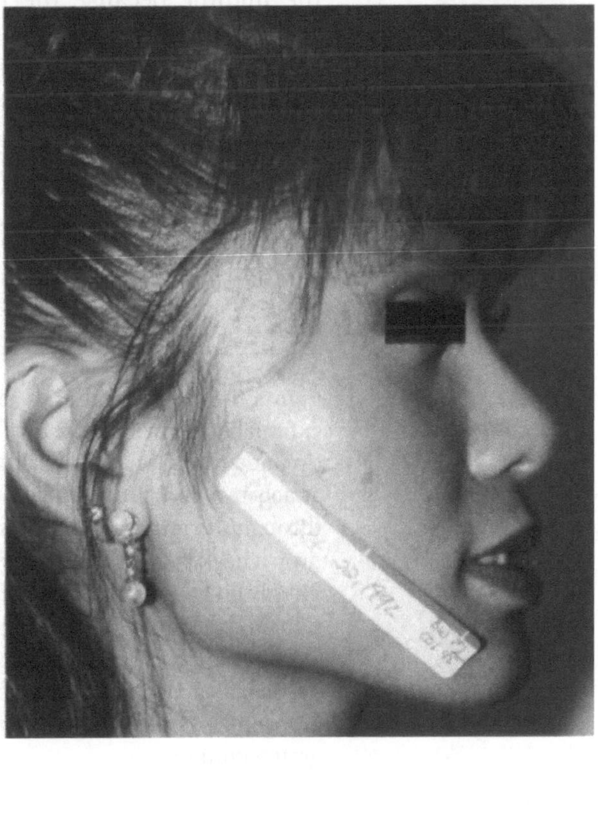

3. Tip grafts remain in place when they are sutured directly. It is easy to add another suture if the graft begins to wobble.
4. There is no problem regarding the reinforcement of struts or "spreader" grafts. Scoring the septum is not as easy, but the mucosa does not have to be opened from below to do it.

The worst problem with this technique is that its proponents use it in all patients. In many cases the result is too up turned or too tall after this procedure. Few individuals have, or can carry off, that high tip. On the other hand, the open suturing of LLCs is the best way to approach the broad, flat-tipped nose.

Are "spreader grafts" a fad? Oscar Ramirez uses them in 50% of rhinoplasties in teenage patients. I use them only for the rare secondary repair of a pinched dorsum.

The scar on the columella due to the open technique is not a major problem, but it is wise to incise at the *base* of the columella in African Americans and Hispanics. Rollin Daniel found that only 2% of the midcolumellar incisions were "unacceptable." Only 12% of Rollin's incisions were visible to the casual observer. Technical point: Use a deep chromic suture in the center followed by 6-0 nylon sutures in the left and right corners. Fill in the spaces between with 6-0 tacking sutures.

For some secondary repairs, only the septum and vomer can be squeezed to the midline because the mucosa is all scar tissue. Establish the airway by out-fracturing, cauterizing, or removing the inferior and middle turbinates.

It is not accurate to say that all the poor rhinoplasty results can be blamed on the fact that they were done endonasally. Furthermore, even the most vehement supporters of open rhinoplasty are slowly decreasing their percentage of open procedures.

(Text continued on page 191)

Figure 8-6. A fascial graft can be introduced into the dorsum of the nose without an external incision after the area to be grafted has been separated by placing a small suction tip under the skin and pressing it against the skin edge. Then pass a Keith needle with an attached nylon suture into the barrel of the suction tip so it can be safely withdrawn through the intranasal incision. Hook the graft onto this suture, reverse the needle, and drop it back inside the barrel. When the barrel slides into position, the needle is sheathed. Simply give a tug on the nylon suture, and the needle point will emerge so it can be safely punched through the skin. Pull the graft into position and tie the suture lightly. Hence no excision is necessary to position the graft. We used this technique for the glabella and nasolabial area when we employed dermal fat grafts, which have now been replaced with autogenous concentrated fat, which can be positioned easily and applied via an injection graft technique.

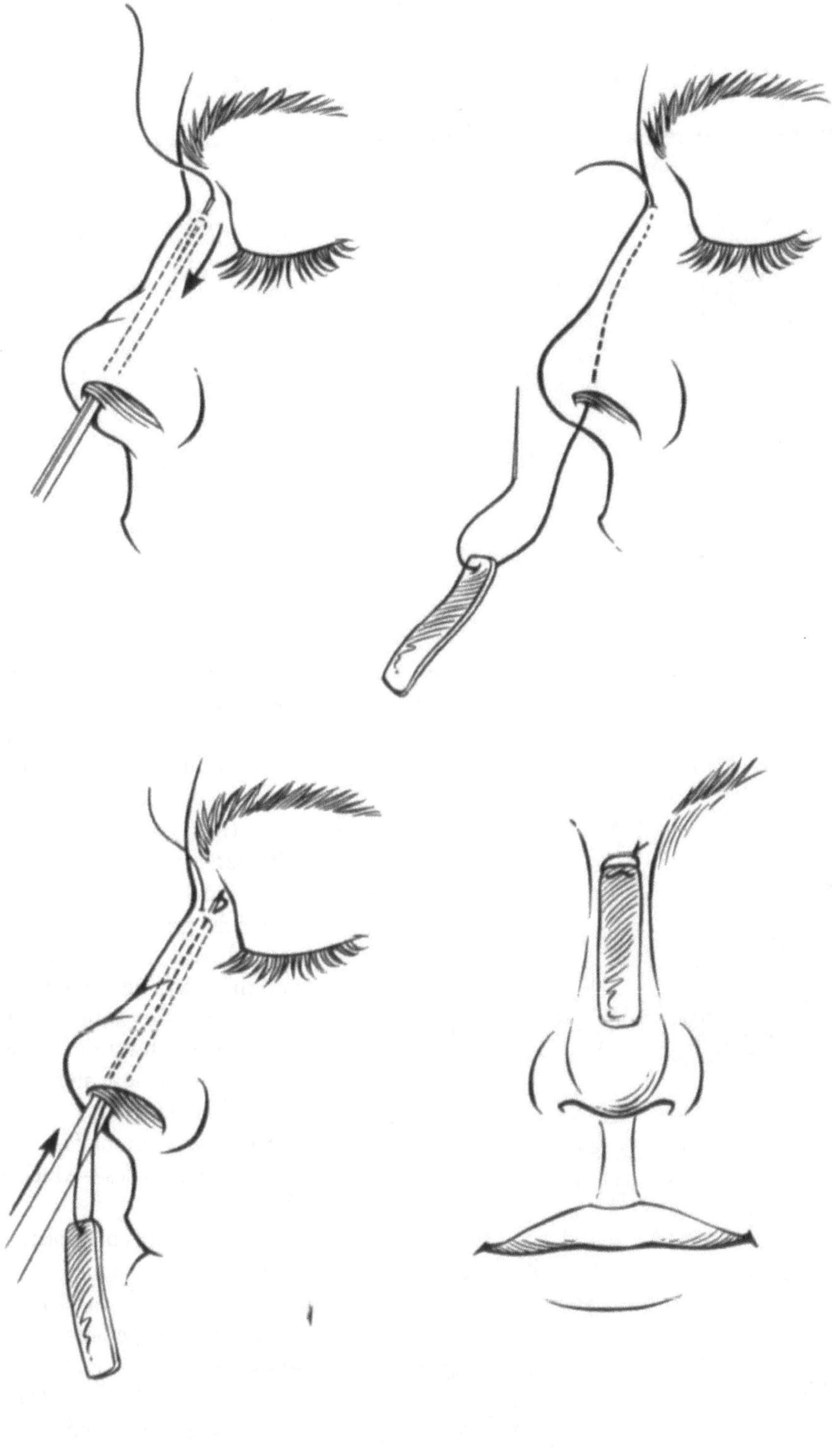

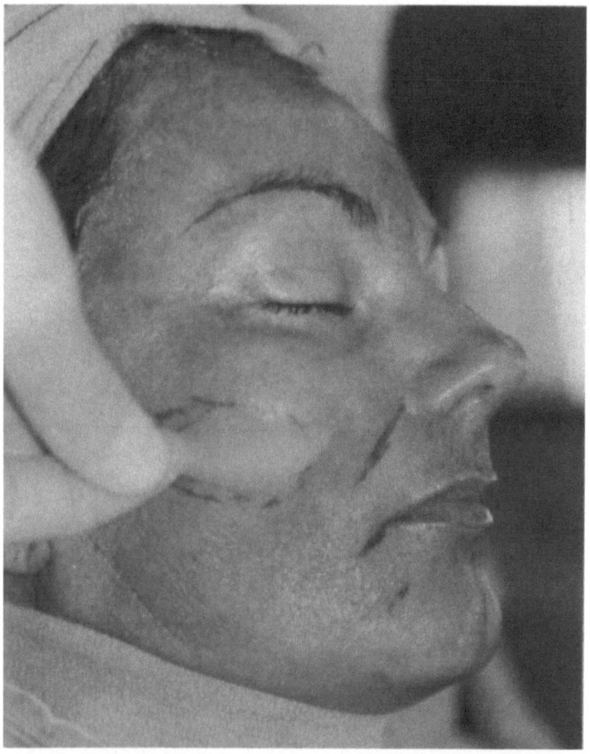

A

B

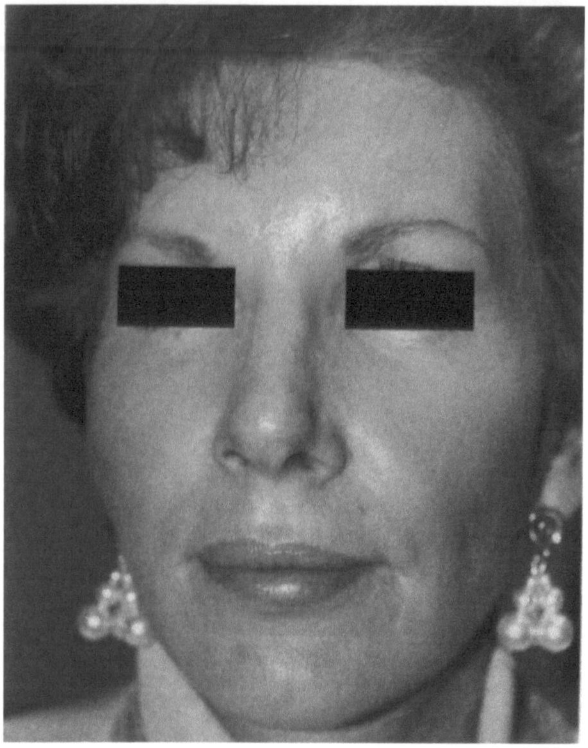

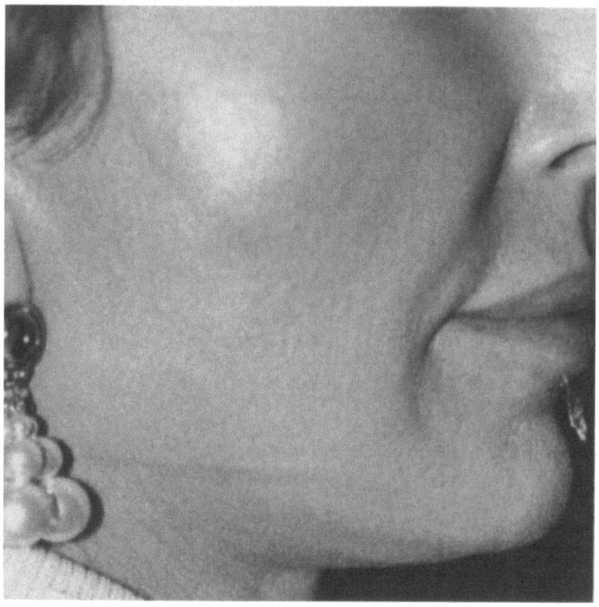

C

Figure 8-7. It is important to start nasal massage as soon as the splint is removed. I prefer soft aluminum splints taped over a tape-shaped nose. After 10 days, have the patient retape the nose and reapply the splint at night. The nose *must* be massaged twice a day. Gentle pressure, a "three-finger" upward run from supratip to bridge, smooths out bumps and holds down the supratip.

(A–C) These measures worked well in this case. The patient is in full makeup 14 days after blepharoplasty, malar implants, rhinoplasty, nasolabial and glabellar fat grafts, and complete rhytidectomy and submental tuck. She massaged the new pretragal groove and the jowl line as well.

Note the submalar implant that gave her the midcheek restoration. Note also the slight swelling of dorsum of the nose and in the areas along the nasolabial zone where fat grafts have been placed. She no longer has the hollowed-out midface, and there is an attractive curvature on both sides—which is what we mean by subtle differences.

If a number of implants are available, and you have a good idea of the shape you wish to achieve, the result may have more to do with trial and error in the operating room than with preoperative planning. We like to think we know exactly the effect of each prosthesis, but sometimes it is best to stand back and take a good look. You may want to exchange one "medium" for another from a different manufacturer just to get a subtle difference in projection or size. The same applies to the selection of chin prostheses.

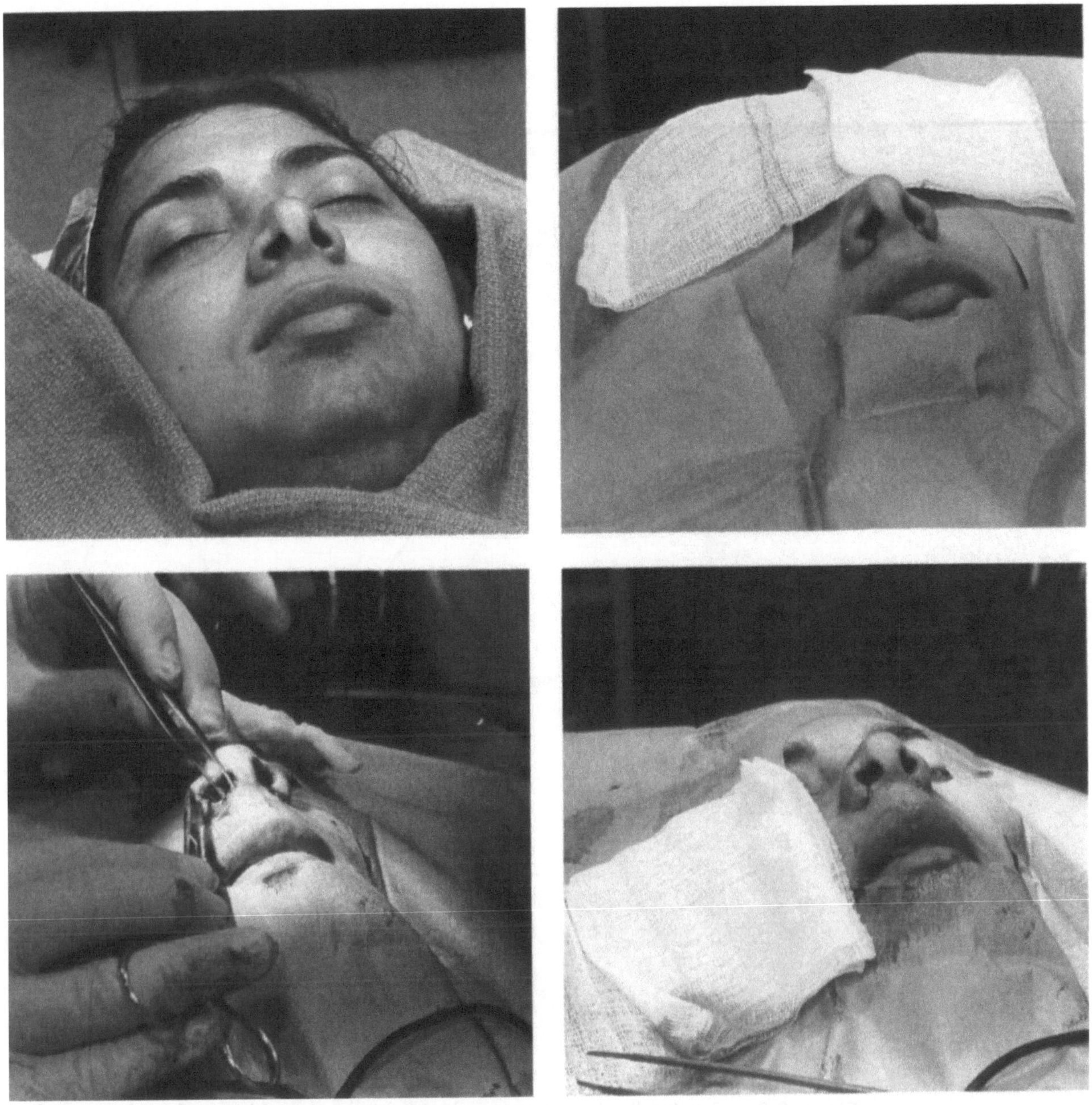

A B C D

Figures 8-8 and 8-9. Alar reduction. What should be a relatively simple procedure that we use in association with many rhinoplasties can be a great asset, or it can leave a noticeable scar. Paying attention to some technical points can determine the outcome.

Figure 8-8. (A–D) This patient has excessive nasal spread, a common recurrence after reducing the height of the nose.

Figure 8-9 appears on the following page.

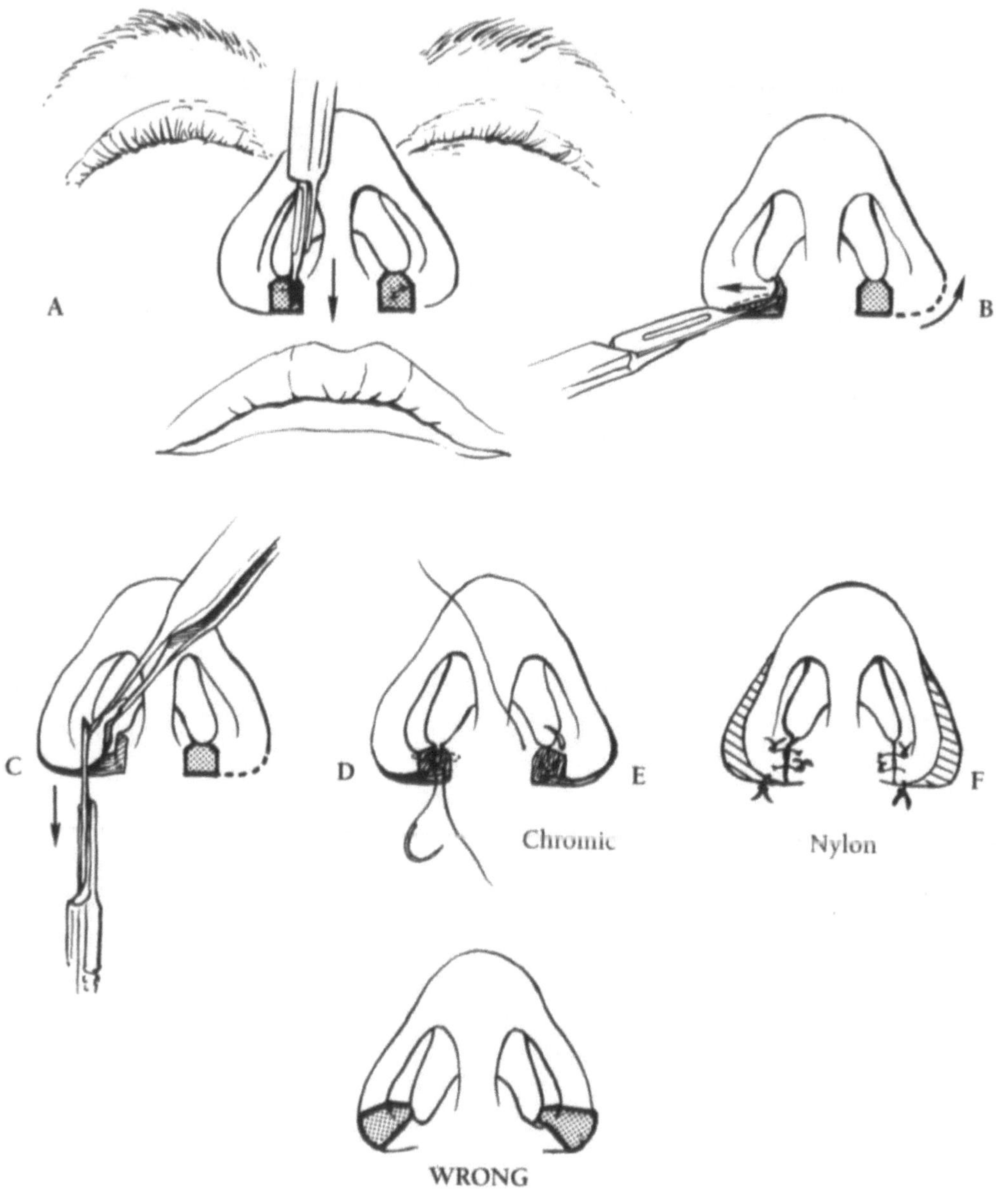

Figure 8-9. Curving lines are drawn at the junction points. Placing these lines too far laterally or on the ascending curve results in a visible step-off. Be sure to make the cuts deep enough and square enough that the two edges join exactly in all dimensions. One way to make them fit is to angle the posterior portion backward (**A**). This posterior triangle can be closed with a single surface suture. It is important to undermine laterally; it not only relieves tension on the closure but allows the alae to drift into natural position. Note also the squared-off edges inferiorly at the level of the alar crease. (**B**) Placing a deep suture is essential. Turn your hand far backward so the chromic sutures needle enters at a right angle (**C**).

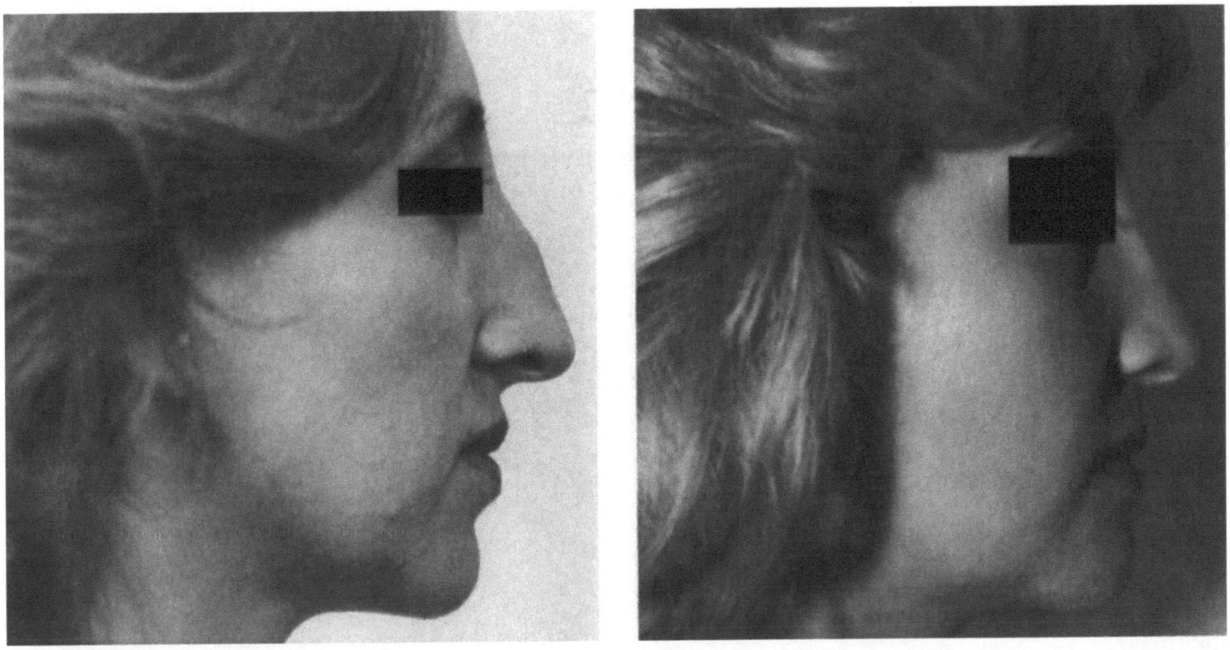

A B

Figure 8-10. **(A&B)** For the patient with an ethnic nose: Have patients bring in photographs that show the *type* of profile they like. More importantly, have them include the type they *dislike*. Keeping a high bridge, as shown here, may not suit someone else, but it was perfect for retaining some of this woman's Hispanic appearance.

Reoperating a Saddle Nose

One of our Oriental patients asked that the tip of her nose be elevated but that we not disturb the silicone implant in the dorsum. Using an open technique we were able to rotate the LLCs up and sew in a tip graft. The thickness of the nostrils was reduced and the floor brought inward with a weir-type advancement. She still was dissatisfied as now she was more aware of the movement and the shape of the carved Silastic implant. I proposed replacing it with a carved Porex or even a folded fascial graft. Fascia, ear cartilage, or Porex seem to work well for *small* problem areas. She, unfortunately, did not return for the surgery.

It is difficult to challenge the use of bone grafts for the dorsum of the nose because they are discussed in all the textbooks. Are bone grafts, however, the best choice, with their history of resorption, difficulty of fixation, and so on? Let us assume that it is a good operation because it works. The question, then, is the best site for obtaining donor bone.

There is currently interest in using cranial bone for these small grafts. Darryl Hodgkenson, an Australian colleague, has presented a strong argument against cranial bone grafts. He pointed out the morbidity and danger associated

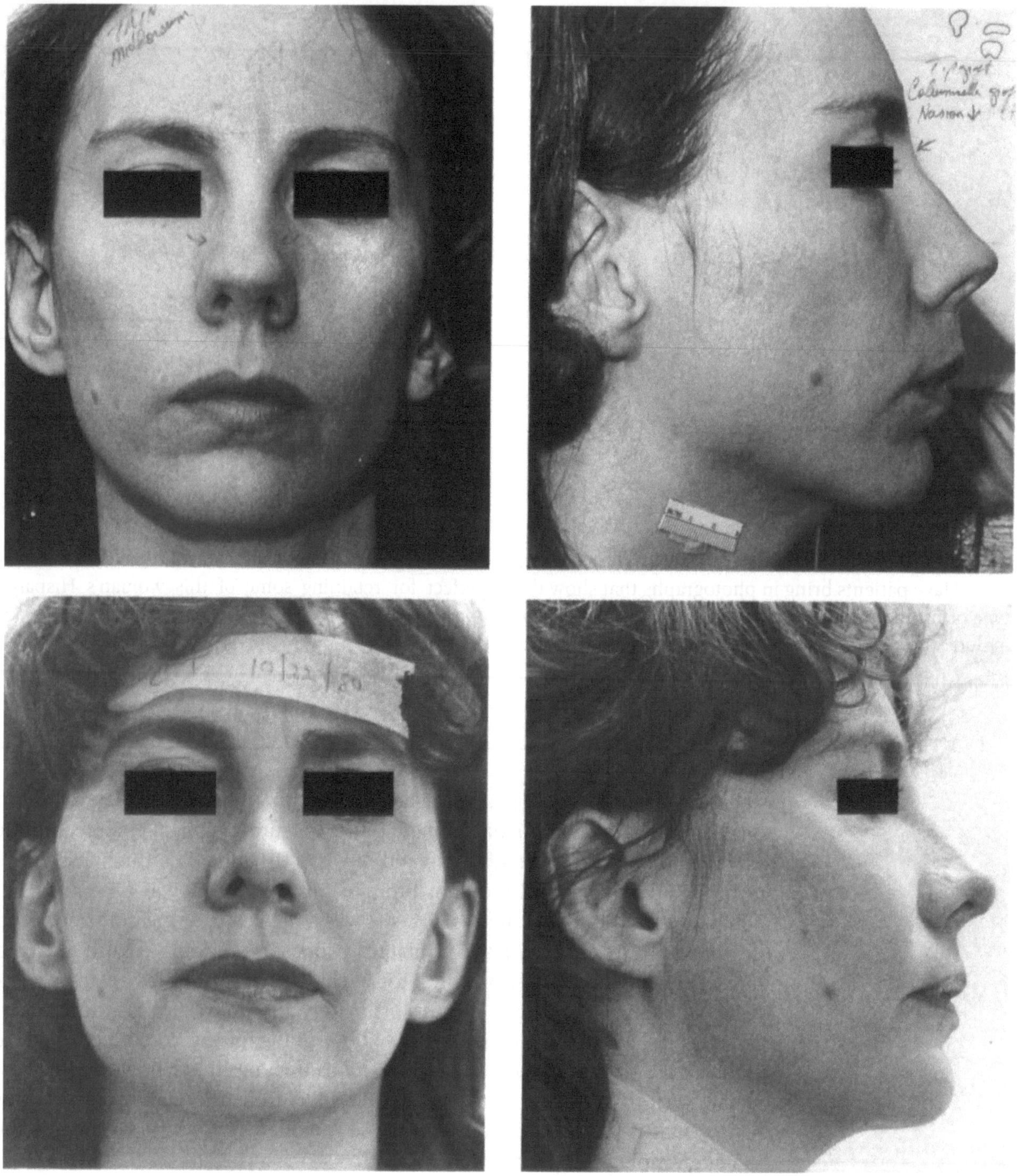

Figure 8-11. For this underdeveloped tip, correction was with a chevron tip graft, a columellar base graft, lateral LLC trim, and a malar implant to lessen the visual impact.

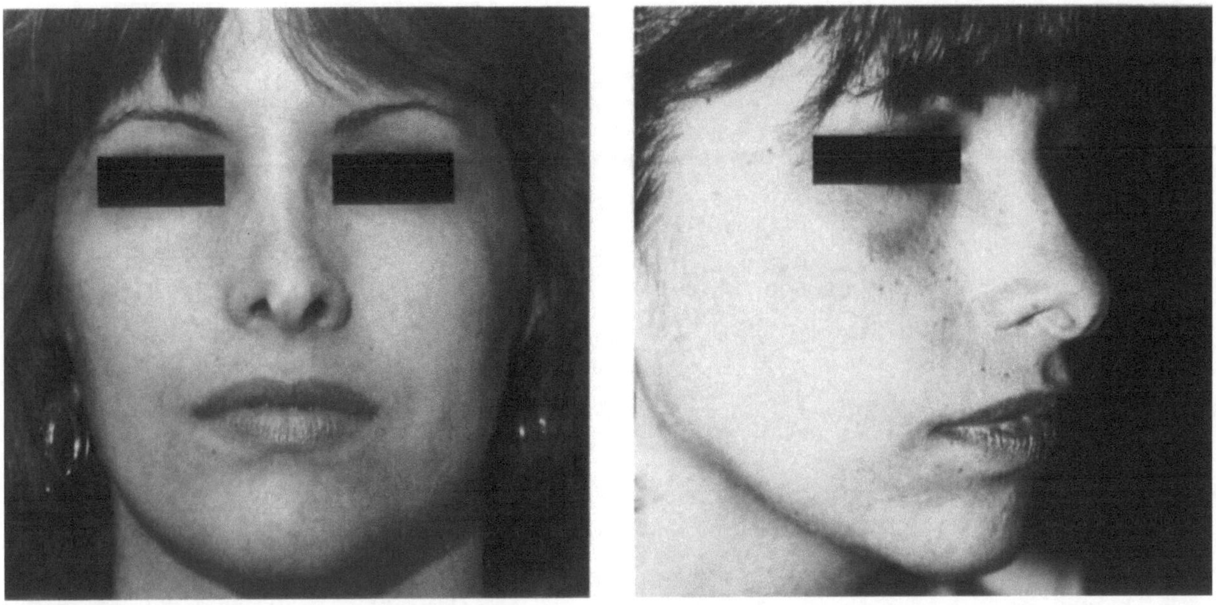

Figure 8-12. This correction was difficult without using an open incision. I grafted the postsurgically retracted dome, resected the excess lower limb of the LLCs, and eliminated columellar "show" by suturing the LLC to the septum.

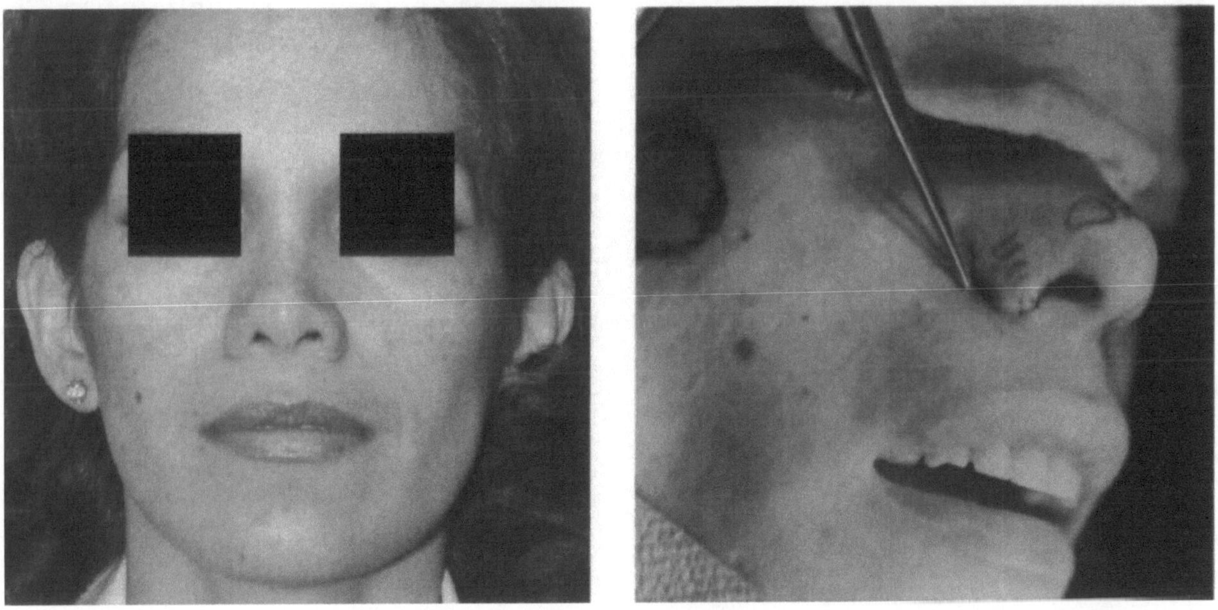

Figure 8-13. Square alae. During previous surgery an alar wedge was removed too high, and the nose has the flat nasal floor and square perpendicular alar takeoff from the cheek. After correcting the rest of the nose with tip grafts, I defatted the nose, trimmed cartilage, and deepithelialized the excess ala. I then tunneled under the nasal floor and rotated that position into the tunnel and anchored it there. The cheek was undermined and advanced up to the new alar edge. Technical point: Attach the cheek skin to *deep* tissue with buried suture, not to the new alar curve. It then cannot distort by retraction.

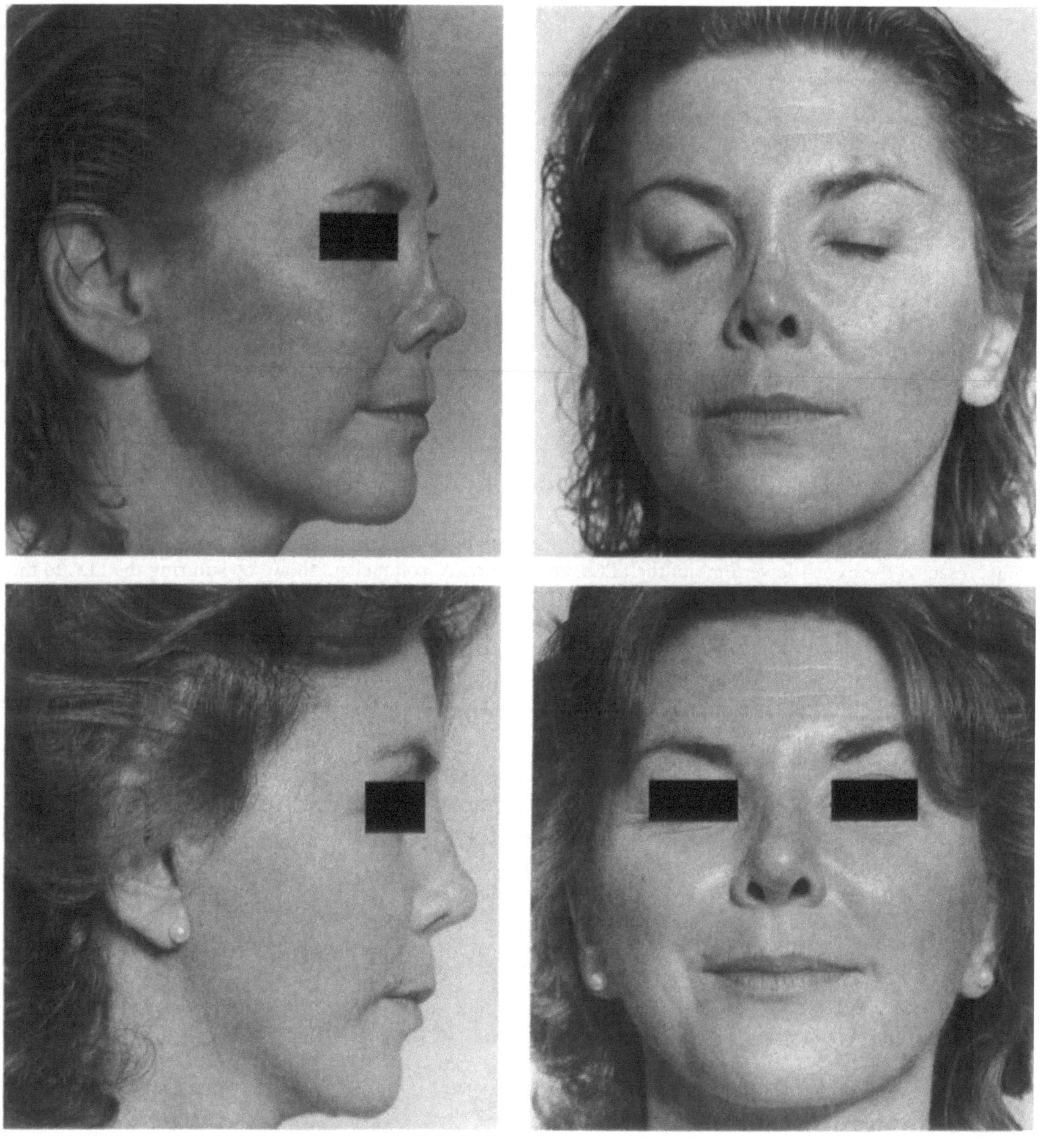

Figure 8-14. Most surgeons prefer not to use bone grafts in the nose. Cartilage and fascia are sufficient grafts with far fewer problems. In the case shown here, nasal collapse followed a self-inflicted intranasal *Pseudomonas* infection after rhinoplasty. Her nose felt "funny" so she poked hairpins up inside. She was so pleased with result of the cartilage and temporalis fascia grafts she would not let us do further revisions.

Originally, she was a plastic surgery nightmare. She had contracted a *Pseudomonas* infection 4 to 5 days with its use and suggested using bone from the elbow. A small incision is made on the undersurface of the forearm and a wedge of bone removed from the ulna. Hodgkenson reported being impressed by the success rate using ulnar bone; he largely attributed its success to the density of the cortex and the ease of harvesting.

With the forearm flexed, a 3 to 4 cm incision is made directly over the proximal ulna. A subperiosteal dissection is then used to expose the width of bone. From this point, harvesting is straightforward. The postoperative scars are acceptable.

Changing Fashions in Rhinoplasty

"Fashions" in rhinoplasty come and go. Francisco Ojeda (Mexico) first described a septal flap to achieve more projection of the tip in 1974. Visualize the septum and an L-shaped cut made just proximal to the tip. Ojeda rotated this L-shaped piece of cartilage, still attached to the tip of the septum, upward and secured it to give even further projection to the overlying LLCs. This appearance, though striking, is certainly different from the current "American fashion," which is more natural, with conservative reduction of size and width. In the past, pinched, small noses were preferred. Now we are passing through another fashion, adding tip grafts to practically every case.

Howard Gordon rarely uses tip grafts and advises us to undermine only enough of the dorsum "to do what you want to do." What about the fashion of doing all of the ULC dissection extramucosally? Gordon thinks it makes little difference. The only major error, he says, is to remove too much bone. The major cause of doing so is "the technique we were taught in our residencies," that is, using a hand saw. Beginners especially should use the dorsal sanding technique that allows slow removal of bone.

Another standard technique now out of fashion concerns passing the chisel on the long side of the septum and then out-fracturing the nasal bone after

---

after rhinoplasty, partly from falling into contaminated water and partly from an unexplained tendency to poke hairpins up her new nose. In any event, it took some time to correct the infection, which left her with a severe saddle nose deformity. Temporary splinting was done 4 years ago with a Silastic strut placed behind a "blocking" tip graft of cartilage. Needless to say, the strut extruded after several years, leaving the deformity. She adamantly refused surgery until the time came for a face lift.

Jose Guerro Santos proposed wrapping nasal grafts in temporalis fascia. The latter gives additional bulk without the risk of absorption, and it blunts the outline of the nasal graft. In this case we finally managed to convince the patient to undergo this procedure and proposed that the best approach would be directly through the anterior nares. The result was satisfying beyond our initial hopes. Note the restoration of contour, smoothness of profile, and practically invisible anterior vertical incision.

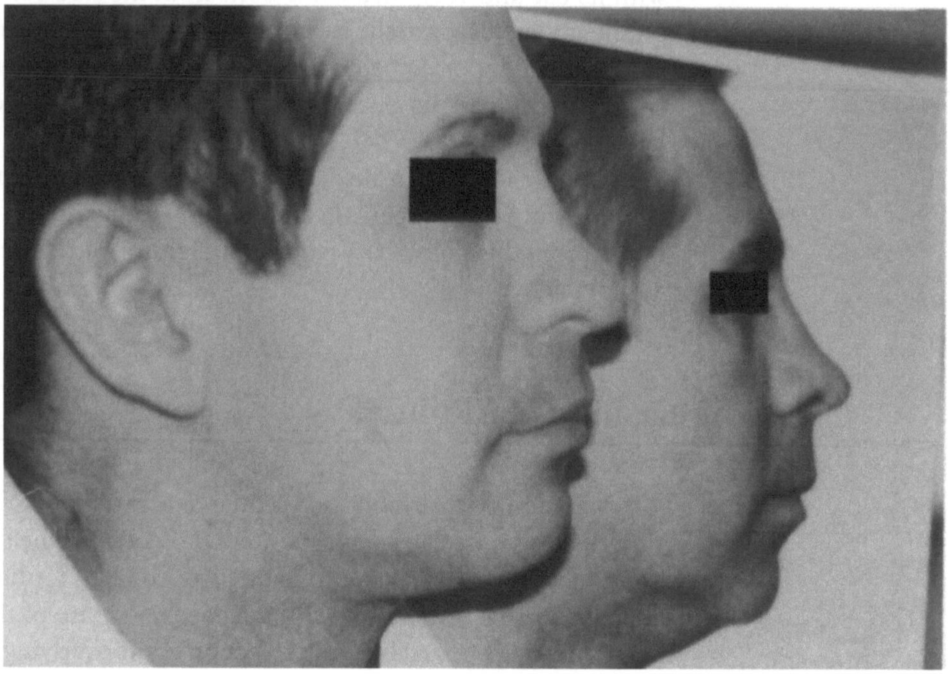

Figure 8-15. Closed nasal revision with alar rim grafts. The technique of applying an alar rim graft to reduce the retraction that may occur following rhinoplasty is a simple improvement but makes a major visual impact. The retracted alar rim shown in the photograph held by this patient is approached through a V-Y incision inside the alar margin. With blunt dissection, a pocket is created beyond the rims of the V-Y for a cartilage graft from either septum or postauricular sources. Once the graft is firmly seated, the V-Y is advanced and closed internally so no tension is exerted on the graft. Note the reduction of the supertip, the presence of a crushed cartilage graft in addition to the middorsal depression, and the beneficial effect of liposuction and submental repair with a chin augmentation. In male patients, sufficient skin retraction occurs following platysma resection and suturing in the midline that skin resection, as done for a face lift, is not required.

separating it from the malar junction. We do not use that technique much anymore. Most of the malar cuts are made only partially through the attachment and the bone is in-fractured only distally. The goal is to make the nose look as natural as possible by conservative removal of cartilage and bone and minimal in-fracturing. Elevate the tips only for those noses that really need elevation.

Comments and Commentary

1. During a presentation on open rhinoplasty, Ron Gruber touted the benefits of hydrocortisone 100 mg IV during surgery. He sometimes also injects triamcinolone (Kenalog) during the early postoperative period to alleviate

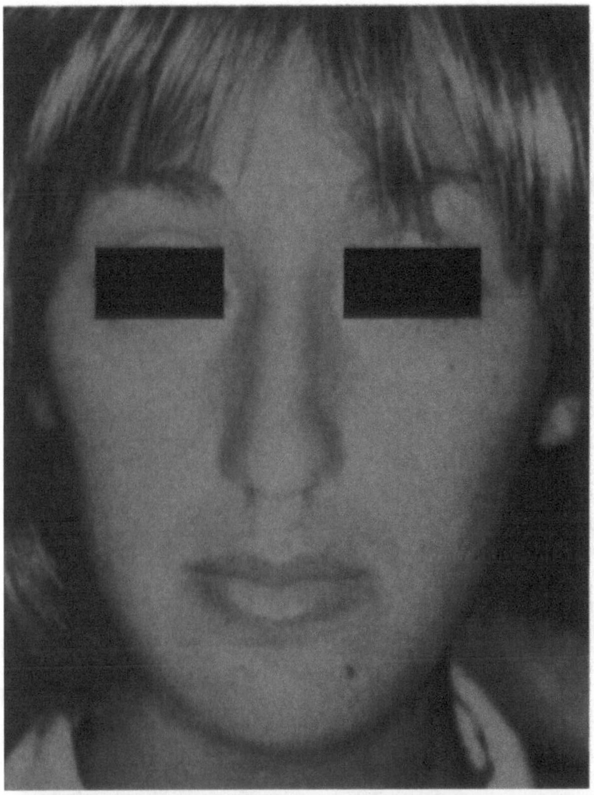
A

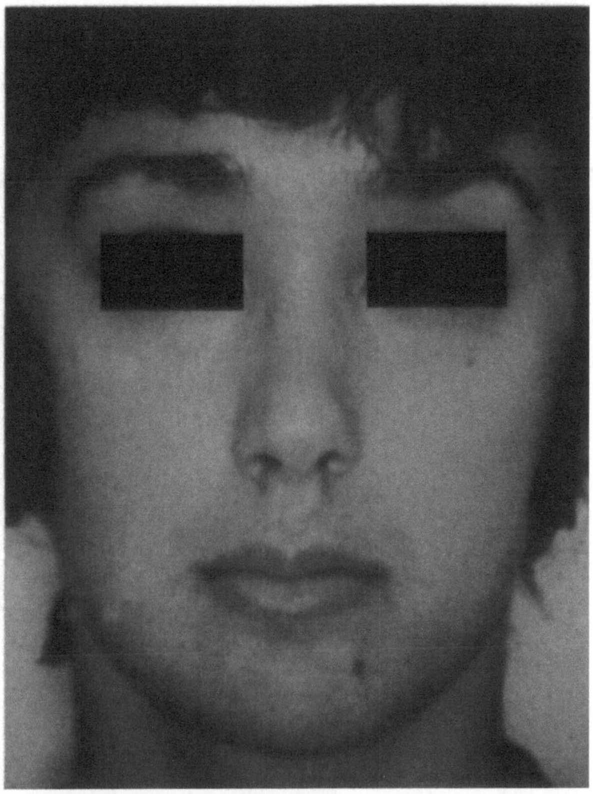
B

C
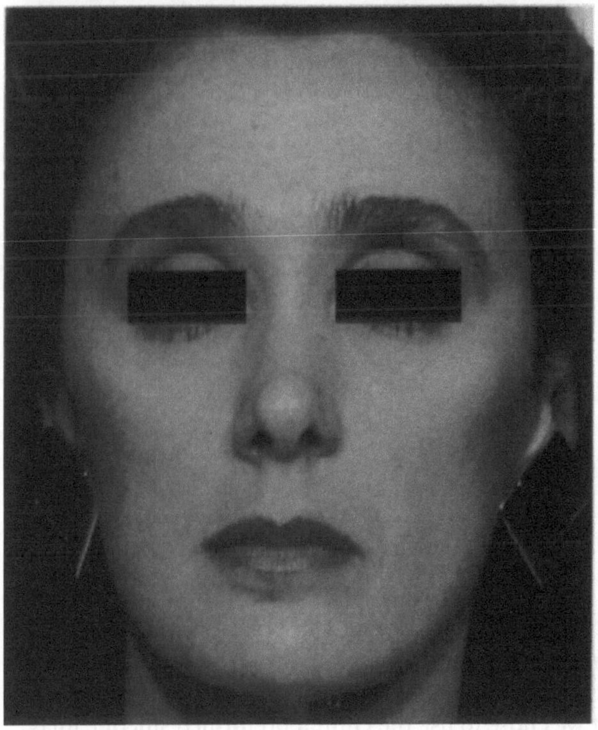

Figure 8-16. Patients with a long middle third of the face (Mona Lisa look) have an unattractive imbalance in the three major elements described by Mario Gonzalez-Ulloa: The midface should equal the segment between the base of the nose and the chin. In some patients chin reduction achieves a visual balancing. In others, such as those with a Mona Lisa appearance, tilting the nose gives the optical illusion of symmetry. (A) Patient is shown in 1979 before rhinoplasty. B is a later photograph, unfortunately taken without the same camera lens. The tip was left full, and the tilt was an exaggerated one so the visual effect would be shortening of the middle third of the face. Even with a 1979 and a 1990 camera, one can appreciate the distinctive look. This professional model has long enjoyed the appearance she chose. The tilt achieved a balance and a striking appearance, which she found acceptable.

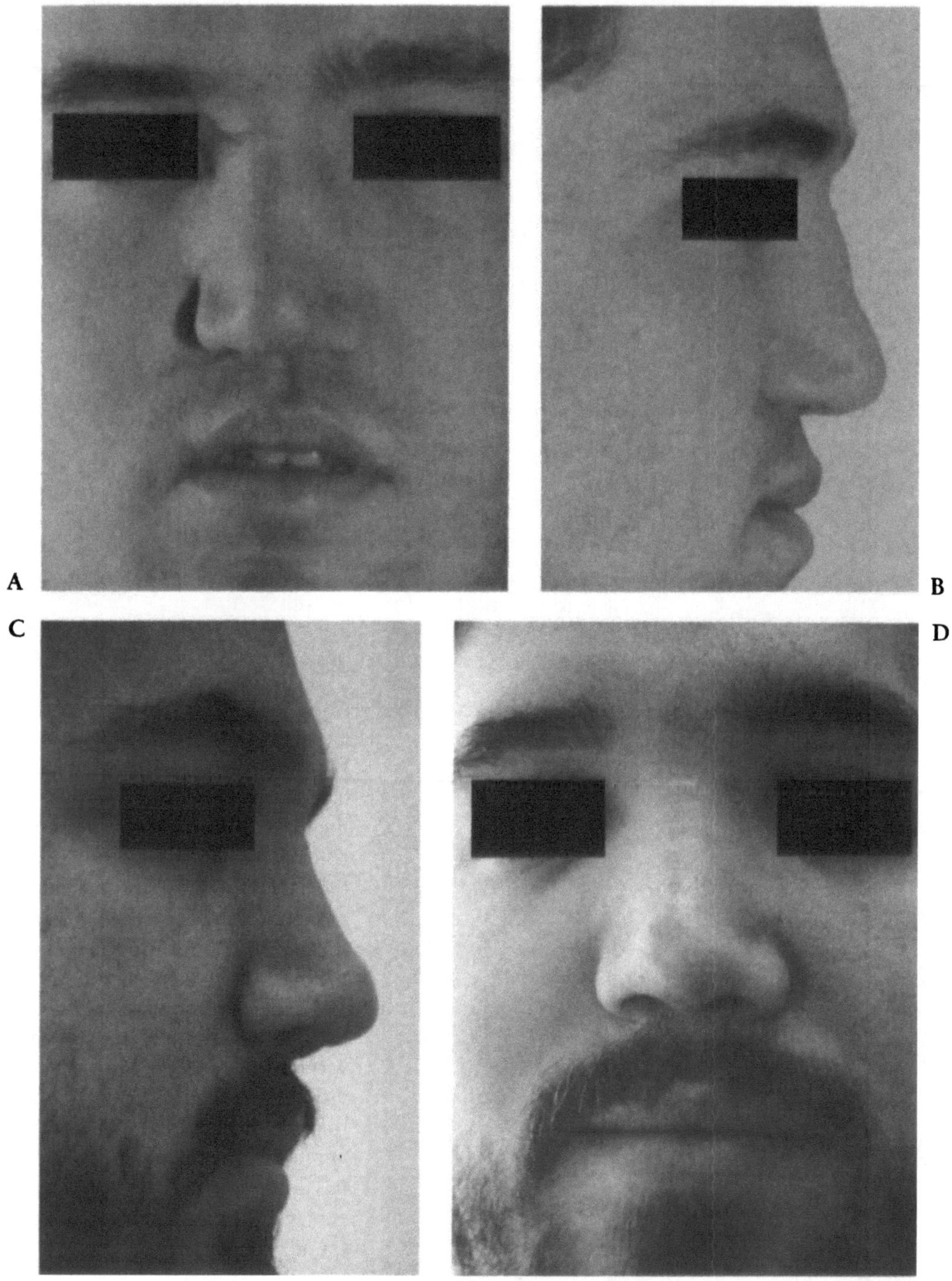

Figure 8-17. **(A&B)** The patient has undergone several rhinoplasties, resulting in a pinched tip, wide base, and complete nasal obstruction. Note the retraction in the area due to overzealous resection of the nasal spine. Cartilage grafts are the traditional method for correcting this area, but we chose to use the Giunta preformed silicone inlay graft below the orbicularis to elevate and project not only the base of the columella but

supertip edema. Others prefer a "weaker" triamcinolone injection (e.g., Aristospan) and begin injections 3 to 4 months after surgery.

2. Surgeons who use "open rhinoplasty" for most of their cases may perform the lateral osteotomies through a buccal mucosal incision "because so much has been done to the nose." Does this approach make sense? No.

3. Although "somewhat controversial", some surgeons with close to 10 years experience in open rhinoplasties perform most of their primary rhinoplasties using this technique. They report no scarring problems with the transcolumella incision, particularly if it is zigzagged, even in African American and Oriental patients. A word of warning about secondary open rhinoplasties: Scar retraction is much more likely to occur than with a secondary closed rhinoplasty.

4. One way of dealing with the concave nose laterally is Ron Gruber's idea of removing the tissue with the concavity, turning it over, and resuturing the LLCs upside down. Concave thus becomes convex.

5. Another useful maneuver for some difficult noses is to raise the alar rim, thereby elongating the nostril. Richard Ellenbogen described this method (*Plastic and Reconstructive Surgery* 90:28, 1992). The technique is simple, but it is delicate. The incision is made on the undersurface, the skin everted, and the overhanging cartilage directly excised. It is even easier to do during open rhinoplasty. The effect is an aesthetic one. You might want to add to this correction, particularly during an open rhinoplasty by making a tighter suture of the descending limb of the LLCs. This suture brings the curve to a higher position, adding to the elevation of the nostril.

6. Little-known facts: (1) The nose is a secondary sex organ. (2) Airflow through the nose is, in principle, the same as fat flow through a suction cannula. You can confirm this claim by examining Benoulli's principle and Poisulle's law. The corollary is that a long nose has lower airflow than a short nose owing to the resistance (similar to a long garden hose and a short garden hose). (3) It is easier

---

the alar wings as well. To narrow the nose a heavy rasp is inserted, and the nasal bone is diminished until it is level with the maxilla. One then proceeds with dorsal reduction, grafting to the midtip depression, and rearrangement of the nasal tip with a full tip graft. **(C&D)** Postoperatively, the sharp nasolabial angle has been eliminated and the columella and nasal wings elevated by the inlaid Silastic prosthesis. The same effect could have been achieved with cartilage and fascial grafts, but the available cartilage was needed for the tip and the middorsal depression. For the amount of elevation required in these difficult cases, Giunta design Silastic is promising.

Tips for insertion: Develop an adequate mucosal flap to allow for stretch and to keep the incision as far from the graft as possible. Once the pocket has been developed with blunt-tipped scissors, pass a Prolene suture percutaneously through the tip of the nose, through the graft, and back out the tip of the nose. This stitch holds the graft in place. Remove it in 2 to 3 days when the tissues have become fixed around the graft.

to detect aromas during expiration. The air is more turbulent then than during inspiration, so more smells float up to the olfactory area.

7. Open rhinoplasty allows easy suturing of freed LLCs in the midline for tip elevation. Central strutting or security is needed in some cases. Why then do so many of the postoperative results seem "overdone"? Perhaps there has been too much elevation.

8. If you want to make the patient who is presented at an international meeting look good, always present three-quarter or oblique views. They are forgiving, particularly with rhinoplasties.

9. A minor disagreement about rhinoplasties in African American patients: Rod Rohrich believes that defatting the nasal tip of these patients is the wrong approach. After considerable experience with the procedure, he concluded that it caused more problems than are alleviated. He agrees with others that tip augmentation is preferable in practically every case and does not hesitate to obtain cranial bone if the septum is not adequate for dorsal grafts. (Is it necessary? Harvesting bone from the skull is certainly more hazardous and time-consuming than harvesting temporalis fascia.) Rohrich prefers the open approach to rhinoplasty in African Americans, as dome plication plays a large role in tip elevation. Most of his patients received a columella graft for central support, one or more tip grafts, plus a dorsal graft.

Concerning the alar incision, Rohrich notes that wide excision of the nostril sill is the procedure of choice in most cases. Technical point: Always place the incision above the alar groove to avoid problems with scar formation. In other patients, a simple alar wedge with tunneling underneath the retracted columella base is better—the Millard deepithelialized advancement technique. These patients have wide interalar distances.

My suggestion is to do a conservative alar wedge and then pass sutures across from side to side to compress the central columella base. Use a V-Y closure to lengthen the columella but place that incision at the nasal floor.

10. Several experienced surgeons who once advocated the use of silicone onlays in Oriental noses have abandoned its use completely. They are back to using galea or temporalis fascia and cartilage.

11. Spraying Polaroid photographs with McDonald's Liquor allows you to draw on them with color pencils. You can thus outline a retouch or adjustment right in front of the patient. Berol Prisma colored pencils are said to be the best for this purpose.

12. Jack Sheen notes that Armenian and Irish men often specifically request that their ethnic characteristics be damped.

13. To add more projection for an "elegant" restoration of the mid-hump, perhaps one could use Jack Gunter's "A-frame" procedure. He does not perform

an ordinary cartilage graft of the dorsum of the nose; he sizes the center of the graft and bends it downward to obtain a V-frame. Fibrotic ingrowth fills in the empty space underneath the graft, making it a permanent elevation. For further stability you can add a cross bar, the A-frame. Furthermore, you can make lateral cuts so the flat graft is now folded into a U shape, obviously called a U-frame. It seems that it would be easier just to place the cartilage and cover it with temporalis fascia until a smooth contour results; or perhaps you could add cartilage in the old, familiar way.

The 1960s may have been the year of the scoop-out, thin nose, but the 1990s have definitely ushered in an era in which reduction/augmentation rhinoplasty is favored. Reduction means less radical removal of the hump usually using the more controlled rasp technique, and augmentation means elevation of the tip or sides with some type of graft material.

We plastic surgeons tend to become rigid in our views. We tend to find one rhinoplasty technique that works, and we continue to use it even though it may mean doing too many tip grafts or too many alar repositionings. The mark of true aesthetic surgeons is adaptability. They choose a technique according to individual features and incorporate technical tricks they think are worthwhile within the limits of their talents and expertise.

14. You probably are resistant to using the Straith paraphernalia, what with those funny looking wings and the elastic that hooks behind the head. You likely say that that much bony pressure is not needed for a routine rhinoplasty, and that patients will hate it because it is cumbersome. These arguments are valid. It is much easier to use a metal splint, one of the hot-water-softened plastics, or even plaster. Sylvan Bartlett has convinced his patients to use the Straith splint, especially those with thick Mexican American noses. Those of you experienced in rhinoplastic surgery know that the biggest problem with African American or Mexican American noses is slow resolution of edema, with frequent occurrence of permanent, fixed edema in the supratip. Bartlett instructs patients to wear the device at night. Once patients get used to the idea and see the definite change in contouring of the nose each morning, they use them until they are worn out. With this particular type of thick nasal skin, you dare not thin subcutaneously along with removal of the nasal fatty tissue, and the Straith device offers an alternative.

15. Our colleagues in Southeast Asia are ambiguous when pressed regarding the extrusion of Silastic prostheses placed in the nose. Apparently nasal augmentation represents a major portion of plastic surgery practice in Oriental faces, as is supratarsal fixation during blepharoplasty. Apparently every imaginable size and shape of prosthesis has been used: L shapes, straight lines, double dippers. One surgeon reported a case in which some enterprising soul carved a toothbrush handle and placed it in the dorsum of an unsuspecting patient's nose.

One lecturer in Bangkok was concerned with "contractures" around nasal prostheses. Apparently thickening of scar tissue near the tip can occur, and a

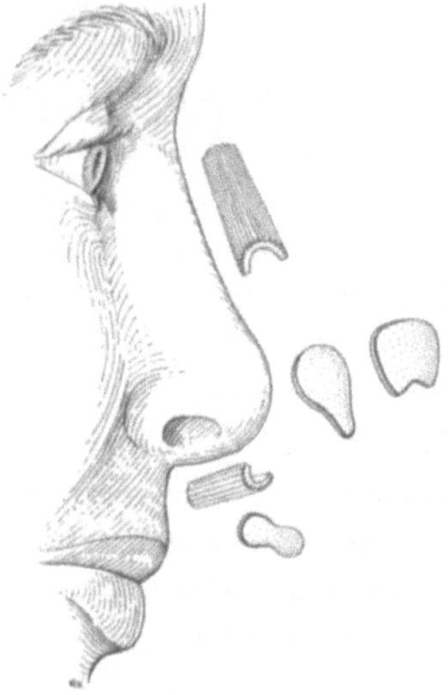

8-18

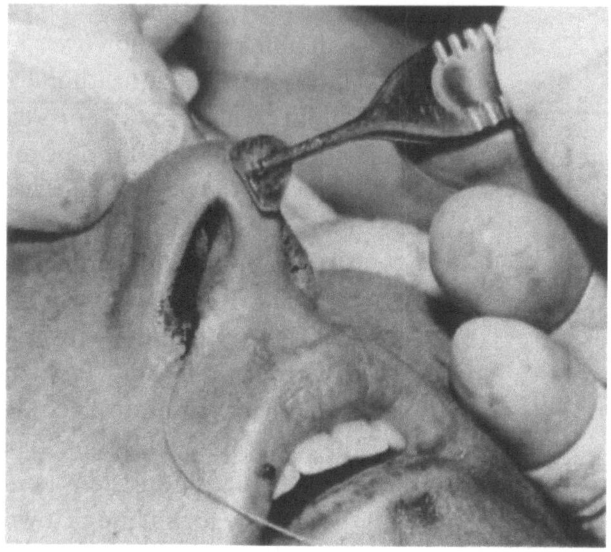

8-19

Figures 8-18 and 8-19. Today it is easier than ever to position a tip graft of septal or conchal cartilage. Most aesthetic surgeons prefer the stiffness of septal grafts (and there is no need for a second incision). For the severely damaged tip, I have achieved remarkably good results by wrapping the graft and the dorsum where the skin has thinned to tissue paper depth. Mastoid and temporalis fascia work equally well. Fat grafts do not work at all. The open technique makes it easy to sew a graft in place, but Jack Sheen and others have taught us to perform the procedure using the closed approach.

Note the difference in the shapes of the tip grafts. The "chevron" is the classic elevating graft for noses with depressed tips **(Fig. 8-18)**. A short extension **(Fig. 8–19)** is needed when the upper columella is flat, or when the projection in a thin nose is fitted into the upper columella for more dorsal elevation.

Note the scoring on the "roll top desk" design grafts for columella or nasal dorsum. Straight scoring of this type provides a natural external contour without the sharp edges of flat grafts. Conchal grafts may be selected for curve and shape, particularly for curved tip grafts of the type shown. We prefer the thicker and easier to obtain septal grafts, however.

In the rare case of an undeveloped columella, the "tennis racquet" shape gives anterior projection as well as tip elevation **(Fig. 8–18)**. Anterior columella grafts of cartilage (or even turbinate bone) can be combined for difficult cases.

"capsulotomy" is advocated as the method of repair. It looked to me as if there was simply excessive scar tissue in the soft areas of the tip and a prosthesis was practically eroding through. At any rate, "releasing the scar tissue" and redraping the tissue apparently comprise the means of correction if one continues to use nonautogenous materials. Practically no one in Asia uses cartilage or bone for dorsal nasal grafting.

16. When trying to make the columella protrude forward during a nasal reconstruction, try a wrap-around graft. Mike Kelly uses a flexible piece of cartilage and attaches it in horseshoe fashion around the leading edge of the columella. This maneuver provides protrusion as well as some stability. Ray Elliott calls it "salami over a piece of bread."

17. Not everyone is enthusiastic about using temporalis fascia for nasal reconstruction. Those who are disillusioned have returned to dermis grafting with all the problems of cyst formation and so on.

18. For the Pinocchio nose, open rhinoplasty is helpful. Flip out the lateral wings of the LLCs, trim them, and shorten them by removing the distal part. The Pinocchio projection then settles back to the face. It is necessary to remove some of the medial LLC footplate as well. Harder to do with closed technique.

19. On reconstructing the nose: If it looks easy, it is going to be tough. If it looks tough, it is going to be near impossible.

20. The trend in rhinoplastic surgery is to avoid gauze packing or at least to use absorbable packing because of the foul odor and pain on removal. Gene Courtiss long ago convinced most of us to use Gelfoam or similar absorbable products. Patients are uniformly comfortable with this measure, and the packing melts without incident after 4 to 5 days. The only problem is that it is difficult to get Gelfoam into the nostril, although we have used judicious "scrunching." Another product is now available called the Rhino Rocket, designed for epistaxis and postoperative nasal packing. It is a sterile syringe with a squeezed-up narrow cell surgical sponge inside. You slide it in the nose and extrude the contents, which is a sponge that expands to $7.5 \times 20 \times 10$ mm. Its drawback is that it is expensive.

21. Is there any single maneuver that we do differently now for rhinoplasties than we did 10 years ago? We reduce the bony dorsum less. Some ascribe this change to the trend of using rasps instead of chisels. It has been said that "old heavy chisels are unguided missiles."

22. Did you know that 80% of normal people have a 30-minute to 5-hour cycle of congestion and decongestion in the nasal turbinates? We know that the turbinates respond to many medications and swell during periods of sexual excitement. Be aware of this biorhythm when explaining to a patient why breathing is easier at some times than at others. Also be aware of those with "low nasal dyspnea." These patients "need" more air flow than you could ever supply. Even without a septum and the widest nostrils in the world, they complain that they are not getting enough air in. These nasal neurotics should be referred to your nearest competitor.

23. Gram Kemsley has encountered the problem of transillumination of dorsal nasal Silastic implants. I cover preexisting implants with temporalis fascia if possible. The safer method is to replace the implant with morselized cartilage. Kemsley has eliminated the problem in his patients by using skin-tone Silastic implants (available through McGhan Medical). Kemsley and his partner Jim

Vollshin prefer silicone nasal implants and have been "very happy with the results over a considerable amount of time" (more than 6 years). Their record is remarkable given the generally poor experience with silicone implants in the nose.

24. In the opinion of many experts in the field, the turbinates are more often the cause of nasal obstruction than the septum. Because there have been cases of loss of vision following intraturbinate injections of steroids, we have looked at other methods to solve this problem. There are several ways to reduce turbinates, exclusive of total resection. I prefer out-fracture combined with cautery, which works in most patients. For some people only scissors excision of the whole inferior turbinate is effective.

25. Why are we still hearing about the Skoog rhinoplasty? One author bravely presented case after case of removing the dorsal hump of the nose, trimming it, and *putting it back in*!! This doctor obliquely referred to the fact that a number of these noses required revision. In other words, a large hump was taken out, a small hump put in, and then several months later the small hump was sanded down. There are many ways to do a rhinoplasty, but this method is not one of the best.

26. Technical suggestion: Use silly putty to simulate add-on grafts for complex open rhinoplasties. The patient can see the grafts and their position, and silly putty can be kept on a side table in the operating room so you can fashion the grafts to the shape you decided on several days earlier.

27. Technical tip for open rhinoplasty: Use a stab incision to separate the ULCs from the LLCs. Ron Gruber prefers 5-0 nylon for tip sutures, whereas others are content to use an absorbable suture such as Dexon or Vicryl. If you are scoring the dome of the lateral cartilages, use several cuts until the tip–septum angle and position are correct. Use more than one suture.

28. New syndrome: Rhinoscleroma, caused by the gram-negative diplococcus *Klebsiella rhinoscleromatis*. Rare in the United States, this syndrome of hoarseness and epistaxis is commonly found in South America and Mexico. Granulomas block the nostrils. For diagnosis, culture the biopsy specimens. Treatment consists of appropriate antibiotics.

29. One survey of rhinoplasties indicated that only 50% of surgeons keep their patients under observation for 24 hours. The rest send the patients home with a family member, whether the rhinoplasty was simple or complex.

30. There may be legitimate shortcuts for any number of aesthetic surgical procedures, but none exist with rhinoplasty.

31. Bob Flowers advises not to score the cartilage if using the "toboggan"-tip graft. Beveling the upper end of the cartilage that is placed in the columella allows it to bend backward and give a smoother, more rounded tip projection than the standard "chevron" or stacked-tip grafts. A percutaneous fixation suture ensures that the upper portion does not waver from side to side with this closed-tip augmentation procedure. Speaking of cartilage grafts in the nose, several surgeons have distinguished between bruised and crushed cartilage to fill areas on either side of the tip. Now that the U.S. Food and Drug Administration has prohibited the sale of Proplast, crushed or bruised cartilage may be the only material readily available to fill the base of the columella or the radix of the nose (assuming that you believe in augmenting rather than reducing).

32. One surgeon reported using 3-mm Proplast grafts above the glabella and at the base of the columella, and crushed cartilage grafts in the radix, tip, and alar curve. He was asked, "Why complicate a basically simple operation by adding all that extra material?" We agreed that the resultant noses were attractive but reasoned that they would have looked just as good without all the extra grafting.

33. An interesting point: After treating several infections after "clean" nasal tip grafts, Jack Sheen now rinses the grafts in lincomycin (Lincocin) prior to insertion. He believes that ear cartilage is "dirtier" than septal cartilage. Certainly bacteria can be cultured from inside the ear, but they should be eliminated by placing a povidone-iodine (Betadine) sponge in the ear canal and using good skin preparation.

34. Bone or cartilage? It is difficult to believe, coming on the heels of evaluating a distraught young woman who had a large scar in her scalp line and draining sinuses from an infected cranial bone graft site, that some surgeons prefer cranial grafts to rib or other grafts for nasal reconstruction. It has been said that, "As the rib graft has replaced iliac bone grafts, cranial bone grafts have replaced rib grafts." It does not mean that these surgeons have given up on cartilage by any means. Jack Sheen prefers crushed cartilage as a superficial liner, backed up by thicker cartilage or vomer bone. Strips of vomer can be used as well because it is usually straight and highly vascular.

There have been some shocking stories about harvesting cranial bone grafts. Some patients have sinus lakes close to the surface, and others lack an appreciable inner table. If you are an expert like Sheen, you can tell from the "ping" of the chisel when the inner table has been reached and if you have gone beyond it. I for one have vowed never to attempt to harvest a cranial graft. Cartilage draped in temporalis fascia suffices for most problems.

35. I share Jack Sheen's enthusiasm for preoperative photographs. He asks patients to bring in pictures of what they consider attractive noses. This also gives him an idea of the reality of their expectations. "Many patients cannot verbalize what they like about nasal contours." In fact, many of the photographs brought in show what we would have called "contour deformities" or, in plainer language, small humps. Sheen would try to convince you that this "dorsal irregularity" gives "strength and elegance" to the nose.

36. Rollin Daniel noted that columellar notching from the open technique is almost always on the side opposite to that where the surgeon is positioned. Solution: Walk around the table to check the incisions and sutures.

37. Technical point: For an open rhinoplasty in African American patients, put the incision right at the base of the columella. This technique makes it more difficult to dissect upward for a longer distance, but the scar is less likely to be hyperpigmented or noticeable.

38. One of our problems as surgeons is that we were trained in reduction rhinoplasty. We now must learn to augment the nose.

39. Technical point: Suture spreader grafts to the septum to prevent migration.

40. If you still use a chisel to remove the nasal hump, remember that the fracture line precedes the chisel by 8 to 10 mm. You might be able to control the chisel, but you cannot control whether that fracture line goes up or down. A wrong move can create an unstable nose.

41. John Penn (Orlando) on nasal tip surgery: Most postoperative tip deformities that appear after rhinoplasty are directly related to deficiencies of lining. The contractures and synechiae that distort the tip of the nose can be corrected in a number of ways, but they should be prevented in the first place. One way to fill in soft tissue is to elevate myomucosal flaps from the sulcus by opening the nasal labial groove. These turnaround flaps on the mucosal pedicles can be filled into the anterior grooves for correcting perforations and a number of soft tissue deficiencies.

9 Rhytidectomy

RHYTIDECTOMY CAN BE EASY TO PERFORM OR THE MOST CHALLENGING and difficult procedure to do well in aesthetic surgery. If you overdo it, the result is an artificial look. If you do too little, the skin begins to sag, and the soft tissues fall rapidly. One of the difficulties with this operation is keeping scars to a minimun and ensuring that they do not become visible because of tension. The dead giveaways of a poor face lift are true stigmata.

Ear lobes can be pulled down and forward, and the fold underneath the lobule disappears. A straight-line scar in front of the ear is made even more noticeable by the difference in color between the cheek skin and the skin covering the tragus. There should be no scars in front of the hairline. There are better ways to rotate the sideburns downward without an external incision, and there are better ways to lift the forehead. Only in the rare case should one place the incision outside the forehead hairline. (An exception is the patient with an extremely high forehead.)

Technique

1. The subcutaneous musculoaponeurotic system (SMAS) must be repositioned. The "interior" should be tight, but the skin should not.

2. Plan the procedure and technical moves not just for the present. Someday, you will face the challanges of a secondary face lift in that patient. Items to which you must pay special attention are as follows.
   a. Tension points.
   b. Patient who smokes tobacco.
   c. Plication versus deep plane.
   d. Suction lipectomy.
   e. Platysma.

   There are a number of ways to do rhytidoplasty. The consensus is that some form of soft tissue plication and elevation is necessary. Many of us firmly believe that dividing the platysma anteriorly with anterior anastomosis and posterior elevation and overlap for tightness is appropriate. Jose Guerros-Santos (Guadalajara) rarely performs anterior plication, preferring to follow Ralph Millard's advice to do anterior resection. Guerros-Santos admits though, that the subplatysmal tissues are infolded with the same suturing that we would use in the platysma, and apparently an identical tightening effect is obtained. Several authors advocate partial platysmal division.
3. Plan the procedure around tension points and areas without tension. There should be no tension above the ear so the temple hair can survive. There should be no tension on the earlobe; it should hang freely. There should be no tension in the apex of the incision behind the ear where it turns to enter the hairline. This area has little blood supply and is therefore vulnerable.
4. Not all smokers are poor candidates, but you have an obligation to warn smokers that they could suffer skin sloughs. Poor technique probably causes more skin sloughs than suction, because of tension in the wrong places.
5. Do not make obliteration of the nasolabial fold a personal crusade. It cannot be pulled out smoothly even with a deep plane dissection.
6. Instead of a deep plane dissection with its inherent risks, attack the nasolabial fold area directly with transnasal elevation, fat grafting, and transnasal suctioning of the fatty mound lateral to the fold.
7. For most patients, limit suctioning to the jowl area and the nasolabial area.
8. If you plan to use a malar implant to fill out the upper midface, be sure it overlaps the malar zygoma prominence and does not lie free in the soft tissues.
9. Ninety-five percent of face lift candidates benefit from an anterior platysma plication and removal of the deep and superficial fatpads.
10. There are techniques that make the inside-the-tragus incision more acceptable because they reduce the bulking and the "open ear"

deformity. It is now our procedure of choice, whereas once it was the procedure of choice only for the young patient, with elastic skin.

11. If possible, prepare the patient's skin with a tretinoin (Retin-A) and α-hydroxy acid (AHA) regimen. Restart the regimen 30 days after the face lift. It keeps the skin tighter for longer and covers up many small irregularities.
12. Avoid creating bleached-out white lips.
13. Fat grafting, light scalpel abrasion, and 35% trichloroacetic acid (TCA) preserve the color and consistency of the senile lip. Phenol and dermabrasion do not.
14. Do not neglect the withered vermilion in the older patient. Fat grafting works well here.
15. Do not discontinue the incision in the scalp 3 cm above the ear. Carry it up almost as far as you would a coronal incision. That length provides the opportunity to stretch out some of the crow's feet areas and takes out the slack.
16. In my hands, a direct attack on the orbicularis oculi has not been worth the extra time and effort.
17. I agree with many of my colleagues that deep plane rhytidectomy and the subperiosteal rhytidectomy are vastly overrated and capable of creating an artificial facial appearance even in experienced hands.
18. Use coronal or forehead lifts sparingly. For most patients the descent of the midbrow has not occurred and will not in the foreseeable future.
19. It is difficult to induce a good hairline to grow around a scalp incision; use of the interspersed tension suture technique may be helpful.
20. If you plan to fill the midface, do not use a malar implant that lies freely below the edge of the malar or zygomatic processes.
21. SMAS plication works just as well as SMAS undermining and resection; and it provides soft tissue to build into a fuller zygomatic area. For the severely hollow face, plication can take place in the midcheek, largely eliminating the hollow look of old people.
22. On the other hand, there are certain face lift candidates with chubby faces who like the effect of lower cheek liposuction with or without a malar implant to accentuate facial planes.
23. Many face lift patients benefit from small, extended chin implants. The Mittleman design is a good idea, but most patients with lateral deficits also need the anterior projection of an "extended" prosthesis.
24. Do not forget to correct the witch's chin. The correction involves some type of rotation or soft tissue buildup in the groove in the submental zone and resection of the overhanging extra fat even if you add a chin implant.

25. It matters not whether you correct the eyelids first or last, so long as you are familiar with the operation.
26. Spraying bupivacaine (Marcaine) mixed with a steroid such as triamcinolone (Aristospan) onto the surface of the cheeks prior to closure is helpful. Bupivacaine blocks at the end of the operation are even more helpful.
27. Drains can remove serum and a small amount of blood. They do not prevent hematomas, but they decrease postoperative swelling.
28. Most postoperative hematomas can be handled with suction through the incision line and compression.
29. It is not necessary to divide the platysma completely. It may be divided anteriorly to eliminate the bands and then sewn in the midline to recreate the angle.
30. Do not interfere with the submaxillary gland. It is a "mine field."
31. Do not hesitate to use judicious small injections of steroid with lidocaine (Xylocaine) to correct small irregularities postoperatively.
32. It is good practice to apply antibiotic cream behind the ear. Perspiration tends to collect in that area, and an infection can make the patient miserable. Stop the antibiotic after 2 to 3 days and change to an aloe-vera-based oil that keeps the skin soft and lubricated. It also helps to loosen crusts.
33. It is ridiculous to forbid face lift patients to wash their hair after the third day.
34. Advise the face lift patient to wear covering makeup between the seventh and tenth days but not to drive for 10 days. (They cannot turn their heads quickly enough to avoid someone racing out of a side road.) The only method better for preventing postoperative swelling than topically sprayed-on steroids are elevation, ice packs, early compression with intermittent release, and oral or intravenous steroids (and of course good surgical technique).
35. Perform dissection of the cheek with curved, flat-bladed scissors: push and spread, push and spread.
36. Do not use nonabsorbable sutures to plicate this mass.
37. I share my patients' dislikes of steel skin clips in the hair. Sutures allow you to adjust tension, and they are not a bother when patients are washing their hair afterward. They are also easier to cope with during sleep.
38. Neurosurgery clips on the scalp during forehead lifts take little time to apply and simplify your work.
39. By all means, interrupt the corrugator muscles and free the periosteum along the orbital rim. You do not need an endoscope.

40. Choose your own personal method for cross-cutting the galea during forehead lifts. Direct undermining of the deep wrinkles in a superficial plane is helpful, particularly if you add a fat graft to fill out the tissue.
41. For some older patients it is wise to dissect subcutaneously all the way to the clavicle to eliminate the extra fold of skin below the thyroid.
42. Consider earlobe reduction in older patients.
43. It is good practice to free the skin on the dorsum of the nose when you do forehead lifts, but be sure to obtain enough traction that the situation is not made worse. It is well to sand off a bump or two—the patient will appreciate it later.
44. Save the extra fat from the submental zone and place it in the marionette depression and along the malar depressions.

Rhytidectomy and the Nasolabial Fold

Peter McKinney and I discussed the problem of the nasolabial fold and agreed that sub-SMAS, regular SMAS, or other types of pulling procedures are not effective in many patients. In fact, patients' responses to surgery vary so widely that the results cannot be gauged by photographs or by the surgeon. We agreed that a direct approach to the nasolabial fold is a valuable adjunct and should be employed in most cases. It involves undermining and adding autologous tissues. Liposuction of the fatpad is equally important.[1] Little fat is removed, but you do soften the "hills" while elevating the "valleys." Raul Loeb[2] noted this point a few years after our discussion of the subject in Brazil. He now uses a flat underminer similar to the one we describe below but unfortunately approaches the nasolabial fold through a direct skin stab incision, which is not necessary. Suctioning and undermining can be done adequately through an area that is hidden to view inside the nostril.

Curettage and SMAS

Curetting the undersurface of the skin to induce contracture may be a good procedure in the "banana peel" area hidden under the buttock or in back folds where one cannot remove excess skin. I do not care for this in the face, or the results presented by its proponents. On the neck, adhesions and subsequent wrinkling spoil what would be a natural neck contour.

[1]McKinney P, Cook, JQ: Liposuction and treatment of nasolabial folds. Aesth Plast Surg 13:196, 1989.
[2]Loeb R: Nasolabial fold undermining and fat grafting based on histologic studies. Aesth Plast Surg 15:61, 1991.

Most readers are familiar with subperiosteal and deep or superficial SMAS undermining advancement techniques, so details are not outlined here. I simply do not undermine SMAS anymore. The "deep plane" rhytidectomy and the subperiosteal rhytidectomy have not met two of my criteria: (1) One must prove that a procedure is *better* than standard plication or superficial advancement of the SMAS. In my opinion, the results of these techniques are the same. (2) Any additional procedure would have to be almost totally risk-free. Temporary paralysis of the lower lip occurs too often with extended undermining, even in the hands of skilled surgeons.

Rotating the SMAS into the malar zone is an advantage of my plication method. Ewaldo D'Souza-Pinto also reported good results with a SMAS rotation flap on a medial pedicle that is folded and fixed into the malar zone. Rather than design a pedicle, I grasp the SMAS tissue with two forceps and move it upward. I fix it with three or four inverted 2-0 Vicryl sutures to highlight the malar prominence. Then I trim excess SMAS in front of the ear and plicate everything upward with more inverted sutures. The platysma, which has been divided in its anterior half, is then repositioned posteriorly and superiorly. The final inverted sutures are in the preauricular area, creating a smooth, taut cheek from the sublobule area to the malar highlight. At the end of the procedure the cheek is taut, lifted, and smooth. A final check often reveals small, fatty blobs that are then scissored away.

If the patient has midcheek hollowing, preliminary infolding in this area is carried out, again with 2-0 Vicryl inverted knot sutures. The direction of the remaining SMAS may be changed to suit individual requirements.

D'Souza-Pinto routinely augments the base of the columella in older patients using cartilage grafts. I must admit I have not seen that deformity in the older patient often, but we do augment that area with fat grafting, which is a simpler procedure. Because D'Souza-Pinto was one of the pioneers of autologous fat grafting, it is interesting that he omits its use in this zone but uses fat grafts freely in the areas we have discussed.

Posterior Closure

Now that the internal repair is done—whether you undermined the SMAS and resected a portion or simply folded SMAS upward to obtain the same effect—and the submental platysma has been resected and repaired from the chin down to the hyoid, you are ready to redrape the skin. Lift up everything and take a look. You may find fascial bands that are still intact, particularly in the lower neck. When the posterior skin was dissected free, it was from the ear lobe incision. I prefer to pass flat-bladed scissors subcutaneously and simply continue to spread the area until the dissection is sufficient. Once the posterior skin flap is lifted, it is safe and easy to divide any adherences under direct vision. This technique also keeps you away from the postauricular nerve. It is important not to overdissect in these cases unless the patient is an old person with loose skin down to the sternal notch. If that is the case, free up this area *after* the SMAS and platysma have been safely anchored in place.

When closing behind the ear, keep in mind the hair position. The first stitch shown in Figure 9-1A ensures that the most forward flap hair sits as closely as possible behind the ear. Note that there is hair anterior to the stitch. Anything anterior is closed later with half-buried mattress sutures to prevent stitch marks. In Figure 9-1B this stitch has been tied down and we are now working forward with half-buried mattress sutures. I prefer these sutures to clips because they allow rotating the flap toward the ear, not backward, which takes the tension off the skin just in front of that first suture, the most vulnerable area for necrosis. In Figure 9-1C it can be seen that this part of the operation has been completed and we are ready for the first half-buried mattress suture, which will cover some of the hair-bearing skin on the flap and some skin without hair. This suture is tied well away from the ear so the suture marks will not be visible. Make sure both the entry and the exit are in areas that have hair. Note that I have not yet resected skin around the ear lobe—that is the last skin to be trimmed. In Figure 9-1D the drain is in place and the skin is resected in front of and behind the ear so the edges touch. Just prior to this maneuver I lifted the temple area with a single anchor suture. It is now easy to judge skin excess in front of the ear and around the lobule. This area should have skin-to-skin approximation with little tension.

There is yet another step to decrease tension behind the ear even more. A 2-0 Vicryl suture is used for the next advancement stitch. It is first passed into the temporalis fascia (Fig. 9-1E) and then into the subdermal area down low (Fig. 9-1F). When this stitch is tied (Fig. 9-1G) it rotates the skin under the ear so the lobule lies free. The skin has been advanced upward and the only tight point is in the most hidden zone midway behind the concha. Figure 9-1H shows the most tension-vulnerable skin now lying against the skin of the ear with no tension whatsoever. The procedure is finished with a few half-buried 4-0 nylon sutures, passing them from the postauricular ear skin into the superficial flap and tying them fairly loosely.

Figures 9-2 and 9-3 illustrates a technique that ensures the posterior scar does not stray from the sulcus, and that stretched white marks do not appear on the mastoid area 1 to 2 years after surgery. An additional advantage is that this technique enables safely taking up that last bit of slack skin without the risk of having the earlobe ride to a forward position or end up plastered to the scalp.

The suture illustrated is 2-0 Vicryl. Half-buried nylon mattress sutures have been placed in the hair posteriorly and at the tragus (not shown) anteriorly. The former align the hair to avoid too obvious a "stair step" hairline, and the latter elevates and fixes the position of the skin anterior to the ear. The Vicryl suture technique as illustrated lifts the skin underneath the lobule and anchors it to mastoid fascia. *The lobule hangs free.* After three sutures are placed, the skin is neatly tucked around the lower ear with *no surface sutures* to form the slowly elongating white marks that are a visible stigma of rhytidectomy.

The next suture further lifts the skin and anchors it to the ear cartilage.

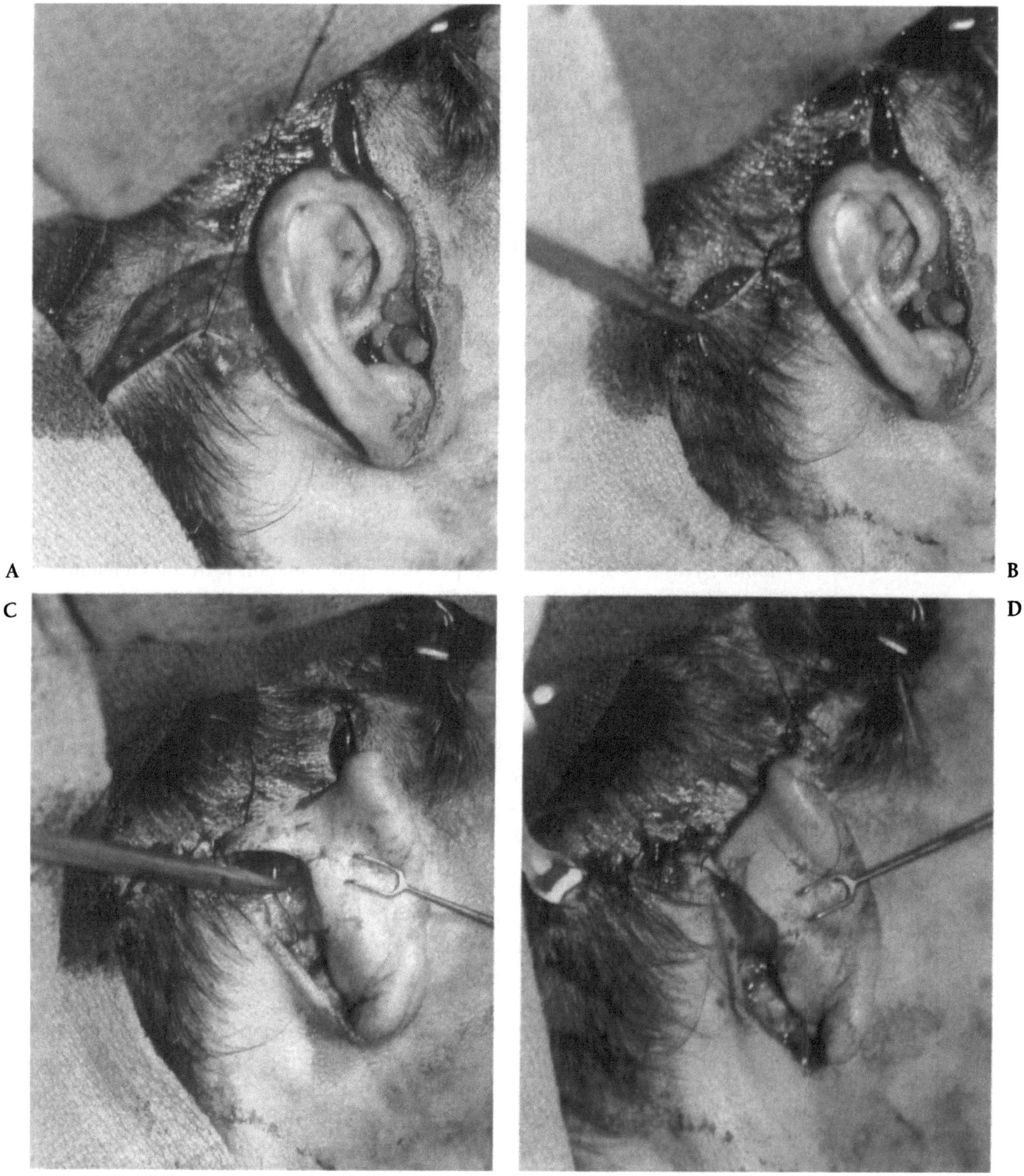

Figure 9-1. See text for explanation.

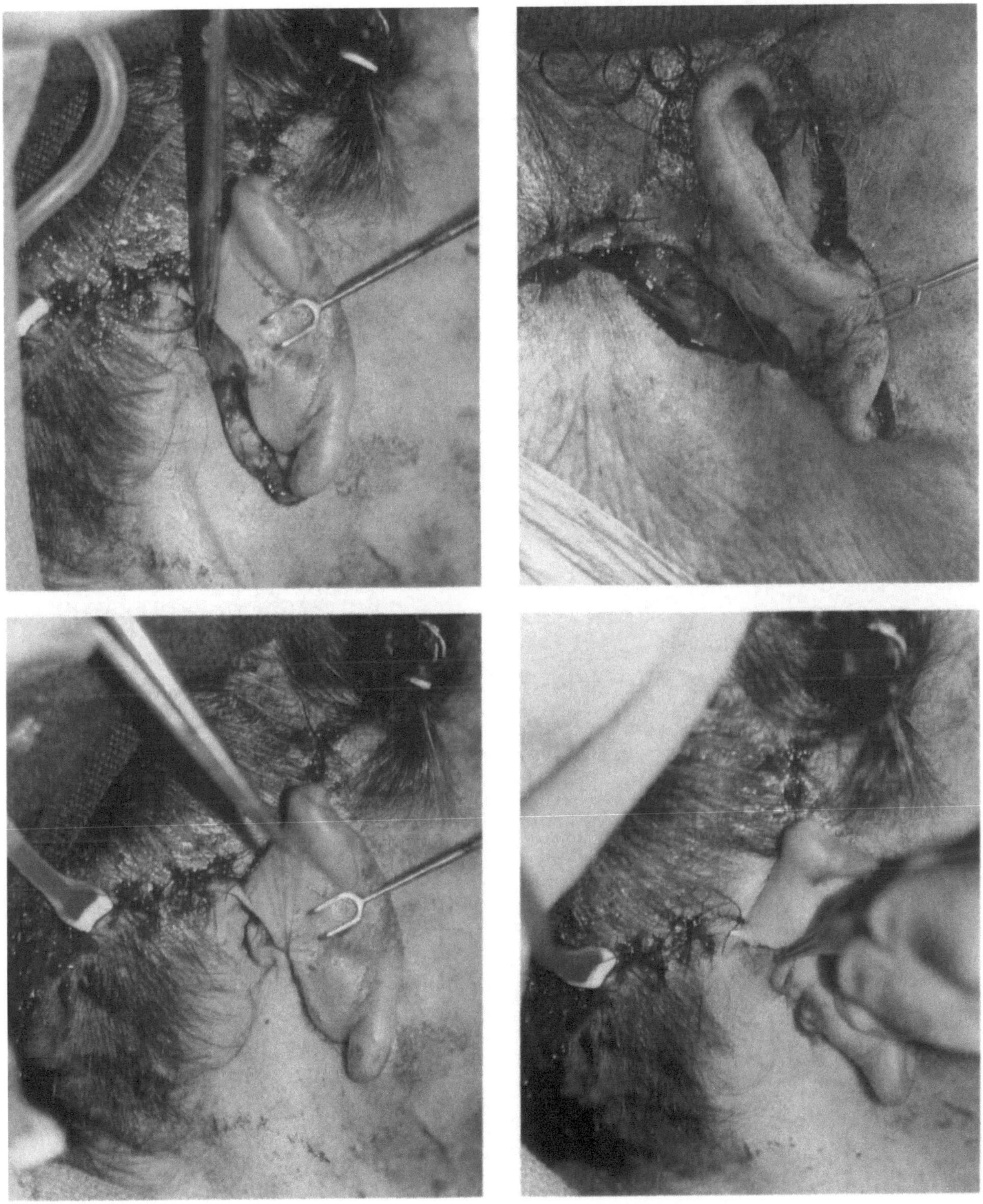

E F G H

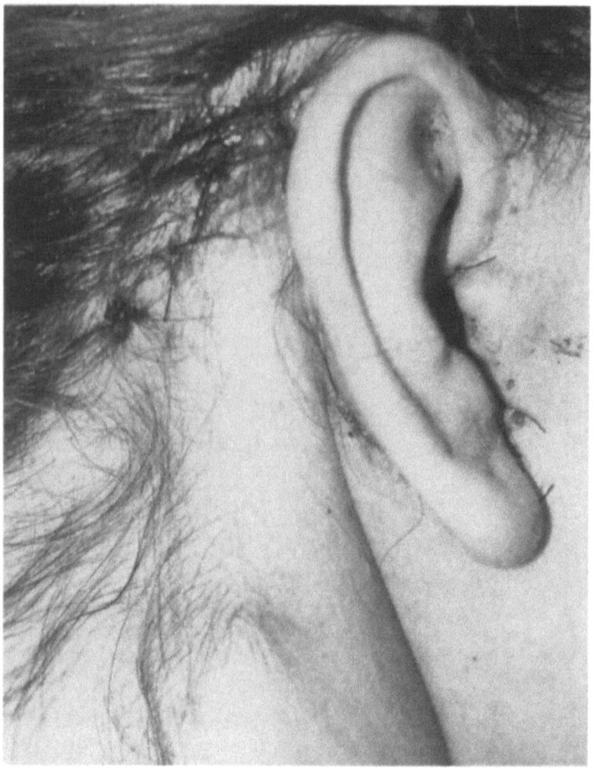

Figure 9-2. See text for explanation.

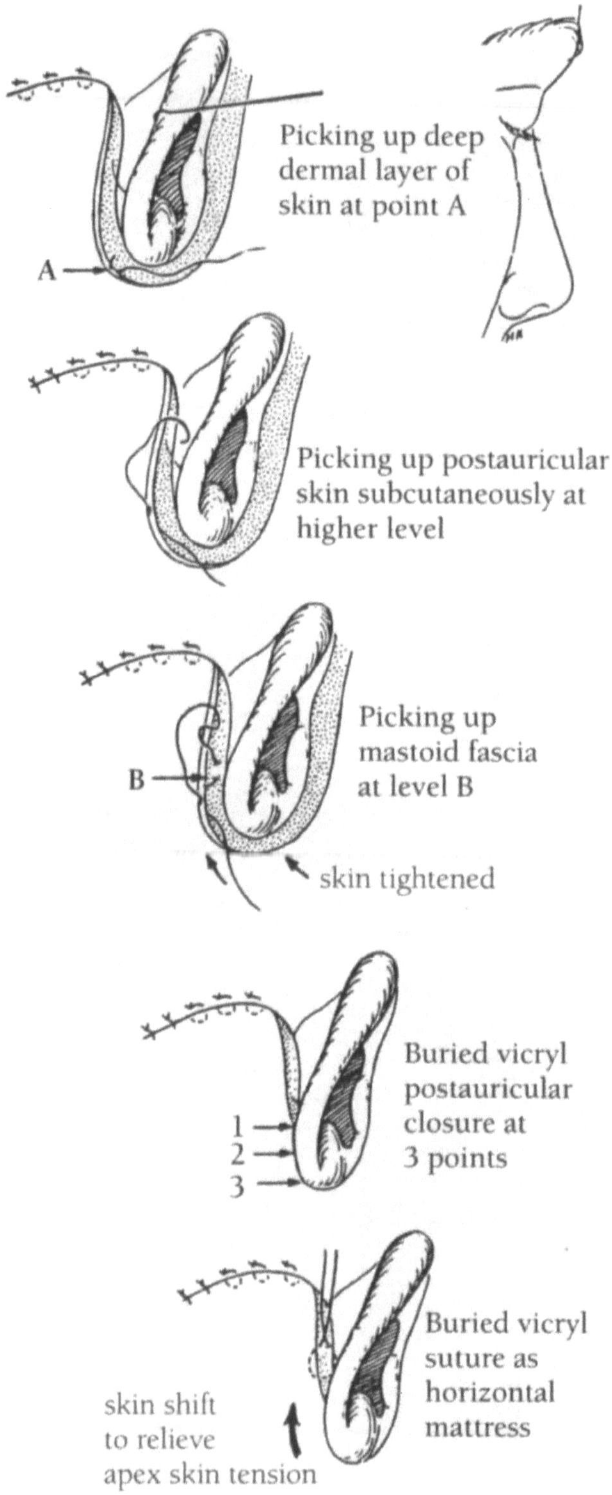

Figure 9-3. See text for explanation.

(Myth of plastic surgery: Never suture to the ear cartilage for infection and necrosis shall fall upon thy head. Nonsense.). Afterward, tacking sutures, half-buried mattresses, or no sutures at all may be used, as the fragile apex *now lies in position without tension.* Perhaps one reason sloughs once occurred in this apex was that with a classic Millard face lift the key suture was placed in the apex.

Several colleagues have advised leaving the area between the lobule closure and apex open for drainage and drain exits.

Anterior Closure

Once the closure is complete behind the ear with the skin flap tightly rotated around the lobule, which hangs free, anterior closure is undertaken. The first step (Fig. 9-4A) is to trim the fat or SMAS from the area in front of the tragus. Note that the tragus has been left clean when the skin was dissected. It must have as little bulk as possible. A trench is now created with the scissors tip. This trench goes down to fascia to recreate the normal fold. Remember that the face lift moves thicker skin upward and over the tragus.

Attention is now turned to the skin flap itself (Fig. 9-4B). Composed of cheek skin that has been moved upward, it is fairly thick and fatty. The area is defatted down to dermis, but only that which will cover the tragus. The next goal is to make this skin a tension free spot.

Figure 9-4C shows placement of a 2-0 Vicryl suture in the trench. The skin flap is lifted and the stitch used to advance everything upward so the skin for the tragus lies in place without tension. For a secondary rhytidectomy, this step allows taking up excess skin in a "double opposing rotation." In those cases, as shown in Figure 9-4C, we rotated hair downward to recreate the sideburn and rotated the cheek upward for the lift. The deep suture helps take up slack. The skin is now closed above and below the tragus with a 4-0 nylon suture that barely catches the deep dermis of the advanced skin (Fig. 9-4D). Because this area is a difficult one from which to remove stitches, three catgut sutures are placed in ear canal skin. They fall out in less than a week, and their sole purpose is to hold the skin over the tragus. Healing takes care of the rest (Fig. 9-4E).

An upper running stitch is started on the ear canal skin as well. This 6-0 nylon suture provides added security in case the patient should do something to break the catgut sutures. Figure 9-4F shows a typical result. The lobule is hanging free. The ear canal is not "open" because the tension is anterior to the tragus, and the tragus is of relatively normal size. The advantage is that skin color blends well into the cheek. This point is particularly important for secondary face lifts, when you are moving discolored skin to a point that is adjacent to undamaged white-skinned tragus.

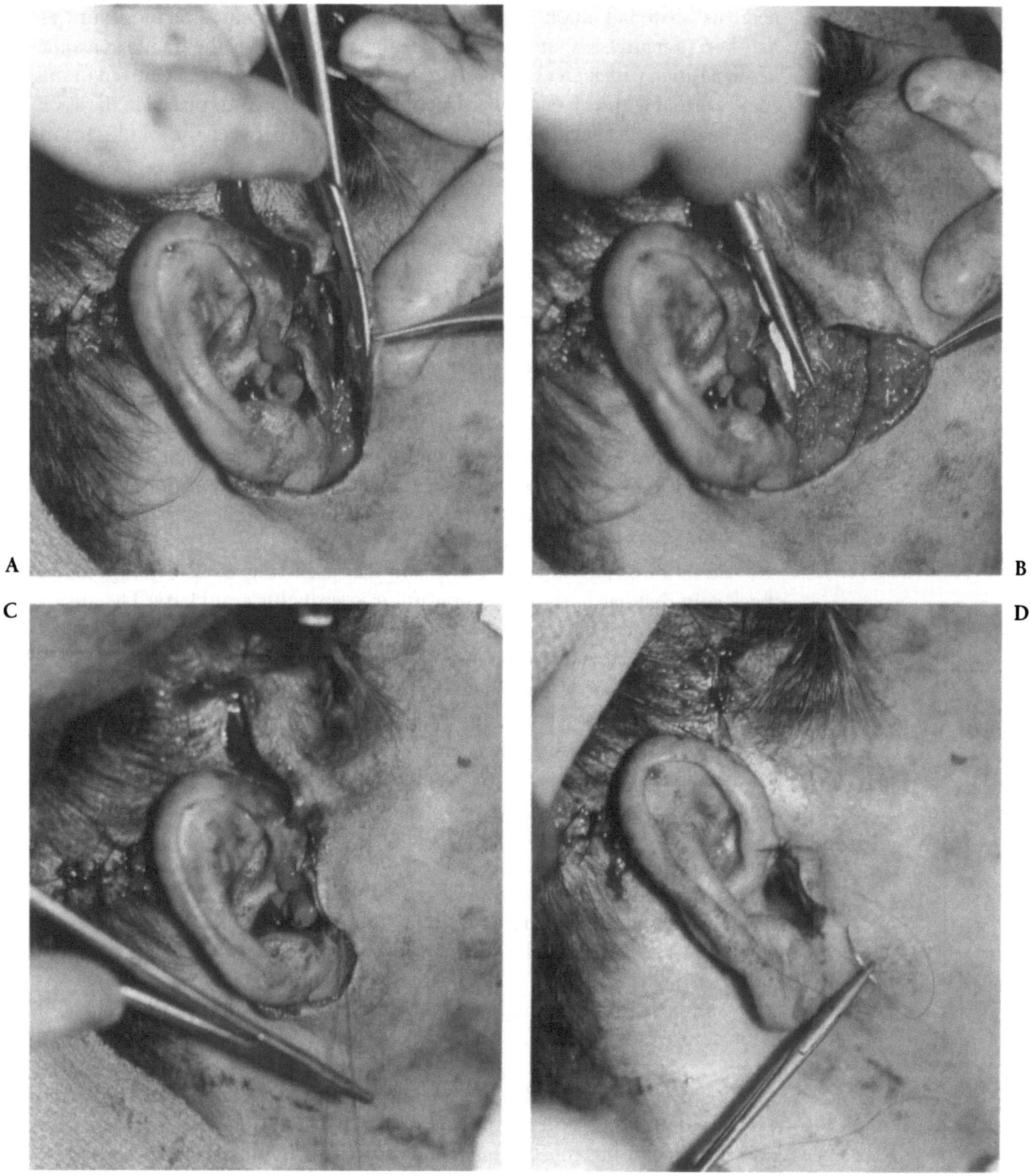

Figure 9-4. See text for explanation.

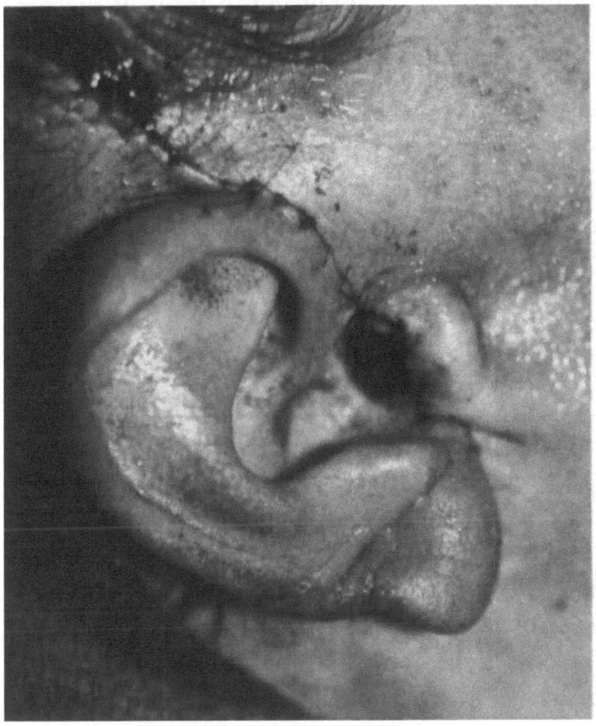

E

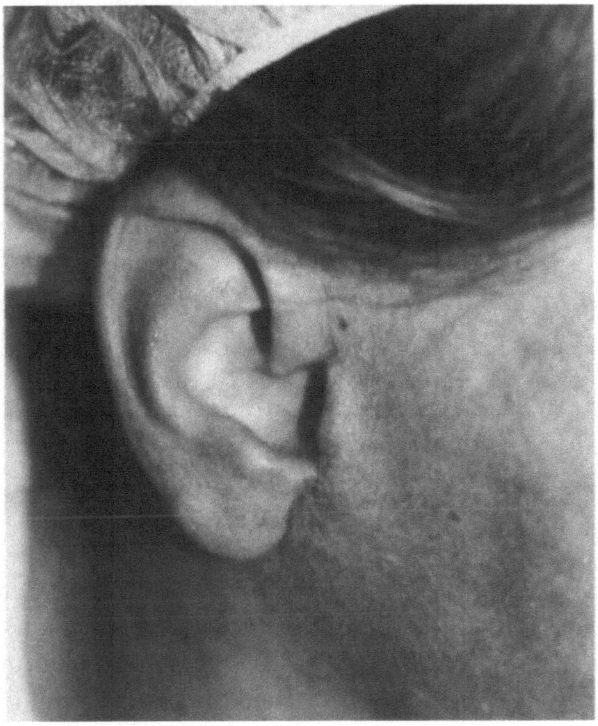

F

Improving the Appearance of Tragal Incisions for Rhytidectomy

A few years ago, the curvilinear preauricular pretragal incision for rhytidectomy was chosen because the W-plasty effect prevents linear contracture and leaves an almost invisible incision line. With a properly performed rhytidectomy, this area is closed without tension. Use of a retention suture of nylon placed within the tragus to the undersurface of the skin flap as a tension reliever has been described. The other advantage of the pretragal incision is that the elevation, color, and shape of the tragus are undisturbed.

Before we found a way to remove tension from the tragus, there were only three cases in which we chose to place the incision within the tragus. The first was a patient with variable skin color, and the second was a young individual undergoing a half-lift. In the first category the paleness of the tragus would contrast markedly with the skin that is brought to juxtaposition. In the young patient, the excessive elasticity of the skin persists in this area, despite the laxity noted in the jowl and upper neck area. Placing the incision within the tragus prevents scar hypertrophy, a complication in a significant number of these young persons. The third patient was a secondary face lift candidate. In such individuals the skin that is now moved upward almost certainly has a different color and texture from that remaining on the tragus.

The disadvantages of the intratragal incision are the change in the structure of the tragus itself and obliteration of natural contouring in front of the ear. Figure 9-5 shows the technique that markedly improves that appearance. Because many patients with poorly performed face lifts require downward movement of the temporal hair as well as upward movement of the skin below the lobule, this curve allows you to take up some of the slack between these points. It might also be necessary to trim the tragus if it is unusually prominent. This small technical maneuver creates a more natural look and is worth the few minutes required.

Reducing Hair Loss

Figure 9-6 illustrates the technique for reducing hair loss along the upper face lift incision. It is not a coronal lift. All of the face lifts performed in our clinic since the early 1970s have this high curve. Most patients have some lateral eyebrow descent, and this maneuver corrects it. After making the scalp incision, the tissues are freed down to the orbital rim and the periosteum elevated. In the past, there was a problem of bald spots in the upper incisions for both the coronal lift and the standard face lift. Years ago Bruce Connell suggested placing one or perhaps two tight sutures and then cutting the elevated flap longer so the skin edges simply touch. First, I determine where the main direction of pull should be. For the patient in Figure 9-6A,B, the lift will be primarily at the center of the eyebrow. For other patients, the clamp is moved lower and the tight spot created at that point for maximum lift of the lateral eyebrow. The cut is made straight to the end of the clamp, and a heavy 2-0 nylon suture is placed there. Once the suture is tied with tension, it is easy to cut the flap so the edges overlap (Fig. 9-6B). The edges can be tacked together with a few sutures. I do not like to use staples in this area because they squeeze the hair follicles, and tight closure is not required. Tension is the problem here, and numerous staples or sutures can cause spotty hair loss.

The clamp shown in Figure 9-6A was developed by Mine Kurtay (Cleveland) and is different from the standard marker. According to Kurtay,

> My clamp is not the same as the D'Assumpcao rhytidoplasty marker, which is the clamp that was devised by a doctor of the above name who trained under Dr. Cronin [Padgett Instruments No. P 390].
>
> This clamp has a similarity, but it is quite different from the clamp that I have proposed. The differences lie not only in the tips, but also the piercing and the locking of the instrument which the precious marker does not have. This is more practical in use and also allows the individual to stabilize and map out the required excessive amount of skin removal without the medial flap sliding, rather, it is held firmly. It shows also the areas of tension, which may be dangerous to the patient regarding its viability.

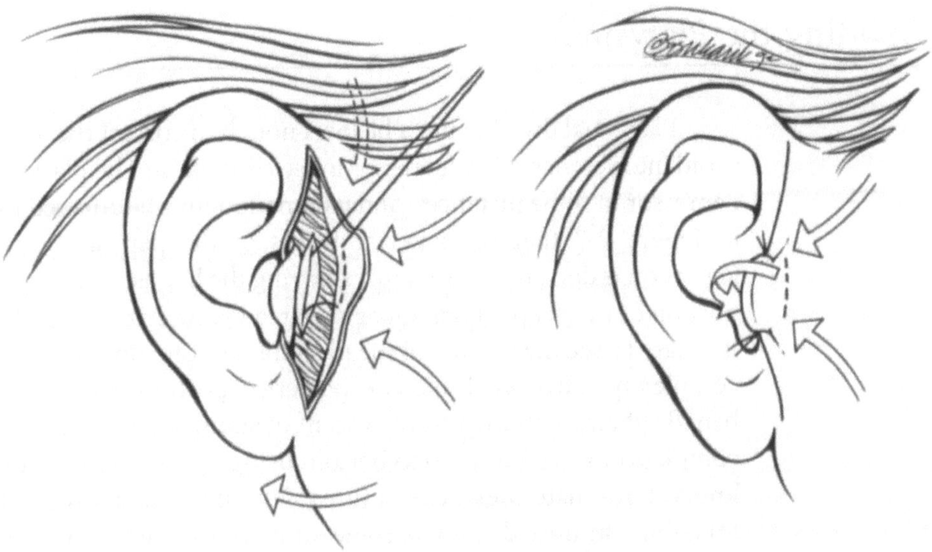

Figure 9-5. See text for explanation.

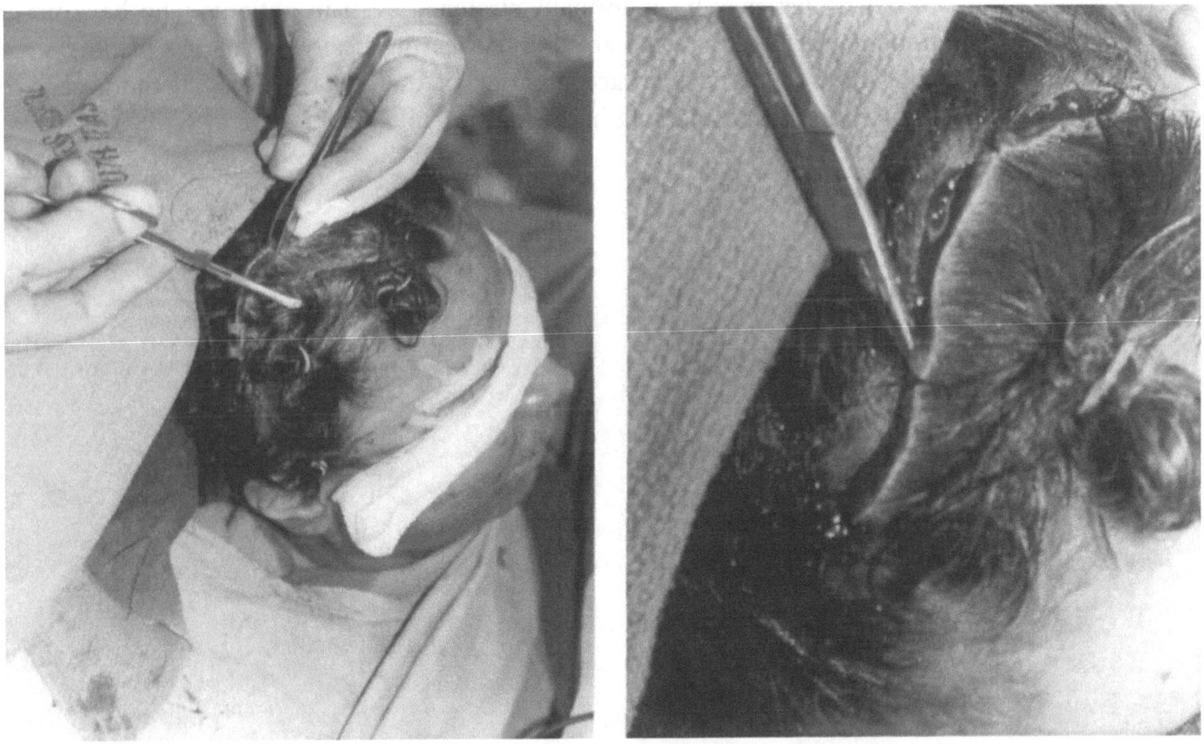

A B

Figure 9-6. See text for explanation.

Dividing the Platysma

Platysmal division must be low enough to correct the visible bands but still avoid interference with depressor muscle function. The platysma blends into the depressor in some instances, and its function may be affected by a high cut. Note in Figure 9-7 that the anterior bands of the platysma have been resected. Resection is done in one swoop, removing the bands, superficial fat, and anterior portion of the deep fatpad. Once the area is cauterized and bleeding controlled, it is easy to see the outline of the platysma. At one time we divided the platysma completely; now we leave the posterior portion intact, which may have a beneficial effect on the future descent of submaxillary glands. Note that there is complete closure from top to bottom using figure-of-eight sutures, burying the knots. I alternate Mersilene sutures with absorbable ones, just to be sure the Mersiline sutures do not become untied. The figure-of-eight sutures are an additional protection maneuver.

Earlobe Sculpture

Earlobes may be abnormally stretched even in patients who have never undergone surgery. Some are due to wearing heavy earrings, and others are congenital or perhaps an accentuation of the aging process. If the goal is to reduce lobule size and length, the incision must be hidden.

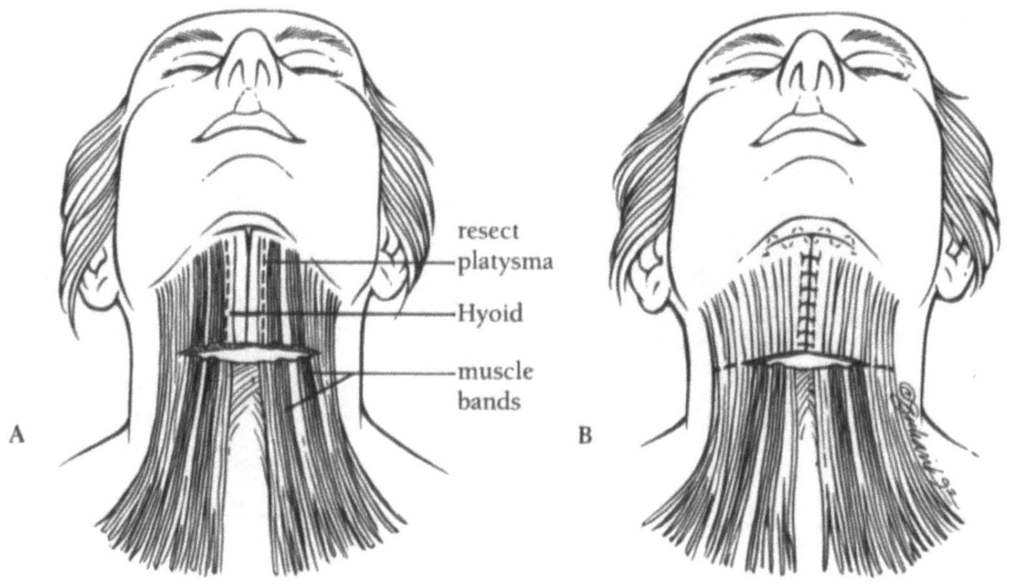

Figure 9-7. See text for explanation.

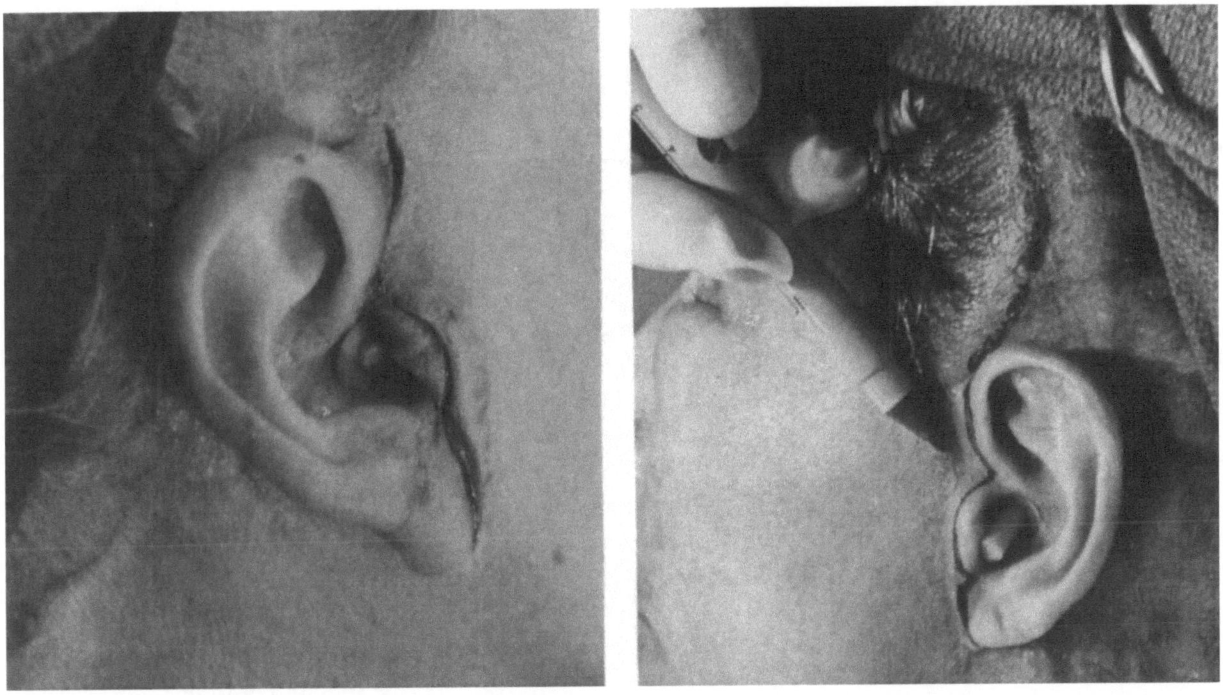

A B

Figure 9-8. If a pretragal incision is chosen, make the incision close to the ear curves and deep above and below the tragus (Fig. 9-8A). The secondary rhytidectomy begins with reopening the old incision anterior to the tragus to facilitate jowl and submental liposuction. The skin over the tragus is later removed and the scar behind the ear advanced upward. Never place a scar outside the hairline for a primary rhytidectomy. Earplugs are used (Fig. 9-8B) to block blood from entering the auditory canal.

The proposed earlobe shape in Figure 9-9A is lightly marked on the anterior skin. The actual skin incision is 2 to 3 mm lower and posterior. A small skin flap is to be created that can be tucked around and sutured on the back surface of the ear.

The earlobe excess has been resected in Figure 9-9B, leaving the skin flap flush with the soft tissue of the ear. This skin is then elevated completely to the line of the new earlobe shape. Scissors are used at this point to trim away the underlying soft tissue until the skin flap can turn under and join the cutaway portion posteriorly (Fig. 9-9C).

The only difficult part is the transition point where both incisions touch the helical rim. Half-buried mattress sutures tied in the back are helpful. They can be left in place for 10 days and do not cause visible scarring. A simple 6-0 running nylon suture approximates the edges and gathers up loose skin. The stitches are removed in 4 to 5 days and the ear coated with collodion for protection.

This operation is simple and technically neat. Patients concerned about long earlobes appreciate it as an added touch in refining their face lift.

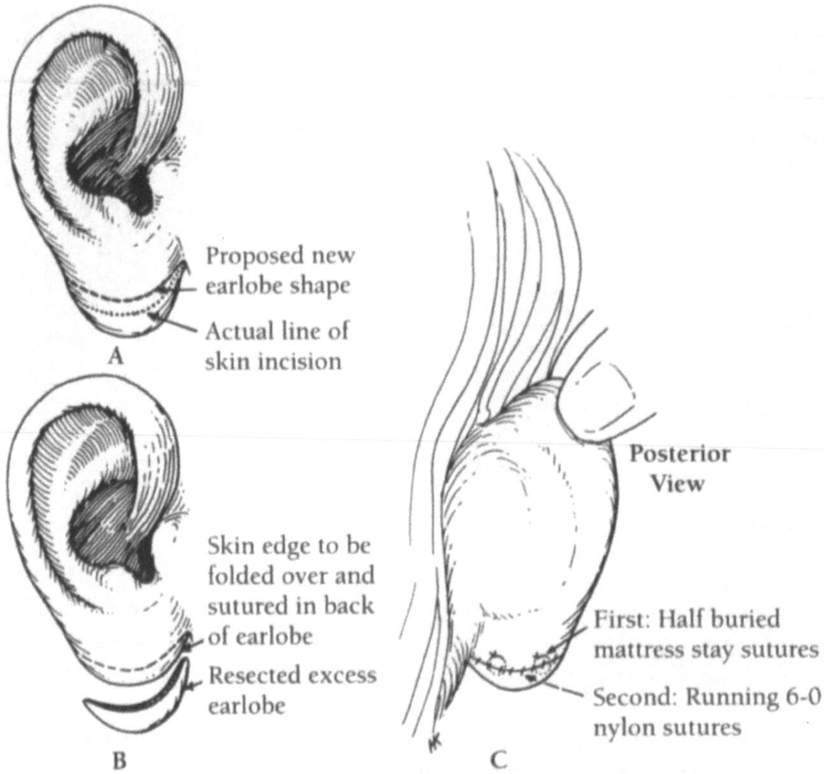

Figure 9-9. See text for explanation.

Effect of Smoking on Face Lifts

Tom Rees and his colleagues in New York finally reported what had been suspected by many surgeons—that the effects of nicotine on some individuals' small-vessel blood flow can cause a plastic surgery disaster. In *Technical Forum* I took early issue with their report simply because the phenomenon of posterior slough in face lifts had become so rare. None of us cautioned the patient against smoking back then. As the years have passed, the evidence has accumulated, reinforced by anecdotes from all areas of plastic surgery. Surgeons have reported abdominoplasty, breast reconstructions, breast reductions, and others to be well healed and well vascularized, only to have tissue loss within hours after a patient resumed smoking.

This situation led one Texas surgeon to promise patients that he would repair any complications of their surgery without charge if they refrained from smoking but would fully charge them for the surgical repair if they did not.

In one case, a fairly routine bilateral subcutaneous mastectomy was carried out through lateral incisions. The area above each areola was simply deepithelialized to allow advancement to a more natural position. This surgery certainly should not have affected blood supply. The patient had been a heavy smoker, was asthmatic, and had been counseled extensively about her problem. Yet she was caught red-handed on the third postoperative day, cigarette in hand with a room full of butts. The dressings were changed immediately, but the area had already begun to turn a darkish color and later sloughed.

Why is it not a universal problem? Perhaps some smokers' blood vessels are not as sensitive to the effects of nicotine, or their vascularity is so cross-linked that tissue survives. Despite initial reservations, no one today doubts the deleterious effect of smoking on plastic surgery results.

I asked Dave Foerster and Tom Rees for comments.

From Tom Rees:

> Our study of slough in face lifts and its relationship to smoking was conducted because we were convinced (anecdotally) that heavy cigarette smoking was a major factor in wound slough. Many surgeons shared this suspicion, especially those doing a large volume of breast flap reconstruction and abdominoplasties. Our clinical study was challenged by some statisticians; yet taking the most conservative view possible, smoking was still incriminated as a major cause of wound slough. A subsequent study of flap survival in hamsters subjected to cigarette smoke compared to controls confirmed our clinical impression beyond a doubt.
>
> The mechanism is still not entirely clear, but the effects of smoking on vascularity are several, ranging from competition for oxygen in which the carbon monoxide of cigarette smoke competes to marked advantage with oxygen for a place in combination with the hemoglobin molecule, to the well-known, long-range pathological effects on the small vessel.
>
> Subcutaneous mastectomy severely challenges the blood supply under normal nonsmoking conditions, and in the chronic long-term smoker there is probably very little margin left. We have all sweated the survival of skin flaps in subcutaneous mastectomy, so it is not surprising that this patient had a problem, most likely accentuated by her smoking. I would think that subcutaneous mastectomy in heavy smokers, especially long time smokers, is risky at best, and perhaps alternative techniques should be considered. The use of immediate implants should be passed over for a second procedure.

From Dave Foerster:

> The problem of postop[erative] slough after flap elevation, be it face lift, subcutaneous mastectomy, or abdominoplasty, does not seem to totally go away and is undoubtedly a multietiology phenomenon with nicotine use playing a major role. Nonsmokers can certainly have sloughs for no apparent reason, and many smokers do quite well in spite of their habit. Postradiation [effects] also can be a factor as can an acute hematoma. And there must be the rare patient who simply does not have the normal collateral circulation to sustain a flap's viability. If you do enough face lifts and enough subcutaneous mastectomies you will get some sloughs. Anyone who never has a slough is a liar or else talks rather than operates. I can remember writing off a prominent West Coast surgeon who bragged about having done

> several hundred subcutaneous mastectomies through inframammary incisions and never having a single slough—I never believed anything he ever said after that.
>
> I have made a very unscientific observation while doing face lifts over the past several years and wonder if anyone else has noticed anything similar. I find that not only smokers but ex-smokers have, as a rule, smaller branches of the external temporal artery than true nonsmokers. This does not necessarily mean that a slough will occur, but when I see this, I tend to be more conservative in my undermining.

A group of Vanderbilt University anesthesiologists may have shed more light on the current plastic surgery controversy about smoking versus nonsmoking and rhytidectomy sloughs than all the protagonists in our profession with this analysis:

Chronic smoking is associated with increased blood levels of carboxyhemoglobin, which causes a decrease in the amount of hemoglobin available to bind to oxygen. In a slightly anemic patient it could make a difference. There is also evidence that carboxyhemoglobin shifts the oxyhemoglobin dissociation curve to the left, resulting in decreased oxygen unloading at the tissues. The important point is that abstinence from smoking for only 12 hours *reverts* these values to near normal. While the patient is smoking, the increased levels of carboxyhemoglobin result in decreased hemoglobin available for binding and unloading. Within 12 hours of the last cigarette, however, oxygen release is facilitated and oxygen-carrying capacity restored. This sequence applies to occasional smokers as well as long-term chronic smokers.

Perhaps those who argue both sides of the controversy are right. Patients who smoke up to moment of their arrival at the surgical center theoretically have less oxygen perfusing the tense skin behind the ear that is to undergo rhytidoplasty. Even with the current techniques that relieve tension behind the ear, it must be recalled that this point is far from its blood supply and would likely be most affected in terms of having access to available oxygen. Some minor technical factors, such as pressure, bleeding, and too tight sutures, could then tip the balance.

Forehead Lift

Forehead lift, endoscopic or direct is the most overprescribed and overperformed operation in facial surgery. It has the most potential for leaving an abnormally bland or abnormally frightened appearance. In one presentation, the surgeon showed a series of male face lifts with forehead lifts included as part of the package. One patient was a Marine officer. In the preop picture, he looked tough, rough, and commanding. In the postop picture, he looked like a pussy cat! Few males with a low eyebrow desire this correction. I always illustrate this point to patients repeatedly, because once the surgery is done there is no turning back the clock.

My standard face lift procedure elevates the outer two-thirds of the brow by freeing and dividing periosteum at or below the medial and lateral orbital rim—without an endoscope! This change is sufficient for most women and gives a pleasing, natural look. For others, it is best to free the forehead completely with a variety of cross-cutting techniques to stretch out forehead creases. The technical points involved for the "coronal" forehead lift are as follows:

1. Always make the incision as a curve that meets with an anterior forward curve in the midline to place the incision farther back than you think you should. It is easier to resect posterior scalp, and patients have a tendency to develop thinning hair over ensuing years.
2. Perform most of the dissection under the galea with blunt fingertip dissection until you reach the periosteum just above the orbital rim. Divide the periosteum and elevate it with a dissector.
3. Try to avoid the subcutaneous forehead lift if possible. Few patients benefit from this variation of the procedure, and the possibility of depressions, wrinkles, and other deformities is great in the average patient.
4. Dissect down to the dorsum of the nose and sand off some of the hump if desired. The wrinkling that occurs late in life is frequently just below the glabella. Destroy the procerus.
5. I prefer Sherrill Aston's technique of carefully dividing the corrugator vertically with a spreading forceps. It allows you to visualize the nerves and still keep the muscle from functioning.
6. Whether you resect a central portion of the galea or simply cross-cut, the results are much the same. I prefer a cross-cutting maneuver, horizontally and vertically, particularly placing the horizontal cuts just above and below the position of the major forehead wrinkles.
7. If you leave some of the fascia intact, you do not need to graft the glabella with fascia. Remember, the temporalis *lifts* the eyebrow.
8. Do not hesitate to undermine the deepest furrows laterally before elevating the flap. Placing a little fat right under the dermis may be helpful, although it is unnecessary for the average forehead lift.
9. When planning the excision, use the Bruce Connell technique discussed in this chapter. Place two "tight spots" sutures on either side of the midline and let the remaining scalp edges touch without tension.
10. Always drain this area. Bruises show up with great regularity even in dry fields.
11. Maintain the smoothness of the forehead with an aggressive skin care program beginning 30 days after the forehead lift. We routinely use TCA peels now at the time of the lift.

(Text continued on page 234)

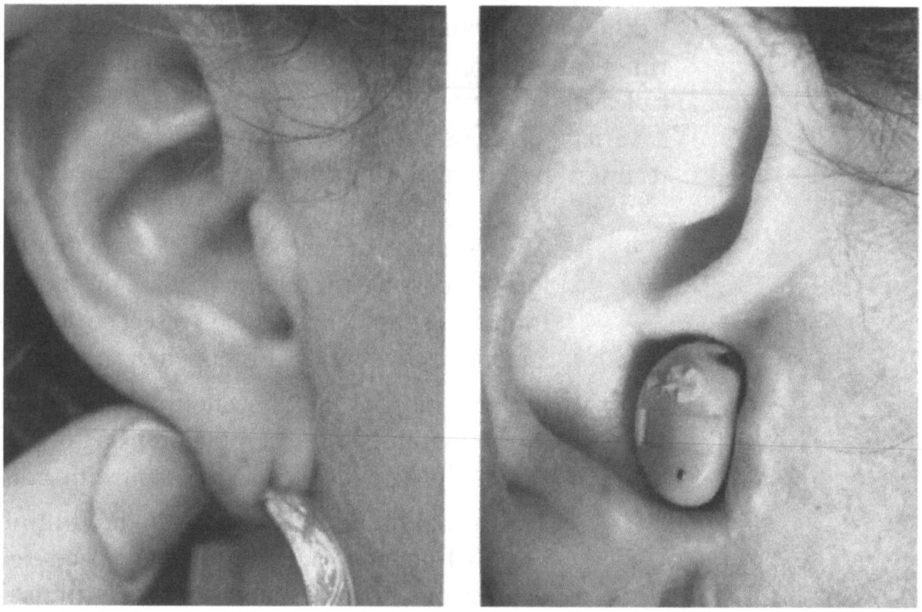

A B

Figure 9-10. Even at best, pretragal incisions are visible, primarily because of the color difference between tragal skin and the cheek skin that is advanced. Until a way was found to prevent tragal displacement forward (open ear technique), this incision was preferred. The Z-plasty effect and curve into ear folds helped disguise the scar. Contrast **(A)** with **(B)**. There is little tragal enlargement, and a pretragal groove has been created.

Figure 9-11. Submental tuck and lower two-thirds face lift is still as good a procedure as it was in 1978. **(A&B)** This patient complained of a "sad" look, with jowl descent and major platysma and fatty neck problems. **(C)** When she was ready for a second procedure in 1992, jowl liposuction was a standard part of our routine. Liposuction and a midface skin lift restored the lost youthfulness. The submental zone remains corrected, 14 years later.

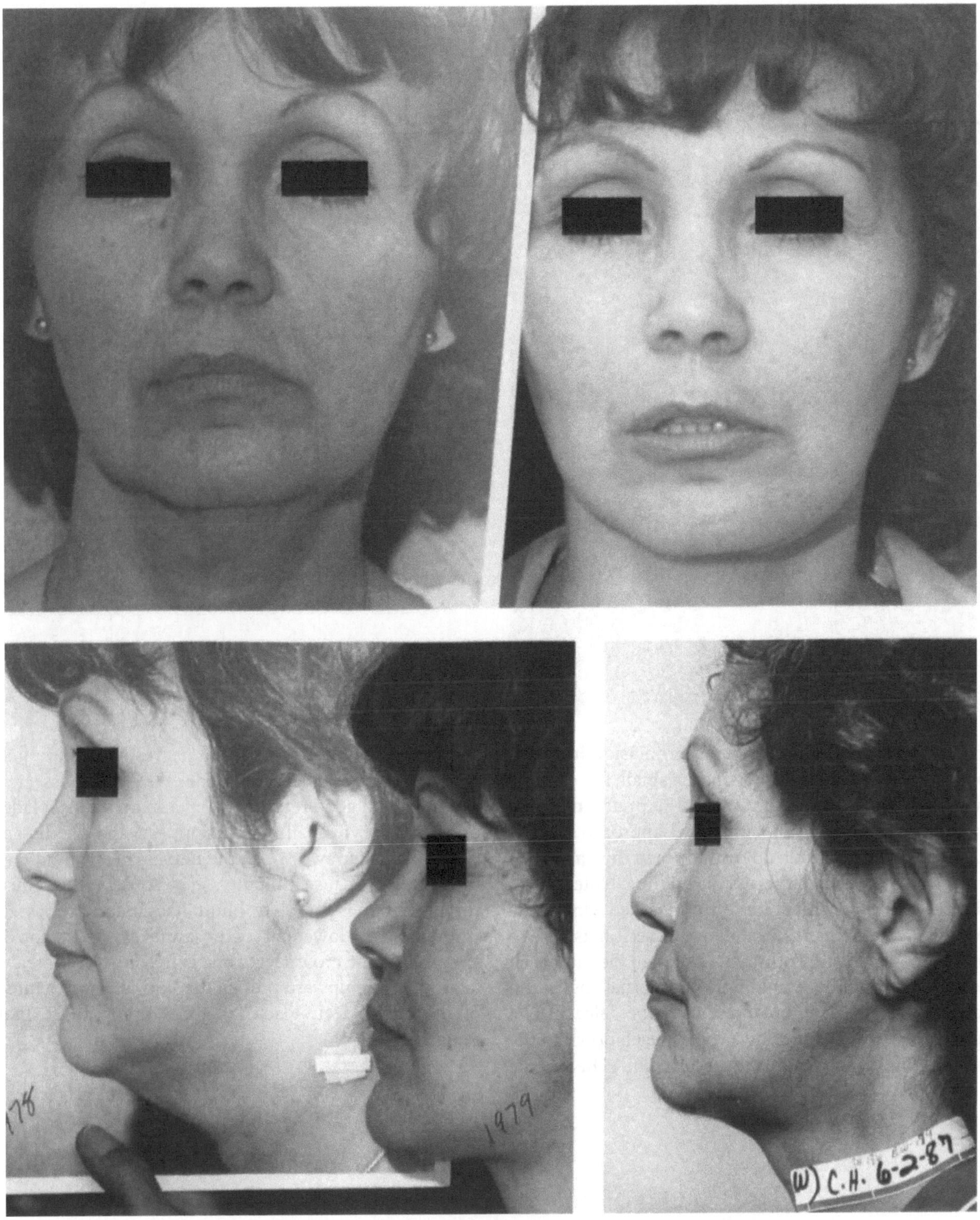

A

B

C

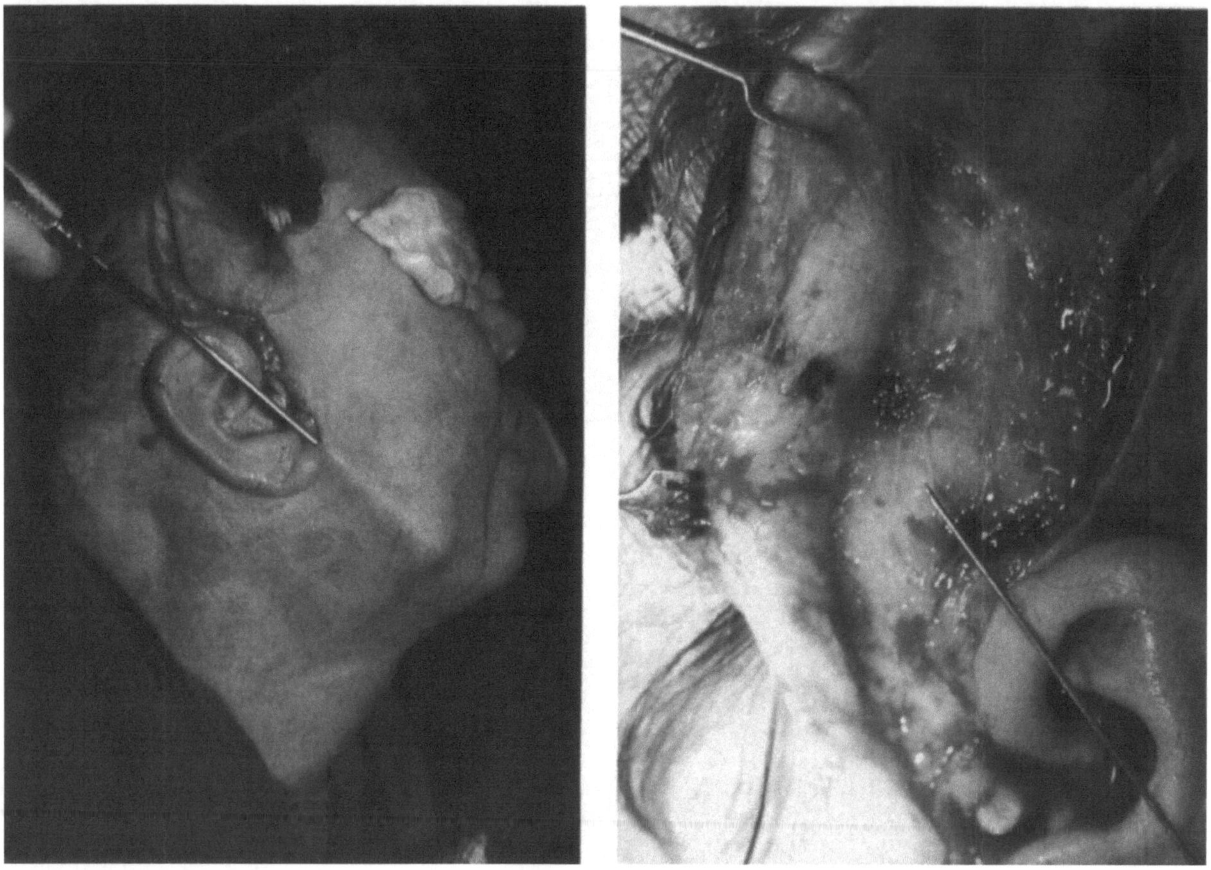
A B

Figure 9-12. (A) Once the anterior incision has been opened and hemostasis is obtained, a small, flat cannula with a slight curve is introduced. I prefer machine suction to syringe SAL for this jowl approach, as it is easy to turn the cannula upward to reach the nasolabial mound and to extend it across the midline. Note that all the areas for suction are carefully premarked. Unless the patient has an excessively fatty lower cheek, it is wise to leave this area alone. Too often, suction in the midcheek results in unsightly wrinkling. (B) Internal dissection far above the ear can be done under the galea. It is a quicker dissection and allows you to reach down to the orbital rim and free up the periosteum. The needle shows the position of the facial nerves, which are just below the fascia. If this area under the skin is dissected carefully with good retraction and a sharp scalpel blade, only one or two small bleeders appear, and the dissection remains far away from the nerves. Even stretching the nerves can cause difficulty, so be conservative. Once this dissection is complete, blunt, flat scissors are passed throughout the lower part of the jaw level with the top of the ear, and the crow's feet zone is freed up. This area is a safe one, and upward pull on the skin can stretch most of the crow's feet. Place fat grafts under those that remain.

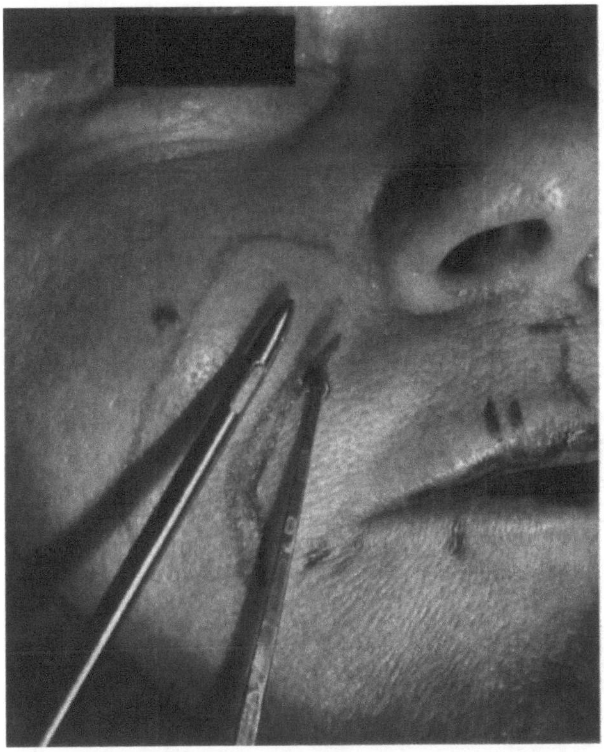

A

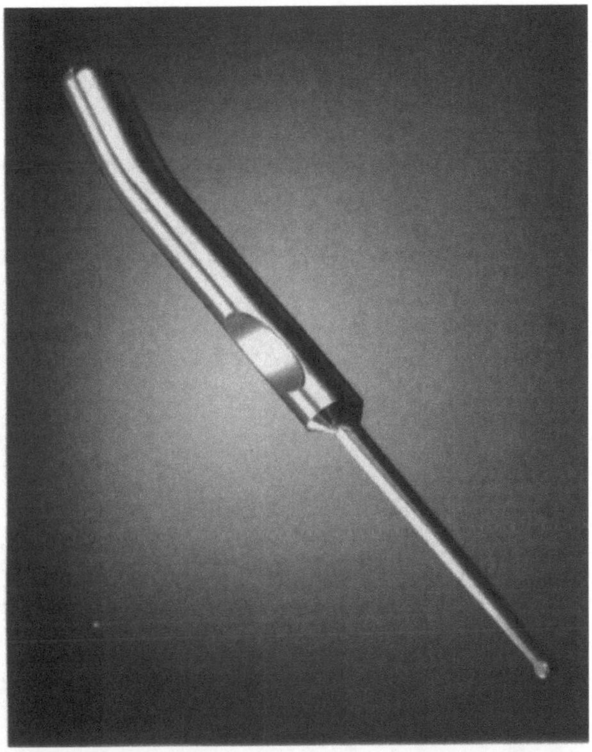

B

C

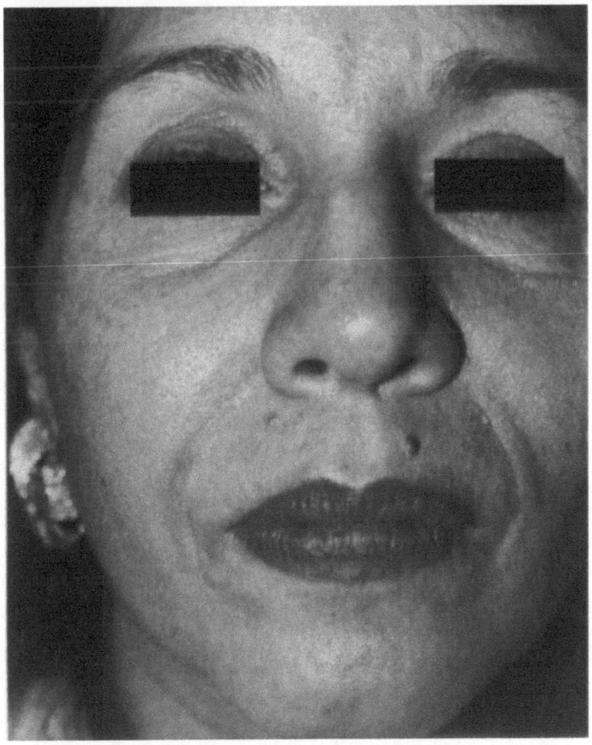

Figure 9-13. (A) Direct attack on the deep nasolabial fold requires two instruments. The premarked fatpad lateral to the groove is best suctioned with a blunt multihole small cannula. This area can be reached from within the nose, from a blepharoplasty incision, or from the submental incision. A separate nasal entry introduces the flat tip of my "rhytidissector" for undermining the crease. (B) (Wilkinson Rhytidissector, Byron Medical). The curved handle gives good tip control, and the semisharp round tip is safe for subdermal scraping. Having a slender tip and good control is more important than the convenience of a combination dissector/injector with which fat can be introduced in one motion without removing the instrument. (C) Wilkinson dissector/injection cannula. Shown earlier in photograph 2-1, is good for minor underminings in the nasolabial area or for the bizarre scar folds shown in which are said to have been from collagen injections. This subdermal scarring can be removed by vigorous subdermal scraping using a syringe-suction device attached to the cannula.

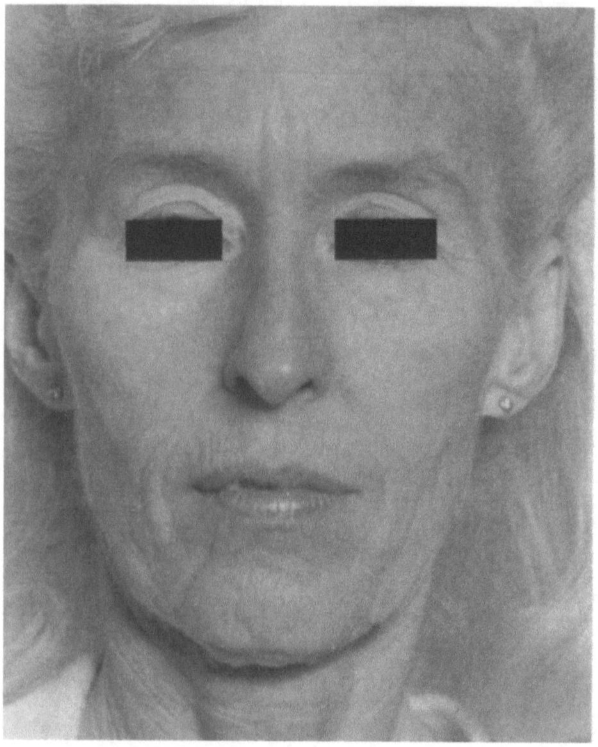

A

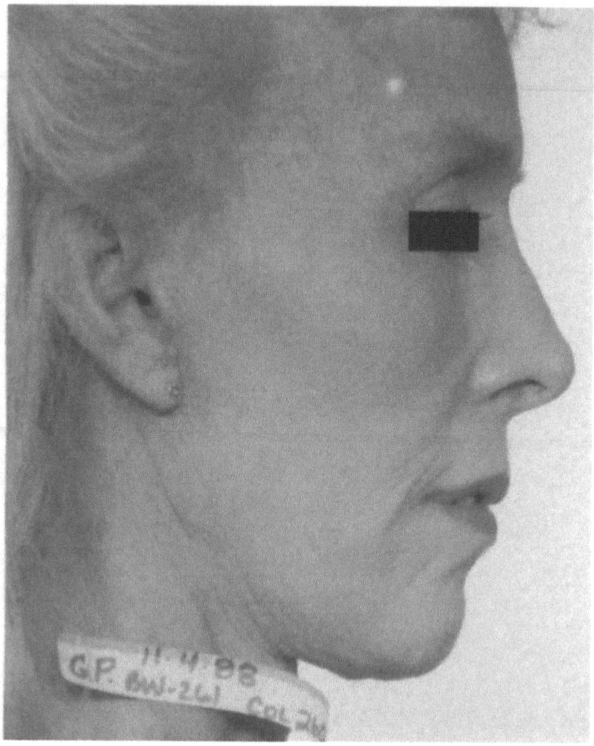

B

C

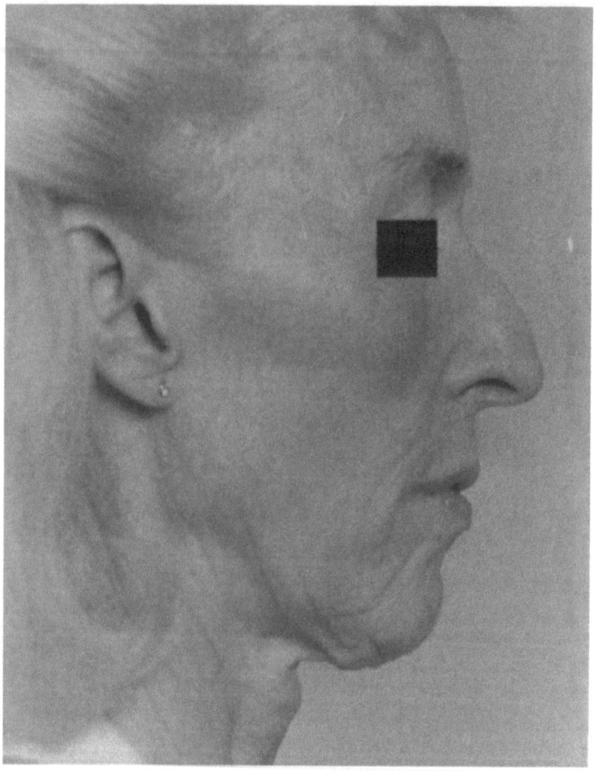

Figure 9-14. (A–C) This woman is one of our three "thirties progeria" patients. The extreme aging changes appeared when she was in her thirties. Each of the three women has had two or more skin tucks during the years following the original rhytidectomy. Fat grafts and TCA peels were repeated as well. (D–F) A reasonable result can be maintained with repeated touchups and a home program of skin care.

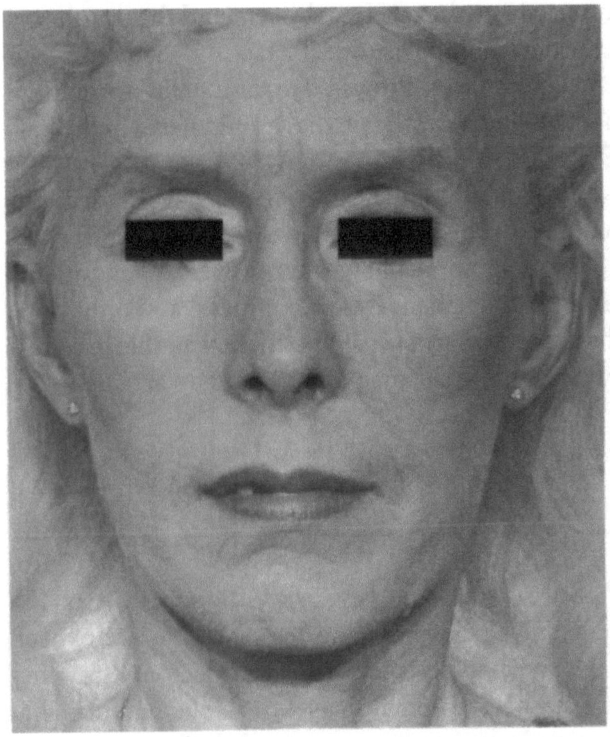

D

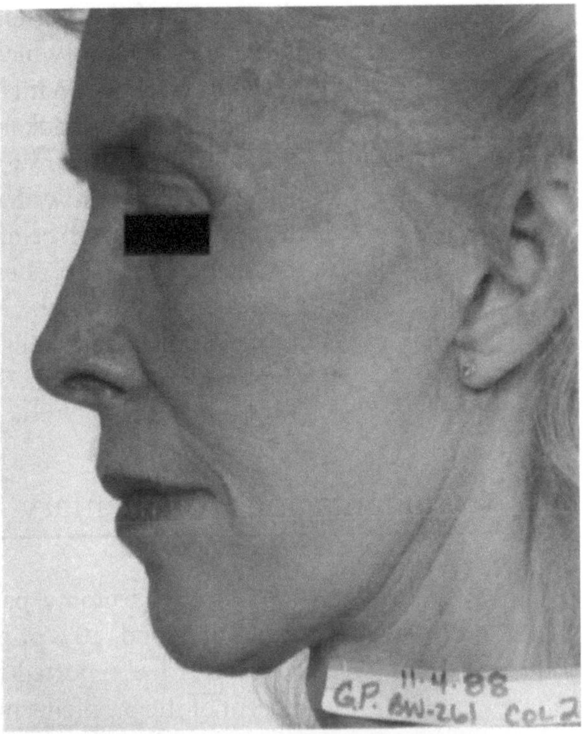

E

F

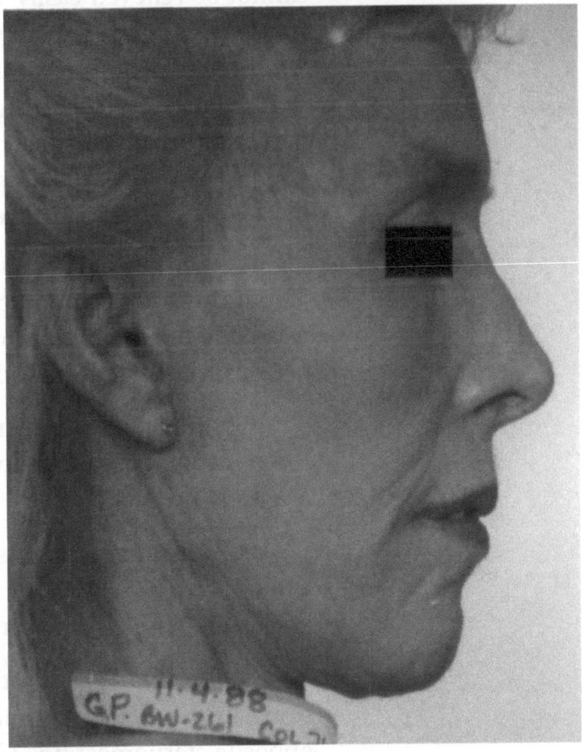

The patient in Figure 9-15A,B is to have a complete face lift and wishes to eliminate the frowning appearance. Note the midface descent and the position of the central eyebrow, which is the determining factor. The face lift was carried out as described above. With forehead lift, the eyebrows were raised, but not enough to make the patient look frightened. She also chose to have fat grafting in the lips, nasolabial line, and crow's feet. Even as early as 2 weeks after the surgery (Fig. 9-10B,C) the eyebrows have a normal appearance and the lips have settled into the position that will be maintained for the next several years. In my experience, the shape of the lip does not change appreciably after 3 weeks. In patients followed for 5 years, there has been little change in the fullness, and only a few are beginning to reestablish the nasolabial groove. This patient was able to return to the classroom within 7 days with the assistance of our makeup artists.

Comments and Commentary

1. Rhytidectomy patients are worrisome because although 90% of the results are good, 10% of patients have a problem and that they did not expect. Tom Baker has reported his extensive experience with rhytidectomy. Seventy percent of the problems in his patients are hematomas, but the hematomas that cannot be relieved easily with simple aspiration or minimal drainage comprise less than 2%. In almost every case the patient with a hematoma had *pain and nausea*, was always *restless*, and usually had *high blood pressure*. If you see this triad, remove the bandages immediately. Tom does not use intraoperative narcotics because he believes they increase the incidence of nausea postoperatively. I use an initial 2-mg dose of butorphenol (Stadol) followed by 2-mg increments. So far we have had few nauseated patients.

2. During a discussion of changing face lift techniques Baker stated, "Plastic surgeons should be clever enough to avoid suture cross-hatching." He was referring to rhytidectomy, but should we not take this advice to heart for breast surgery, abdominoplasty, and other aesthetic procedures?

3. Infections are seen with face lifts occasionally, but there seems to be a lower incidence among those performed at an office surgical center rather than in a general hospital.

4. An interesting case was presented in which the patient had psoriasis extending across the area of the incision. Baker believes there is no risk associated with cutting through such an area.

5. Dick Jones and others use criss-crossing submental platysmal suspension sutures. They extend from the medial upper platysma muscle to the opposite sternomastoid. The pressure of the suture is said to increase the angle between the submental and upper cervical areas and helps elevate any ptotic

A B C D

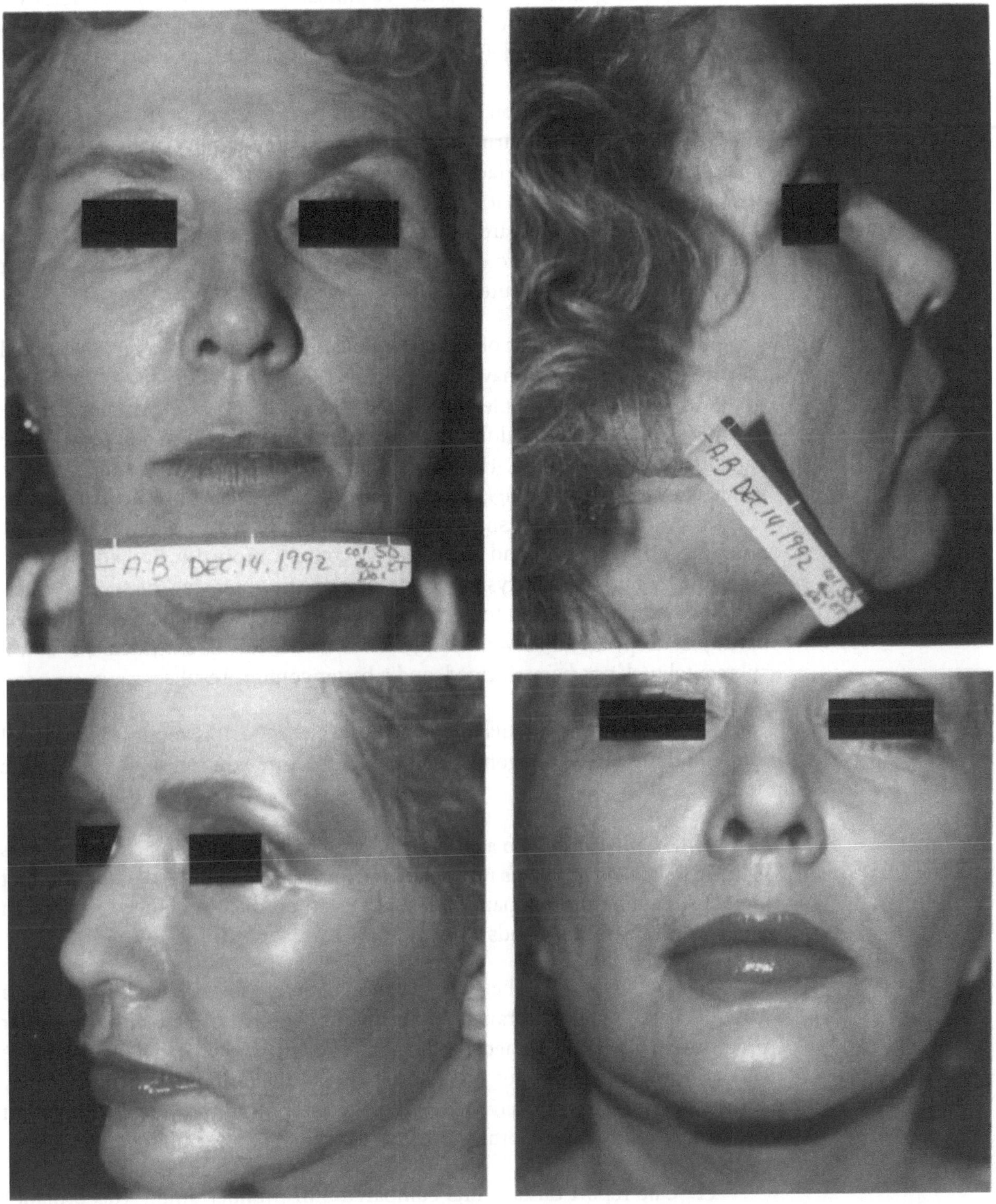

Figure 9-15. See text for explanation.

submandibular glands in the area. Technical point: When Jones removes sections of the corrugator or procerus muscles during forehead lifts he places dermal strips in the defect left by resection of the muscles.

6. There is no question that a face lift is an extensive operation with much internal stitching and repairing of pathology. Therefore physicians outside our specialty who use the term face lift to promote their "suction face lift" are using an inaccuracy. *Suction—let it be said once and for all—is an adjunctive procedure.* It can be used to touch up areas "where angels fear to tread," and it can speed a face lift by allowing you to reach the occasional low cervical fat deposits. It cannot be used as a substitute for the true operation.

7. Gene Courtiss, one of the true innovators in aesthetic surgery, has noted that some individuals do have taut platysmas and small deposits of fat in the neck, usually young people with good skin. Their necks usually can be sculptured with suction alone, but as Courtiss points out indirectly, these patients are the exception. He makes a large enough incision so he can look inside the neck. *Suction lipectomy is remarkably inefficient.* More fat can be removed with three quick snips of the scissors than can be taken with twenty pumping arm motions and with better control. Courtiss has admitted to occasionally snipping a platysmal band and even anastomosing the severed edges onto the midline. The chin to neck angle lies low in these patients and there is usually a deep fatpad as well. If the suction incision is extended 1.5 cm, a submental tuck can be performed, and a better contour results.

8. Beware of the vascular area under the platysma. It is about 1.5 cm lateral to the midline. If you are going to excise fat, be sure you can see what you are doing.

9. One physician who advocates moving "prolapsed" submaxillary glands claimed he had no problems in 40 patients. Readers are reminded of the fact that simply stretching the submandibular nerve can produce prolonged paresis. In other words, leave the glands alone.

10. Oh, just great! The "new" version of subperiosteal face lift has only a 10% VII nerve temporal branch paralysis—in contrast to 20% with the earlier procedure. This "improvement" is not good enough. We agree that the risk of the subperiosteal face lift is not justified by any aesthetic improvement that may accrue. Several surgeons have tried to make the procedure work for them but gave it up for this reason, others prefer it to "standard" face lifts.

11. One report on face lifts compared SMAS undermining (deep plane) and SMAS resection without undermining. Conclusion: they look the same. Why? Probably because the author used wide skin undermining, to the nasolabial line. That helps to smoothe the nasolabial fold.

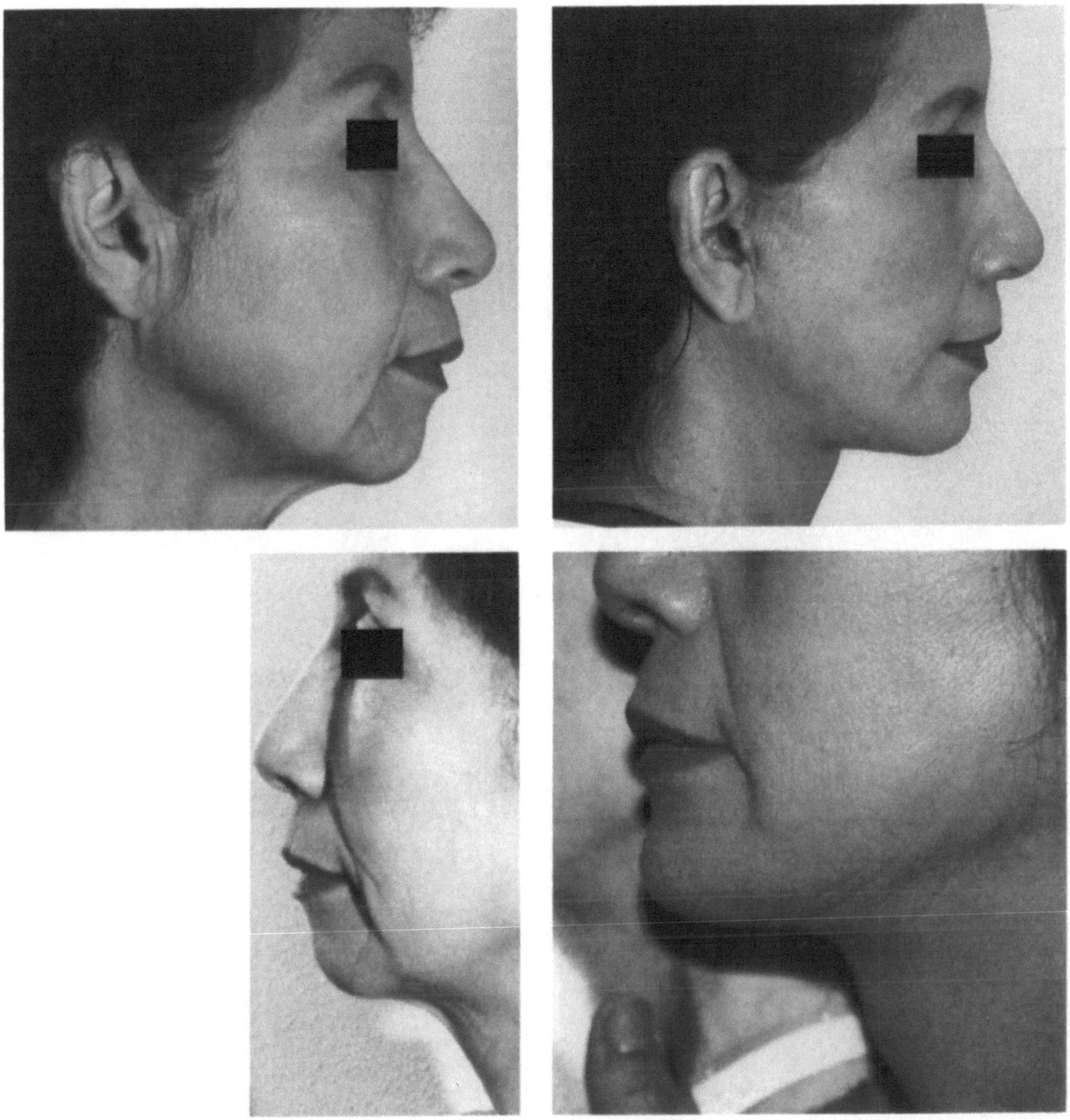

A

B

C

Figure 9-16. Rhytidectomy and submental tuck combined with chin augmentation and fat grafting resulted in a pleasing "soft look" in this patient. Note the relatively minor change in the eyebrow positioning and the sculptured appearance of the eyelid after resection of skin, muscle, and fat. The incision was made in the pretragal area because of relatively similar textures in the tragal skin and cheek skin. Note that the lobule hangs free (**B**) and is in fact more freely positioned than in preoperatively (**A**). The addition of the chin prosthesis plus complete submental platysmal repair and liposuction has given her a natural chin line (**C**) without the artificial, stretched appearance of the early face lifts. Note also that the marionette area has been filled by fat grafting (**C**).

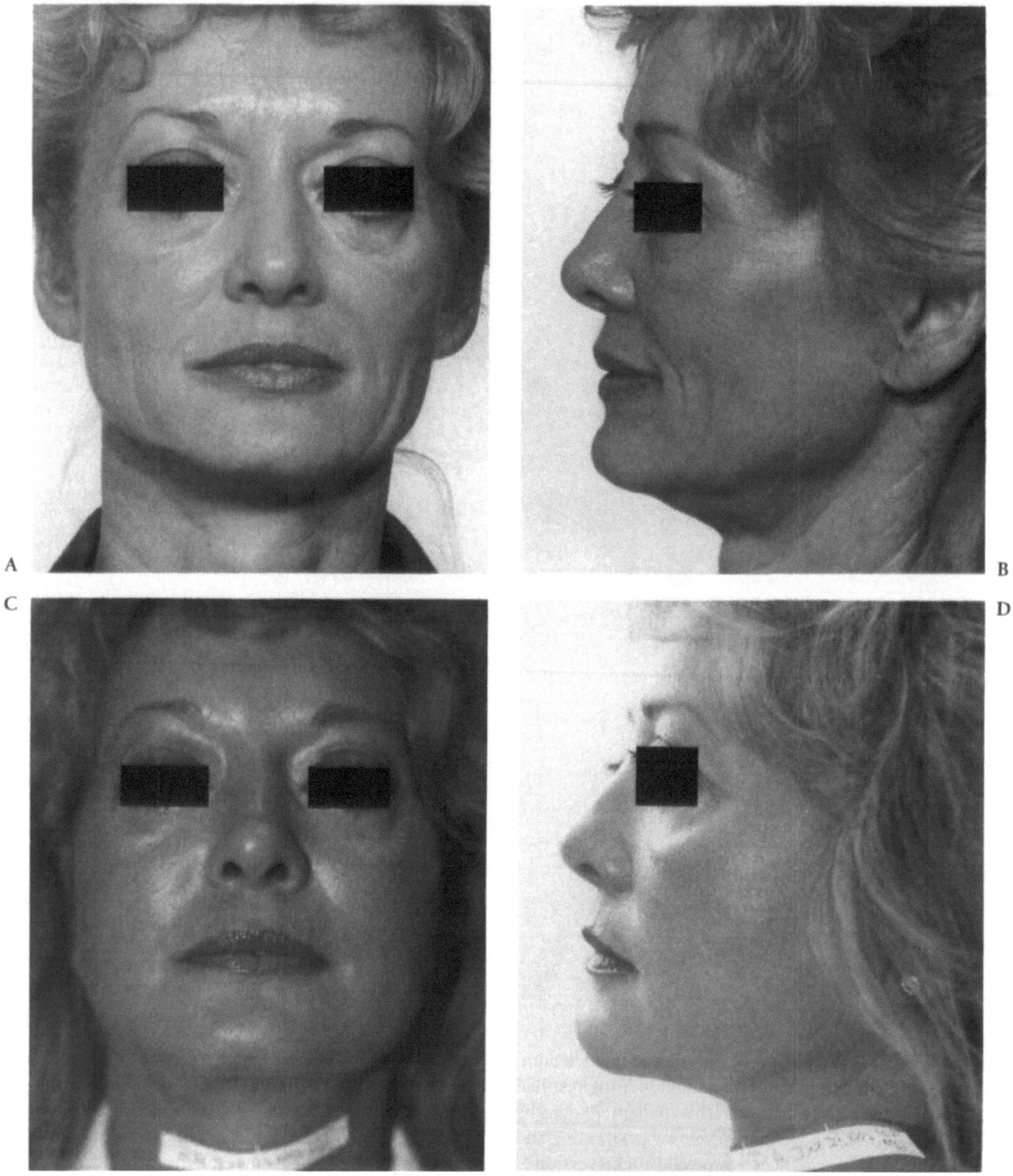
A
B
C
D

12. Bob Flowers (Honolulu) has reported two new implants he likes. One fits below the rim of the orbit for those patients who have depressions, and other fits in the area below the nasolabial fold as part of an extended malar implant.

13. Guerro-Santos' mucosal excisions combined with buccal pad excision is a new approach. There's a place for Bichat pad removal, particularly in Oriental patients, but removal is more often associated with "unnatural results" than are malar implants and liposuction.

14. Many endoscopic forehead lifts presented at national meetings are grossly overdone. How many times have you sat in the audience and watched a "national expert" show patient after patient who looks frightened?

15. Most of us have been under the impression that lasers performs as a "hot knife" and that its tendency to burn the skin edges is a minor but annoying drawback. In the deep tissues it seems to be about as effective as electrocautery, which is less expensive and less difficult to master. We were also under the impression that laser face lift or laser blepharoplasty were gimmicks more than scientific advances. We should not denigrate colleagues for extending the use of their instrument, but we should not be gulled into jumping aboard a slow-moving band wagon.

In "Small Incision Frontal Rhytidectomy," a handout promoting the use of CKP-532 laser for cosmetic surgery, the author would have us believe that frontal rhytidectomy (fore head lift) can be done with a 2-inch incision posterior to the hairline, in which case hemostasis becomes important (although there is minimal bleeding in this area). The incision is made parallel to the hair follicle with a scalpel. The author goes on to say that the subcutaneous approach is easiest, and that the numerous vessels are obstacles to visualization—hence the needs for laser.

Experienced surgeons understand that entering the subcutaneous plane is rarely indicated, and that if one uses the subgaleal plane and divides or resects the galea above the brow area, consistent and natural (not "overstretched") results can be achieved. I agree it would be good to correct an entire forehead through a 2-inch incision; but then the author says, "If an alteration of the brow or forehead

---

Figure 9-17. Facial rejuvenation in the presence of proptosis. This patient **(A)** has had a preliminary course of Retin-A and skin care and is now ready for surgical enhancement. For patients with proptosis, one must reinforce the lateral canthal ligament, the lateral orbicularis, or both but still remove the fatty deposits; one should be conservative when resecting skin from the upper lid. The lateral view **(B)** shows the extension of the blepharochalasis beyond the corner of the eye, the descent and fatty deposits in the submental triangle, and the unchanged texture of the skin. Postoperative photographs **(C)**, **(D)** at 1 year show considerable improvement in skin texture due to an ongoing program of skin rejuvenation with Retin-A and α-hydroxy acids. The fat grafts have corrected much of the shadowing in the glabella and nasolabial area and have added fullness to the upper and lower lips. The proptosis, if anything, is less prominent. This patient will be offered a light chemical peel to the upper lip and face in the future.

is intended, the incision may be lengthened." This statement counters his arguments that promote the advantages of the 2-inch incision. Why incise the skin with a scalpel and then switch to laser to cut through the subcutaneous fat, which bleeds so little anyway? His rapid hemostatic dissection is with blunt scissors in the subgaleal plane, and that too is associated with minimal lateral thermal damage—which obviously is zero thermal damage. This surgeon who is advocating laser forehead lift performs "deep plane dissection" with laser. He justifies his use of laser subcutaneously on the basis that an unknown number of patients show "less edema and ecchymoses on the laser side." In fact, without the use of laser, we rarely see edema and ecchymoses to any degree in our nonlasered patients.

16. According to Claus Walter (Switzerland), eyelid surgery should be performed only in patients 34 or 35 years of age or older, and then only "if the [patient's] profession depends on it." Moreover, he goes on to say that face lifts should not be done before age 40 and that eyelid surgery must be redone every 8 to 10 years.

Face lifting and eyelid surgery depend on the appearance, not the age, of the patient. All plastic surgeons in the United States have seen numerous nonprofessional patients whose eyelids appear ancient even though the patient is between 20 and 30 years of age. Congenital eyelid bags is a good example. People with allergies can develop the loose skin and baggy lids of an older person before age 25. As for face lifts, John Williams spoke for most of us when he emphasized that some of the happiest patients are those whose faces had sagged prematurely by age 30 to 35 and we have helped by performing a face lift. Another example is the acne patient for whom all other measures have been tried and failed; undermining and tightening with an intratragal incision can rejuvenate their skin remarkably.

17. The patient who complains of slowly resolving bruises is a problem. Unfortunately, one method used to alleviate this problem—leeches—causes more problems than cures. According to a recent mailout, leeches are useful on any skinflap suffering from impaired venous circulation. However, the leech produces an anticoagulant vasodilator and a local anesthetic, so the wound made by the leech continues bleeding for days. And they are scary little things.

18. Dressings or no dressing after a face lift? Harold Gunatillake (Australia) writes, "During the past two years, I too have adopted the no dressing technique, and neither do I use drainage tubes. All my face lifts are done under local anesthesia (Marcaine 0.25% with Adrenalin on the first side and 0.5% Xylocaine with Adrenalin on the opposite side). Gunatillake ligates fine bleeders with plain catgut and uses a frozen saline bag on the already operated side while dissecting the opposite side. He says that postoperative swelling and bruising are negligible after 24 hours, and patients can begin shampooing and showering immediately. One of his patients had fainting attacks, which he attributed to the heavy padded dressing, which caused "pressure on the vagal nerves." The heavy bandaging may also compress jugular veins and cause venous congestion in the face.

Those who disagree with these conclusions point out that compression over the cheeks reduces ecchymoses; and the suction drains, although not preventing hematoma, certainly do remove enough bloody fluid to reduce swelling and bruising significantly. Another advantage of a well padded dressing is that if it is carefully applied it does *not* compress the jugular veins, and it holds the patient's head relatively immobile. For pain relief, remember to block the greater auricular area and all of the repair areas with 0.25% bupivacaine (Marcaine) with epinephrine at the *end* of each procedure. This measure keeps the patient comfortable, but it led to a number of male patients becoming too vigorous and breaking internal incision lines. The presence of pressure padding in our hands has been beneficial. It keeps edema pressure away from the vulnerable stretchable skin of the upper neck and submental zone.

19. Joe Naud (Troy) believes we spend too much time working on the SMAS: "that tissue is junk or the patient would not have required a face lift!" He rightfully points out the advantages of platysmal surgery and gets good results with the Guerro-Santos sling. He believes that it minimizes nerve damage, allows conservation undermining, and flattens the nasolabial fold better.

20. Face lift patients usually follow the general rules for skin behavior if they have had adequate internal repair and good submental plication. Most patients are ready for skin tightening 5 to 10 years after the original surgery. Skin care with Retin-A can prolong this period as does the light chemical peel.

Occasional patients develop submental stretching when the rest of the face is holding well. Moreover, a number of face lift patients continue to age at such a rapid rate you can barely keep up with them despite Retin-A treatment. Others do not withstand the edema of surgery, and touchups are needed on the lower lids, the corner of the upper lids, or under the neck.

When these problems occur, there are three treatment choices: The first is to inject a dilute steroid [triamcinolone (Aristospan) mixed with lidocaine (Xylocaine)] into the firm tissue underneath. Frequently the problem is an old, organized hematoma or permanent edema. Another treatment is to take a small V tuck (not a full inverted T scar that is so objectable) to delete some of the loose skin. The third treatment choice is a full skin face lift, which would be done at an earlier date than you or the patient wants.

21. Today we add submental muscle surgery to practically every face lift. This procedure used to be reserved for the true "turkey gobbler" neck. Now we are seeing another group of patients, those who have had suction of the submental area and still have platysmal banding and a neck deformity due to the positioning and bulk of the muscle. These people require the submental repair we described during the mid-1970s.

Two experienced aesthetic surgeons discussed the problem.

Bernie Kay (Jacksonville):

Regarding the length of time a face lift lasts, this is the way I explain it to my patients: I tell them that in one sense a face lift will last indefinitely. If a patient had had an identical twin sibling who did not have a face lift, the patient would look better than that imaginary sibling for many years, perhaps indefinitely. On the other hand, in contrast to a rhinoplasty or augmentation mammoplasty or augmentation mentoplasty, a face lift is not a permanent operation. No one knows how to stop the clock.

I go on to tell them that if, for professional or personal reasons, one wanted to look as good as possible, it is not inconceivable to think of a renewal of the face lift procedure in modified or full form as early as a year or two later. Why? Because a year or two later they will not look quite as good as they did 3 or 4 weeks after the operation. If one wants to continue looking as good as possible, then the next interval between procedures could be 5 to 7 years. If someone followed this schedule, they could look almost the same over an approximately 15-year period, whereas their contemporaries would look 15 years older. Finally, I point out that there is nothing about the operation that would make the skin age any faster, and that even if they did not do any renewal operations, they would look better than they would have looked otherwise.

Exceptions to this would be people who have waited a very long time, or who have some intrinsic connective tissue disease (such as a forme fruste or Ehlers-Danlos syndrome). I have seen one of the latter types of patients. I did her procedure, and 2 months later she looked almost as if I did not do anything for her. She looked older than her stated 41 years of age prior to the operation. Subsequent to the operation she told me that she was the youngest of eight siblings and looks the oldest. The latter is a retrospective clue to her condition. Incidently, she also had hyperextensibility of her joints.

Tom Biggs (Houston) says he does not know how to prevent early stretch.

As for plication of the platysma in people with loose neck tissues, I have not given any kind of objective analysis as to whether or not I'm doing them any good. I feel that if I am, I'm giving them a tighter, more secure lift, but I've not honestly observed any kind of long term effectiveness.

22. Initially tissue expanders to enhance face lifting seemed like a good idea to some. Frankly, it is difficult to become enthusiastic about a new procedure when the results shown are worse than your own. It brings to mind the adage, "If it's not broken, don't fix it!" Some say the expander damages the skin, especially in older people.

In a preliminary study Tom Baker emphasized that tissue expanders were not used for the purpose of taking out more skin and that their use needs more study. There may be a place for them, but Baker and I are undecided about it. Patients in the 65+ age group sometimes quickly stretch with the inevitable edema of rhytidectomy, and they are ready for their first "skin tuck" within 12 to 24 months. Baker indicated that this group of patients *might* benefit from immediate tissue expansion. If tissue stretching will not result in a peculiar brow position, it might be worth the time and effort for some patients.

Technique: Rather than using saline, Baker places a small expander near the temple under the crow's feet as well as a crescent-shaped expander and expands each for a 1.5 minutes. Some studies indicate that tissue collagen expansion is complete within that time. The air is then evacuated, and the surgeon proceeds to the next task. Early studies show extra skin removal—more than one would think. Some of our colleagues use the procedure, whereas others vociferously call face lift expanders a waste of time!

23. A Brazilian surgeon tries 20-minute tissue expansion for all face lifts. Although he is enthusiastic, many irregular lines remained in the patients' faces. One patient had severe anterior migration of the preauricular scar. It was easy to conclude that these face lifts were not as acceptable as the one done by standard methods. Furthermore, no one's mind was set at ease by his statement that, "we had no problems with paralysis; but if we did, it was because of this SMAS dissection."

24. There are a number of ways to do rhytidoplasty, but the consensus is that some form of soft tissue plication and elevation is necessary. Many of us firmly believe that partial platysmal division with anterior anastomosis and posterior elevation and overlap for tightness is the preferred method. Jose Guerros-Santos (Guadalajara) rarely performs anterior plication, preferring to follow Ralph Millard's advice to perform anterior resection. Guerros-Santos admits that the subplatysmal tissues are infolded with the same suturing that we would use in the platysma, and apparently an identical tightening effect is obtained.

Sherrell Aston (New York) and others believe that this central undivided portion keeps the submaxillary gland from descending. Others disagree and believe that the low divided platysma, which is elevated upward anteriorly and posteriorly, acts as a supportive sling.

Jose Guerros-Santos does not divide the platysma completely but, instead, removes superficial strips of muscle to thin it and aid its repositioning; he also removes local bands. Several European colleagues apparently pay no attention to the fat or musculature of the neck whatsoever. There are advocates of platysmal division with anchoring of one portion superiorly and one portion inferiorly, sort of a Y elevation stretch.

These many choices of technique present a dilemma. The simple answer is to do what works best in your hands. If you can adequately defat the area above the platysma, with a resulting tight neck, that is the way to do it. It takes a certain amount of experience and skill to obtain a good anterior repair, but this repair makes defatting so much simpler by placing the platysma under tension. Short of removing a ptotic submaxillary gland, you should consider leaving the central part of the platysma intact.

Howard Gordon (Miami) says that his group does not use midline sutures as much as they had in the past, and he believes it makes little difference if the platysma is sutured posteriorly. He agrees that the low platysmal division keeps the submaxillary gland in place. Interestingly, their group performs few SMAS plication elevations unless the patient has an "exceptionally loose and floppy cheek." Bruce Connell shares my view that plication in the cheek is the most important part of the entire lift.

I expect that in a few years we will know which technique is best, but I suspect that equally good results are obtained by a variety of means in most patients.

25. U.S. surgeons disagree with the use of a suction curette for facial resculpturing, preferring either open suction or direct scissors excision. Neither appears to be dangerous in the hands of a skilled surgeon. Frankly, some of the patients shown by those advocating curetting had large jowl pads remaining after rhytidectomy, and others had bizarre neck skin contracture.

26. Occasionally the postoperative picture looks worse than the preoperative picture. We refer to the bold maneuver of total regloving of the upper half of the face in order to correct the senile orbit by adding redundant tissue. Not only is this maneuver an unparalleled example of overuse of surgical talent, but the results are a step backward.

27. Other advocates of midface lifts in patients under 45 are Frances Ottenni (Strasburg) and Larry Reed (New York). They believe that the obvious benefits of midface plication advancement and resection of the stretched facial skin should not be denied just because the patients have not reached a preconceived age.

28. It seems that few who serve on panels have directly discussed attacking the tissue around the nasolabial fold during rhytidectomy. It does improve the quality of the rhytidectomy.

Some say that the half face lift is a difficult operation, and that in most cases it ends up being almost a full face lift anyway. I disagree. A number of patients have tight necks and no descent of the forehead, but there is undue laxity and midface descent. I correct this problem with the so-called half lift. The operation is a full internal repair but through a shorter incision, limited simply by the available excess skin. Because these individuals have more loose skin than many older patients, the incision must inevitably be extended above the ear, behind the ear, or both to take care of the excess. In combination with suction or facial fat injection, the internal plication provides a pleasing result in these 35- to 40-year-olds.

29. Bernie Kaye (Jacksonville) says that the *pre*tragal incision for rhytidectomy is still the best. He also is an advocate of *pre*rhytidectomy suction, a problematic maneuver unless you limit the suction to the jowl and nasolabial fold zones.

30. David Connelly (Montgomery, AL), commenting on editorials in *Plastic and Reproductive Surgery* that decry the practice of suggesting alternatives for additional aesthetic procedures to patients who seek consultation: "Our job is to give an aesthetic evaluation." David goes on to say that we should advise patients about whether their initial point of interest is worth considering and point out to them other areas that could be corrected in relation to the problem, for example, the patient with a large nose whose appearance would still be less then acceptable if the eyelid bagging or weak chin were not included in the correction. David admits that the patients must make the final determination, but he notes that they come to us for our opinions and advice. Hopefully, none of us falls into the trap of talking someone into an operation. Any ethical aesthetic surgeon knows the difference between advice and coercion.

31. James Gates (Camp Hill) says he is not in favor of SMAS undermining. He thinks that simply pulling up the fatpad complex and suturing it into its proper position on the parotid fascia can accomplish just as much as undermining and resecting. We may be fooling ourselves when we undermine the SMAS and lift it. As soon as it is separated and undermined, it immediately retracts, giving the impression that you are doing a great deal when you pull it up for resuturing. Many of us still believe that plication in the cheek by the techniques that John Lewis taught so many years ago can provide equal, comparable, or even superior facial repair during rhytidectomy.

32. Bruce Kaplan, commenting on subtotal resection of ptotic submaxillary glands, noted: "If you run into bleeding, stop. It's not worth the risk." He went on to explain that some submaxillary glands simply must be resected. The operation is technically difficult, and it is best if the gland can be simply elevated by the partial divided platysma during a face lift. The problem is different if the patient is in the group Kaplan classifies as "severe prolapse," meaning that at least half of the gland is in the visible area and can be palpated at least three fingerbreadths below the margin of the mandible. He approaches the gland through the sternocleidomastoid edge and gently teases out the lobules of the gland to avoid damage to the nerves and related structures. It is important to close the capsule of the gland over the area after resection when you are finished.

Technical point: Approach from below by incising but not elevating the platysma. Tease the gland downward. "Stop and control, tease, stop and coagulate." Close the gland's capsule with a lock stitch to decrease the risk of draining saliva. Suture-ligate the raw surface of the gland.

33. Some patients come to the plastic surgeon with a load of guilt. In each of these cases someone in the family or a friend has told them they do not need plastic surgery. Others, in addition, believe that God is probably going to punish them for having such impious thoughts about self-improvement.

34. Bruce Connell admits he is "too timid to suction under the platysma" from an external stab wound. I agree.

35. Beware of postauricular sloughs due to extreme neck flexion. Raymond Faries (Houston) presented a case in which a patient fell asleep after a rhytidectomy. If you measure the distance between the clavicle and the postauricular fold with the head upright and the increase in distance with the neck flexed on the chest, as when one is deeply asleep, you can see that tension results from the extreme neck flexion. This added tension converted a good result to a skin slough. The tension also reduces venous return and by stretching the skin makes venous blood travel over a longer distance. Faries and colleagues write strict postoperative orders that patients with face lifts are not allowed to use pillows for 48 hours. Positioning is diagrammed for them to demonstrate proper elevation without neck flexion.

36. Joe Bongiovi (Las Vegas) also says SMAS undermining is overrated particularly when compared with less extensive undermining or plication. He has tried both procedures (minimal undermining and plication) unilaterally in the same patient or alternating patients and sees no difference. I agree.

37. Are you convinced that you should resect the levator muscle to keep older patients from developing a "sneering expression"? There are better ways to correct an acute nasolabial angle and soften the nasolabial fold. Don't do it.

38. Ivo Pitanguy (Rio de Janeiro): "The surgeon is a creative artist. The creativity is only limited by the form and rigidity of the body."

39. Removal of nasolabial fat was discussed recently by Ralph Millard (Miami). I differ with Ralph Millard only in that I believe it is not necessary to make a percutaneous incision to elevate or to graft material under the nasolabial fold. I wholeheartedly agree that subcutaneous dissection plus SMAS tightening can be equally effective as deep plane dissection. In fact, it results in a more natural appearance. Many surgeons report long-term smoothing of the nasolabial folds by attacking them from the rear (subcutaneous dissection up to the edge), flattening the lateral folds (suction lipectomy), and elevating them from their deep attachments (dissection underneath the fold and autologous fat grafts).

40. Some experts advocate suctioning the nasolabial fold area only when there is excess soft tissue, whereas others ignore this area. Why not undermine the nasolabial crease and add autologous tissue (fat, SMAS, or fascia) at the same time you are suctioning the lateral bulges? No complications.

41. A transverse incision is sometimes used, just below the sideburns, after face lifts, particularly in men. It is not necessary, and it is visible.

42. Extensive subperiosteal dissection is a new hot topic separating periosteum down into the midcheek. One is reminded of Bernie Kaye's diplomatic discussion of this procedure. Essentially, he said that one case of facial paralysis after this subperiosteal dissection was enough to convince him that it was not only unnecessary but perhaps dangerous. My impression is basically the same. Why should you expose a cosmetic patient to a long, hazardous procedure? The prolonged anesthesia required is enough to give one pause.

43. A most unusual forehead lift is the no-scalp resection technique. Several surgeons describe a subperiosteal forehead lift in which suspension sutures do all the work, and no scalp is resected. One might argue that the reasons for not resecting scalp (e.g., hair loss, paresthesia) are not valid with a properly performed forehead lift, but it is fascinating to see the effect achieved with periosteal release, with or without sutures connecting the forehead, skin, and fascia to underlying deep fascia for elevation.

44. If any of you go to movies, you probably have noted poor results from face lift. You see the scars extending from earlobes to the cheek, earlobes tacked down about an inch below where they should be, fat underneath flaps and in the neck, and jowls saggy. It is for these reasons that I emphasize skin fixation in rhytidoplasty, making the earlobes free, and so on.

45. Technical point on the incision above the ear in rhytidectomy: Bruce Connell prefers to make it curve, i.e., project forward. He says that suturing it prevents upward rotation of the hairline. The suture can be removed at time of closure. Fix the hair position first!

46. After three presentations about Bichat fat pad excisions, Dick Goulian (New York) spoke for the audience thusly: "In looking at your before and after photographs, I do not see one case in which the result justified the risk of the procedure." I agree. Assuming you may be approached by a jowly patient some day, two techniques for fat pad removal are as follows: (1) During rhytidoplasty, approach the pad with careful blunt dissection. Cauterize lightly as the pad is teased out for removal. (2) Incise from within the mouth just below the maxillary reflexion. Tease out the pad using external pressure of a finger over the pad.

47. A warning on facial suction from Greg Hetter: Flat cannulas tend to peel the fat off the face. Round ones provide more margin for prevention. Hetter does not like most facial suction devices because they are too heavy. Technical point: you may leave ridges if you use a 4 mm suction cannula for the face. Something smaller is better and easier to control.

48. For a patient with a deformity due to silicone injections, try removing it with a triple-hole suction cannula. Those who have tried it think it works better than the standard ones.

49. Hematomas after face lifts almost never occur in patients who are normotensive and free of nausea and pain. Technical points: Avoid preoperative narcotics, and use intraoperative narcotics sparingly [I recommend intravenous butorphenol (Stadol) in 2-mg increments]. For the mildly hypertensive patient prescribe usual antihypertensive medications according to their schedule. Premedicate with chlorpromazine (Thorazine) 25 mg IM or 2.5-mg IV increments, or sublingual cardizem.

50. "Hematoma is the penalty incurred by the efficient surgeon owing to the rapid completion of the operation."

51. I do not agree with direct excision of perioral skin folds.

52. The best approach to the corrugator and procerus muscles during forehead lifts is still being discussed. Sherrell Aston (New York) noted that cutting the muscles with cautery is not the best way to do it. If you spread the muscles you tear away the muscle fibers without damaging the supratrochlear nerve. Everyone who has spoken on the subject recently has had a different way of handling the frontalis and the galea. Sam Hamra (Dallas) likes to cut a 1-cm grid on the undersurface and does not remove tissue. He cauterizes the center of each island. Others remove a wide stripe of galea and then suture it down over the glabella, theoretically to prevent the muscles from reattaching. It seems odd that these muscles could reattach if they have been so extensively spread and stripped, but who can argue with success?

53. Anthony Sokol (Beverly Hills) has had some success with an eyebrow suspension in which he turns back a flap of soft tissue and imbricates it. Apparently the wider space of soft tissue (the flap is based superiorly and is a square measuring 2 to 3 mm in each dimension) provides more permanent adherence and holds the brow in its new position above the rim. Sokol says the eyebrows then stay there.

54. Malcolm Paul (Fountain Valley, Calif.) on his technique of anchoring eyebrows via a blepharoplasty exposure:

> In answer to your question in terms of descent of the eyebrow, I also have seen that occur to varying degrees. You will note that my last patient is several years after the procedure was performed and does have some hooding, but the result is overall still quite satisfactory. I think the most important part of the procedure is actually excising some of the orbital portion of the orbicularis oculi muscle and the suborbicularis fat to correct the hooded portion of the eyelid. The brow fixation to the periosteum is helpful and I have overall been quite pleased with the follow-up. I do feel, as you do, that there will inevitably be some descent of the brow due to gravity and frontalis motion.

55. Technical point on coronal lifts: Cut through the periosteum and free everything from the periorbital ridge. You can still preserve the nerves, but binding down is not seen during the immediate postoperative period. This also can be performed by blind dissection from a stab wound in the hairline, or with the assistance of an endoscope. (Endoscopic forehead lift is a new hot topic. In my opinion, the minor differences in results do not justify the time required, or the expensive new equipment. But, we all love new toys!) Freeing the midzone where the supra-orbital and supratrochleal nerves live is the least important. Separate corrusator, procerus, and medial and lateral periosteum with or without direct visualization.

10 *Secondary Rhytidectomy*

UNFORTUNATELY, EVEN GOOD SURGEONS SOMETIMES CREATE problems for rhytidectomy patients. Most of the problems are due to poor planning and poor execution of the procedure. Other stigmata come from placement of incisions outside the hairline and failure to shape the internal structures of the face. When I was a resident in plastic surgery we were taught a procedure that today we call a skin lift. The distortion of the earlobes, widening of the scars, and visible hatch marks that result from this operation are the subject of this chapter. The addition of liposuction and fat grafting and the acceptance of the platysmal surgery during the early 1970s have largely eliminated the problems we discuss here. Nevertheless, some patients still have these problems, and the techniques to correct them make a fascinating story. For example, the aesthetic surgeon must frequently simultaneously move hair downward into the sideburn area, rotate skin upward toward the tragus, rotate skin underneath a newly released lobule of the ear, rotate hair foward from the back of the neck, and rotate skin upward in the opposite direction. The term "double opposing rotation" was coined to describe the procedures in which one rotates tissues in seemingly incompatible directions.

Technique

The technical points of second rhytidectomy are as follows.

1. Hair position is important. The first maneuver is to move hair into the sideburn area and as close to the postauricular area as possible.
2. After rotating and securing the hair and eliminating bald spots in the temple, one can proceed with subcutaneous musculoaponeurotic system (SMAS) plication or resection, liposuction, and other maneuvers.
3. Most second rhytidectomy candidates have not had a complete platysmorrhaphy, nor have they had liposuction of the jowl or the nasolabial fold.
4. Patients undergoing a secondary face lift are older and often demand impossible results.
5. Be sure to recommend skin rejuvenation programs for these older patients because it not only makes them more comfortable but happier with the overall result of a second rhytidectomy.
6. All secondary rhytidectomy patients have less skin to remove and frequently more difficult or complex internal repairs.
7. These are generally thin-skinned with little subcutaneous tissue patients, so be extremely cautious with liposuction, directing it only into the jowl area.

Prevention of Problems Around the Ear

Prevention is far more important than correction. The technical maneuvers described in Chapter 9 are designed specifically to prevent the deformities that we illustrate in this section. Correction of these deformities involves almost exactly the same technical maneuvers that should have been used in these patients.

In Figure 10-1, the scars are visible as white lines contrasting with dark pigmentation. The sideburn hair is separated from the upper portion of the ear, and there are stitch marks as well as a tied-down earlobe. To prevent this problem, it is important to place the two hairlines together without tension just above the ear. The incisions should have been closer to the skin of the helix and should have been hidden totally within the ear canal. The rotation with posterior tacking that we discussed in posterior closure in Chapter 9 would have left the earlobe hanging free over the advance skin flap.

In Figure 10-2 the incision lines are too low and have been allowed to drift outward. Hatch marks should be avoided by using subcuticular placement of all

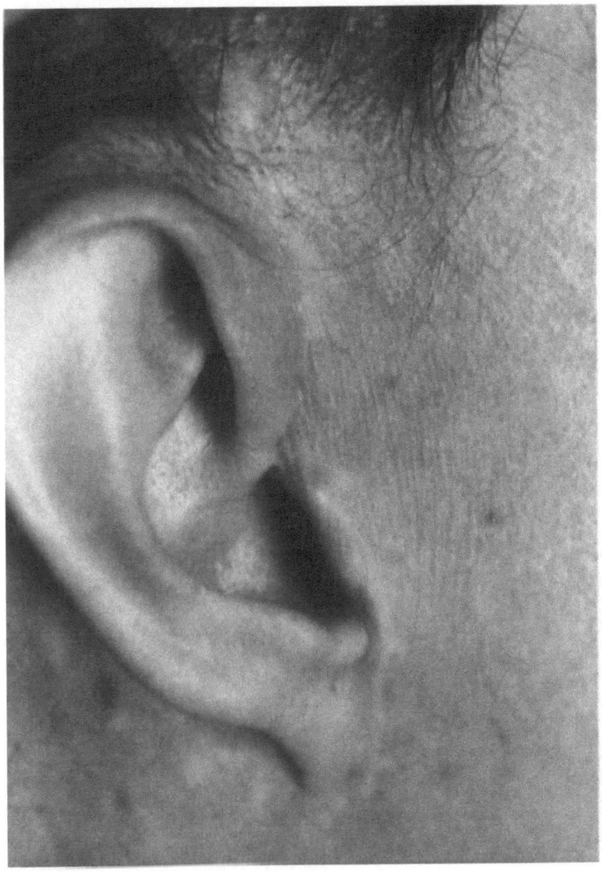

Figure 10-1. See text for explanation.

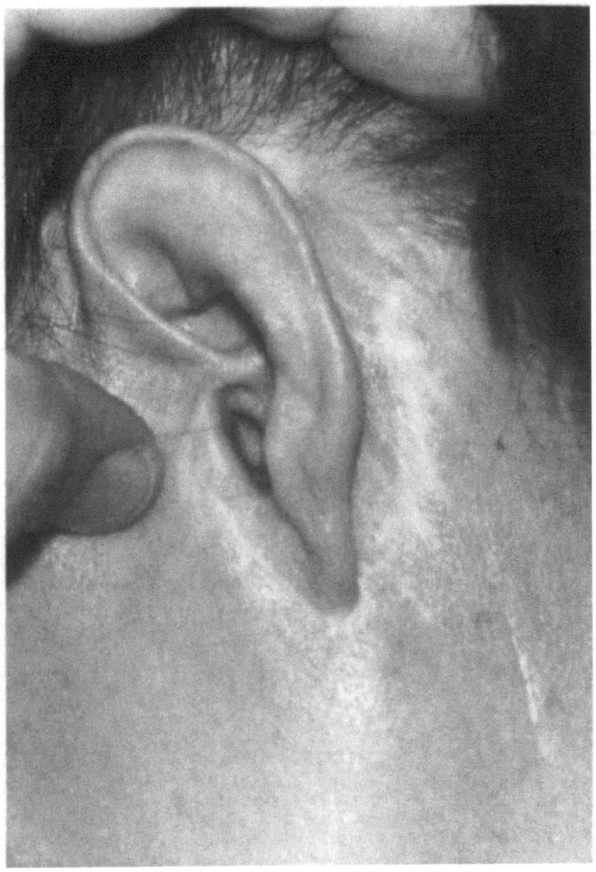

Figure 10-2. See text for explanation.

sutures in this zone. The advancement and tacking maneuvers with the "ae" stitch that anchors the advancing skin flap to the mastoid fascia would have prevented this type of skin relaxation.

In Figure 10-3 the earlobe is attached in a vertical position, and the original incision was placed too low. This incision should be 2 cm higher than is shown and, with the advancement from posterior to anterior, it should lie in position without tension. The tension points, as we discussed, are within the hairline and at the mastoid fascia attachment posteriorly at a level of the tragus.

Figure 10-4 shows what happens when all of the principles are ignored. This patient has undoubtedly suffered vascular embarrassment in the entire zone. Proper placement of tension points far above the temple would have prevented the thinning of hair. Attaching the sideburn hair with a single tacking stitch at the top of the ear would have kept the hair in position and prevented this upward migration. The low incision with the big hatch marks may have been

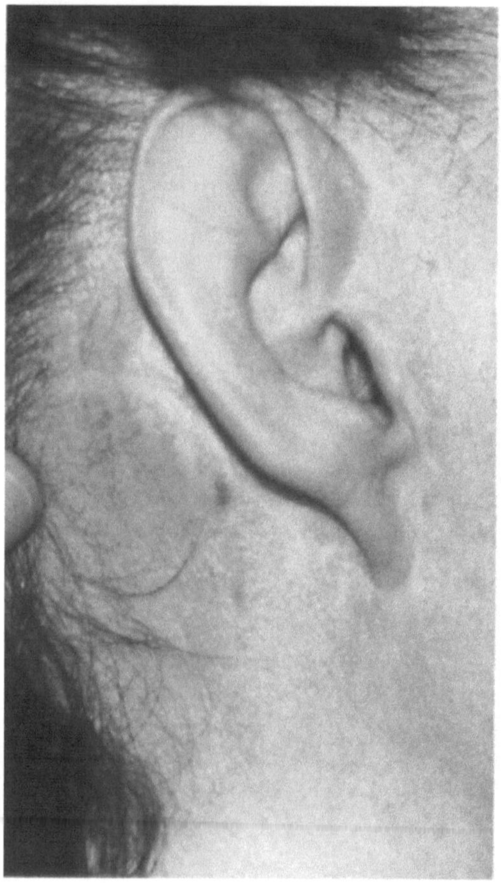

Figure 10-3. See text for explanation.

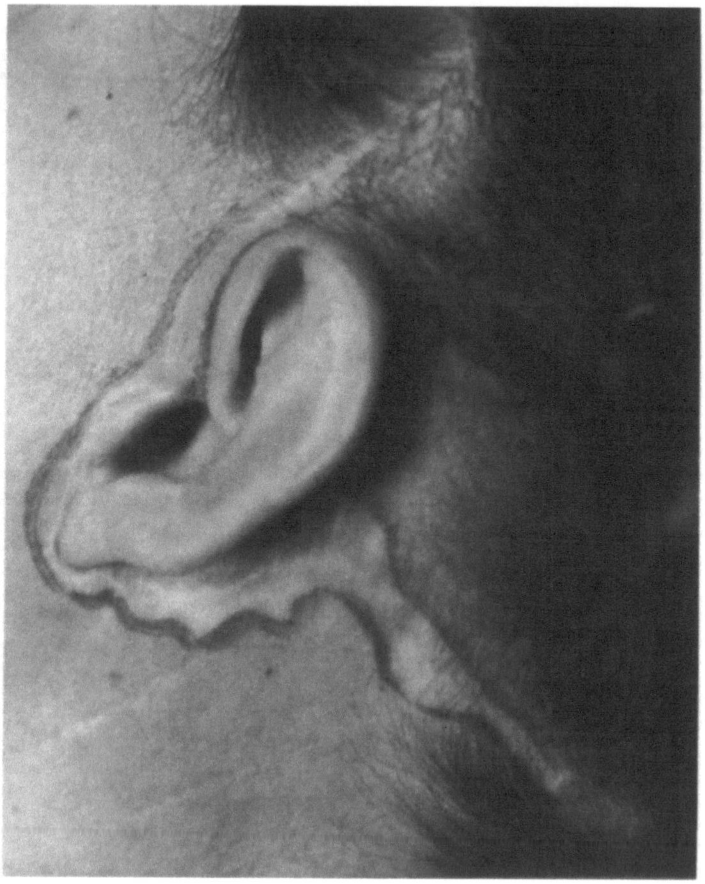

Figure 10-4. See text for explanation.

designed to prevent tightness on the advancing flap, but it defeated its purpose. Half-buried mattress sutures at wide intervals, mastoid tacking sutures, and all of the rotation advancement techniques should have been employed here.

Face Lift "Stigmata"

Secondary rhytidectomy should address the stigmata shown in Figure 10-5A–D. First, a bald spot should not be created in a visible area above the ear (Fig. 10-5A,B). The posterior incisions are far too low. The ladder stitch and extensive undermining down to the clavicle were required to move that skin up. Scars in front of her ear are not highly visible on the left, but on the right they

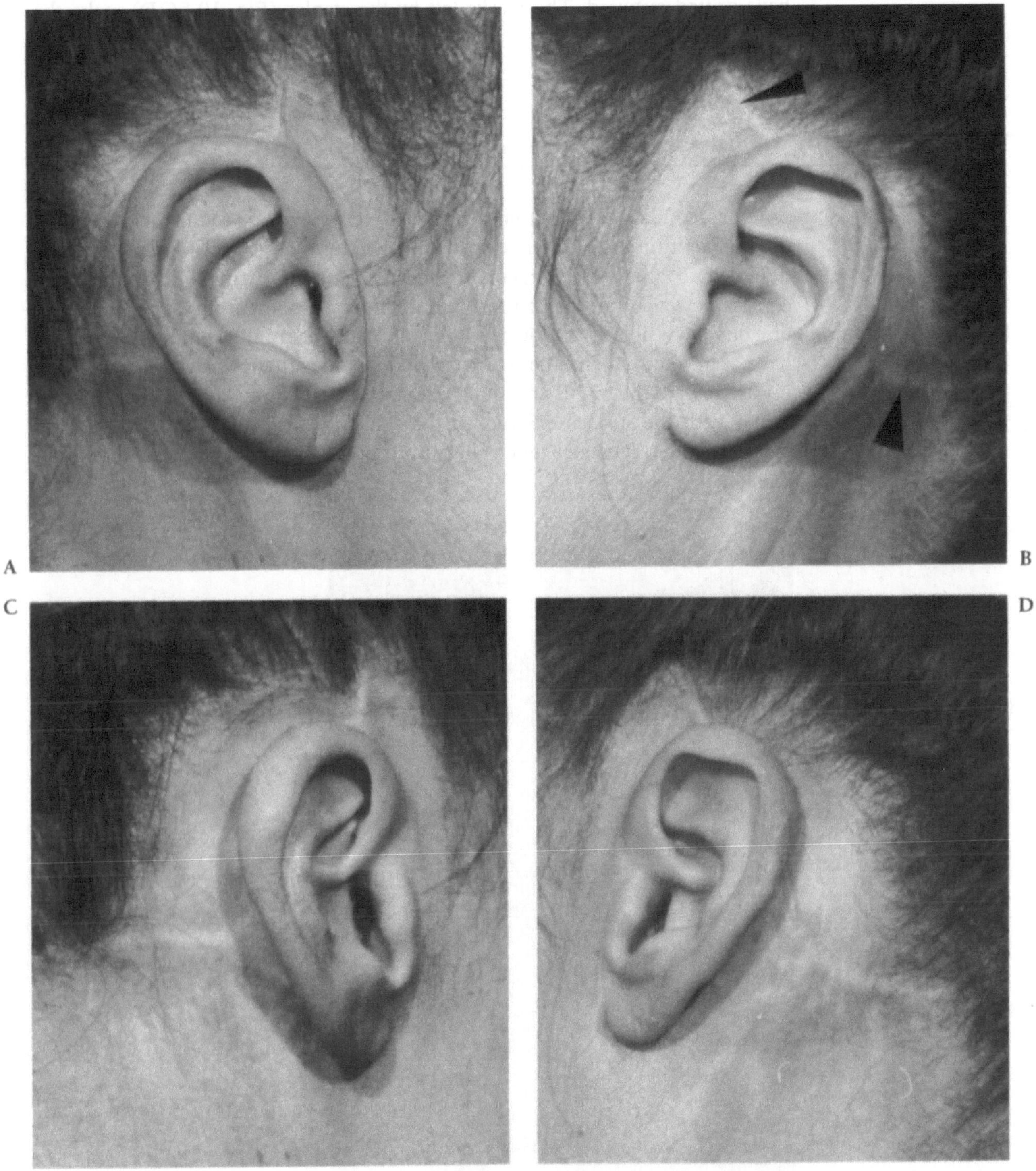

Figure 10-5. See text for explanation.

have drifted outward. The marks left by the staples (Fig. 10-5C,D) make the repair more difficult.

Minimizing Color Contrasts

In secondary rhytidectomy, the skin that is moved up to the ear usually is a different texture and different color. The procedures described in this chapter are designed to allow the surgeon to cover the tragus with skin of the same consistency and limit the contrast to the junctional point at the upper ear, a less obvious and visible area. Note in Figure 10-6 that the running sutures on the skin have been removed and the two 4-0 nylon tacking stitches placed to bring skin inward toward the tragus are still in place at 8 days. The advancing Vicryl suture underneath the surface has tucked the skin into the new groove so the skin overlying the tragus can touch the suture points inside the ear canal without tension.

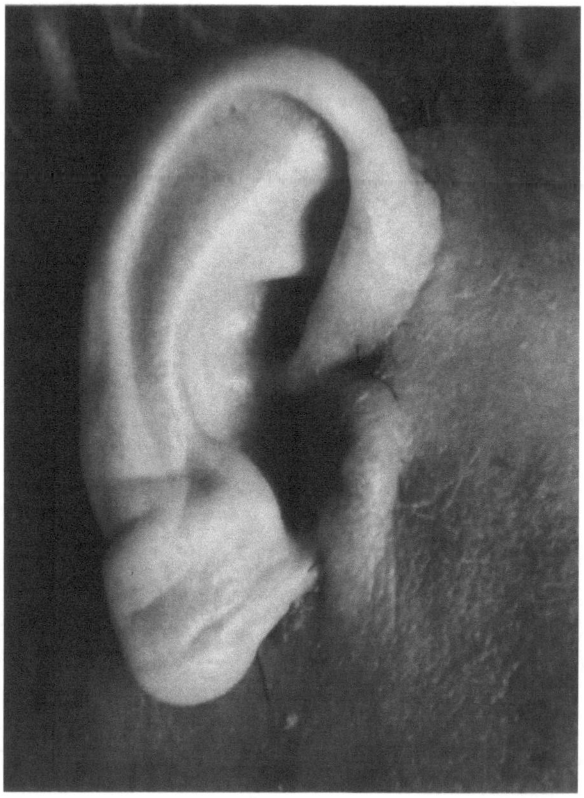

Figure 10-6. See text for explanation.

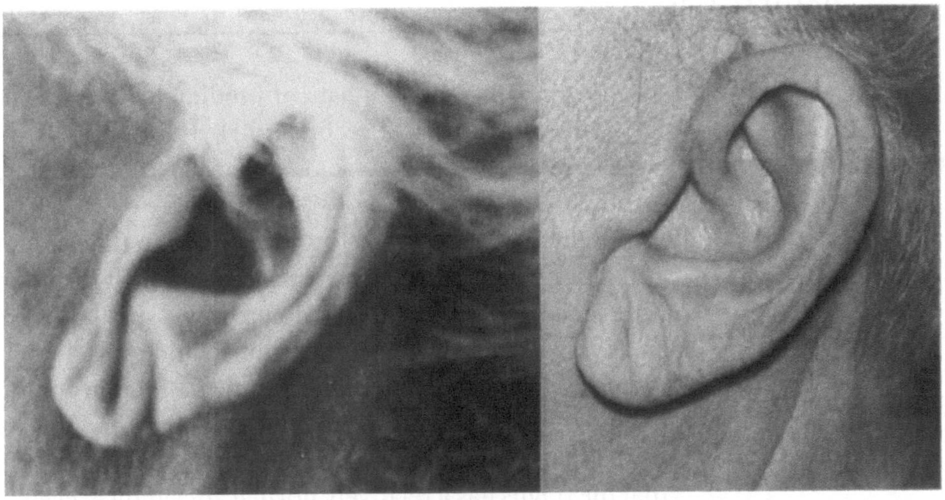

Figure 10-7. In the older patient, the color contrast of preauricular and tragal skin is an obvious stigma of prior face lift. Note the color contrast in the preoperative photograph (left) the patient is holding in front of her face. Also note the wrinkled earlobes. We injected fat into the earlobes, which helped. More importantly, the upper and lower preauricular incisions now hug the line of the ear. We have also been able to use the double rotation technique to bring hair down into the temple and from posterior to anterior behind the ear.

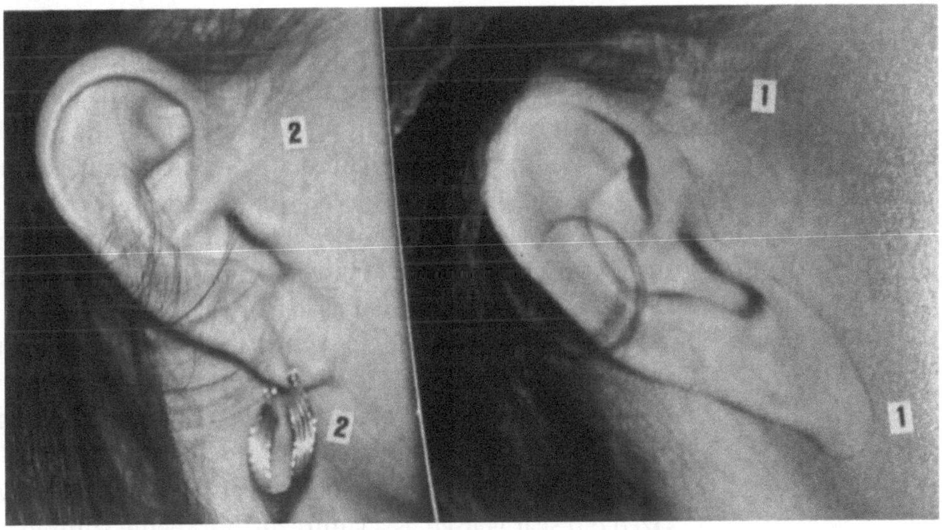

Figure 10-8. See text for explanation.

Slanted Ear

Figure 10-8 shows a patient holding her preoperative photograph next to the corrected ear. For a secondary rhytidectomy of this type, hair position is already established, and one must take care not to raise the short sideburn. The skin is stretched mostly at a point 2 cm above the helix.

When the ear is as distorted as it was in this patient, one must shorten the earlobe as well as tuck the skin underneath with the double opposing maneuver. The sideburn has been moved down only a small distance, but in the crow's feet areas skin has been widely undermined and moved upward. The skin below the lobule has been rotated upward into the fixation points in the mastoid fascia behind the ear, allowing the earlobe to hang freely. The excess skin in front of the ear has been contoured around the tragus. The incision is intratragal. Note also that the tragus has a relatively normal appearance, even though it is now covered by cheek skin. The problem with the slanted ear in this patient is different from that which results purely from distortion of the lobule due to ear tension.

Tension Relief with Subdermal Deepithelialized Flaps

For the secondary rhytidectomy portrayed in Figure 10-9, the problem was rather difficult to solve. The original surgeon had placed all the scars in front of the hairline and left the patient with a tied-down scarred earlobe as well (Fig. 10-9A). Referring to Figure 10-8, the plan was to attack point 1 first, point 3 last, and then rotate good skin under and around the earlobe. In Figure 10-9B the arrows indicate the different rotations. A back-cut was made parallel to the curve of the ear to allow hair-bearing skin to slide forward and downward. At the same time, a Z-plasty effect was achieved by a second straight back-cut at the upper arrow in Figure 10-9B. This maneuver allows even more rotation downward. The goal was to move hair as far forward as possible.

The area of the old scar was deepithelialized in the temple area, after which I undermined backward toward the occiput. This maneuver allowed moving this hair as far forward as possible. If it had not moved enough, I would have made a straight vertical cut far back into the hairline. Moving the front edge forward creates a gap, but it closes spontaneously in less than 2 weeks. The deepithelialized old scar is used as a suture anchor, being sutured tightly under the temple skin to reduce tension.

Next to be addressed was the scar that was left on the neck (Fig. 10-9C). It also was deepithelialized and used as a deep anchor to subcutaneous tissue underneath the undamaged hair. This maneuver at least can bring unscarred skin up to the hairline without tension. No tension was transmitted to the hair-bearing skin that could cause hair loss.

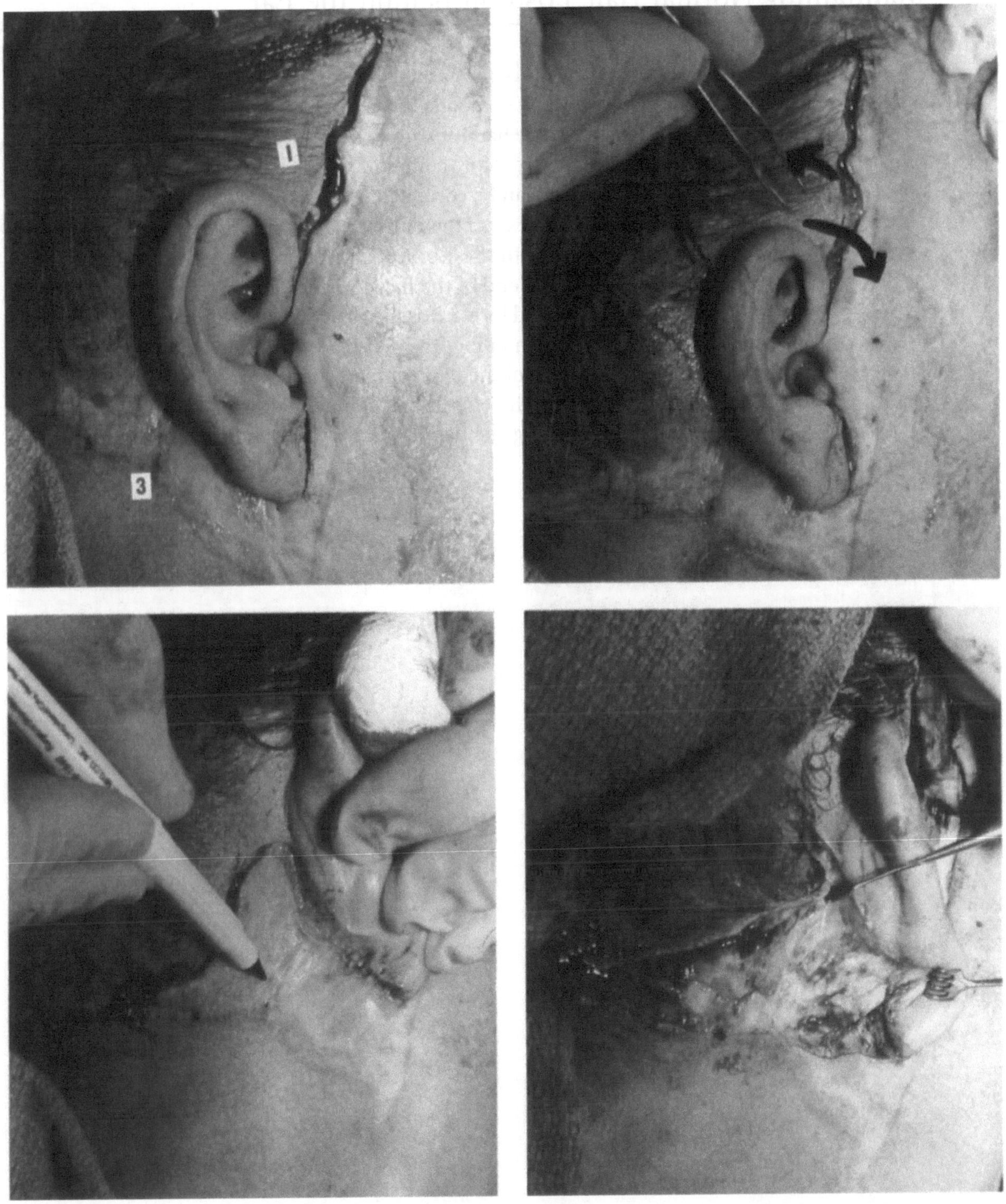

A B C D

Figure 10-9. See text for explanation.

Maintaining Normal Hair Position Behind the Ear

One of the problems of the early rhytidectomy was the resulting absence of hair behind the ear. Many surgeons made the incisions outside the hairline. At least, we can advance some hair forward to help hide incisions and allow patients to wear different hair styles. More commonly, spot baldness resulted from suture tension. Either problem can be corrected.

First (Fig. 10-12A) excise the old scar and make a back-cut well into the remaining hairline. After the rest of the dissection is complete and the flap is freed far backward, at the end of the incision and down into the neck there is a free area that can be moved forward as much as possible. This maneuver spreads out the back-cut, as shown in Figure 10-12B. Use a single nylon suture that just touches the undersurface of the flap 1 mm beyond the last remaining hair. That spot is the anchor point. Then insert half-buried mattress sutures from posterior to anterior, always moving the flap forward, which reduces the tension on the initial fixation stitch.

A

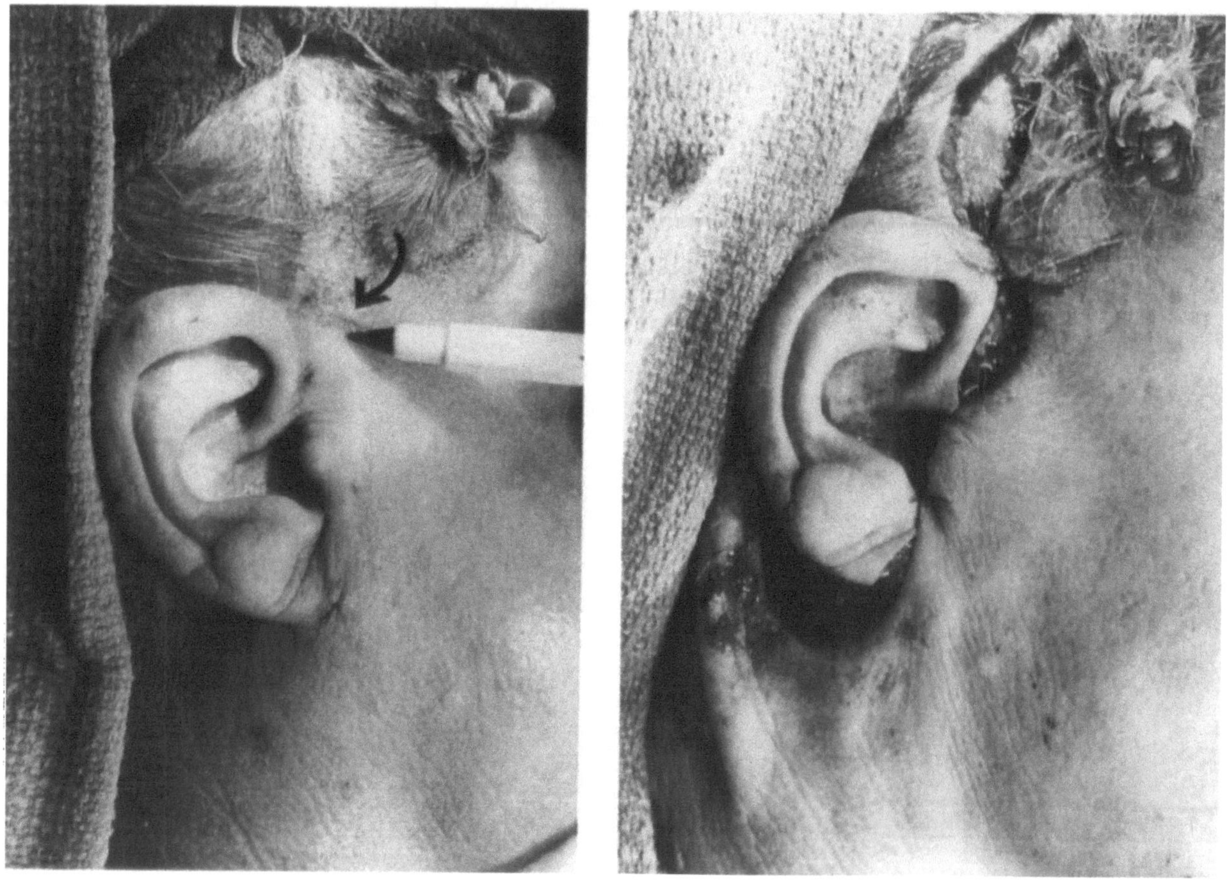

B

Figure 10-11. When the old incision is outside the hairline, all one can do to improve the situation is to rotate hair forward and elevate the postauricular scar to a less visible position. I use half-buried mattress sutures to avoid skin marks. (I prefer mattress sutures to buried subdermal sutures, as the latter may embarrass a tenuous blood supply.) The sutures are left in place for 20 days.

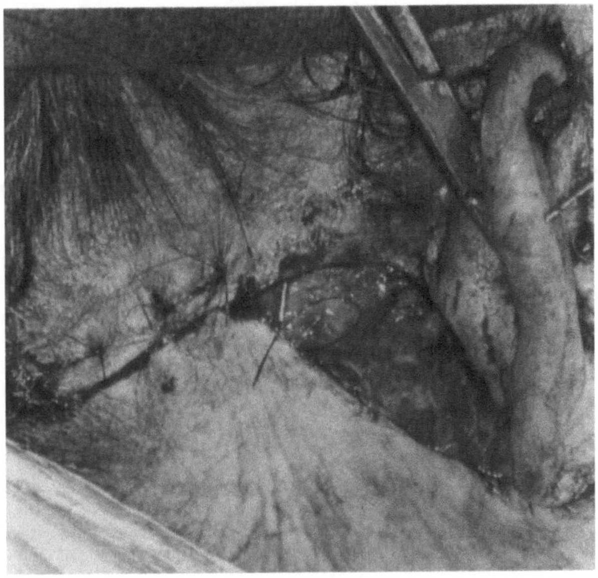

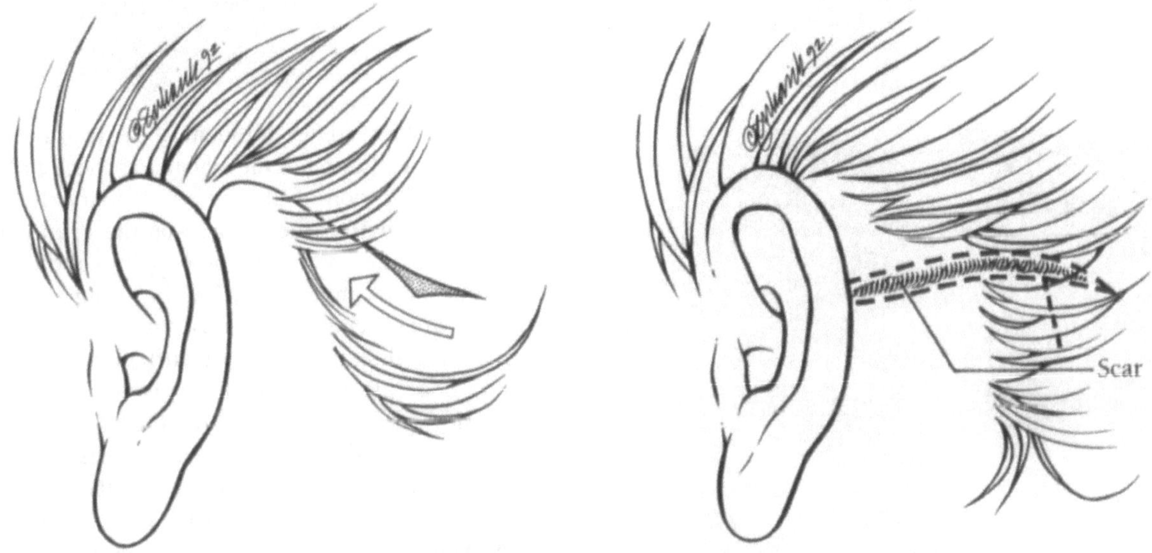

Figure 10-12. See text for explanation.

Figure 10-10. This patient presented with an unusual combination: baldness above the ear and a cluster of hair anteriorly. The intervening bald area parallels the straight-line incisions made by the original surgeon (A). This area will be excised first followed by downward rotation of the hair (arrow). A back-cut will be made above this zone from the old scar forward, so the hair can be rotated into the temple and fixed. (B) The wrinkled skin has been largely removed around the tragus. Postauricular subcutaneous advancement sutures will bring the skin flap up to and around the ear posteriorly, so the lobule is not distorted by tension. This series of advancements is similar to the ladder stitch that we use posteriorly. The two skin edges from the tragus upward will then meet without tension, and the hair will be in a normal position.

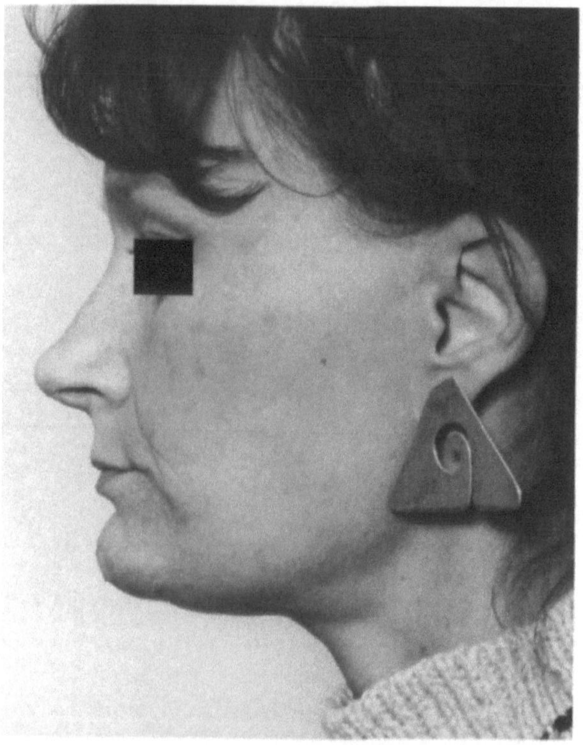

A

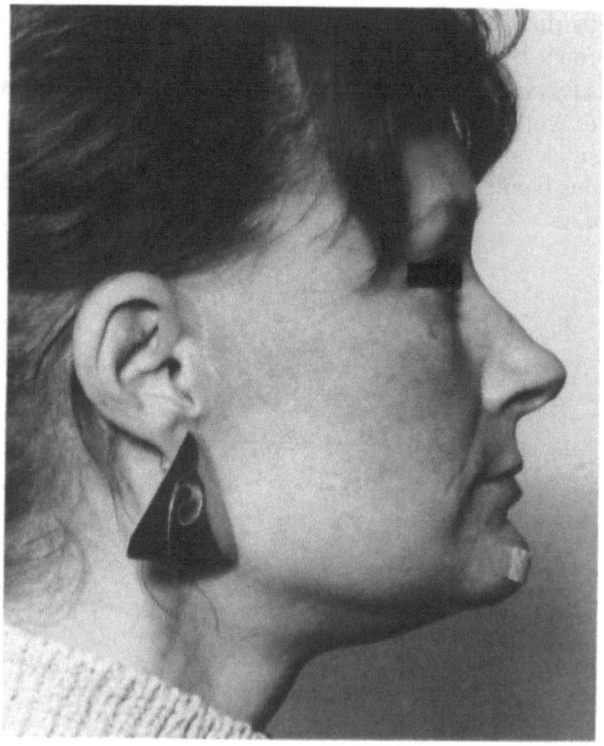

B

C

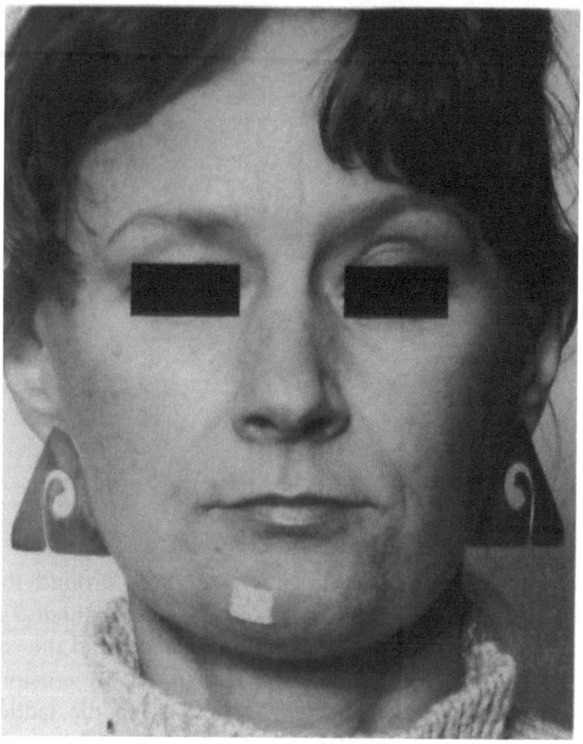

Figure 10-13. Prior to development of the technique for preauricular anchoring of the advancing cheek flap, a common complication of placing a secondary rhytidectomy incision within the tragus was the open ear deformity. Note the extremely poor skin condition **(A–C)**, which was improved with our program of Retin-A, α-hydroxy acids, and creams. Note the contrast between the tragal skin and the preauricular skin, as well as the poor placement of the incision. We also addressed the high hairline anteriorly and posteriorly. Fat grafting was used to fill the deeper lines in the glabella and nasolabial zone and lips, and liposuction plus retightening the platysma corrected the lower face. The result **(D&E)** was pleasing with the exception of the tragal position. With the technique described in this chapter, the advancing sutures placed at the base of the tragus eliminate tension on the covering skin flap. The technique is also applicable to primary face lifts when good skin turgor might result in an open ear deformity.

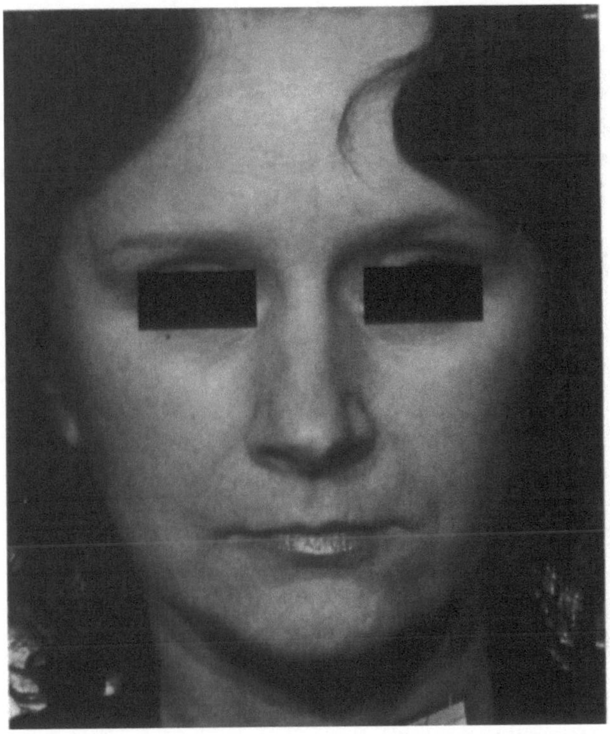

D

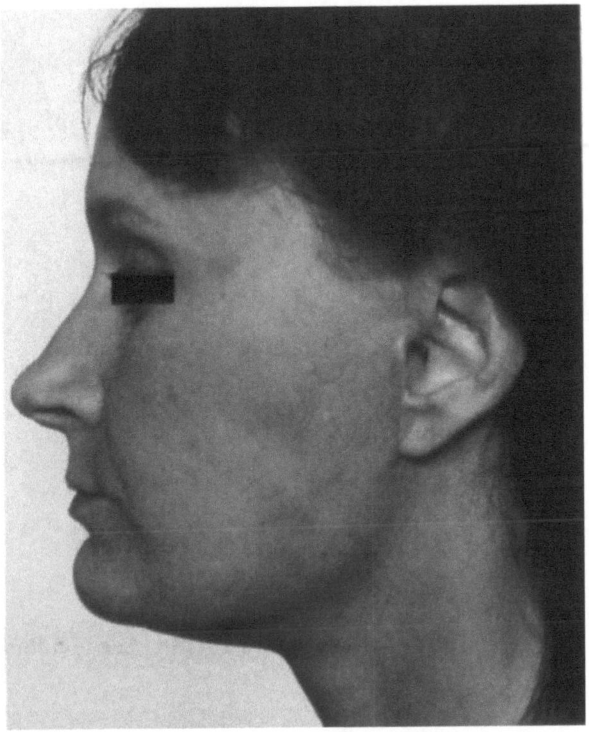

E

Lost Sideburns

A common problem with secondary rhytidectomy is the need to restore hair in the sideburn area while still elevating the corner of the eyebrow. It requires rotating the skin of the eyebrow *upward* while rotating what little hair remains above the ear *downward*. This maneuver is the "double rotation advancement" (Fig. 10-14). First, make the new incision inside the tragus in order to remove extra skin. Once the old scar is excised, make a hidden back-cut as shown in Figure 10-14. When the hair is moved downward, it is fixed in place at two points: just above the tragus and just at the curve of the ear. Those two tight spots leave the hair in its lowest position but do not exert any tension on the temple hair-bearing scalp. Skin tightening is avoided here. To elevate the eyebrow, place the "tight suture" in the scalp far above this point. In these cases, it is more important to preserve sideburn and temple hair than it is to achieve the desirable lift of the crow's feet area. Because the crow's feet area is undermined subdermally from above, flattening is already in effect. Ideally, the crow's feet triangle is stretched in two directions. Note, however, not to overdo the pressure on skin.

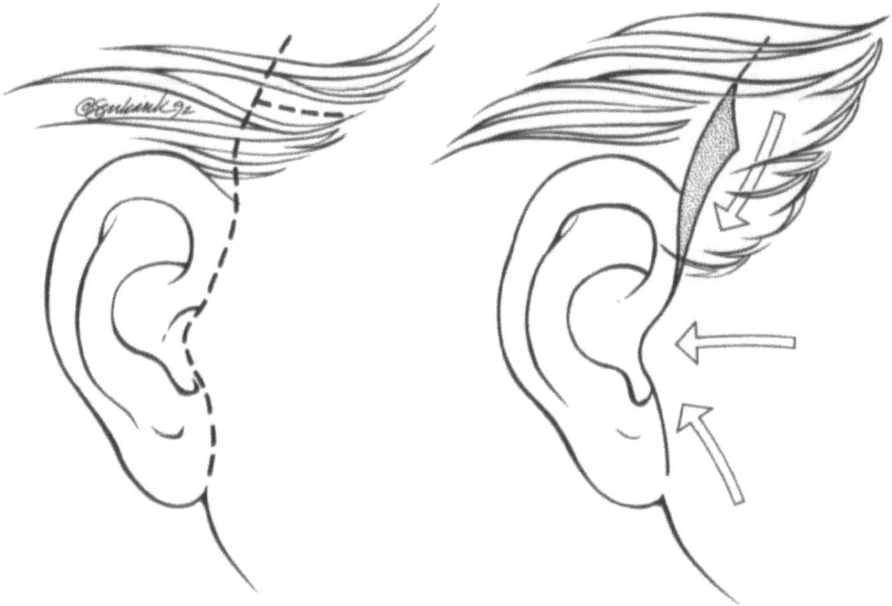

Figure 10-14. See text for explanation.

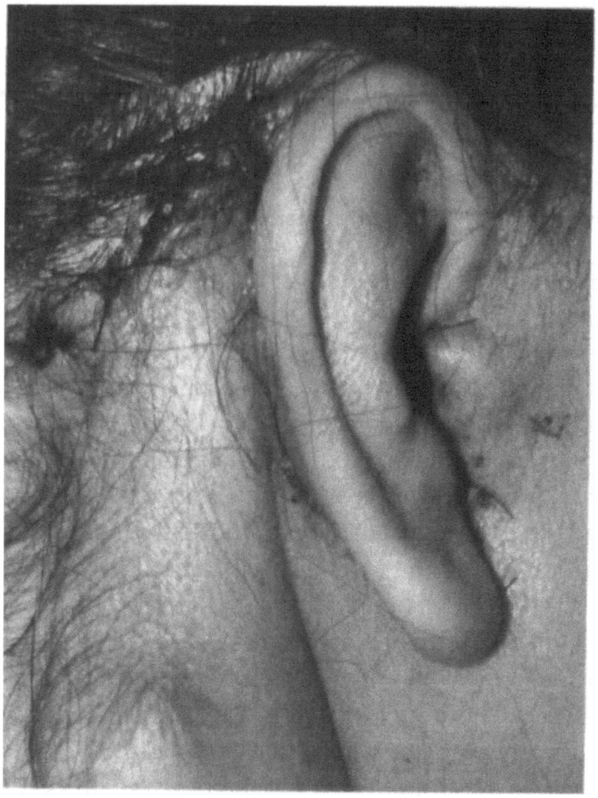

Figure 10-15. See text for explanation.

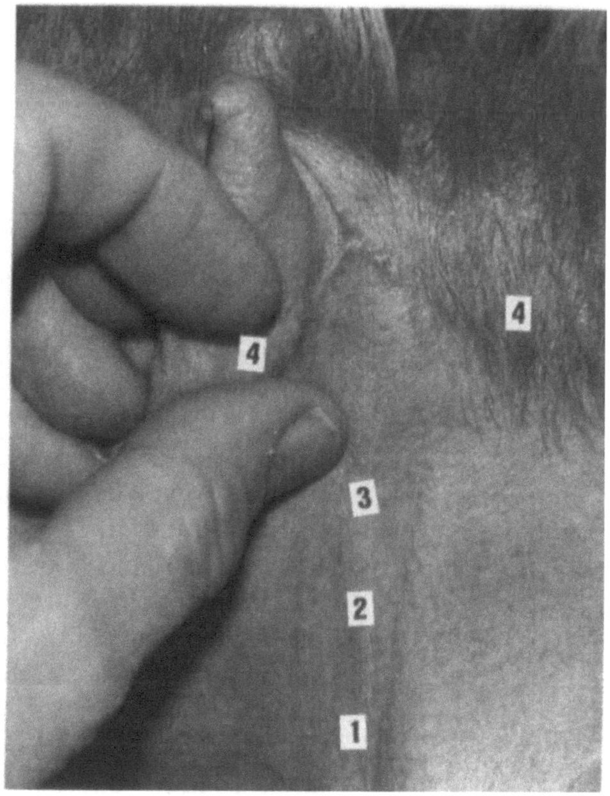

Figure 10-16. See text for explanation.

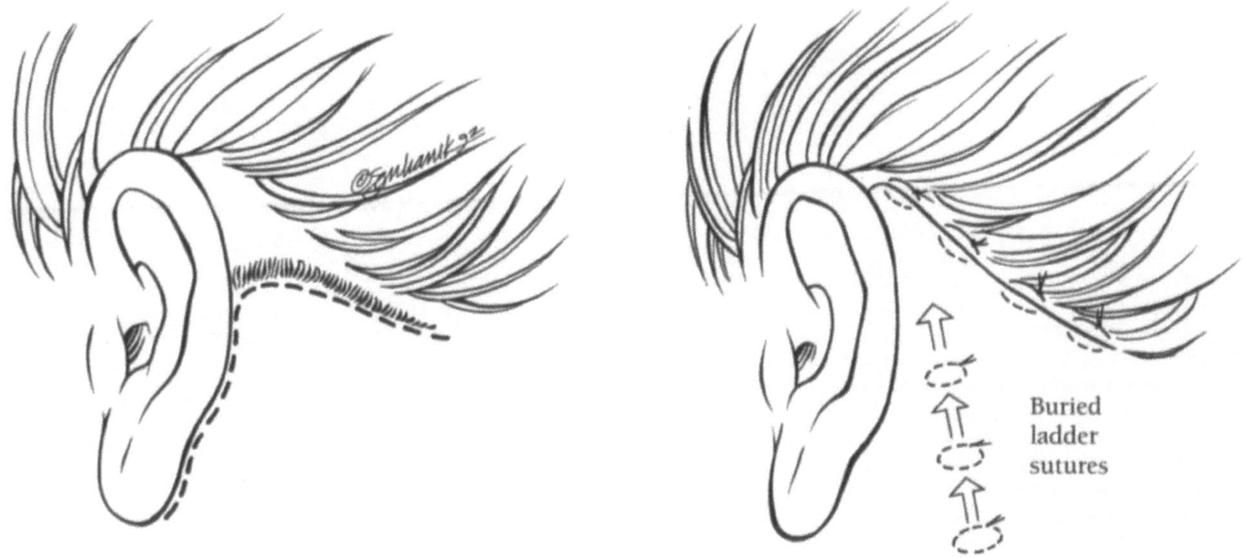

Figure 10-17. See text for explanation.

Ladder Stitch

There are methods for reestablishing a more natural hairline in a patient who has had a face lift with a low postauricular incision. A buried ladder stitch is used and begins low in the neck after undermining almost to the clavicle. These absorbable 2-0 sutures hold the skin in an upward position (Fig. 10-15). Note the bunching of skin from these deep sutures. They are placed at points 1, 2, and 3 in Figure 10-16. Hence the skin between the two No. 4 markers (Fig. 10-16) is without tension and can be extended upward to a more desirable position. This technique can be combined with forward rotation, as shown in Figure 10-17. The essential point is that there is no tension behind the ear, and the original incision can be marched upward to a more hidden position.

11 *Midface Rhytidectomy*

CHANGES IN THE TYPES OF PATIENT REQUESTS AND THE NEW techniques of skin rejuvenation make the midface lift worthy of a complete chapter. The typical face lift patient has inelastic skin, bowing of the submental triangle platysma, jowl fat deposits, and general deterioration with descent of eyebrows, midcheeks, and even the neck to the clavicle. The candidate for the midface lift is a young individual who has practiced good skin care. The changes are simple removal of jowl fat deposits with a "slide" of the subcutaneous musculoaponeurotic system (SMAS) area of the midcheek. Many candidates have no loose skin under the neck, and others have only a small amount, which can be corrected by extension behind the ear. The patients generally follow instructions for postsurgical skin care. We have been able to maintain the tightness in younger individuals for many years longer than the average full face lift patient with our home programs and light chemical peels.

When discussing the options with these patients, we mention that certain individuals can have the upper face corrected by simple insertion of a malar implant, suctioning the nasolabial fat fold, and fat grafting into the nasolabial groove itself. Some young individuals have aged so little in the midface that isolated submental platysmal repair with liposuction of the midjowl and face is adequate to restore youthfulness. Few of these defects can be corrected with liposuction alone because of platysmal bowing; yet liposuction plays a role in all

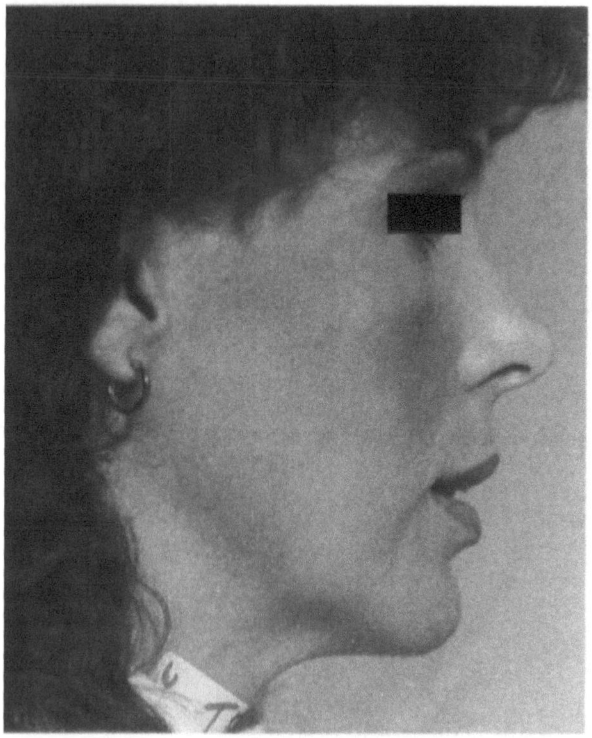
A

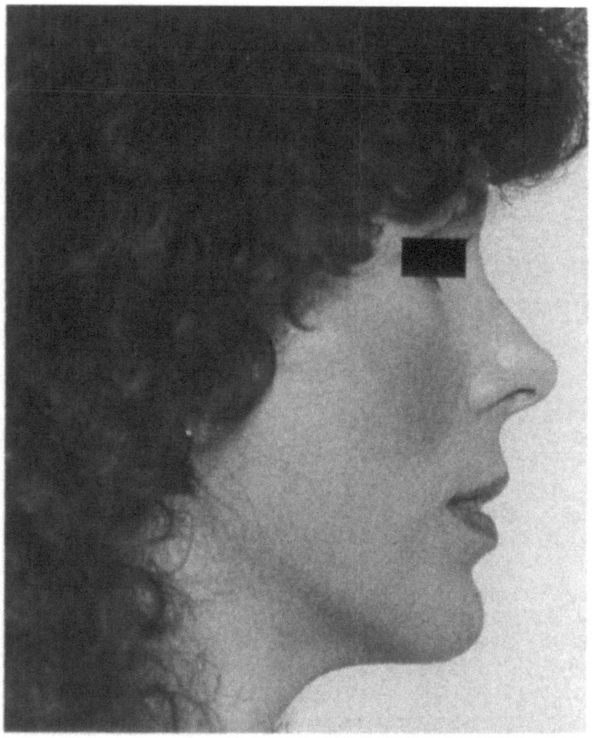
B

C
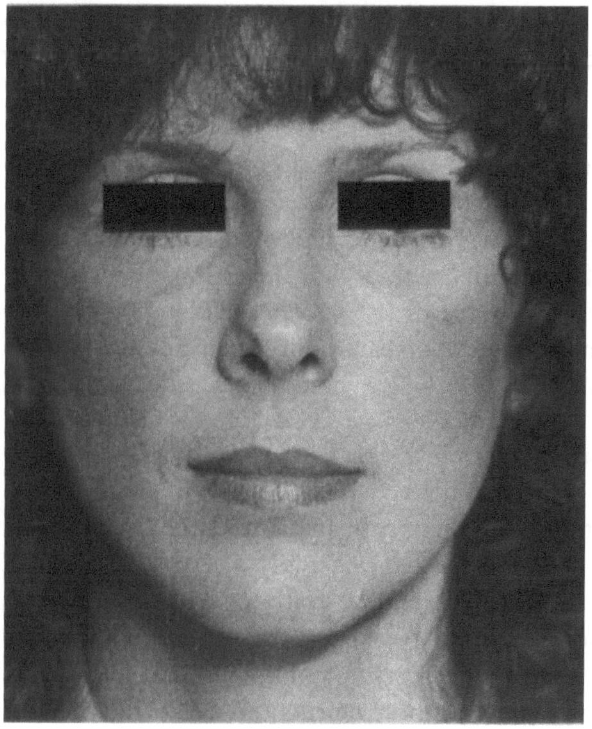

Figure 11-1. A fresh, "natural" rejuvenation is effected by the half-lift. **(A)** This patient's blepharoplasty was done 6 years before this photograph. **(B&C)** The postlift photographs show the smoothing and softening effect of midface surgery.

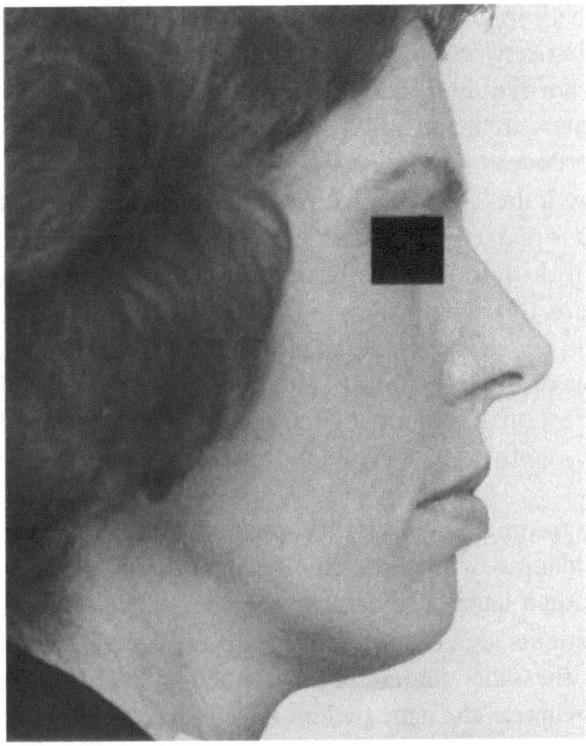

A

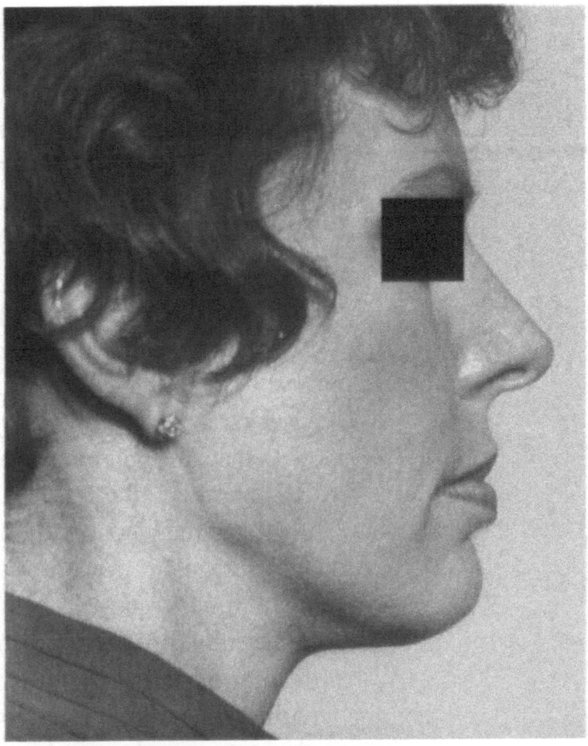

B

C

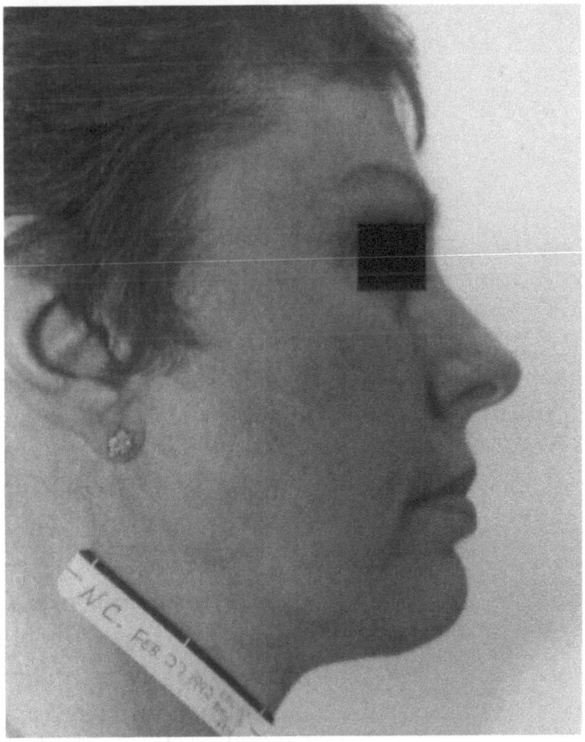

Figure 11-2. (**A**) This patient was operated on before liposuction and fat grafts became a routine addition to the half-lift procedure. She chose blepharoplasty and chin augmentation *without* a forehead coronal lift in 1982. In 1985 she asked for correction of her "angry" look and this time accepted my suggestion of a forehead lift. Note the eyebrow position in 1992 (**C**) compared to the preoperative position (**B**).

categories. Others show such dramatic improvement in skin quality with the "jump start" of light acid peels followed by a home program of tretinoin (Retin-A) and α-hydroxy acid creams, or mixed or trichloroacetic acid (TCA) peels that excision of skin is not required. Each option is discussed with the patient, and the recommendations are made based on the anatomy, not the age, of the patient.

In general, men do well with the lesser procedures. The skin contours well to the neck when the platysma is reattached; and when the jowls are suctioned, the cheek contours well. Men do not show early midface aging as often as women; the few exceptions are those with a vague "Clint Eastwood" look: folding of skin in the midcheek, which is considered desirable by some patients and undesirable by others. Two or three sessions of fat grafting into the central cheek may be adequate for correction. In other patients, a midface lift, combined with malar augmentation and fat grafting just beyond the area of dissection, is the best choice.

Because most patients requesting early face lifts are young, one must take precautions to prevent scar widening or hypertrophy. Early face lifts (in those aged 30–45 years) last longer than later ones because the connective tissue is inherently stronger and the patients are committed to healthful living. Overall healing also is faster than in the older patient. Fair-skinned individuals are vulnerable to skin stretching, whereas the acne patient have less stretching but derive greater benefit from skin tightening.

For a number of young patients, malar implants and fat grafting may be as effective as the half face lift. Those who wish hollow cheeks are usually chubby individuals who believe their "baby faces" are a hinderance. Liposuction from a three-point approach and with tiny cannulas can diminish this facial chubbiness and create a submalar shadow, which would not be as visible in these individuals after malar augmentation. The malar augmentation lifts the upper part of the nasolabial groove and provides a lifting effect as well; it is particularly effective when combined with undermining and fat grafting of the nasolabial groove itself.

The same principles apply when evaluating the submental triangle in these young individuals. Age is not a factor. Many young individuals have low-lying hyoids, stretched-out platysmas, and fat in both superior and deep zones. They should be offered the submental tuck discussed earlier in the book. Others can be offered a reprieve of a number of years with simple liposuction across the midline. We offer this option to everyone who is having a midface lift, even if there is only a minor fatty deposit. The procedure takes only a few minutes and is a small bonus for the patient.

Does smoking play a role in these patients? Probably. There is evidence that smoking decreases the blood flow to the lips and face, but it is probably not as important as the mentality that drives some young women to be sun worshippers during their teenage years. The delayed effect of sun damage is the prime factor in midface descent, although heredity may play a role.

Technical Points

The approach to the midface is difficult because of the limited exposure. Moreover, closure must be in two layers because of the inherent elasticity of the skin.

1. Always place the incision inside the tragus. We did not do it in many early patients, and a significant number developed wide or visible scars.
2. Always reinforce the skin closure above the tragus with a buried suture as well as the surface tacking sutures.
3. Keep the incision short, only in front of the ear if possible. Even though it is difficult, this exposure is adequate for suctioning and internal plication.
4. Suctioning from the edge of the mandible downward and into the jowl area is useful. In many of these individuals, a direct attack on the nasolabial area is essential.
5. Grafting fat or SMAS into the nasolabial groove, along with transnasal

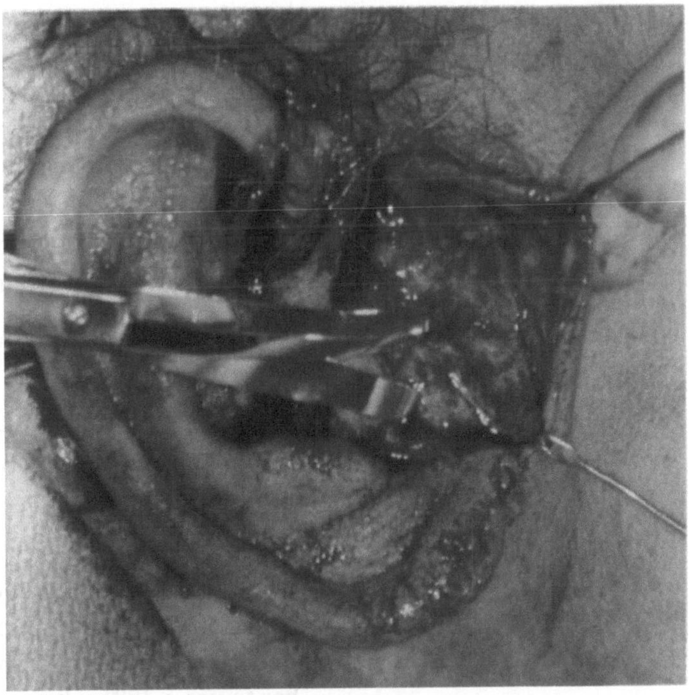

Figure 11-3. Technical point regarding the half-lift: Because of the limited exposure, half-face SMAS plication would leave a redundancy immediately in front of the earlobe. Excise it. This tissue also makes good graft material for lip enhancement or the nasolabial fold.

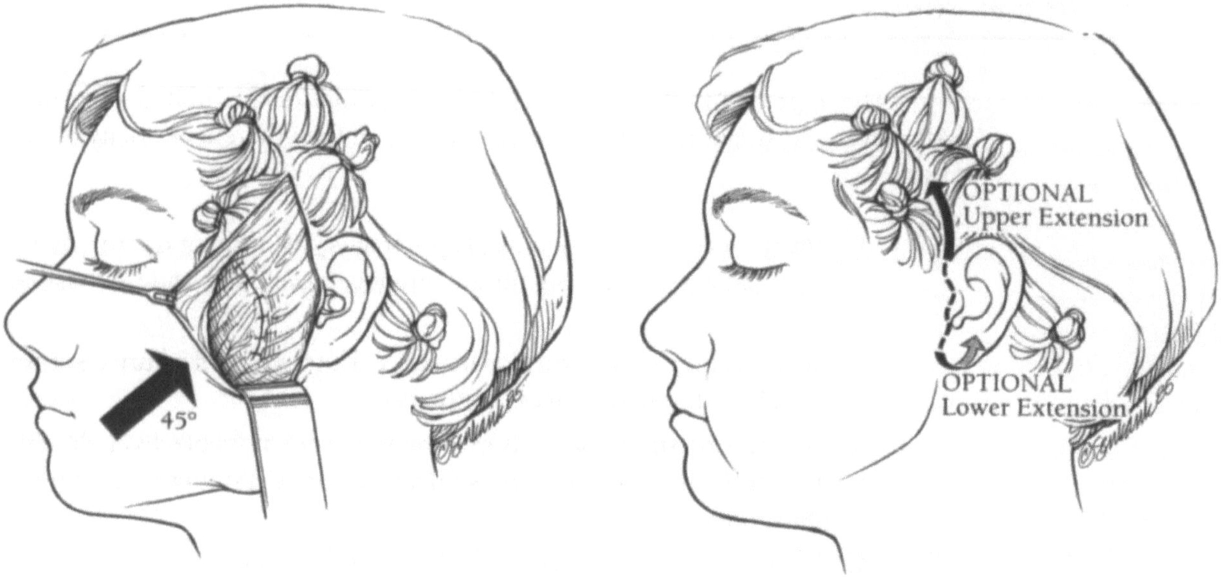

Figure 11-4. The half-lift is more difficult for the surgeon than complete rhytidectomy owing to limited exposure, but it spares the patient. Correction is limited to the midface, with SMAS plication upward and backward. To accent malar fullness, a more horizontal plication would be done. The optional extensions for candidates with early laxity of skin are at the crow's foot zone or below the jawline.

suctioning of the fat lateral to the nasal groove, makes a smooth transition.

6. I prefer SMAS plication in these individuals rather than undermining. I plicate upward in the first row of sutures to give prominence to the malar area and then backward in front of the ear to smooth out the soft tissue. Once the plication is accomplished, scissors dissection is used to trim away any fat that is irregular.
7. If there is loose skin under the neck, free this area completely and extend the incision around the tragus and at least halfway up behind the ear. Try to avoid the visible area, even if it means leaving a small amount of wrinkling behind the ear, as in these individuals it smooths out rather quickly.
8. Crow's feet are a problem in a few individuals. Direct undermining of the skin at the crow's feet and an extension of the half-lift incision into the temple allows one to spread this skin, thereby diminishing the crow's feet.
9. It is safe to peel the forehead with TCA and even to peel the lower lids at the same time as performing a half-lift. Because there is not complete undermining, this peel should also cover the crow's feet area. Remember to use a 35% solution rather than a stronger one.

10. Fat grafting is most successful in young patients, and the half-lift patients are prime candidates. Most of our half-lift patients have had fat grafting in the glabella and nasolabial area, and often into the vermilion of the lips. They seem pleased with the fat grafting because the half-lift simply "refreshes" the face.
11. Although none of these patients achieves dramatic changes, the changes that do occur are visible.
12. These individuals are some of the happiest patients in our practice.

General Advice

Without being redundant and repeating much of the information that is given in Chapter 10 on the complete face lift, it is well to remember that these patients are unique. They are usually well read and highly critical of minor problems that might be easily dismissed by the older patients undergoing a complete face lift. For this reason, it is essential that, for example, one create a groove in front of the tragus. Using a 2-0 Vicryl suture here is a better choice than a smaller suture because of the elasticity. As we said earlier, do not hesitate to reinforce subcutaneously in these patients. Their tissue does not swell as much; their skin is more elastic and therefore does not balloon as easily.

Emphasize early mobilization, steroids to reduce edema, early massage of the scars with aloe-based oils, and early skin care and makeup consultations. The average half-lift patients progress to full makeup and are able to drive safely within 5 to 7 days. Because a complete platysmal sling has not been created, the patients need not be cautioned against the danger of driving on modern expressways with a tight neck. It is well to emphasize to these people that long-term care is in their best interest. If they cannot avoid the sun, at least establish a Retin-A regimen that allows them to enjoy their active life style while still protecting and tightening their skin. Insist that they wear a facial band for at least 5 days so edema does not settle in the neck area. (Even though you have not dissected in that area, the skin there may be vulnerable to stretch.) A tennis headband is a good addition after the fifth day. Because it covers the ear incisions, it allows the patient to resume an active life. We do caution them not to engage in vigorous sports until at least 14 days after the operation.

When I first presented a paper on the midface lift, I asked the question, "Is it catering to Yuppie anxiety?" My answer then and now is "Certainly not." These individuals are convinced that facial appearance is essential to career advancement and enjoyment of life.

Midface lifting is now an accepted part of the plastic surgery armamentarium. It is well to point out that if the lower neck does not require repair, why use a long incision that will have to be repaired later. If the forehead has not yet fallen and the eyebrows are in normal position, they may remain so another 10 to 15 years. Why "repair" them now with a long, unnecessary incision?

I strongly believe that my obligation to the patient far outweighs any question of propriety. We must not talk them into surgery; we must simply point out the aging changes and advise which ones can be corrected with peels, which ones with "bone structure" alterations, and which ones with internal and skin repair. Let the patients make their own choices. With modern surgery, the half-lift, in combination with the other procedures that we have discussed in this text, offer a valuable service to a certain segment of the patient population.

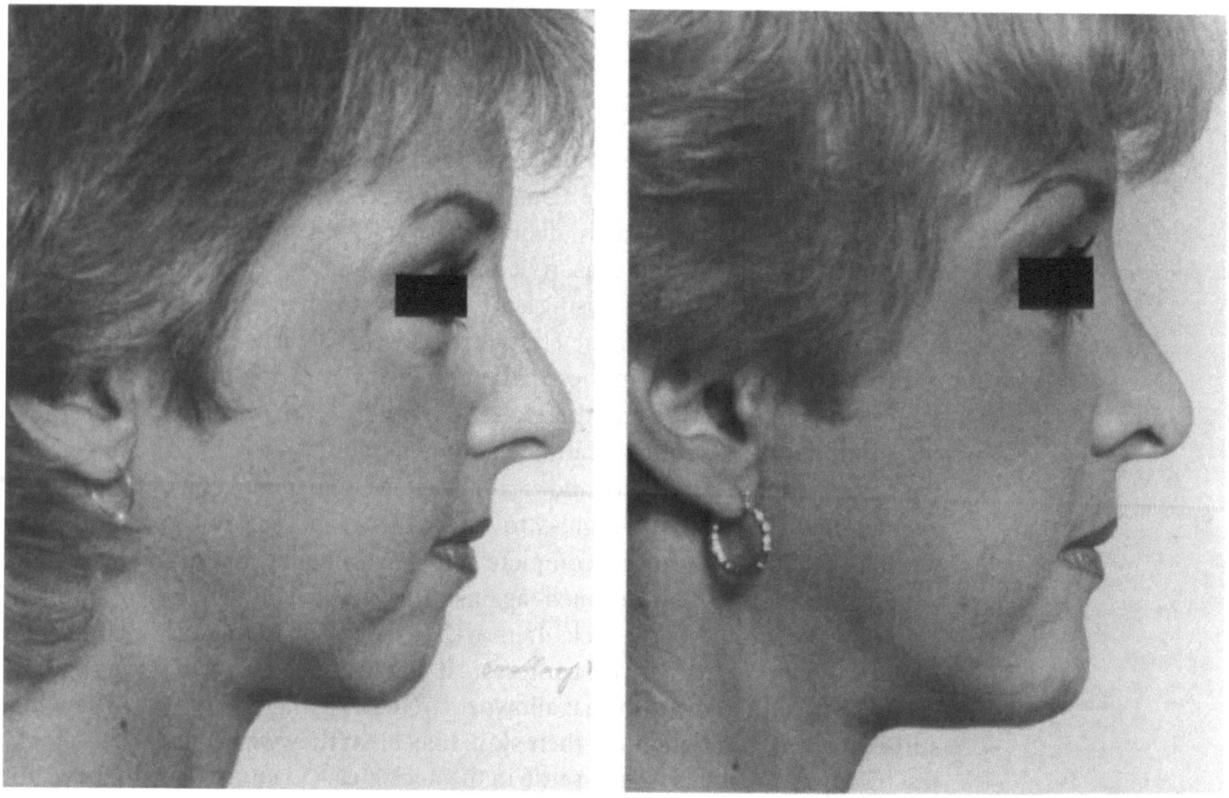

Figure 11-5. This patient illustrates the beneficial effect on the submental zone by adding a chin implant. During the preliposuction years, direct intervention would have been required. Shortening the nose adds balance to V-shaped faces. Note that liposuction and fat grafts would have helped here, particularly in the jowl area.

Figure 11-6. **(A)** This patient is shown in 1977 before blepharoplasty (SMF type) and rhinoplasty. There has been no facial descent. **(B&C)** By 1983 only the midface has changed. For minor skin excision in the submental zone, the incision must be extended behind her ear. **(D)** Two years after a half-lift and revision of the nose, her face is "refreshed." Such patients do not require liposuction of the nasolabial or submental areas.

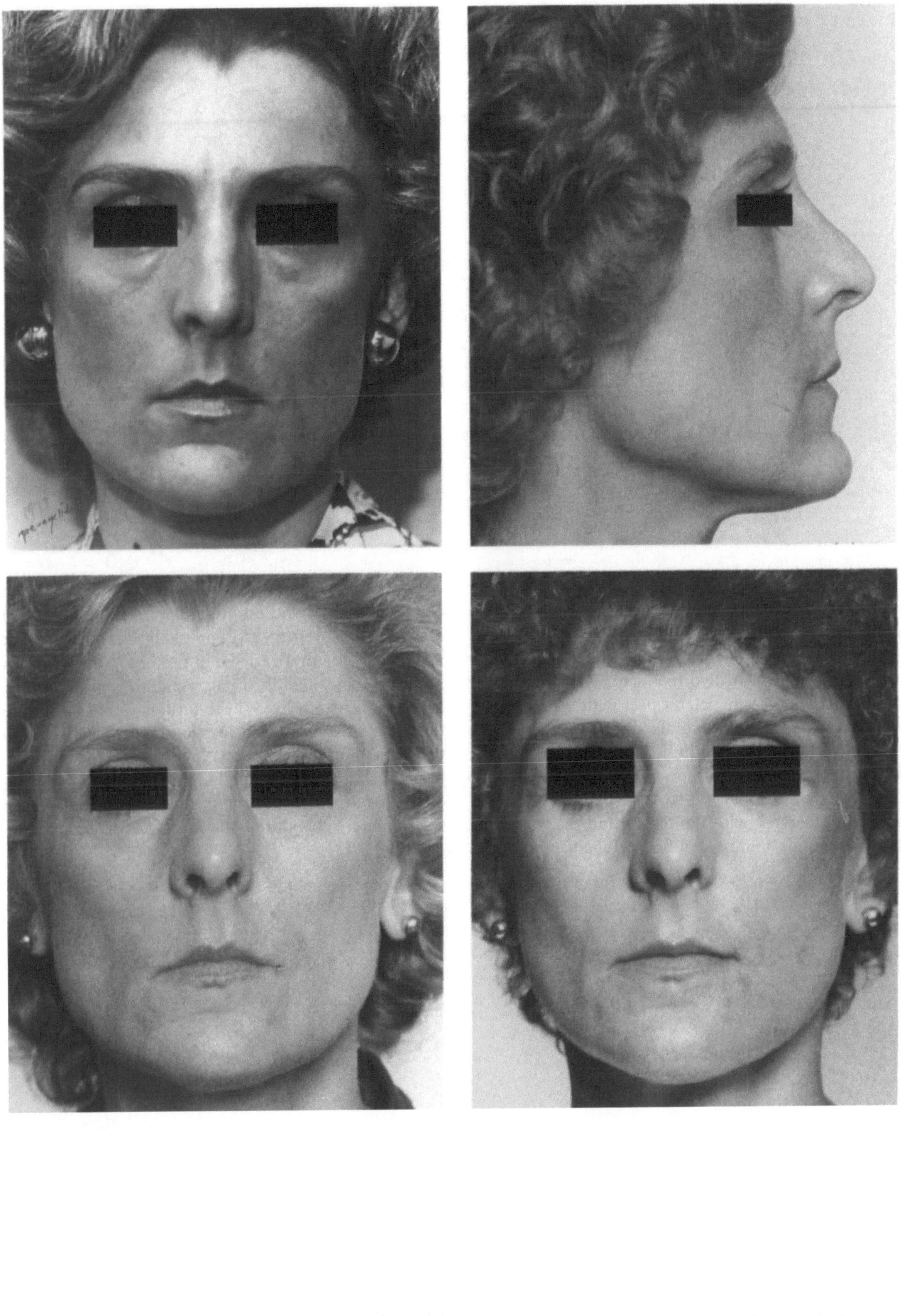

A B

C D

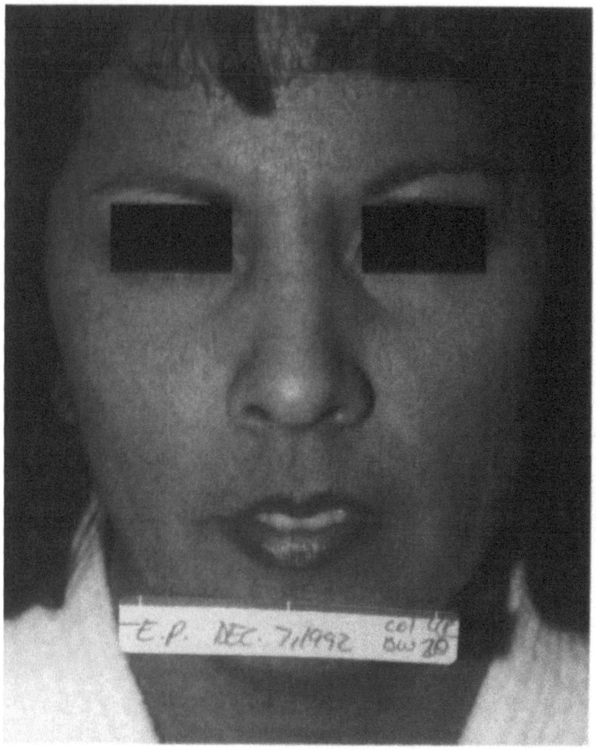

A

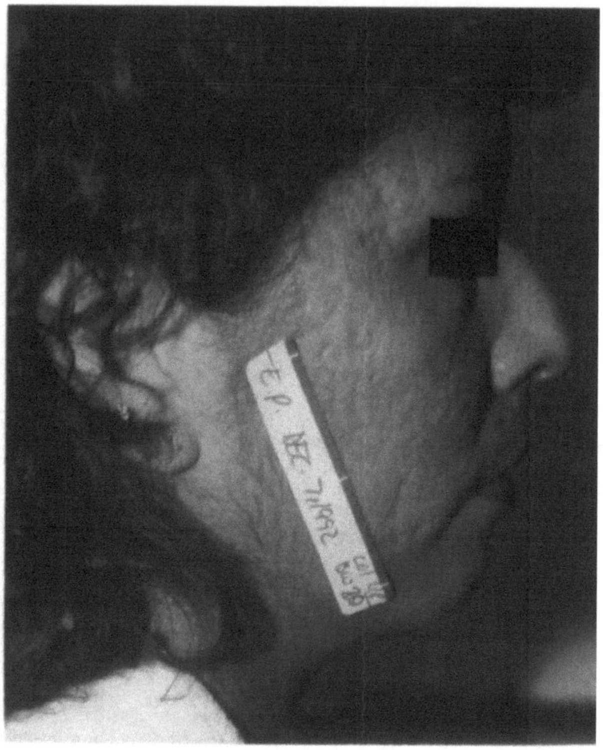

B

Figure 11-7. **(A&B)** When counseling a patient such as this woman, it is important to mention all of the modalities that can be used for the acne patient. They include consultations with an aesthetician for cleansing, steaming, a Retin-A/α-hydroxy acid (AHA) regimen, and perhaps the aesthetician's peel with 40% glycolic acid. We also propose the combination of "mixed peel" (which includes fat grafting), TCA peel, and light dermabrasion over the deepest scarring. This patient chose to have the upper half-face lift, which gave her the most improvement with the most rapid recovery. For the type of undermining required here, plication of the SMAS is not as important as full skin undermining at the corner of the eye and into the upper forehead. **(C&D)** Note the improvement at 14 days. She has been at work for 1 week with proper makeup and has returned at this point for removal of the final two sutures placed in the high temple extension. These sutures were essential to the procedure because the acne scarring extended into this zone. Simply overstretching this area with appropriate tacking maneuvers eliminated much of her obvious deformity. In the future, she will consider lower face surgery and will continue the Retin-A/AHA regimen.

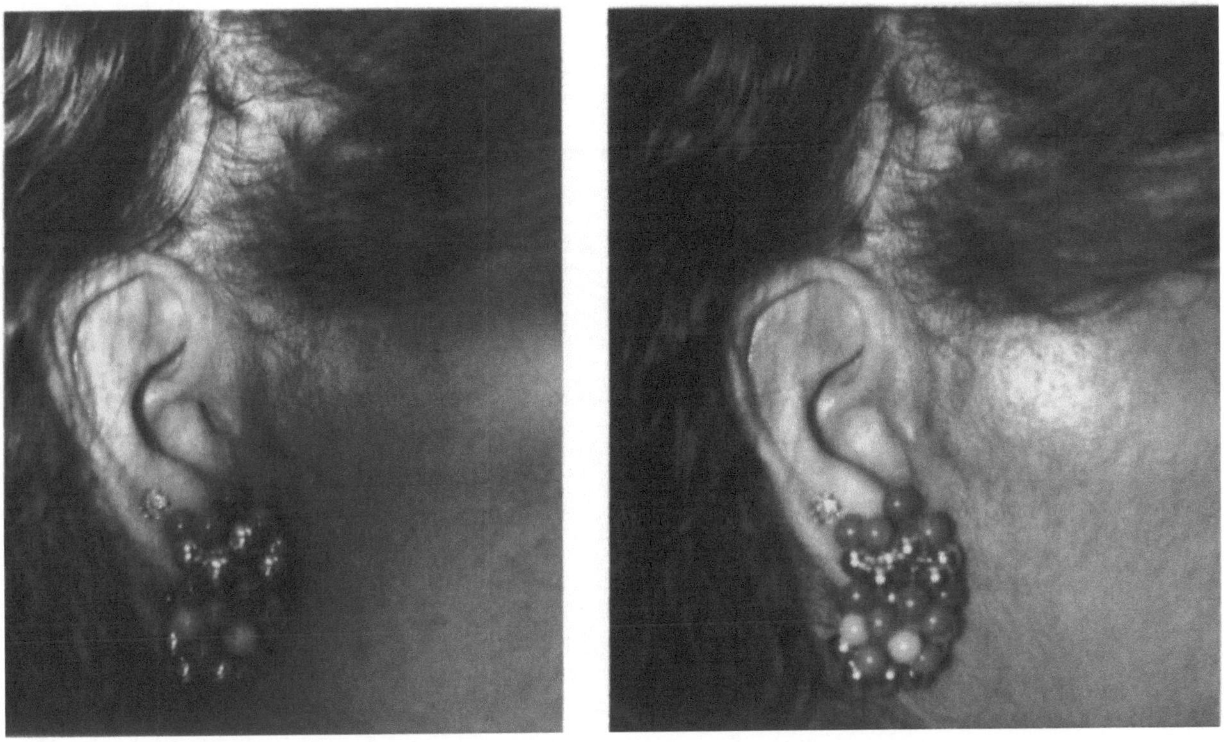

C D

PART TWO

The Body

Introduction

MANY OF THE PROCEDURES THAT WE ONCE PERFORMED FOR body sculpturing have been radically redesigned, with great improvement in the aesthetic results. The addition of liposuction to breast reduction, mastopexy, abdominoplasty, and hip and thigh reduction was a major change. Progressing from a relatively crude procedure in 1982, the sophisticated application of liposuction today involves smaller cannulas, multiple tiny incisions for criss-crossing in several levels, elevation of skin depressions, "cellulite" removal with fat regrafting, and using liposuction as an adjunct to the other procedures.

Too often we see rippling and dimpling due to overzealous resections or areas that did not respond to the original suction lipectomy. The new techniques not only should prevent this problem but they are useful for the corrective surgery. An intensive postoperative program of skin care and exercise is emphasized.

The pseudocontroversy surrounding breast augmentation is addressed as well. Conditions that we consider complications today were considered triumphs 30 years ago. Our standards have changed. Breasts should be as natural, and the changes as undetectable, as possible, and of course the operation must continue the excellent safety record that has been established over the years. We discuss how changes in composition of breast prostheses were stimulated by discussions between manufacturers and surgeons and how the complications that were so frequent during the early years are rarely encountered today. The choice of procedures and prostheses, the nonoperative correction of problems, and the new techniques of internal repair for the mechanical complications of breast augmentation should be part of every surgeon's armamentarium.

The emerging methods for controlling bacteria are but one factor in our increasing success rate. When a silicone implant is used as a lens replacement in the eye, as part of a pacemaker or cardiac valve, as a replacement for wrist or finger joints, or in the testicle, brain, or intraabdominally, bacteria do not play a role unless they are transmitted through the bloodstream from an infective source elsewhere in the body.

The breast is different from other areas. It must contend with fibrocystic disease, stress, trauma, pregnancy, and gravity; hence we must devise methods for continued upgrading of the procedures and restoration of normalcy. This subject leads us to a discussion of the "internal" mastopexy using circumareolar principles. A new use of these principles lies in breast reduction. Again, liposuction plays a critical role.

For abdominoplasty, the basic principles of short incisions with upturns to fit within "French line" bathing attire and liposuction to prevent "dog-ears" and to remove flank fat and recreate natural folds are discussed. We also apply the principles of "limited" abdominoplasty to patients who require a full abdominal repair from xiphoid to pubis. Because liposuction is employed liberally in these individuals, the techniques to diminish tension on the closure become of paramount importance.

In the chapter on miscellaneous topics, I discuss unusual procedures and those with which I have little experience, such as buttock implants and calf implants. I also comment on the many foibles and problems of modern plastic surgery.

12 Breast Augmentation

IN 1983 *TECHNICAL FORUM* CONDUCTED A SURVEY ABOUT CHOICES and techniques for breast augmentation. We received more than 300 replies—about 90% of those to whom the questionnaire was mailed—with some strong opinions. In 1983 we were trying axillary incisions and double-lumen implants, and a few surgeons were still working with saline implants. At least 50% of the first 300 respondents to the survey said that they had abandoned the axillary incision, primarily because of scarring and the inability to create a central and medial pocket, a message repeated at our national meetings. I looked at several presentations on axillary surgery and was not impressed. However, when I performed the next dozen or so periareolar incisions, I asked myself if I could have created that space, lowered the inframammary fold, or cauterized bleeders from the axilla.

In 1983 only 20% of our correspondents were using saline implants, and 40% said they had used them at one time but abandoned them. They mentioned deflation, "a crackling" feel (particularly in double lumens that had deflated), and visible wrinkling. We still have that problem today.

A number of us still use steroids in the pocket. After experiences with the heavier particles of Kenalog and some of the problems that call for thinning, most surgeons have changed to methyl prednisolone (Solu-Medrol), triamcinolone (Aristospan) or some other steroid that is mixed liberally with saline or bupivacaine (Marcaine).

A number of colleagues prefer the submuscular augmentation that was popular during the early 1980s because it "reduced the number of contractures." It did not, however, reduce them enough. With the current emphasis on physical conditioning and aerobics, women do not like the sensation of the implant under the muscle, and they report much more pain than do those with subglandular implants. Today the submuscular position is not as popular. We use textured implants exclusively now, not just in taut fibrotic breasts. A saline implant is used for the primary augmentation and a textured gel implant for the ptotic breast or for replacement. At one time I believed strongly that one should leave the upper part of the pectoralis muscle intact so as to cover the upper pole of the implant in thin patients. I rarely do it now. The activity of the muscle too often pushed the implant into a lower position, producing a ballooning or overstretched effect for the lower half of the breast. In 1983 Louis McCraw (Portland) summed up the consensus opinion: "There may be fewer contractures with submuscular implants, but the overall problems are as great. The contractures are more troublesome. It is difficult to obtain symmetry, and minor degrees of ptosis will require mastopexy." There is also a major problem in that a closed release cannot be done in a submuscular placement. The implant cannot be used to stretch fibrocystic bands with the submuscular placement, whereas the subglandular placement allows it. On the other hand, contracture of an implant in the submuscular condition is not as noticeable and perhaps can go undetected by the patient, if not by the physician. This is still true.

At the time of this writing "activists" are claiming that plastic surgeons have suppressed data on the complications of breast implants, and that little or no research has been done to assess their safety and biocompatibility. This assumption is patently untrue.

As a medical student and intern at Duke University, I witnessed large incisions for the insertion of solid *foam* implants—no other materials had been successful. These implants looked good for the first few months. (Perhaps our profession is guilty of overenthusiasm over early results.) As everyone knows, these 1961 foam implants have all been replaced because of fibrous ingrowth.

The first *silicone* implants in 1962 were "bricks." Wide incisions were required to position them and to ensure that the Dacron patches held the breast in the right position. Little did we know that the breast tissue would slide over the implant and ptosis would occur in a certain number of women despite the so-called internal support by the implant. The breasts were hard, but at least the body was not rejecting them. They were followed by the softer implants without Dacron, then implants without any attachment features at all, and finally saline implants. It soon became obvious to those in the field that the softest breasts were those in which the suture that held the implant in place had torn loose and the implant was free to move. It also became obvious that certain breasts would become ptotic with time because they were ptotic and less fibrotic at the beginning. Other patients—those whom we describe shortly as type A—had firm, flat breasts. Implantation in these patients gave a fuller, firm breast that never changed. Now we are told that hardness is a major complication that should have been "disclosed!!"

In 1970, Dick Jones and I began working with a periareolar incision for gel implants. It was apparent that saline-filled implants were not the best choice. They just did not have the natural feel of the newer gels. Soft implants that were in wide use during the early 1970s until about 1980 were well accepted. The complication rates dropped. We learned how to control infection with appropriate antibiotics, double-lumen prostheses with steroids and antibiotics, povidone-iodine (Betadine) irrigations, and so on. We then began to observe double-lumen prostheses with problems, including deflation of the outer portion. It was not an overwhelming problem unless the surgeon had used a saline injection to balance the size of the breasts. When we only used 20 ml of saline and combined it with antibiotics and steroids, the deflation was not noticeable unless of course the implant folded on itself—which it often did. We then went through a period of adding triamcinolone (Kenalog) to the outer lumen instead of within the pocket. Kenalog is a thick, granular steroid. When it settled into the lower part of the breast or the double lumen, there was thinning of breast tissue, the so-called "blue holes." That problem led to some rather ingenious methods of turning up pectoralis muscle flaps and capsule flaps for internal repairs. The problem has now disappeared. Many still believe that steroids in the pocket help to decrease fibrous capsular contracture by stopping it early. It is an effective method only if you dilute a "thin" steroid such as Aristospan or Solu-Medrol with Marcaine for comfort and dispersion.

During our routine operation, just prior to closing the subcuticular portion of the incision I inject 20 ml of Marcaine, 20 mg of Solu-Medrol, and 250 mg of cephalothin (Keflin) through a catheter placed inside the pocket. I then pull the catheter out and finish the closure. The patients stay comfortable, and *perhaps* the antibiotics and steroids are useful.

These agents were certainly useful in one case. Despite our written materials and counseling, one of my patients called the day after surgery to complain that fluid was running down her chest. "But you told me I had to get out of bras in a hurry." She had forgotten that we emphasized protection for 3 days because of the Marcaine. She had no pain, so she decided to go to a dance the day she got home. She wore no brassiere, someone hugged her, and the incision on one side split. We were able to close the incision; and despite the wound being open for 24 hours, there was no infection thanks to the amount of Betadine and Keflin that was still within the pocket. This case supports the argument for antibiotic instillation.

Technique

There are several important technical points regarding cosmetic breast surgery.

1. The periareolar incision is almost invisible in 98% of my patients. It is technically more difficult, of course, but it is worth it. There is good visualization for hemostasis and dissection.
2. With a periareolar approach, the breast can be expanded with the fingertip and a retractor once the implant is in place. It is amazing how much stretching can be obtained by thus enlarging the pocket and breaking up some of the fibrous bands in the parenchyma.
3. Irrigate with povidone-iodine (Betadine). It stays in the tissues for weeks and helps to control the bacteria that live within the ductal tissue. (These bacteria play a role, perhaps a major one, in capsular contracture.)
4. Those of us who have used steroids over the years have been through ups and downs with them, but we are still believers. Mixing Solu-Medrol 20 mg with a generous 30 or 40 ml of Marcaine ensures that the steroid is well distributed.
5. For patients with smooth implants, the installation of Marcaine allows them to begin pressure massage without discomfort the next day. For patients with textured implants there is the advantage of general comfort. We also add an antibiotic, either Keflin or gentamicin (Garamycin). We are not sure it helps, but it certainly does not hurt.
6. There are reports that cefazolin (Kefzol) can cause an acute fibrous reaction, stimulating scar contracture around the prosthesis. It is also true of tetracycline. Tetracycline is used to eliminate seromas; do not put it in a breast pocket.
7. Sharp dissection to lower the inframammary fold is necessary for practically all breast augmentations. The fold attaches too high and makes the breast appear ptotic. It also restricts expansion of the breast envelope. Bleeders may be encountered, but they are easy to control from a periareolar incision.
8. Do not hesitate to put in a drain if there is unusual bleeding. Such bleeding is rare, but it does occur.
9. Offer to pinpoint-cauterize hairs that grow around the areola. It is effective in about 75%. We use a 30-gauge needle and the usual electrocautery apparatus.
10. If you expect a patient to wear a brassiere for 10 days to allow a textured implant to settle into place, be sure to supply her with creams and ointments to keep her comfortable. Otherwise she may renege. We also supply soothing oils for her bath. Textured implant patients are allowed to shower with a brassiere on at 5 days and to bathe without the brassiere at 10 days.

Choices for Breast Augmentation

Numerous prostheses are available today, each with major advantages and minor disadvantages. Some surgeons prefer double-lumen prostheses because antibiotics or steroids can be added. Others have discontinued their use because the outer lumen sometimes deflates (not seen with "reverse double-lumen" types) and the transient effect of steroids on secondary breast augmentation. The only consensus is that textured implants are advantageous when replacing a prosthesis in a patient who has had multiple open or closed capsulotomies. These patients are different from most: Their breasts are more fibrotic owing either to fibrocystic processes or a reaction to the old prosthesis, which "sweated" liquid silicone. The "misdirection" of collagen fiber by the textured cover seems to make a difference. For a first-time patient, however, neither of these implants is probably worth the extra cost unless the breast is small and taut, and the patient is nulliparous.

In laboratory models there seems to be no great difference between the types of implant in terms of the appearance of contractures. Early clinical reports were prefaced by a reference to the contracture problems reported for the pre-1982 series, but such statements do not help us understand the current dilemma. One author, promoting immediate expansion during breast augmentation, judged his success against a "30% to 80% recurrence rate." It is not a valid comparison because there are few patients today who require an open capsulotomy, regardless of the type of implant used. The manufacturers of the "open"-type textured implants (McGhan, Misti) claim that their implants are superior to the less open type (Siltex). My statistics do not support this claim, but recent studies support this advantage.

In fact, if you look at the literature and ignore the references to past problems, practically every surgeon is reoperating 2% to 3% of patients. There are differing opinions on this subject.

Greg Hetter:

> It seems to me that no particular technique of breast augmentation is a perfect technique. All have advantages and disadvantages. At this particular point in time, I believe that smooth-shelled, water-filled, or double-lumen implants containing antibiotics in the subpectoral position in properly selected patients give excellent results. I have a 3% reoperation rate in these patients over an average follow-up time of about 4 years. In the prepectoral position, I believe that textured implants of similar type offer the best long-term result.

Many readers did not agree that textured implants are an advantage for stretchy "type B" or "type C" breast augmentation. Their belief was based not on the fact that more contractures can be released without surgery, but because there have been fewer problems in these groups using any type of breast implant.

By now many surgeons are reassured that textured breast prostheses do not limit free movement of the breast. Hence textured surfaces are an advantage and comprise the implant of choice for most plastic surgeons.

A number of us were outraged by an article appearing in a newspaper quoting an ASPRS member on the advantages of submuscular breast augmentation: "They are less likely to change shape, a leading expert says. His new study found that 2% of women suffer complications or disfiguring changes compared to 25% suffering disfiguring scarring around the implants with conventional subglandular augmentation." Those figures are inaccurate and do not address the major problems.

Richard Toronto:

> "The statistic of 2% contractures was in patients followed for 1 year. Two percent of breasts equals 4% of patients, and their follow-up at 1 year was only 70% of those operated. They used steroids in bi-lumen implants. We learned years ago that steroids give wonderful results early on. Submuscular placement of a prosthesis offers no great advantage. Contracture bands occur across the breast, and there is very poor cleavage in a large number of patients."

It is not appropriate to comment on polyurethane implants because the parent company of Surgitek took them off the American market. However, when polyurethane-covered implants were available, in the improved form, contracture problems in our patients practically disappeared. We were able to reconstruct breasts with immediate expansion and easily place an appropriately wide and large polyurethane implant in the position desired. Latissimus and TRAM flaps were not necessary. The large polyurethane implant, placed under the muscle after "immediate expansion" for mastectomy reconstruction, acted like a koozie ball. It slowly pushed itself up and expanded the breast from within. Aesthetic surgeons were satisfied with these reconstructions, which did not require expanders or flaps. It is unfortunate that the manufacturer yielded to legal pressure of threats, which ignored the scientific data on safety. Fortunately for our patients, both gel "smooth" and gel "textured" implants are available for breast surgery.

It has become apparent that we do not need submuscular placement to reduce the risk of contracture. Contractures occur both submuscularly and subglandularly, and the incidence figures are identical now that textured implants are available. We do not know exactly why the textured implants work. No one believes today that they adhere for an extended period, but they do influence the way the collagen is aligned in the capsule. Capsules form with textured implants, but they are easy to release if subglandular.

Opinions are currently divided as to the value of textured implants. The only clear statement that can be made is that saline implants that are textured seem to have less tendency to leak, possibly owing to tissue ingrowth around the valve.

To be perfectly fair about the submuscular–subglandular controversy, we should point out that a number of prominent surgeons still prefer total muscular coverage of an implant and others perform various releases to prevent implant migration too high or down to the middle of the chest. Such migration was the main reason I abandoned submuscular augmentation during the mid-1980s. We treated too many women with "stretch-out" problems that had to be corrected using the internal mastopexy technique. In others the implant sat so high the patient described herself as feeling like a weight lifter. There was also the problem of inadequate cleavage centrally. This problem does not occur subglandularly because one can dissect closer to the midline and stretch the breast tissue manually.

Mark Mandel:

> "The subpectoral implantation of implants does, indeed, cause distortion in women who are fairly muscular. This is a problem in Southern California, where many of the patients actively participate in exercise and body building programs. . . . Until recently . . . all of my implants were positioned subpectorally. Approximately 12% of all of the patients developed some degree of mild distortion, especially in women who had well developed pectoralis major muscles."

In regard to Mandel's statement, the 12% figure of distortion following pectoral implantation appears to be low. In addition, I found that at least 15% to 20% of all of the submammary implants develop some degree of capsule formation, especially in Oriental patients.

Clyde Litton:

> "Relative to breast contractures, it has been my experience, and in conversation with fellow plastic surgeons, that if an honest survey was made of silicone implants for augmentation breast surgery, that anywhere from 15% to 20% would represent an accurate figure. How do authors claim that the submuscular approach is so superior and his contractures are so few? Other people cannot repeat these same results. If the submuscular approach was so dramatic, why hasn't everyone gone to this route in the past? Why can't others produce the same results?"

Another voice in the swelling tide against submuscular breast augmentations, Ed Terino, clearly points out the dynamic deformity of the submuscular implant and the limitations of space. "The late deformities are horrendous."

It all goes back to the basic principles of breast augmentation: Create a wide enough pocket, increase massage, and keep the overlying tissue soft and stretchable. The muscle just does not stretch that way. Those of us who use submuscular implants for breast reconstruction are pleased that the augmentation patients do not have the complications and problems of muscle tightening, adhesion, and displacement of implants inferiorly.

It has been said that one of Tom Cronin's most famous quotes is as follows: "Because you know how to do an operation doesn't necessarily mean you should do it." The subject came up in a discussion of whether latissimus flaps were always necessary during breast reconstructions. Reconstructive surgeons had frequently performed breast reconstructions using myocutaneous flaps in which there was more than adequate chest wall skin.

Presad Sureddi has reported patients who have back pain following submuscular breast reconstruction. He insists that the capsular contracture rate is less for cosmetic patients (most authorities agree that they are exactly the same for submuscular or subglandular reconstructions). We agreed that the problems are fewer with submuscular placement. The unusual cases involved detachment of the serratus muscle from the rib cage all the way to the posterior axillary line. When the contour deformity and the late discomfort were evaluated, it became clear that the pressure of the implant against the insertion of the serratus musculature in the inferior angle of the scapula was the source of the pain. Thus excessive dissection of the serratus anterior muscle should be avoided during the initial surgery.

John Hartley (Atlanta) said, "I have not been putting implants submuscularly, although there seems to be a lot of enthusiasm for this approach [in 1983]. It is nonanatomical. Many patients have experienced discomfort while doing exercise and athletics. I have actually removed some from the submuscular position and placed them subglandular in patients from other surgeons. It is hard for me to imagine that there would be less contracture around implants in the submuscular position." It still seems to be the case after 10 years. The contractures are still there but they are more difficult to control.

Safety Controversy

The following descriptions are in sequence and illustrate well the astonished, amazed, and totally unprepared reaction of the plastic surgery community to junk science "charges" that breast implants cause cancer, scleroderma, rheumatoid arthritis, or chronic fatigue syndrome.

It began with rat experiments. Silicone balls cause sarcomas in rats. Of course these rats form sarcomas with any type of implanted material, whether it is glass, steel, wood, or whatever. In 1992 the scientific community responded in anger to the media and "studies" relying on rat experiments. Practically everything is carcinogenic in Fischer 344 inbred species. In fact, rats that live in nature do not have malignancies.

It continued with the panic about polyurethane implants containing carcinogens. We pointed out that 99.9% of the polyurethane remains in the patients and does not break down, releasing TDA. This breakdown product of polyether and polyester urethane that can be produced only under extreme laboratory conditions. No one thought to point out that polyurethane is used in many medical implanted devices including pacemakers, and that the latter have an excellent safety record.

The 20-year experience with polyurethane breast prostheses was reviewed. The early models were poorly accepted by our patients because of tissue ingrowth, calcification, and the inherent rigidity of the prostheses. Several of my patients developed infections, as did patients of other surgeons (in 1984 and 1985), but virtually no infections were reported after 1987. Soaking the prostheses in Betadine and our greater familiarity with their use may have made a difference, or there may have been more careful sterilization by the manufacturers. Jack Fisher's editorial was excellent: "Why is our society responding emotionally to a *presumed* threat? Why believe that an artificially created chemical product will induce human cancer if the 'studies' are based on an entirely invalid evaluation model? We have allowed science and good medical practices to be manipulated, misquoted, and condemned by the media hungry egoists and greedy legal practitioners."

Let us begin this discussion with an excellent summary by David Wood, who sent the following letter to the Director of the Food and Drug Administration (FDA), whose bureau allowed nonscientists to make their claims public.

Dear Dr. Kessler:

I am absolutely appalled at the lack of straightforward honesty and correct reason and logic in the recent breast implant panel's recommendation. Their recent decision to hold off implants available to women for purely cosmetic reasons for the examples and excuses given is coercive. By the panel's own concession, there is no true scientifically demonstrated link that the so-called immune diseases are causally related to the silicone breast implants. How in the world are they safer for "reconstruction" than "cosmetic" reasons? They are still silicone implants. Such syllogistic reasoning is not even worthy of children. For a panel to arbitrarily make a decision between "reconstruction" and "cosmetic," as their announced reason, is disgustingly illogical and demonstrates a colossal bias, though poor excuse, which is intolerable.

I am old enough to remember the *free injection of liquid silicone* into women's breasts. Extensive complications of scarring and deformity resulted from those injections. I do not recall any report blaming such injections for *any* diseases.

Certainly you know that all silicone forms result from the amount of catalyst added to the silicone material. The basic silicone is thinner than water, but with added catalyst all grades of viscosity, from the thinnest to the hardest of hard rubber consistency, is achievable. To allow *saline implants*, which have a form of silicone shell, and not allow the silicone shell around the silicone gel doesn't compute. By the same token almost all devices implanted in the human body have some form of silicone cover because of its proved inertness. It is interesting that little concern is voiced for the silicone covered cardiac pacemakers, the brain shunts in neurosurgery, the testicular and penile implants of urology, and the joint replacement prostheses of the hand. However, any attack upon all these politically unimportant devices would be just as spurious.

The worming of political considerations into the medical-scientific field is insidious and harmful. I, for one, vigorously oppose it. This politically motivated attack is spawned by private interests pushed by attorneys and must not be allowed to deny women their right of choice.

In their desire to assuage the anger of those who are convinced otherwise, the panel is willing to hinder unabashedly the true right for choice of women who can, when totally informed, make a value judgment in their own behalf without the pious position of this committee's ban ("recommendation"). This is nothing more than a cheap political compromise. By contrast, if the panel had true concern for people's welfare, then they and the whole American public should screamingly demand removal of cigarettes and alcohol from the societal scene because of their *known* causes of human misery and death.

I personally feel, and my medical profession collectively feels, sadness for any woman inflicted with the so-called immune diseases, which are claimed by some women to be related to implants. The concomitant occurrence of implant complications at the same time that rheumatoid arthritis (or other adjuvant disease) is diagnosed is not a valid reason to withhold breast implants for the population.

Complications do not equate to diseases!

If silicone should be a cause of a so-called adjuvant (immune) disease, then it is worthy of scientific investigation. We encourage this, and ASPRS (American Society of Plastic and Reconstructive Surgeons) is setting up a central registry. However, even the claimed incidence is so low that your restriction on the whole population is truly unjustified.

David Wood, M.D., F.A.C.S.

Fallacy of Statistics for Analysis of Complications

As director of a large cosmetic surgery center, I evaluated the complications of breast augmentation in our own practice and in a large referral group. My experience with this survey refutes many of the tenets of breast augmentation based on statistics that do not reflect the true nature of the operation and its effect on patients.

The impression that submuscular prostheses have relatively equal complication rate with subglandular prostheses has been supported by a national survey that was requested through *Technical Forum*. Published statistics indicate that contractures occur more frequently with subglandular augmentation. Although this may be true, the erroneous impression is that these patients require frequent surgical correction. We have evaluated our patients and those referred to us with intractable contractures. We evaluated only those contractures that could be released *only by surgery* and could not attain Baker's 0 or Baker's 1 softness. Contractures in submuscular prosthesis patients almost always require relief by surgical intervention, whereas the opposite is true for contractures in patients with subglandular prostheses. Since the mid-1980s, our reoperation rate has been approximately 2%, whereas our closed-release rate is 10%. We believe that a program of repeated massage and testing by the operating surgeon can control 98% of "smooth wall" contractures, thereby avoiding surgical correction. These statistics give the true impression of the differences between the procedures.

Patients with subglandular prostheses are more comfortable, have a more natural contour, have more natural ptosis, and can be sculptured surgically to specifications desired by the operating surgeon. Such has not been the case with submuscular augmentation. Changing from submuscular to subglandular placement and to textured prostheses has been successful for us.

A second fallacy of statistical reporting ignores the fact that most patients have asymmetry with a difference in thickness and elasticity. Even with offsetting size augmentation, the thick breast is never as resilient as the opposite one. If one were intent on making a case for contractures, these thicker breasts could be labeled Baker 1 or 2, when in reality there is no evidence of contracture.

In other words, density, hormonal response, fibrosis, trauma, pregnancy, and even stress cause changes in breast softness. The capsule may contract as a consequence. Closed compression in "modern" (i.e., 1984 onward) implants can safely and effectively expand *extracapsular* tightness, another advantage of subglandular placement.

Polyurethane Implants

Because a substance biodegrades does not mean that it is dangerous. Most sutures biodegrade, including silk and nylon, but they do not then migrate through the tissues. Neither does polyurethane. According to investigators, polyurethane stays "remarkably well preserved in its foam structure" even at long-term follow-up testing. It becomes incorporated into the fibrous capsule. When the capsule tissue is digested away, practically 100% of the foam is still there.

Why then did mice get sick when fed the by-product of polyurethane, TDA? In fact, those mice were fed pure, concentrated TDA in high doses. When the same type mice were fed polyurethane foam, there was no carcinogenicity at all. In other words, rats who ate implants did not get sick. What about the implantation results in three "lifetime" studies? Animals with implanted foam showed no malignancies. The evidence seems conclusive in cancer-prone animals.

What about the question of carcinomas in implant patients? It has been implied that the presence of an implant makes detection of a carcinoma impossible. Can it be true? In women with *palpable masses*, the carcinomas were at earlier stages in a group with implants in 1993 reports.

Experts agree that modern x-rays allow one to examine the breast adequately. A better examination is obtained in flat-chested, augmented women because the breast has been lifted away from the chest during the augmentation. One group of investigators stated that they have no diagnostic trouble with women who have implants—submuscular or subglandular—even when standard mammography is used for diagnosis. The key word is "diagnostic," which infers the use of multiple views and enhancement, and often thermography, and sonography.

Human Adjuvant Diseases

There is no recorded instance of "human adjuvant disease." Adjuvant disease *can* be produced, but only in rats and only by injecting mineral oil and extracts from tuberculosis bacilli. The myth all started with Japanese patients who were given injections of paraffin and others given injections of liquid silicone and some type of industrial solvent designed to create inflammation. They did indeed become ill. The investigator who reported this study said that it "reminded him" of the syndrome that was produced in rats by tuberculosis bacilli extracts, so he took it upon himself to label this syndrome (the reaction to industrial solvents and paraffin) "adjuvant diseases."

Laymen immediately jumped to the conclusion that silicone must induce strange syndromes, and therefore women who have vague complaints must be suffering from "human adjuvant disease." In a subsequent report, our Japanese colleague described breast implant patients who had back pain, knee pain, bursitis, and arthritis and claimed that these problems were related to the silicone—with no scientific data to support his claim.

In all the laboratory studies to date, silicone has not been shown to produce an immunologic response, even in rats. Interesting point: In rats who had adjuvant disease induced by the tuberculosis bacilli, stress made their disease worse.

Informing Patients

A number of colleagues have suggested simple homilies that can be used to discuss patients' concerns about polyurethane and silicone. First, point out that those who gave the media information on these substances did not tell the whole story. The investigators doing the research had already placed modern polyurethane microimplants into three rat generations, and all the rats lived to a ripe old age of grandmotherhood. The same result come about when another set of rats were forced to eat massive amounts of polyurethane.

Point out that silicone has never elicited an antigenic response in the laboratory or in humans. Point out that if someone wants to flush silicone through their body, they can drink a bottle of Digel or Gas-X, either of which is almost pure simethicone. Once swallowed, it is absorbed but does not result in illness. (Injectable collagen is different. It is an antigen, and humans do develop antibodies to it.)

Point out that the patients who had silicone injections in their breasts had problems related to migration or had reactions to the materials practitioners added to the pure silicone to keep it in place. Recent studies show no increased incidence of systemic diseases in this patient population.

Point out that more than 1 million women have had breast implants or lens implants as a treatment for cataracts in the eye, some of them since 1964. They have been studied from one organ system to another, and there has been no untoward incidence of gallbladder disease, breast cancer, hair thinning, premenstrual syndrome, or other diseases. Nor is there a problem in men who have testicular prostheses.

It is true that the early implants leaked silicone, but the damage done was never more than the creation of fibrous tissue and scarring. It scared a few individuals, but it never made anyone sick. The only reason we are reluctant to do closed releases in patients with the older implants is that the implants are thinner and less solid than modern implants.

Point out that this scare tactic is brought to you by the same people who tried to convince Texans that eating steak can cause cancer. The manufacturers of Alar, the chemical used to help apples ripen, were victims of the same type of media scare. It too was based on totally irrelevant "scientific" data.

In some cases the women who appeared on television had had 14 or 15 operations. Their problems likely were with their doctors, not their implants. A good number of subcutaneous mastectomy patients had multiple surgeries. Our surgical experience during the early 1970s did not produce the results we obtain today, and the implants were of a less forgiving nature. Nevertheless, even these individuals, who are "surgical cripples," can be salvaged with textured implants and tissue expansion.

Today we are better surgeons, and it is surgeons with experience who are doing most of the operations. Point out also that women are blaming *all* surgeons for problems, when rightfully they should be blaming *untrained individuals who practice outside their specialty*. Of course, there are a few "bad apples" in our own specialty who just cannot perform adequate breast surgery. It is much easier for these physicians to blame an implant for failure than it is to blame his or her own inadequacy or the developing surgical technique. Many of us work hard to make breast reconstruction a viable operation, and when it is not successful we suffer along with our patients.

Panel Discussion on Silicone Implants

A recent panel discussion on silicone implants and their possible relation to disease states provided reassurance about several things. First, the rebuttals concerning the silicone scare have been made to the FDA. Moreover, the campaign of medical misinformation from the "activists" has been answered again in a calm, reasoned, scientific way. For balance, the ASPRS allowed several individuals with reasonable credentials to present their thoughts on the matter. They had implied that there was something unknown about human reactions to silicone. Is there a small subgroup of individuals who respond to silicone with an allergic phenomenon? Each presenter stressed the fact that this question may never be answered, but evidence to date does not support this possibility. Nevertheless, investigations are continuing and rightly so.

An eager rheumatologist from Florida reported that he had acceded to the wishes of frightened patients and recommended implant removal in those with chronic fatigue syndrome (CFS) and in a small number of patients with true autoimmune disease (six with rheumatoid arthritis, lupus erythematosus, or mild scleroderma). One did get better but was on steroids. Of this CFS group, the only ones who seemed to improve were those who could be said to have had a placebo effect, which was transitory at best. What he did not say was how unhappy the patients were to find that they still had fatigue and muscle aches but no breasts. He also did not mention the recent finding of "foamy viruses" in patients that are linked to CFS. Because there were no changes in his patients' erythrocyte sedimentation rates (ESR) and other exotic studies after implant removal, and only 27% of this entire group seemed to be improved after 6 months (placebo effect), we were relieved to hear the panelists agree that breast implant removal *cannot be supported* at this time. Why then was he quoted in the press implying the opposite?

A *Newsweek* article stated that there was a "safer method" for breast implants. Either the "researchers" or the science editor must be seriously lacking in knowledge. The article started by saying that we need to improve the safety of breast implants because the silicone "is opaque to mammography x-rays." It neglects to say that any competent radiologist can order triple-views and so view all the detail that needs to be seen. The original fear of hidden malignancy in breast implant patients was based on a series in which a radiologist unfamiliar even with the appearance of capsules was looking at some severely contracted breasts—and the patients presented required capsulectomies and repairs first.

Other researchers presented a paper recently in which they showed that it is difficult to obtain a good picture in a flat-chested woman. The conclusion that submuscular implants were easier to visualize was also based on an erroneous series. Radiologists tell us that the size of the breast makes no difference whatsoever. With submuscular placement of a prosthesis, the patient is at a disadvantage when performing a two-handed breast self-examination. This is a major advantage for the subglandular placement patient, far outweighing any theoretic disadvantage with early detection by radiography.

The thrust of another article was on an innovative experiment performed by a plastic surgeon at Washington University. He was looking for an implantable substance that "would be biocompatible with the human body." Apparently the authors evaluated a number of oils and found that ordinary peanut oil "provides what seems to be a superior substitute for silicone." New materials currently under evaluation may prove to be as effective as silicone gel without the disadvantages of gel, saline, or oils.

The oil is encased in a silicone envelope so thin that it does not prevent x-rays from detecting tiny masses. A shudder must have gone through the plastic surgery community at that point. How many times have we had to repair patients whose thin-walled implants broke after only minor trauma? How many of us want to deal with the foreign body reaction that would occur when an oil is liberated in an unsterile environment such as the breast? Moreover, how could these individuals conceivably think that oil implants would be less likely than silicone implants "to turn unpleasantly hard"? They seemed to think that a broken prosthesis would cause an "arthritis-like inflammation." This question has been investigated extensively. To date there is no evidence that oral ingestion of simethicone, intravenous infusions of silicone from coated blood bank products, or broken prostheses have any relation whatsoever to arthritis. Many factors are at play within a breast that will not concern those who implant silicone products for heart valves, ureters, or whatever. The breast is a mobile organ, often bounced about or physically abused in sports and other activities. We do not fault investigators for looking for new products, but we do fault them for reporting their rabbit findings to a gullible press.

The *New York Times Service* has finally published something of benefit to plastic surgeons. They have reported the largest study yet of chronic fatigue syndrome (CFS) and they do not blame it on silicone implants. The first documentation of chronic inflammation in the brains of patients with CFS were not specific enough to be used for the diagnosis. The evidence does not establish that herpes virus 6 is the absolute cause of the syndrome. Some abnormality of the patient's immune system may have reactivated a virus that had been long dormant in the body. Fatigue patients have immunologic and hormonal differences, so it is certainly not a true psychological disorder. It usually begins with flu symptoms that are followed by months or years of lethargy and other mental changes. The scans pinpoint areas of swelling or loss of nerve sheaths in the central nervous system in most patients.

Do Breast Implants Cause Cancer?

It has been stated by a misinformed physician that breast implants hide the development of cancer. It is not true. First, subglandular augmentation cannot hide anything because all the breast tissue is in front of the implants as it is for a submuscular augmentation. The important point is that augmentation patients must continue to have breast examinations or undergo xerography. The two-handed self breast examination technique, although easier prior to augmentation, can still be done. The implant is soft and moves away from the fingertips; it is therefore good practice to hold the bottom of the breast between the thumb and forefinger or between the fingertips of the two hands, feeling for lumps. Breast implant patients are at the same risk as everyone else.

Garry Brody has brought us up to date on the Los Angeles statistics used to rebut claims that augmentation increased cancer risk. He and his colleagues traced their patients in the Los Angeles area 15 years after their initial breast augmentation. Starting with patients who had prostheses, various agencies and rosters were used to be certain the patients were still in the area. Fortunately, there is a good cancer registry there, so names of breast cancer victims could be cross-checked against the names of patients who had had augmentations. In 37,000 "women years of risk," the control group had 48 cancers, about the national average. The augmented group had fewer cancers, only 32. There was a difference in the stage of the malignancy for augmented and nonaugmented groups. Augmented patients' were smaller and in earlier stages.

It is satisfying to have one's beliefs reinforced by scientific data.

Lateral Drift

An increasingly common problem in women who have soft breast prostheses is lateral drift and occasionally the difficult "loaf of bread" breast that results from medial drift. Some of these cases are due to overexpansion during the breast augmentation procedure. It is difficult to achieve good cleavage with submuscular placement, and some surgeons overrelease the muscles. Muscle activity then moves the implants too far medially. Submuscular implants usually do not become laterally displaced. The main complaints of these patients are the change in breast shape when the pectoralis muscle is flexed and flatness in the axillary area. These problems are easily corrected by replacing the implant in the subglandular position, although then you must then deal with gravitational changes.

After a number of years, patients with curved rib cages often have a slow drift laterally, and when they lie down there is a space between the implants that did not exist before. There are two corrective choices here. One is to use a large implant and maintain the space exactly as it is. The second is to use the same size implant or a smaller one that has *texturing* to hold it centrally and then close off the lateral groove. Whether closing off medially or laterally, do not try to sew capsule to capsule. It does not hold. First, cauterize the capsule, then fold it on itself, and close in layers. By the time the textured implant loosens, the repair is solid.

It is possible to reduce the size of a breast implant while maintaining central cleavage. First, perform a complete capsulectomy if there is any chance of silicone leakage (and hence tissue reaction). If not, remove the capsule except in the lateral groove, but cauterize it lightly in spots in this area. A textured implant is then placed in a central position. The texturing holds it there long enough so it does not slip laterally and press against the repair. Close with heavy sutures (e.g., No. 1 Dexon) using figure-of-eight stitches. On each pass, pick up the *entire depth of the lateral groove.* Once the suture is tied, it disappears. (If you seal it from above, the sutures inevitably give way and the space is still there. The capsule does not adhere to itself.)

Inframammary Fold Scars

At best, scars in the inframammary fold are unpredictable. The best procedure is to close everything with a subcuticular closure. Even a single crossover stitch can leave a white mark that stands out like a beacon on tanned skin. Today's bathing suits are cut higher and higher, and no one wants a visible scar. The technique of deepithelializing an old scar and using deep dermal scar tissue to hold the deepest stitches is a good method. First it must be decided if the old inframammary scar should be anchored in the fold or the fold lowered for symmetry. If the fold is lowered from within, the scar then sits on the breast but on the undersurface of the curvature. The next decision regards skin tension, which will determine what to do with the deepithelialized area. A useful maneuver for scar revision is to use the deepithelialized zone, 1 to 2 cm above the incision line, as an anchor to the deep dermis. The technique is as follows.

First, deepithelialize the scar, and then cut back along the skin edges on both sides so they evert. (When the second-layer closure is done, those skin edges should pop up in the air.) The edges should just touch. The final subcuticular closure with 5-0 absorbable sutures makes sure they stay there long enough so the scar does not widen.

The only decision is whether to prepare the deepithelialized scar tissue as a tuck-under flap for the incision or to anchor it with three or four stitches to the pectoralis fascia. With a normal fold position and no tension on the skin, split the scar tissue in the middle of the incision. First, place a deep layer of stitches to close off the capsular tissue and breast tissue. Then place a series of 2-0 Dexon sutures in the deep portion of the deepithelialized scar. When these interrupted stitches are tied, the skin edges come together. Finish with a running subcuticular 4-0 Dexon suture. (I almost never use Vicryl any more because many sutures were splitting.) Technical point: Bury the first knot as far away from the surface as possible, then back-track and finish the subcuticular running suture with a continuous bite from side to side. When you get to the end, do not try to bury the knot, as it will reappear in 50% of cases. Just pass the suture through the skin, tie a loop knot on the surface, and clip if off 3 to 4 days later.

Effect of Pregnancy

The effect of pregnancy on breast augmentation patients is not always bad. For example, one of our patients, with type A, flat, thick, fibrocystic nonstretchable breasts who had undergone breast augmentation a year before, had a 12-week pregnancy that ended in miscarriage. For patients with breasts of this type it is usual practice to use a textured implant, but in her case we had thought she was stretchy enough that a standard gel implant would work. Examining her a month or so after the miscarriage, we found that the breast was more natural, thicker, and had more of a mature appearance than in her old photographs. Hence the pregnancy seems to have had a positive effect on her breasts.

When advising a patient who is pregnant, be sure to point out that the breast can "turn to mush" under the influence of the new hormones. Practically, then, she should wear a brassiere day and night, use creams, and perform a pressure massage at least once daily even with a textured implant. We teach patients to reach around the lower pole and slide their fingers together along the rib cage. That keeps the thicker upper half of the breast "honest." A little pressure every day seems to prevent extra thickening or contracture.

Some patients do not look as good after pregnancy as before. The breast may stretch and become distorted, but generally stretch marks do not appear because the tissues have already been loosened. We do, however, see a few women each year who have lost so much breast tissue with pregnancy that the implant is no longer large enough, and a simple replacement is indicated.

Ptosis

One of many goals of the aesthetic surgeon is to correct deformities with minimal visible scarring. Between the desire to create a youthful, uplifted breast to replace an atrophic ptotic breast and the wish to avoid skin scarring, we must choose an acceptable compromise.

With certain types of mildly to moderately ptotic small breasts, surgical techniques can create the illusion of an uplift utilizing only a short periareolar incision. In effect, an illusion of normalcy is achieved by lowering and filling the breast envelope internally rather than reshaping with highly visible skin incisions of conventional mastopexy.

The primary advantage of curvilinear periareolar incisions for breast augmentation or subcutaneous mastectomy is that they blend into the junction between loose, pigmented, areolar skin and taut, less pigmented, areolar skin. To preserve this highly important advantage, the incision must lie exactly in the junction. To transgress onto the areola leaves a contrasting and thus permanently more noticeable scar. In most of our patients, periareolar incisions are, for all practical purposes, invisible. In my opinion, the only alternative that is superior is augmentation via an abdominoplasty incision.

Periareolar incisions have additional advantages. The central location affords easy access for medial sharp dissection, which creates "cleavage" with breast augmentation. Achieving hemostasis and fully developing the submammary space by sharp dissection are greatly facilitated. With augmentation from an abdominal incision, suction drains left in the submammary space prevent blood clot layering on the raw surface, probably a factor in preventing future capsular contracture. Drainage and pressure are effective in almost all instances, and the position of the inframammary fold can be created at the appropriate level.

Certain types of breast require only areolar repositioning, rather than complete mastopexy envelope reduction, to achieve a shape consistent with popular concepts of normalcy. Another advantage of the periareolar incision is that of excising adjacent breast skin for areolar repositioning with the same hidden scar.

The plastic surgery literature portrays detailed designs for mastopexies, often illustrated with breast types that, in my opinion, do not warrant mastopexy. The devastating emotional impact of unpredictable mastopexy scars is not emphasized. As our standard idealized breast, we are taught to choose the uplifted breast typified by Venus de Milo. Our patients, however, are more attuned to the standards of our society.

Twelve years ago, I wrote the following summary. It is even more appropriate today.

> Contemporary motion pictures depict the physical attractiveness of the "older woman" including mature breast shapeliness. Current role models include women whose attractiveness is not diminished by moderate ptosis. Also, in today's world, clothing is worn openly, covering less of the breast and chest, areas often traversed by mastopexy scars. The ultimate arena of female appreciation, the men's magazines, invariably display glamorous women with mild to moderate, or even severe ptosis.
>
> Our patients express the desire to look normal and attractive for their age group and social standing. Most of our group C patients are in their late twenties or thirties, and ptosis is acceptable if the shape is pleasing. When asked to choose between photographs of the compromise corrected breasts we have described and the uplifted breast with mastopexy scars, the reaction universally is dismay and rejection of the latter. *We do no disservice by bowing to our patients' wishes*, even if we are simply providing several years of scar-free happiness in certain instances. Weighed against scarring and distortion that frequently mar results of mastopexy, the illusion of mastopexy created internally is an acceptable alternative.
>
> Contemporary standards of attractiveness of female breasts in lay persons is often at variance with traditional plastic surgery concepts. "Repair" of mild to moderately ptotic breasts with various mastopexy incisions often creates greater problems due to the presence of long scars on breast skin often accompanied by permanent loss of sensation. Eminently satisfactory breasts may be created by technical maneuvers confined to incisions hidden at an areolar edge and internal adjustments of size and position.

Tubular or Conical Breasts

In 1983 I discussed a simple way to correct the tubular or conical breast. Before John Williams showed us how to correct the "Snoopy" deformity, some of us were simply expanding the capsular space underneath a "Snoopy nose," or tubular, breast and inserting an implant. Although it is agreed that many of these patients require exotic releases and transfers or resections of the subareolar tissue, others can attain an acceptable result with augmentation alone and certainly without the need for external excisions except that for the periareolar augmentation.

When the patient in Figure 12-1 was first evaluated, the current mode of therapy was to incise completely around the areola and reduce it by undercut-

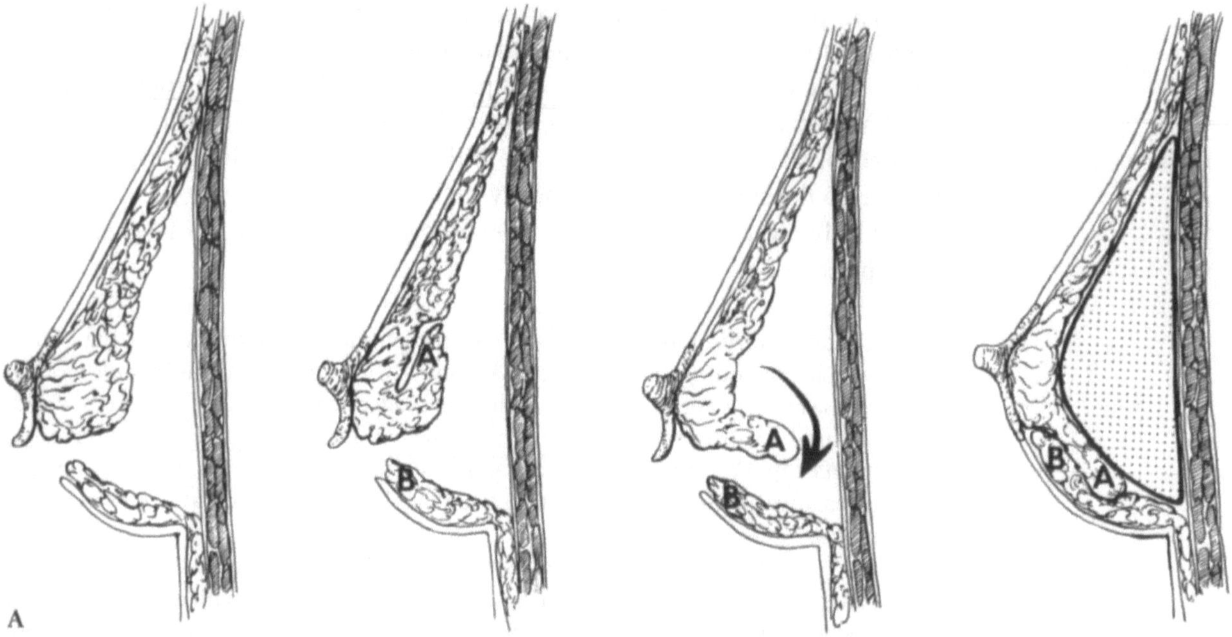

A

Figure 12-1. Snoopy deformity. John Williams has advocated excising periareolar skin and inverting the nipple underneath, or infolding the nipple itself, to reduce the overhang during augmentation in such patients. Others have reported various external incisions. (B–E) In this patient, I simply expanded the undersurface of the breast with my fingertip and used a fairly large implant. The long-term photographs show that the snoopy deformity had smoothed and the breast was now conical. (A) A second maneuver that should be employed in cases with more deformity. Careful examination of these patients reveals a deficiency in soft tissue below the areolar edge. Approaching through a periareolar incision allows you to turn down a flap of soft tissue. This maneuver not only reduces the excess subareolar mass, but reinforces the breast from below. Importantly, there is no external incision. The flap shown has been useful in other situations as well, such as in patients with scar breakdown due to infection or trauma. The "unfurling technique" that Charles Puckett described a few years later is essentially the same operation, although the flap is made somewhat longer. There is no external scar except the periareolar incision, the lower portion is reinforced, and a conical breast results.

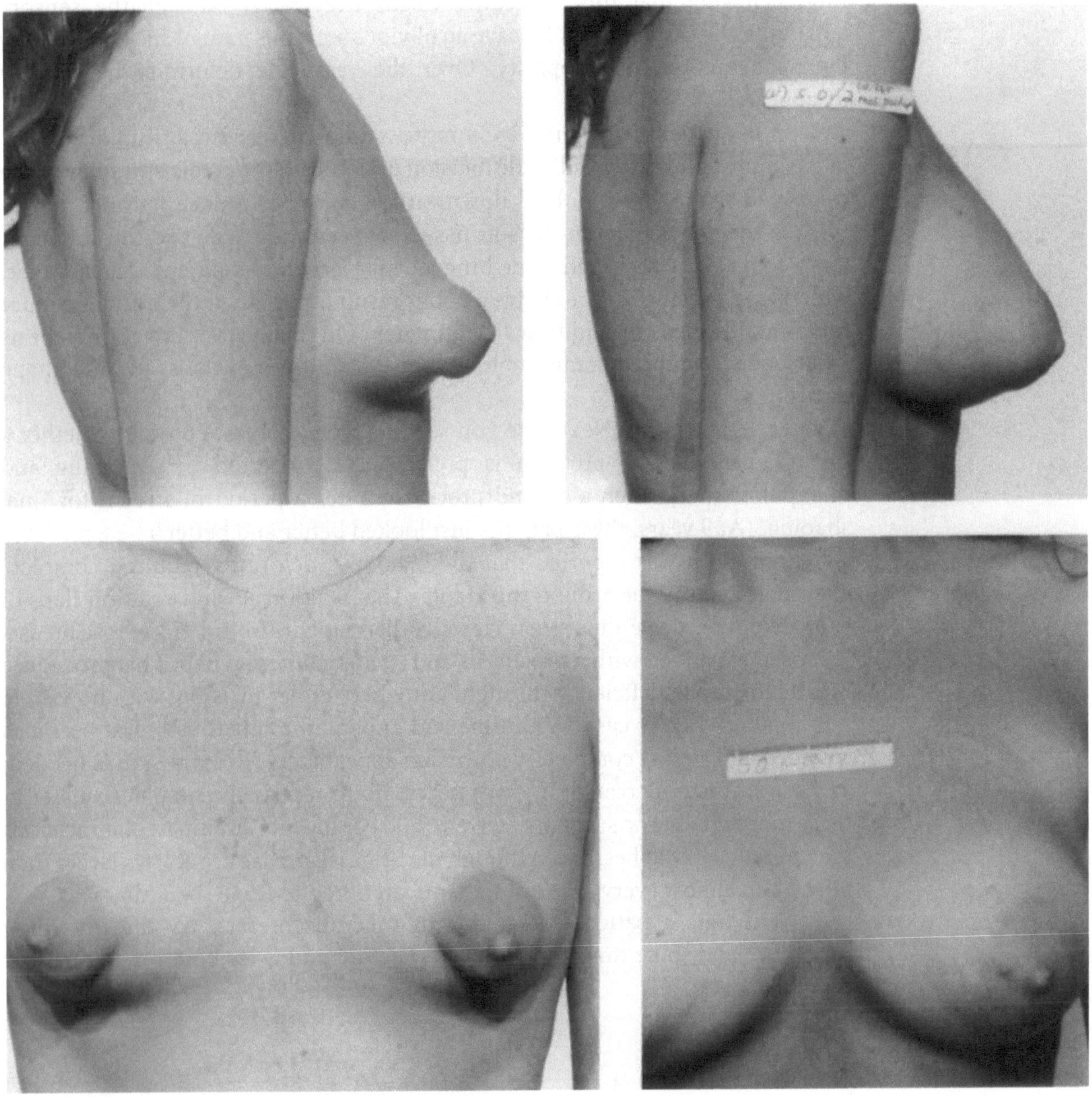

B C

D E

ting. Believing that this procedure might irreversibly damage the sensory apparatus and certainly would leave an obvious scar, this patient was treated only by augmentation mammoplasty. Over the years the deformity has largely disappeared.

In the patient in Figure 12-2 a more natural areolar expansion developed later simply because we had made incision underneath the areola and some of the thickened tissue was unfolded downward as a flap to reduce its bulk and to thicken the deficiencies in the soft tissue between the areola and the submammary fold. With time and stretching, it may become apparent that a larger, wide-based prosthesis would give a better result especially if the inframammary fold was lowered an additional centimeter. Originally this larger prosthesis would not have fitted comfortably within the confines of the space and shape available.

Technical point: Next time you see this type of breast consider whether a direct attack on the problem is preferable to a period of stretching and manipulation and then a second procedure after a period of stretch for final shaping. (At 9 years, these patients just looked better and better.)

In 1988 it was reported that the "Snoopy" deformity required complete excision of soft tissue around the areola. That is not true, and rotation flaps of skin are not needed either. We reviewed other patients from 1971 whose breasts had been expanded with a prosthesis and a simple internal flap. This procedure repairs the tissue deficiency through a tiny periareolar incision, with no visible scar in almost every case. With time and gravity, the tuberous breast becomes rounded and almost completely normal in appearance. No extra skin is needed, and a T scar is not created. It is not necessary to reduce the nipple diameter in these individuals. The scar is a deterrent, and completely circumareolar incisions are unpredictable at best. Even though the original areolae are always larger than normal, in almost every case our patients preferred to leave them that way.

Next time a patient presents with tuberous breasts, try the unfolding procedure and some time and patience. The method is far better than one that produces a scar.

Uneven Periareolar Incision

Almost any scar can be camouflaged by avoiding straight-line incisions. The periareolar margin, on close examination, is not a straight line but, rather, diffuse and serpiginous. A straight line scar draws attention to an otherwise highly concealable scar. Therefore it is sensible to make an irregular incision when performing breast surgery using this approach (e.g., augmentation mammoplasty, breast biopsy, reduction mammoplasty, mastopexy, nipple–areolar reconstruction).

When elevating the areola during an augmentation procedure, it is helpful to excise a deepithelialized ellipse superiorly around the areola. The distance

(Text continued on page 308)

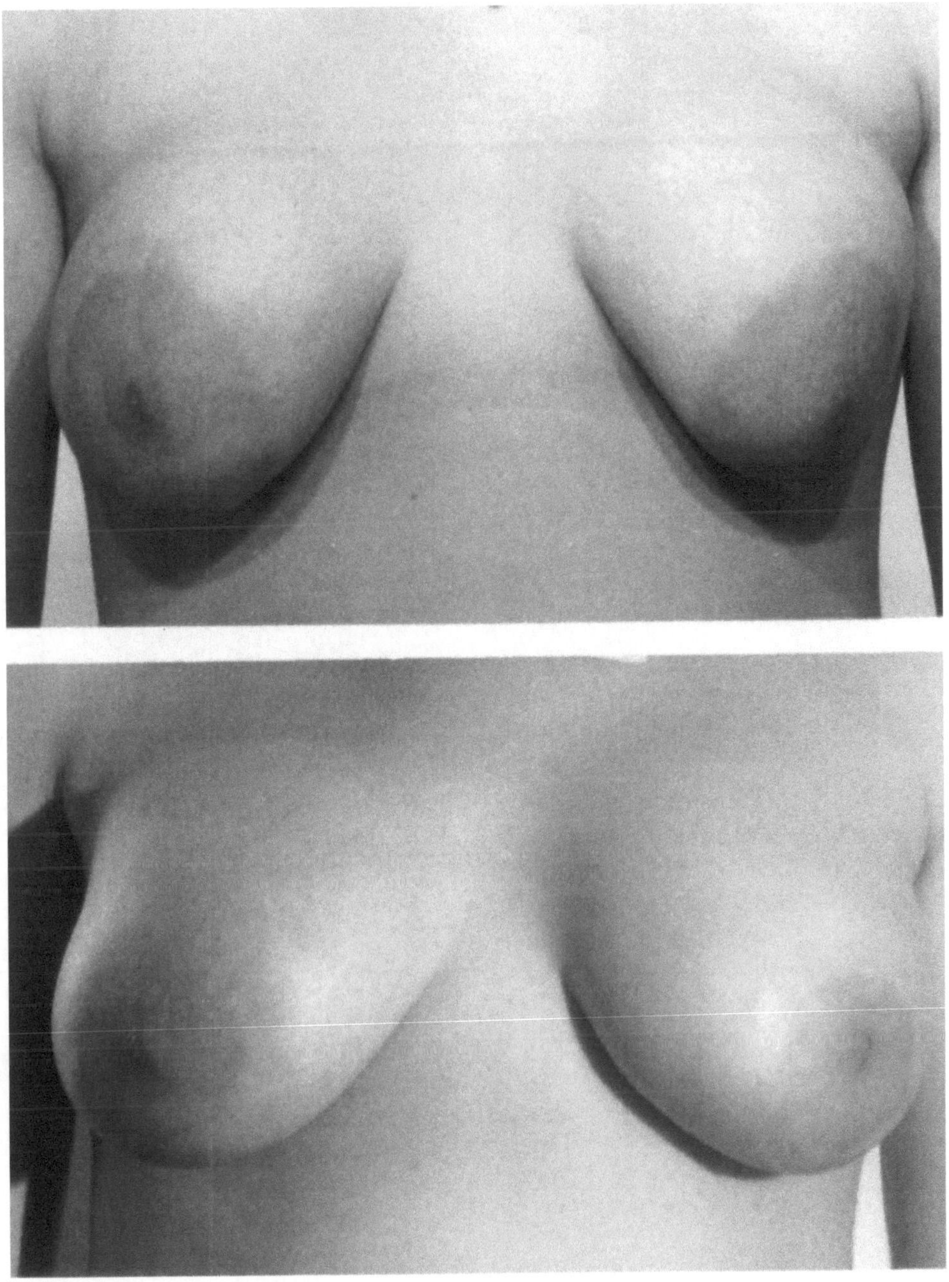

Figure 12-2. This patient had a "Snoopy" deformity with a small, extremely narrow-based projection from the chest wall that was almost entirely areola. **(A)** Her appearance 2 years after correction with an unfortunate side effect of contractures on both sides. These patients are good candidates for circumareolar mastopexy with a secondary reinforcing rotation flap. Full expansion and lowering of the inframammary fold play a role. **(B)** At 3 years postoperatively the areola scar has not spread thanks to the double Benelli suture. The breasts are soft, and there has been no further descent during these 18 months.

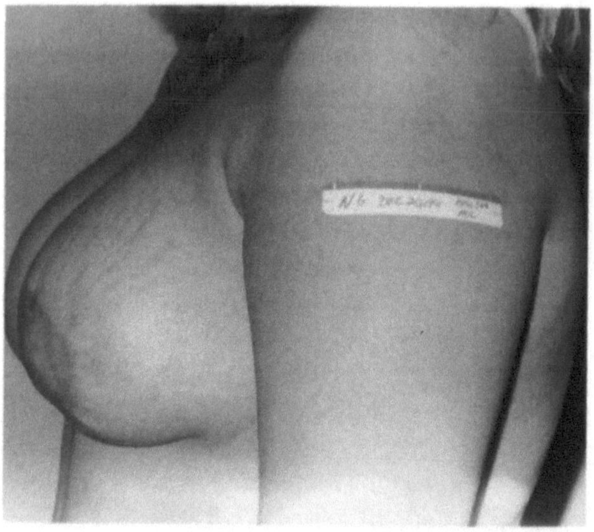

A

B

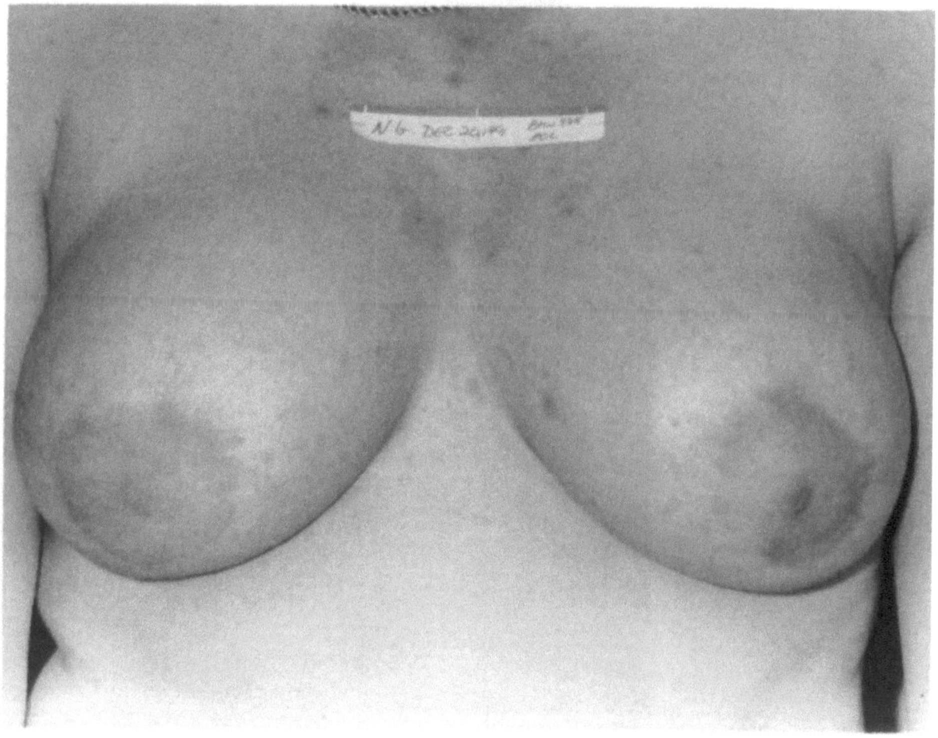

Figure 12-3. "Snoopy" deformity with circumareolar reduction. In such cases **(A–E)** when the areola is giant-sized to begin with, the circumareolar technique is used either as a primary or a secondary procedure. For these unstable breasts, secondary stretching of the areola and descent are not unusual, and one should be prepared for a revision within the first 18 months. **(D&E)** This revision should include overcorrection of the lower half of the breasts because stretch is unavoidable in this area.

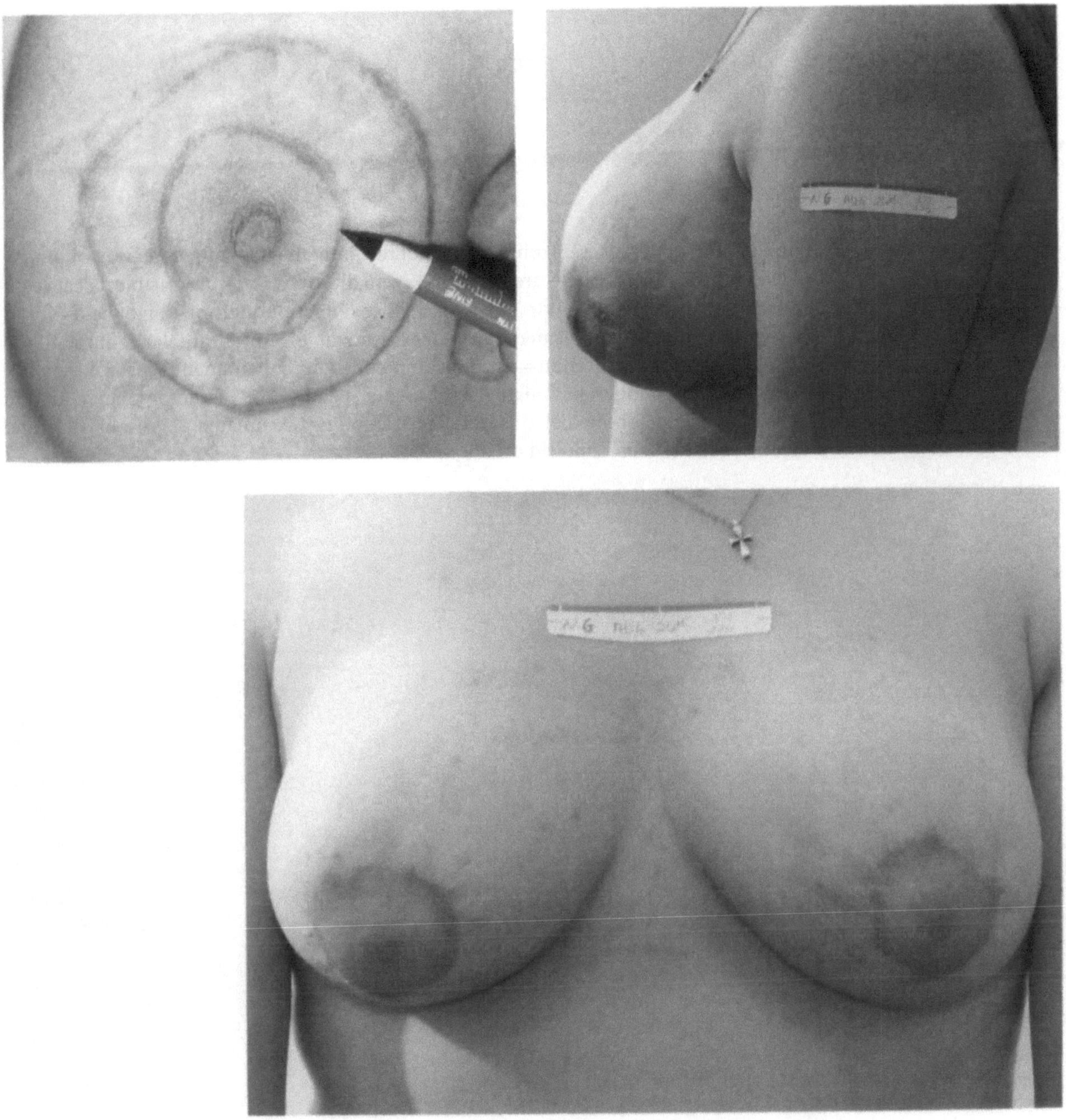

C D E

For this type of circumareolar reduction with retention of the same breast prosthesis, the left-to-right overfolding maneuver is done after the inferior flap of skin and subcutaneous tissue has been reflected. The double Benelli advancement sutures bring the surrounding skin to the base of the areola as described. Internally, the soft tissues have been repositioned at a higher spot, and a left-to-right overfolding has reinforced the breasts between the areola and the inframammary fold.

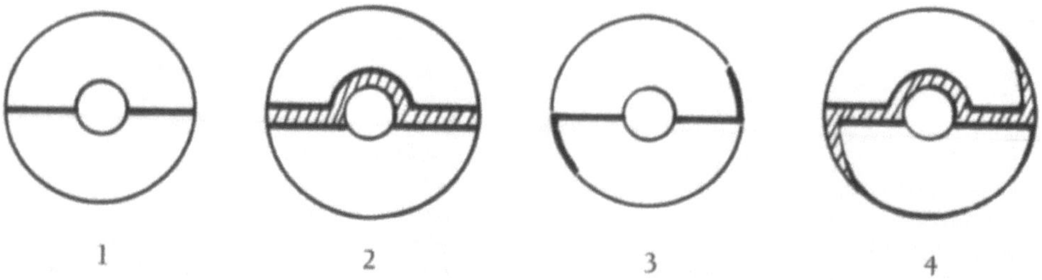

Figure 12-4. (1) Transareolar incision—not recommended for augmentation or biopsy because bacteria-filled ducts are cut, and even the best scars are visible because of contrast with areolar skin color. (2) Transareolar reduction incision—may be useful in cases where a biopsy is indicated or a request is made for minor areolar reduction. (3) Extended transareolar incision—once recommended for subcutaneous mastectomy but associated with a moderately high risk of areolar necrosis. (4) Transareolar reduction extension—useful for medial or lateral repositioning. A greater degree of skin and subcutaneous tissue is removed on one side as needed.

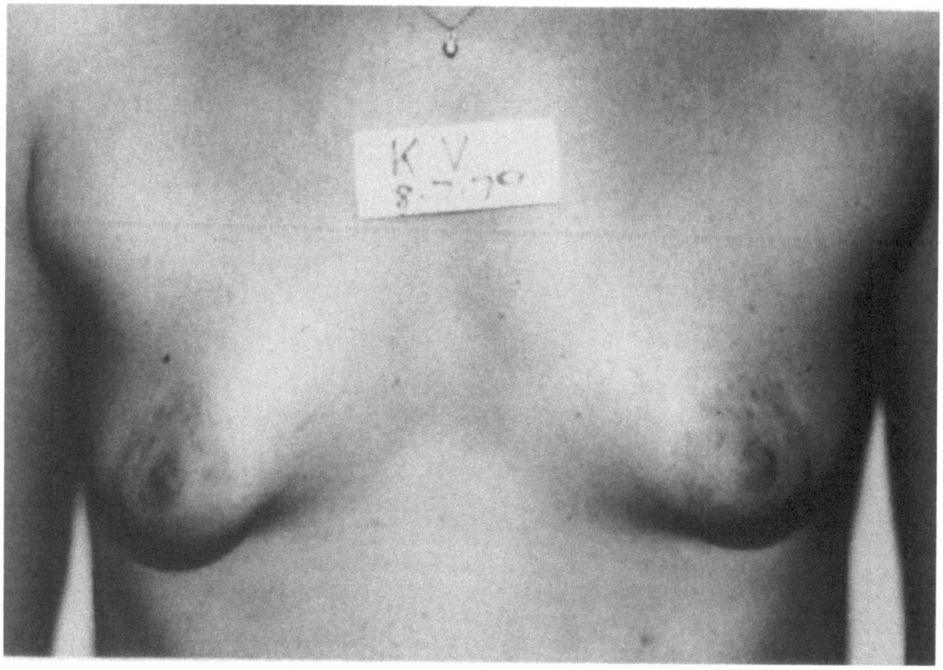

Figure 12-5. (A–D) Even in 1979 we were aware of the value of internal stretching maneuvers and lowering of the inframammary fold. Stretching is done with the fingertips or a temporary expander if you prefer. Sharp dissection must be limited in order to protect the innervation. Lowering the fold in these type C breasts is important, even if small arteries just below the pectoralis major origin are troublesome. The periareolar incision allows full visualization.

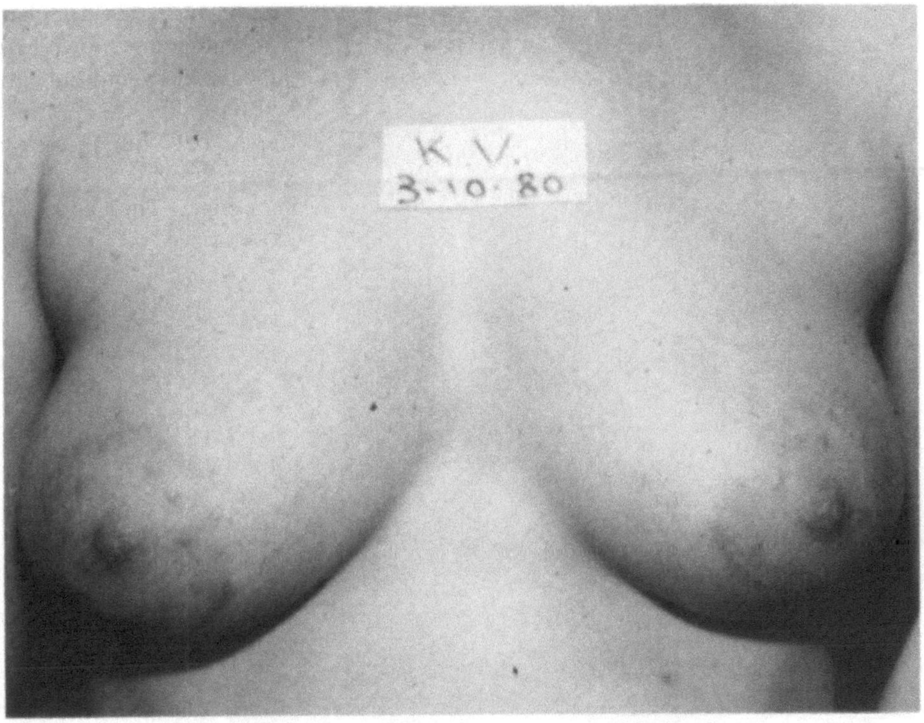

B

C

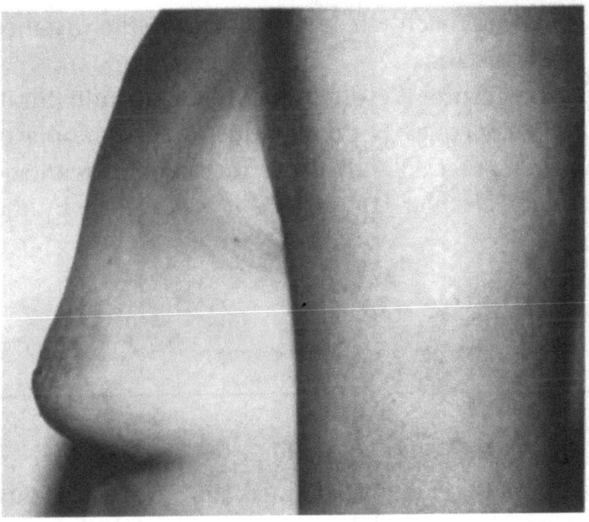

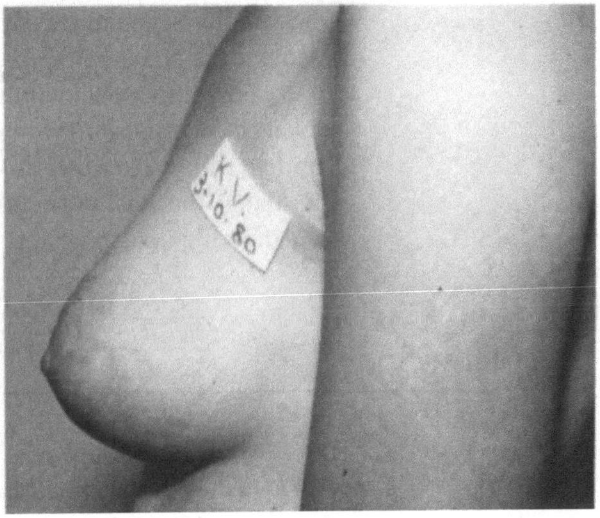

D

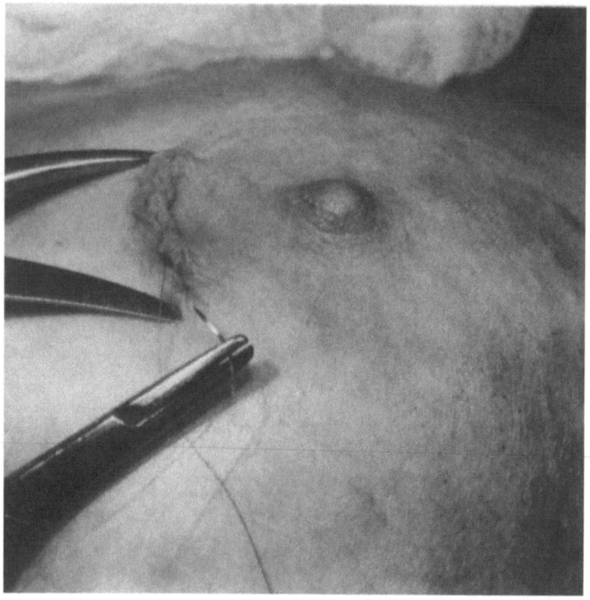

Figure 12-6. Periareolar incision for augmentation. The techniques shown here for skin eversion and deep subcutaneous and subcuticular suturing to diminish scar visibility are applicable to many aesthetic procedures. The skin is back-cut, so the inverted Dexon sutures provide a "shelf" of firm support while everting skin edges. The end of the 5-0 subcuticular suture is exteriorized.

along the straight upper margin of this excised area is much longer than the periareolar segment. A curvilinear approach effectively elongates the distance around the areola to equalize these distances.

For reduction mammoplasty, results are often marred by an unnatural, even circular incision with sharp, clear edges. For both reduction mammoplasty and mastopexy, try the same uneven periareolar incision. Yet another advantage is that if there is any tendency for circular contracture it is lessened by the meandering incisional approach.

Thin Spots

With the changeover from the supersoft, stretchy prosthesis envelope of 1971–1979 to the thick-walled variety widely used since 1982, we are seeing patients with minimal contractures who can feel the edges or folds of the implant through the skin. It is less of a problem with the smooth-surfaced implant than it is with the textured or saline implant.

In one case I reopened the capsule to do some minor releases and found that only one thin spot required an internal capsular turnover flap. Other patients may have normal breast thickness, and for them the problem is contractures. These "thin spots" are not the same ones we saw during the early 1970s, when it was fashionable to place Kenalog inside a double-lumen implant. They were *real* thin spots. Internal reinforcement by turned-down flaps of pectoralis major,

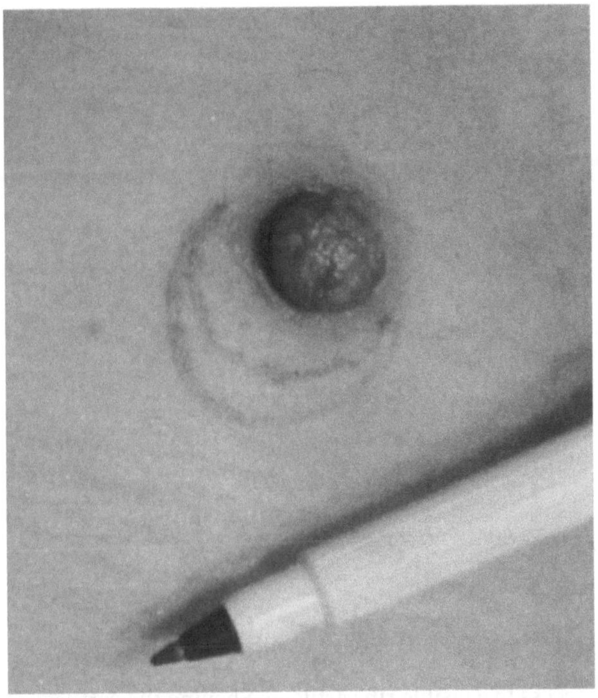

A

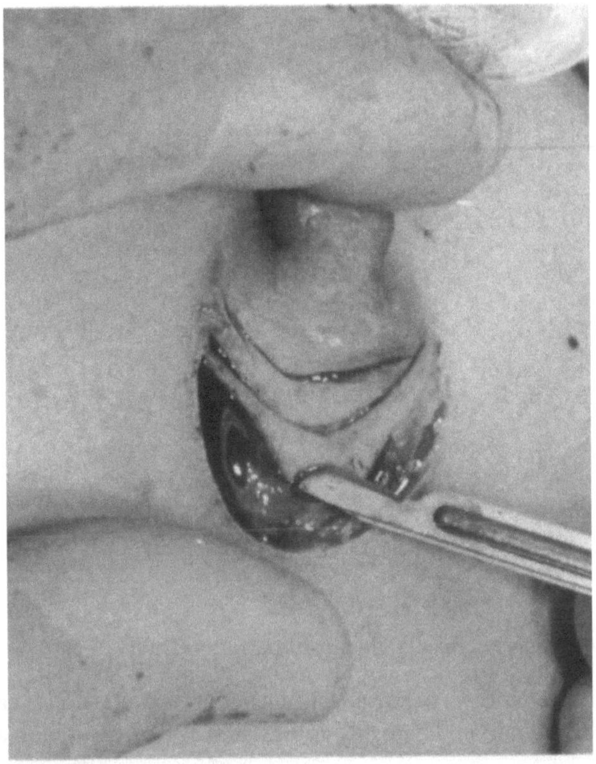

B

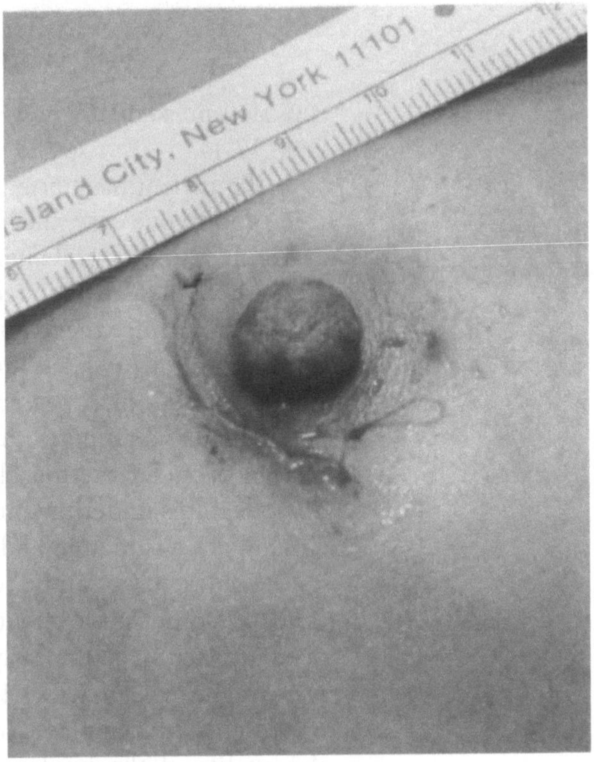

C

Figure 12-7. How often have you calmly discussed breast augmentation with a patient and then looked at an areola the size of a dime? Reluctant as many of us are to use an axillary approach or to place a scar on the unmarred skin in the inframammary fold, one still may proceed with a periareolar approach using the following technical points to protect the delicate, soon to be traumatized edge of the areola. (**A**) Draw a double line beyond the areolar–cutaneous junction. The longer lower line marks the incision into the subcutaneous tissue and is adequate with stretching for breast augmentation. (**B**) Note the mark at the edge of the areola that will eventually be the closure line (**C**). Deepithelialize the central zone. The microareolar skin is advanced over that deepithelialized zone and anchored to the edge of the deepithelialized area to expand the size of the areola to attain symmetry between the superior portion and the inferior portion. Leave the bottom ellipse attached: It acts as a buffer against the retractors. When the implant is safely in place, remove the bottom ellipse, advance the areolar skin over the deepithelialized middle ellipse, and proceed with a subcuticular closure. Exteriorize the last knot. An additional point: by moving farther away from the areola, there is less likelihood of interrupting the nerve supply to these tiny nipples.

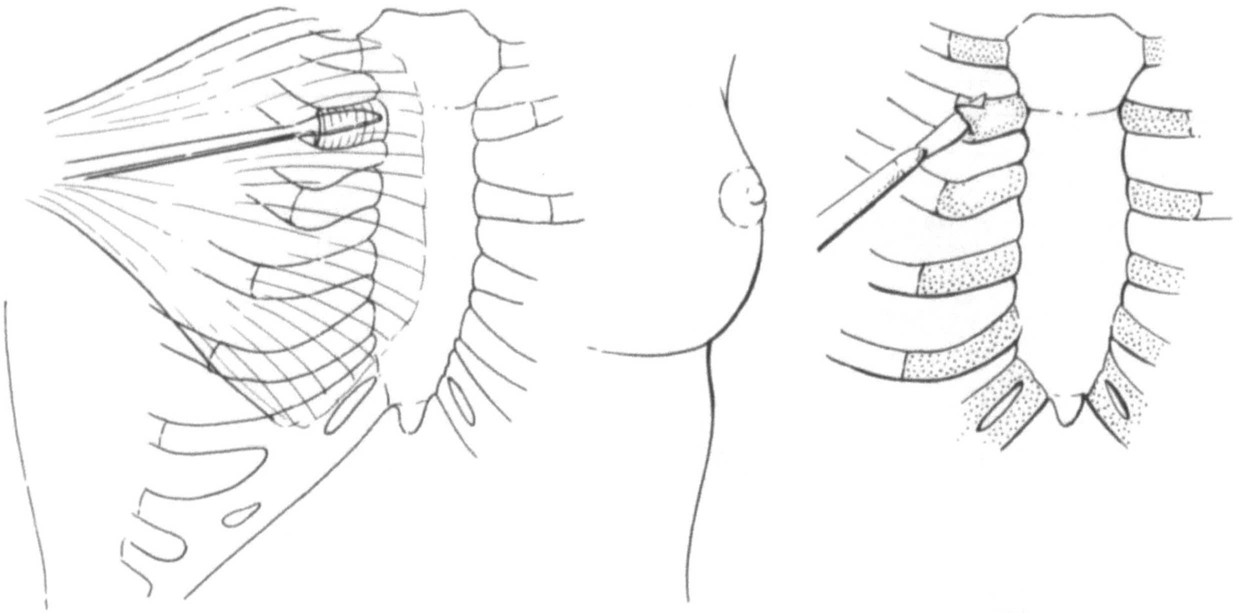

A) Push Pectoralis off rib subperichondrially

B) Shave cartilage until flat

Figure 12-8. An advantage of a periareolar incision is easy access to a visible rib cartilage. Shaving the cartilage is not difficult and is highly appreciated. Offer this option at no charge to the women who have this problem.

capsule, and so on are now a lost but not regretted art. We rarely see it anymore (Fig. 12-1).

If a patient has normal thickness and a minor contracture, it is not a true thin spot. In one case, the breast did not "relax" until the patient had finished a 3-month course of oral vitamin E. With minimal pressure we were then able to stretch out the capsule *and the tissue above* the capsule, and the "thin spots" disappeared. Once the textured implant was restored to its original position, the folds in the thick-walled implant (which the patient had been able to feel with light palpation) disappeared.

This case supports the argument for placing implants under the breast instead of under the muscle. If a minor contracture occurs, it may not be as obvious if it is under the muscle, whereas subglandular implant patients would certainly be aware of it, and have it released earlier.

Contractures can be released easily in 95% of cases. There is a new rule, though: Do not perform closed releases on old implants. An implant that has been in place since the early 1970s has probably worn thin and is fragile (they were fragile to begin with). I have no hesitation about performing a closed release on patients with implants inserted between 1984 and the present time because the quality of the implant is known. Contractures occur infrequently now, although mechanical, fibrocystic, hormonal, and traumatic problems remain.

Closed Capsulotomy

Is closed capsulotomy dangerous? The FDA thought so initially, but they withdrew their prohibition when faced with the overwhelming evidence that it is a useful procedure that avoids surgery. Of course, there is a right way and a wrong way to do it, and there are reasons not to perform a closed capsulotomy at all. An important reason for not doing it is if the implant was manufactured before 1984. Those implants are thin, and some contain small amounts of liquid silicone. A closed capsulotomy can cause a major problem with tissue reaction. Even if there is no liquid silicone, we know that the gel eventually breaks down and creates the type of foreign body reaction called siliconoma.

For most closed capsulotomies I use the locked finger technique. It is important to continue this procedure until certain that the entire capsule is free; if it is not, the capsule will simply readhere. Work the complete area—across the bottom and across the top—until you are satisfied. If it takes a great deal of pressure, stop the procedure (that much pressure could break the implant, could create scar tissue and bleeding, and does not produce a good result). Moderate pressure is the key. Then prescribe vitamin E (whether you believe in it or not. Many patients in our practice are believers, and if they stop taking vitamin E their breasts become stiff). Start with high doses, perhaps 3000 units/day, and gradually decrease the dose over 6 weeks. Be sure the patient performs hand massaging and hand squeezes twice a day every day. Examine the patient again at 10 to 12 days and at least once or twice a month thereafter until the situation has been stable for several months.

Patients' exercises are as follows. They are instructed to put one thumb on the sternum and one at the rib cage and close that hand forcibly around the base of the breast; do the same thing at the top; then do it with two hands together. These exercises elevate the central areolar zone and keep the capsule from reattaching. Within a few weeks the new capsule has formed in the gaps. We found that patients only rarely require a second closed capsulotomy if this exercise regimen is followed. Others, particularly those with recurring fibrocystic disease, must have capsulotomies every 2 to 3 years; they are not surgical capsulotomies but they accomplish the same thing.

Implants today are practically impossible to rupture with closed capsulotomy. One can therefore summarily reject the conclusion that "closed capsulotomy several years after implantation should be performed with a maximum of care and a minimum of pressure," as stated by Dutch colleagues.

Our breast clinic follows patients rather intensively, and our series is large enough to draw certain conclusions. Prior to 1980, gel implants were uniformly thin-walled, and the gel was not "cohesive." Many American surgeons reported siliconomas that derived from intact prostheses and broken prostheses discovered by routine xerograms or at the time of replacement to vary the size or shape. One would certainly use caution during closed capsulotomy in the presence of a pre-1984 gel prosthesis.

To say that one should not use pressure to completely release the capsule is ridiculous. A timidly closed capsulotomy invariably and inexorably recurs. Experienced plastic surgeons know that pressure is needed to "crack" the capsule in four directions and to completely release the final pockets of resistance in both the capsule and the banding within the breast tissue, a variant of the classic Cooper's ligament.

Technical point: If a patient has a minimal contracture or even a fairly extensive one, do not hesitate to use the pressure necessary to obtain a full release.

Technical point: Intensive, close follow-up and recompression are a must. The capsular releases sometimes tend to stick again, so use five or six consecutive minimal compressions. In at least 99% of our cases, there is a point at which the breast remains soft and the contracture does not recur.

Mammography

To date there have been more than one million breast augmentation patients. Long-term surveys show that the incidence of breast cancer in these women is the same or less than that for the general population. We believe that if there is a lower incidence it reflects the fact that most of the women are small-breasted, although it may be only a statistical variation.

It has been stated by a California group that death rates were increased in breast implant patients because of their augmentation, but it has not been proved. In fact, an opposite conclusion was drawn from a larger survey in California showing that death rates have not changed since the introduction of silicone. Undeterred, the press was told by the same Californians that "augmentation patients have given up access to state-of-the-art breast examination." This statement is far from the truth. They certainly have not given up their right to self-examination or to adequate xeroradiographic assessment. Garry Brody gave a semiofficial rebuttal, first pointing out the small number of patients in the "study" on which the press statement was based, the false generalizations, and the release of inflammatory and incorrect conclusions to the press before subjecting those conclusions to analysis by those with knowledge of the field. He then discussed the study in Los Angeles County that showed breast cancer rates among patients who had undergone breast augmentation. Unfortunately, the argument was not put to rest as conclusively as it should have been.

The main reason for delayed detection and advanced cancer is ignorance—ignorance on the part of the physician and the patient. Self-examination by women with breast prostheses can be done thoroughly using the "hand under the prosthesis" technique. Studies tell us that routine screening mammograms should not be ordered on a more frequent basis for breast augmentation patients

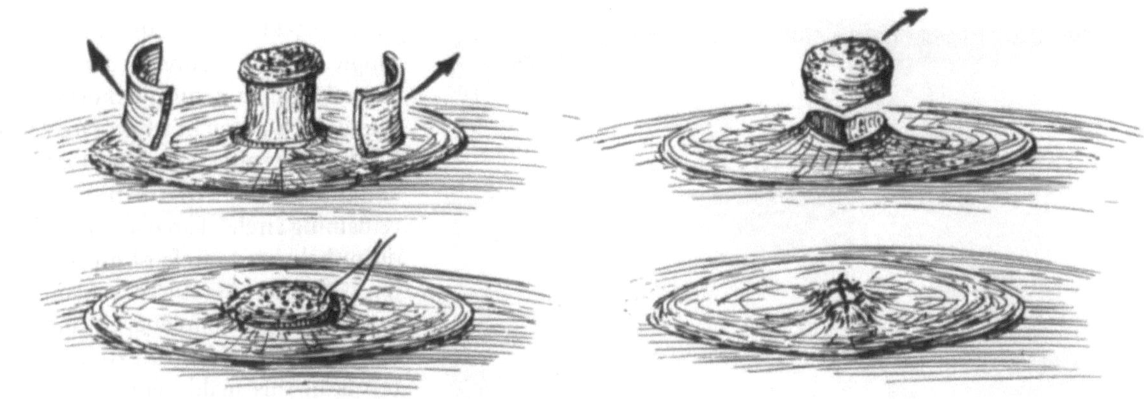

Figure 12-9. In the past we were rarely called on to *reduce* a prominent nipple; much more often we were asked to increase the projection. Today we advise the method illustrated here for young pre-child-bearing patients. In essence, the dermis and epidermis are removed laterally so the stalk can be invaginated. Minimal undermining and mattress sutures are required. The ductal system is entirely preserved. For the older patient we prefer the simpler technique of mid-ductal wedge excision and closure.

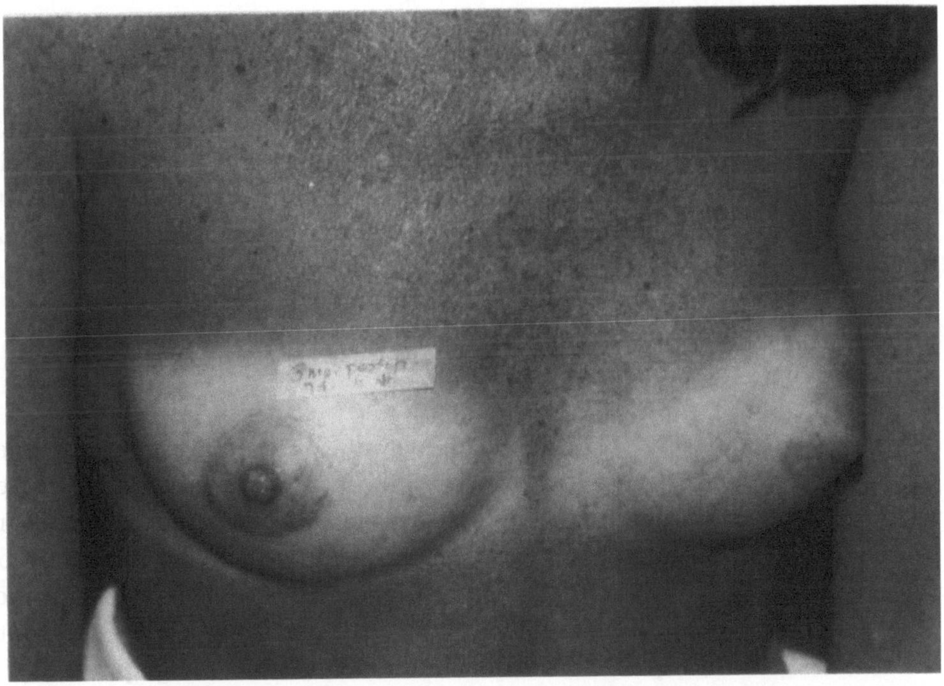

Figure 12-10. Deflations do occur, perhaps less so with textured saline implants. This woman, 3 months after textured saline augmentation, awoke one morning to find that her right breast felt "like a bag of water." Even though she waited longer than I would prefer, replacement was completed before there was any change in the capsule.

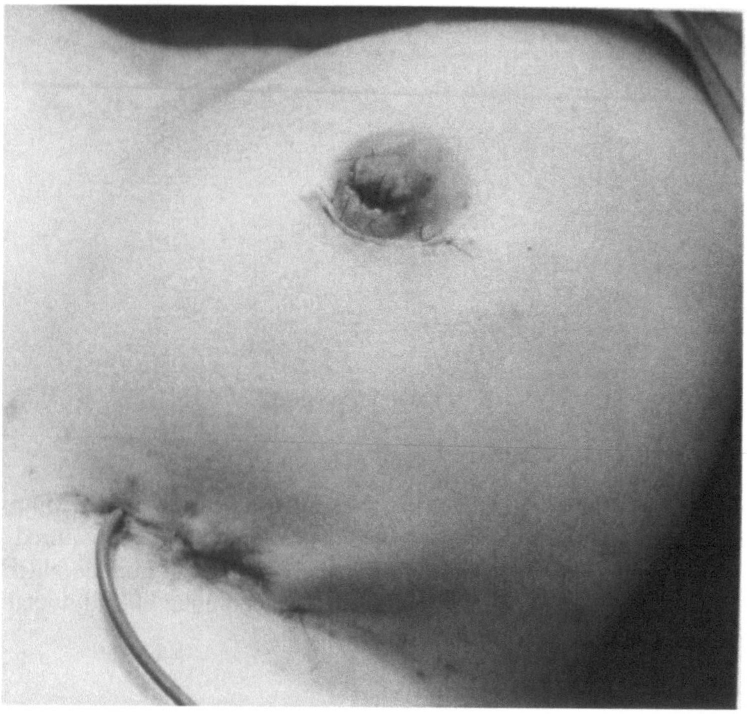

Figure 12-11. When the entire areola is nipple, create a mound by converting the central skin to a full-thickness flap. In this case, a segment of periareolar skin has been deepithelialized to form a base and turned under. We then stretched the remaining circle of areola outward over a deepithelialized circle of greater diameter. A "modern" textured implant is used to replace older implants because of the frequent occurrence of extracapsular fibrosis in this maldeveloped group. Because an inframammary incision was present, we used it to tack the deep subcutaneous tissue to pectoral fascia. This maneuver tucks the scar out of sight under the new breast curve. Note the subcuticular Dexon suture closure with exteriorization of the distal knot. Do not try to bury the distal knot—they emerge too often. Also note the catheter for instillation of Solu-Medrol, Keflin, and Marcaine.

than for other women unless there is a positive family history or changing nodularity. In the report released to the press the lesions had appeared 6 months to 15 years after breast augmentation. Few of these patients had had routine screening roentgenograms during the interval, and apparently none had been taught self-examination.

Value of Mammography

The debate on the value of mammography continues. Surgeons have been accused of overusing the procedure in order to increase their incomes by performing unnecessary biopsies based on questionable mammography results. Plastic surgeons might be lumped in the same category. Others have been chastised for their resistance to this valuable screening procedure. The American Cancer Society has "no ax to grind" in regard to this controversy, and summary of their evaluation of the status of mammography today. We use it as a basis for recommendations in plastic surgery.

Obviously, young women do not require mammography; on the other hand, there is no disagreement that patients with a positive family history of malignancy should undergo mammography on a regular basis. What about the older patient who is scheduled for reduction mammoplasty? Perhaps she falls into the same category as a breast reconstruction candidate, for whom we would not hesitate to order a xerogram.

It was estimated that 130,000 new cases per year of invasive breast cancer would be diagnosed in the United States, and more than 5000 cases of in situ cancer. At least 30% of women with invasive cancer ultimately die of their disease. To date, no one has any idea how to prevent breast cancer. There are ongoing trials with low dietary fat, and several chemopreventive agents seem to work in animal models. The only factor that definitely reduces mortality is early intervention. Investigators in one study concluded that a screening program substantially reduced breast cancer mortality among women age 50 and older, and it suggested that young women may have benefited as well. Mortality was reduced about 50% at 5 years and 33% at 10 years. X-rays were not the sole method of detection; more cancers in this survey were discovered by physical examination than by radiography. Yet in the 50- to 59-year-old group (those at greatest risk) 42% of the cancers were detected by mammography alone.

Two major institutions have totally different ideas on who should have radiography. The National Cancer Institute would restrict x-ray screening among young women to those at high risk, that is, with a personal or family history of breast cancer. The American College of Surgeons, on the other hand, recommends a baseline roentgenogram for all asymptomatic women aged 35 to 40. They also recommend screenings every 1 to 2 years for asymptomatic women age 40 to 49, and the American College of Radiology supports this view.

Most physicians agree that mammography is useful, but few had recommended it to asymptomatic patients. We worried about the risks of radiation, the incidence of unnecessary biopsies from overdiagnosis, and of course the cost to the patient. The costs have been reduced, and radiation levels have declined dramatically. In an early study the average skin dosage for a mammogram was 7.7 rad; currently for mammograms it is 1.2 rad. The American College of Surgeons has concluded that the radiation risk is negligible. Other large-scale studies have shown that screening for breast cancer did not result in overdiagnosis—merely in earlier detection of cancers that would ultimately have surfaced on their own. Some argue (and I disagree) that biopsy specimens showing "minimal cancer" are cancers histologically only and do not qualify on the basis of their biologic behavior. This judgment does not make sense. If a lesion is malignant, it is going to remain malignant.

What then constitutes good practice for plastic surgeons? For the older patient scheduled for breast surgery who has not had mammography since age 40, it is wise to do a screening test. If cosmetic augmentation is being planned it is helpful to identify a suspicious area so it can be removed before the augmentation. The x-ray may also identify cysts or fibroadenomas that can be easily disposed of to avoid potential problems later. For older cosmetic surgery and reduction mammoplasty patients, this procedure is a must, particularly for the reduction candidates. Physical examination reveals little about large breasts, particularly those with severe fibrocystic changes. Hence it is to the patient's

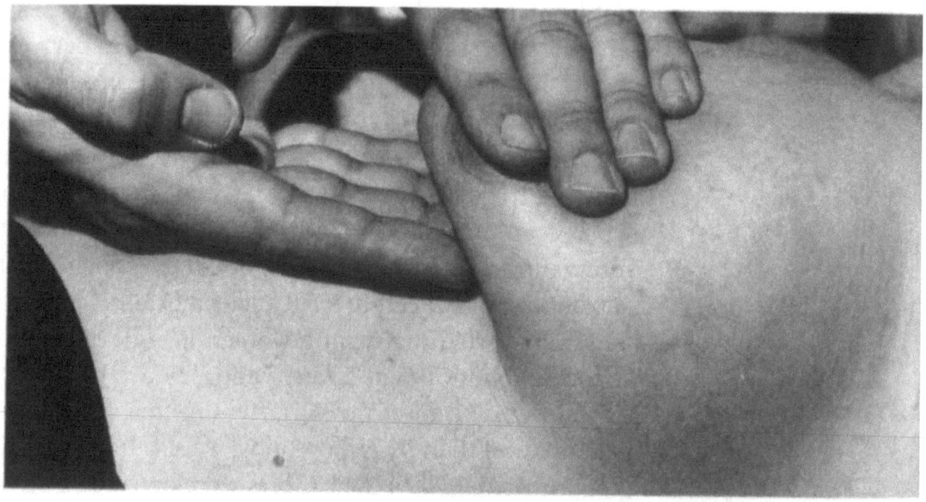

A

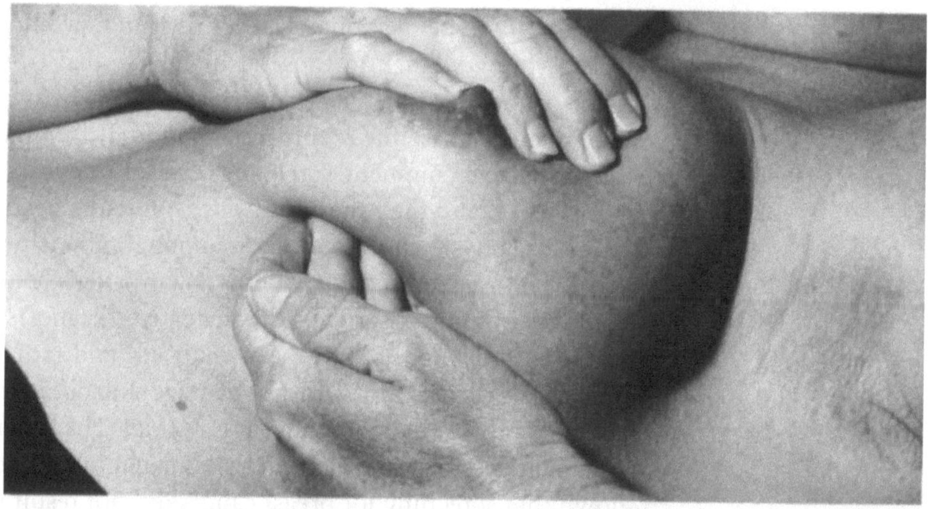

B

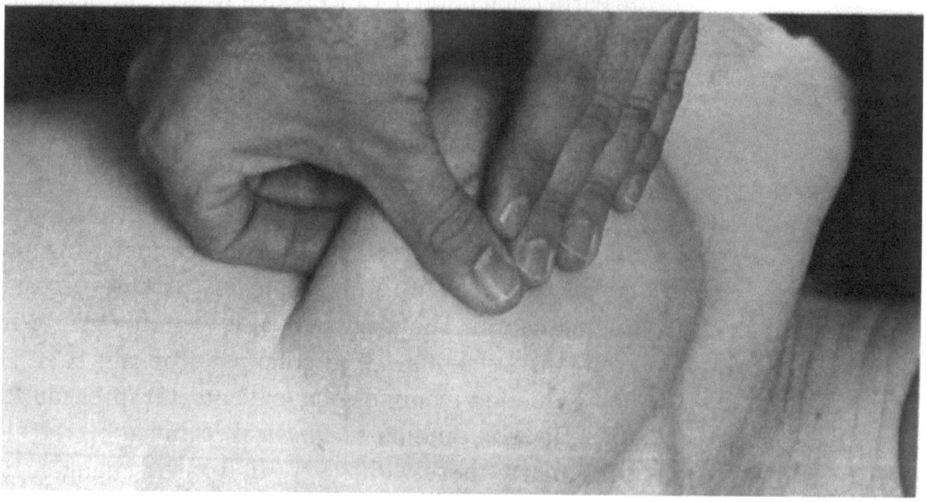

C

D
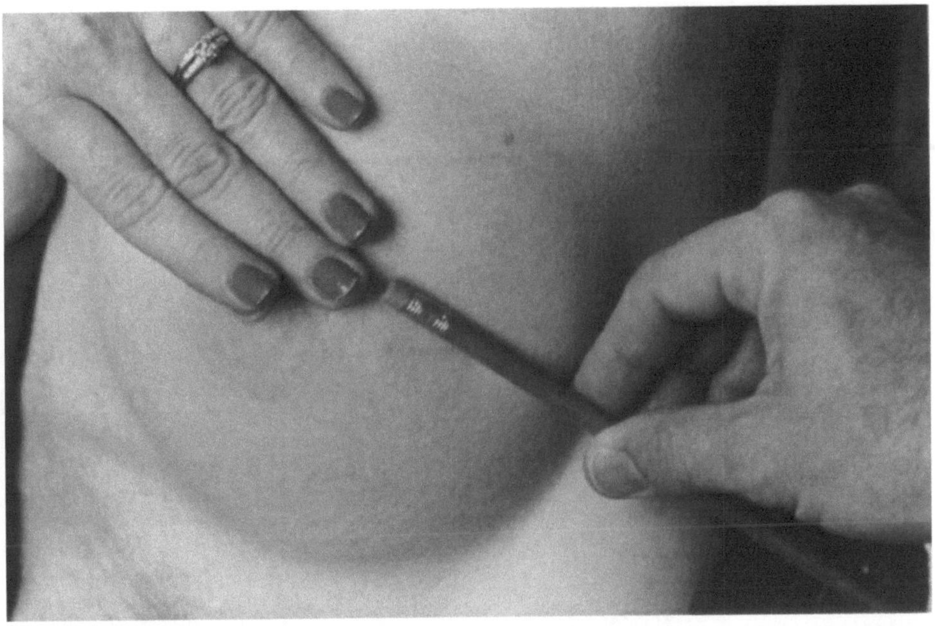

Figure 12-12. Teaching the breast augmentation patient to do a thorough breast self-examination. With the current rise in incidence of breast cancer in the United States, emphasis on self-examination should be part of every surgeon's postoperative instructions. Having a breast prosthesis certainly does not protect the patient against malignancy, but it does not induce malignancy either. Explain to the patients that they have the same risk as everyone else and that they must do a monthly self-examination like everyone else. With the technique described below, they can do it more completely.

Before subglandular augmentation, the breast was attached to the pectoralis muscle. Self-palpation can only reveal lumps in the upper portions of the breast, unless they are more than 1 cm in diameter. Once the breast is "floating" above a prosthesis, the bimanual technique can be employed, and the patient can feel the bottom surface of breast tissue as well.

(A) First, have the patient go through the standard fingertip surface self-examination technique and then show her the two-hand technique. **(B)** Ask her to place one hand in the inframammary fold. The second hand is used to stabilize the breast above. By curling the fingers of the lower hand upward and gently stroking the undersurface, she can feel the lower surface and "trap" any lumps present between the hands. A number of patients have been able to discover small lumps or cysts arising in the undersurface of the breast or deep within the breast in this manner. **(C)** After using this maneuver around the periphery of the breast, the thumb and fingers technique may be employed, particularly if she has long fingernails. The object of the maneuver is to ascertain that the breast parenchyma is soft and uniform. Trapping tissues between the two examining fingers is an easily learned and valuable technique. Emphasize that she must repeat this maneuver on a monthly basis for the rest of her life. This instruction makes the patient aware of your concern as well as relieving her mind about the risks of hidden malignancy. Perhaps widespread use of this self-examination technique will establish a new surgical principle: Breast augmentation can reduce the overall mortality from breast malignancy. **(D)** Another good way to illustrate how malignancies feel to use a pencil-tip eraser for the standard fingertip self-examination. Feel for something this distinct.

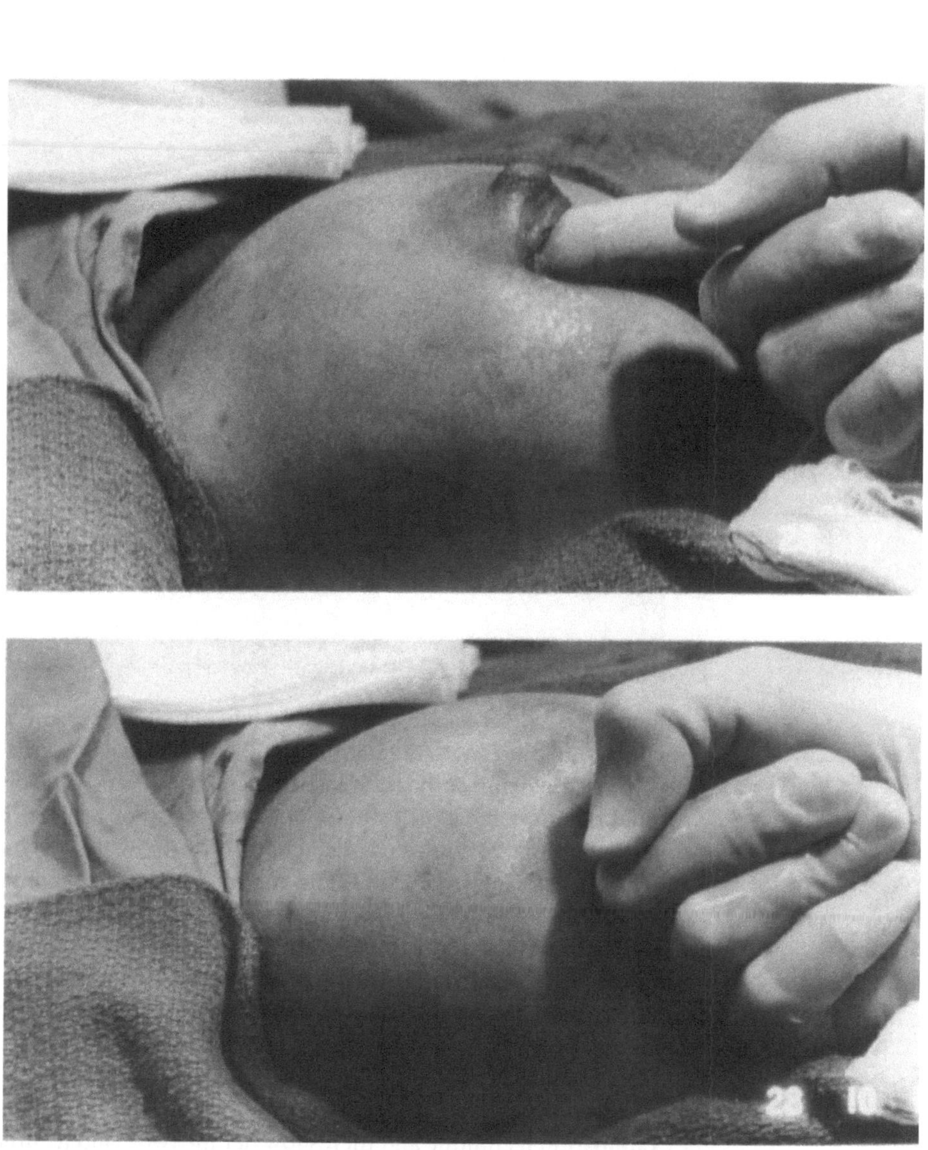

A

B

Figure 12-13. Breaking internal capsular bands. Once the prosthesis is in place, it is essential that capsular bands in the entire breast are released with manual pressure. **(A)** Note how tight the breast appears to be. Once a finger is inserted, these bands, which resisted breakage earlier, are easily "popped." We always use a retractor to pull upward and outward before inserting the implant, but this method is only partially effective owing to the elasticity of the breast. Once tension is established by the presence of the implant, it is easy to press in all directions. The release is obvious, and the breast settles easily into a more natural position. I believe this maneuver is important for preventing future capsular contracture, and is an advantage over trans-umbilical placement. **(B)**

For cosmetic breast augmentation, always break up the internal breast bands *after* the prosthesis is in place—yet another advantage of the periareolar incision. An implanted breast that is taut and round settles into a normal configuration as you press outward around all points of the compass. Those bands and fibrocystic thick spots are now less likely to cause future problems.

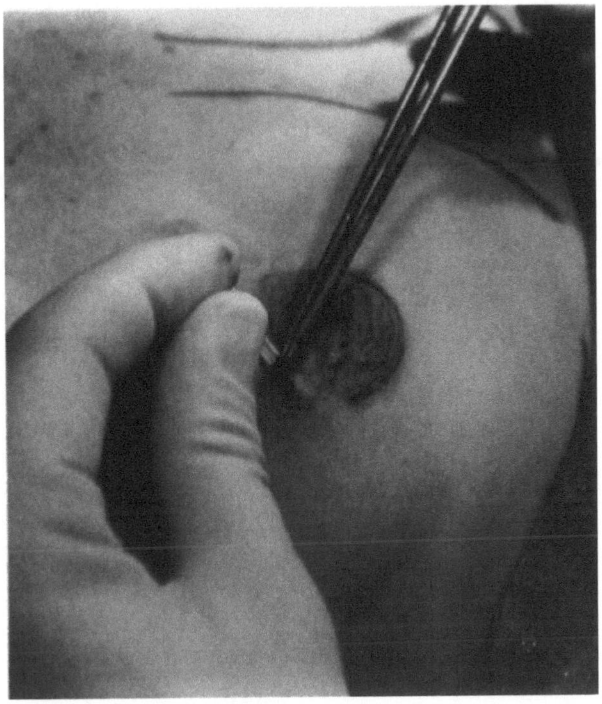
Figure 12-14. Use a 30-gauge needle and cautery to eliminate hairs around the areola.

advantage that the area be "cleared" by preliminary xerograms. Breast cancer reconstruction patients should have periodic evaluation of the opposite side if they decline subcutaneous mastectomy.

Some radiologists advise us to obtain a screening mammogram on all women over age 30, regardless of whether there is a significant degree of fibrocystic disease. Most 35-year-olds who have any degree of fibrocystic disease must have a baseline. One point worth remembering: If calcifications of the benign type are present, they mean little; but if these calcifications increase with time, there is at least a three times greater risk of developing breast cancer.

Dense breasts are difficult to examine radiographically, as is a dense breast with augmentation. The most difficult is the breast with an old calcified capsule—one of the reasons I recommend resecting the entire capsule and replacing it with a modern prosthesis.

It has been flatly stated that among all patients except those with very small breasts better visualization was obtained in those with submuscular implants. What was not said was that most of this reported series comprised old calcified subglandular implants. That situation certainly affects the ease of mammography as well as totally skewing the statistics.

This issue does not focus on subglandular versus submuscular implants. It is an issue of the competence of radiologists as new techniques evolve. Excellent evaluations can be obtained in both categories. Balanced against the known

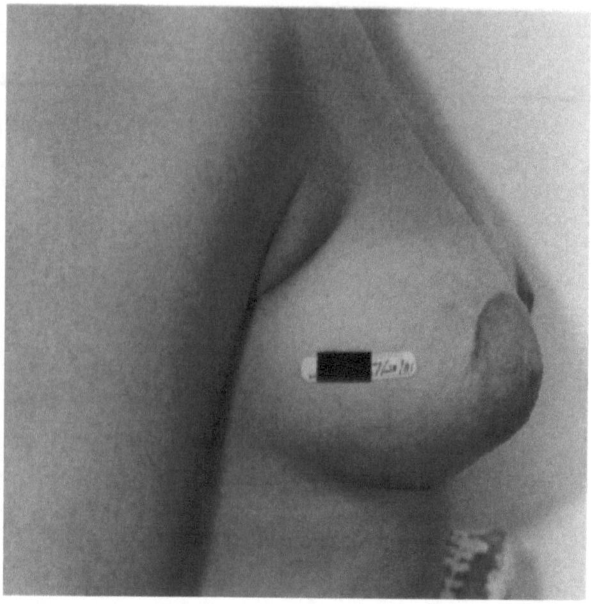

Figure 12-15. Another advantage of periareolar incisions. Lifting the areola to a central position while augmenting the breast through the *same* incision creates the illusion of mastopexy without the scars. **(A)** In this case, the inframammary fold was lowered from within, and both areolae were repositioned. **(B)** In another case the fold on the right was already low, and the distance between the fold and the areola would have been too great. Only the right areola was repositioned.

B

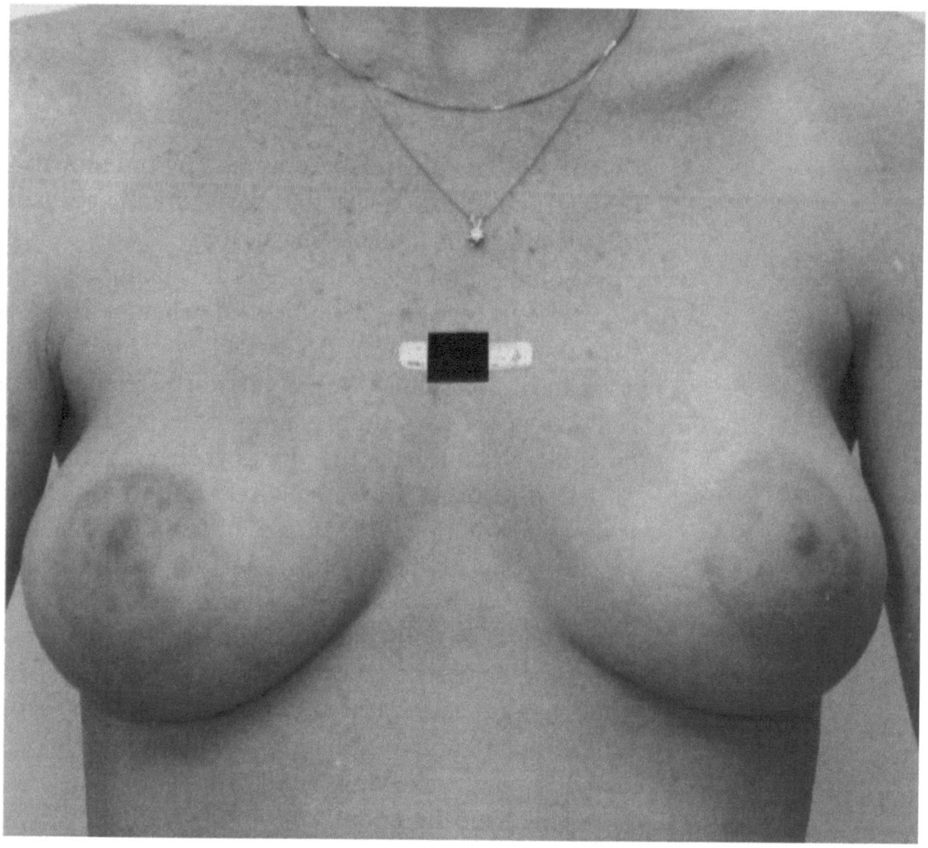

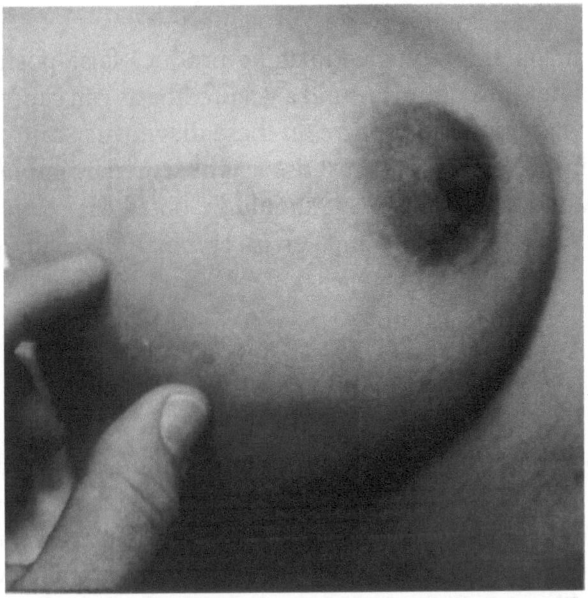

12-16

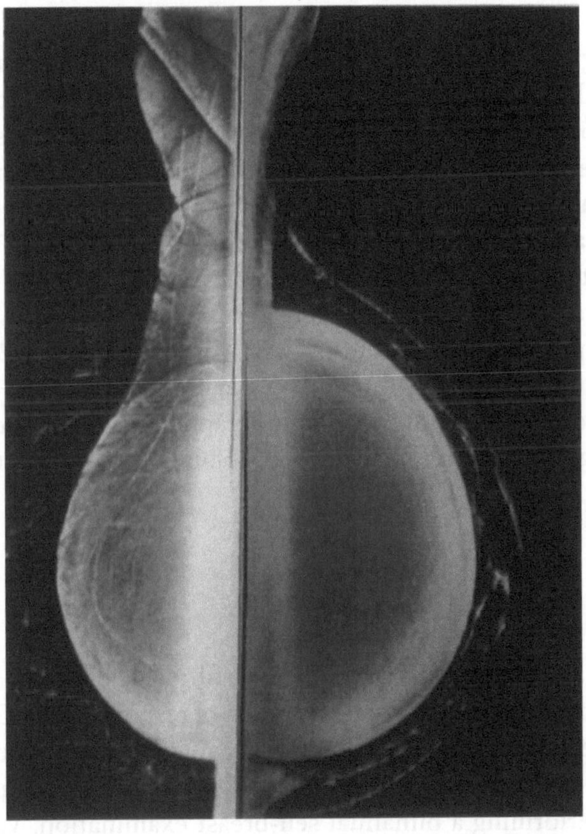

12-17

Figures 12-16, 12-17, 12-18. Mammography and silicone tissue reactions.

Figure 12-16. Unusual surface reaction of a patient with a broken prosthesis and a tissue reaction following trauma. Whereas we once advised patients with broken implants to leave well enough alone because contracture would be the only complication, we believe now it is advisable to have the prosthesis replaced before scar tissue forms. In this case, removal of the silicone foreign body reaction tissue must be followed by local rotation flaps of capsular tissue to reinforce and repair the defect.

Figure 12-17. Obvious silicone migration from a broken prosthesis. With the older implants, this situation may have occurred with minimal trauma. The radiologist completely missed this diagnosis. Fortunately, the material that was removed was of watery consistency, and there was no tissue reaction (the most worrisome aspect of traumatic implant rupture). If the material reaches the axilla and tissue reaction occurs, as it inevitably does, a major disability might result.

Figure 12-18. Typical small isolated siliconoma, characterized by a swiss cheese appearance and hard consistency on palpation. All small masses are lifted up by the prosthesis, so they are easily detectable. Even though the diagnosis is obvious, the material must be removed and examined microscopically to be certain of the diagnosis.

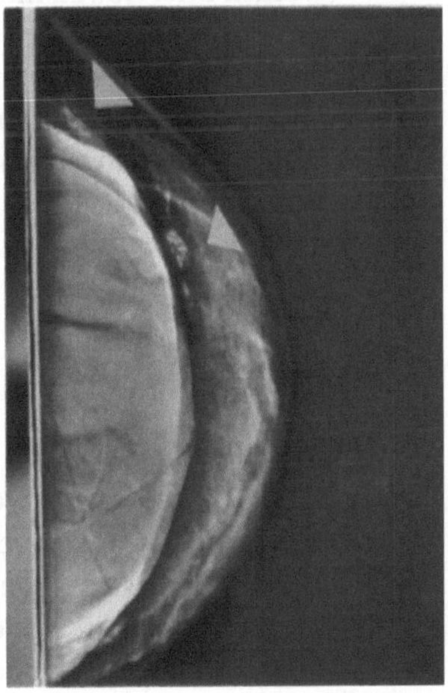

12-18

problems of submuscular augmentation (pain, movement, upward or downward displacement), it should be a moot issue.

Ultrasonography and magnetic resonance imaging produce false-positive results in some cases. Moderate contracture around a gel prosthesis can cause an unfolding of the prosthesis that mimics a rupture on these diagnostic scans.

Let us try to take a balanced view. That breast tissue is obscured by implants may be valid for certain individuals. However, it should be noted that patients with breast implants discover significantly smaller carcinomas through self-examination.

Screening Mammograms

"Diagnostic" mammography usually includes a combination of Xray and thermogram and is more expensive than the usual mammogram. Are those mammograms helpful to the overall picture? According to a 1987 study, survival of woman with minimal breast cancers detected by screening mammograms was more than 90% at 10 years. These malignancies were classified as intraductal, in situ, and "invasive less than 1 cm." The early fears of radiation-induced changes have proved groundless.

Media-based campaigns in Texas increased our participation in screening mammography dramatically, and this experience has been repeated in other states. Of the more than 64,000 women who had screening mammograms in Texas, at least 90% credited media publicity for their decision to be screened even though 60% had seen a physician during the preceding year. Perhaps the physicians were not emphatic enough about the need for screening tests. The women interviewed indicated that cost was a major factor, as was the lack of the physician's enthusiasm. The bad news is that women 50 years and older were not participating in screening programs: In a state-by-state comparison, only 30% had had a screening mammogram. Even though we plastic surgeons are not primary care physicians, we can inquire about mammography during preoperative consultations and suggest strongly that one be obtained before elective surgery.

Needle Aspiration

Small cancers can be associated with large, benign, fibrocystic lumps. If a needle biopsy is negative, that does not relieve the surgeon of responsibility. Cyst aspiration is good practice unless the cyst recurs, indicating the presence of another process. I recently had such a case. The patient discovered a 2-cm lump in the axillary tail while performing a bimanual self-breast examination. With one hand on top, she had pushed her fingers under the breast implant and had trapped the growth between her fingertips. It was not palpable from the surface.

(Three of my patients within the previous month had found tiny carcinomas during self-examination that would not have been found at this early stage had the women not had breast implants.) I discussed open biopsy with her. She brought up the question of needle aspiration, and we declined. During surgery, the large cyst was surrounded by a dense growth of fibrocystic disease. Aspiration would easily have missed the cyst and left her with a growing lesion. Fortunately, all of the tissue was benign, and we were able to reconstruct that area and slip the implant back in during an office "twilight" procedure. There was no extra scar, no long recovery, no recurring problem. General surgery colleagues often prefer needle aspiration if it gives a positive diagnosis: They can then plan reconstruction and mastectomy if needed. There are a few reports of puncturing implants with the aspiration needles.

Update on Breast Cancer and the Precancer Question

A review of breast cancer statistics is important to plastic surgeons, as we deal with the normal breast on a daily basis, and many of us are involved with "subcutaneous mastectomy. According to the late Leonard Koch, insurance companies want us to change the terminology. Koch had a case in which the company refused to pay for a "subcutaneous mastectomy" but would pay for a "total mastectomy." There is little difference between the two procedures. Leonard cored out the central ductal system but left the areolar skin intact—making it a "total mastectomy." We could have easily labeled it a "subcutaneous mastectomy" or "preventive" mastectomy.

One of every ten to fifteen American women develop breast cancer according to different sources and only one-fourth of them have a positive family history. Thus in at least 75% of patients the malignancy appears suddenly and unexpectedly. Currently, 92% of diagnosed breast malignancies have progressed beyond the in situ phase. Note that mammography is detecting a large number of in situ carcinomas—now 24% of the total breast cancers diagnosed by screening. If we are to increase that number so most carcinomas discovered in asymptomatic women are still in the in situ phase, we must order more mammograms.

Should one be done in augmentation patients before or after the operation? We suggest before *and* after. If the patient is at least 35, the film can be helpful for finding an area that may need a biopsy at the time of augmentation and can be removed if suspicious. On the other hand, the preoperative screening mammogram gives little information that can be used in the future. For that purpose, a film should be obtained after the augmentation. Therefore request a screening x-ray on any patient over age 35; if you then proceed with breast augmentation, reduction, or other procedure, obtain a second film a year later and use it as a baseline.

A radiologist has shown mammograms of normal unencapsulated breast augmentation patients and reinforced my belief that an adequate examination can be carried out by any competent radiologist. Gilbert Eklund reported an ingenious "compression film" in which he simply pulls the breast tissue away from the implant and obtains an additional view from above. Using a sort of "grabber paddle," the breast comes under the x-ray cassette while he pushes the implant back against the chest wall. He also had some ingenious focal compression devices that can be clamped around a suspected area to give a blow-up of any calcification spotted on routine films.

Fibrocystic "Disease"

We should be pleased we have so few problems, compared to those encountered by ophthalmologists and urologists, who do not have to contend with changes due to hormones, stress, local bacteria, sex play, and fibrocystic "disease." The latter is responsible for more complaints of "tight" breasts today than is true capsular contracture.

Some facts you may not know about fibrocystic "disease" are as follows. In 1977 we were fairly certain that breast cancer was at least three times more prevalent in patients with *severe* mammary dysplasia and at least seven times more prevalent in patients with the microcystic variant of fibrocystic "disease." Vincent Pennisi further reported that during the period 1968–1973 the incidence of breast cancer rose at a rate of 1000 cases per year, from a total of 28,000 per year to 32,000 per year. This figure increased the total new cases of breast cancer from 65,000 per year to the present 88,000 per year. Pennisi's statement that "early detection should mean detection in the preinvasive stage" is worth pondering. It is one of the reasons that many of us advocate subcutaneous mastectomy in patients at high risk, particularly those with cancer of the opposite breast and a strong family history for cancer. This severe form of fibrocystic "disease" occurs now in only 10% of women in the United States, but we know that practically everyone who walks into our offices has some degree of fibrocystic changes. In other words, it is not a "disease."

The lesions that are most ominous on biopsy are (1) intraductal hyperplasia; (2) papillomatosis; and (3) lobular hyperplasia. The latter is practically indistinguishable from lobular carcinoma in situ, which is a preinvasive form of breast cancer. Among the 711 cases Pennisi studied extensively, 24.5% had lobular carcinoma in situ. An additional 5.5% had adenocarcinoma that was not detectable preoperatively by the usual screening devices. In the midst of all these discouraging statistics is one bright point. The fact that among the 850 patients who required subcutaneous mastectomy only one developed invasive carcinoma during the postoperative period is reassuring. Incidentally, "apocrine metaplasia" on a biopsy specimen is not considered pathologic today. We once thought it was a strong precursor for breast carcinoma, but it is not; neither is a family history of cancer in a member over age 65.

Nipple Reconstruction

There are several ways to reconstruct a nipple, with the choice of the procedure based on the surgeon's experience and sense of aesthetics. Tattooing of course is the easiest method, but tattoos, in my opinion, have never looked good enough. Full-thickness skin grafts give the best appearance, but they fade with time, so you probably have to tattoo them anyway. Someone once suggested smearing some of the tattoo pigment on the dermal bed and allowing it to seep through, but that method seems hazardous. Charles Puckett has discussed nipple reconstruction using an "inch worm flap," which is basically a large VY flap. The problem with all of these techniques for elevating—whether by a double VY flap, a triangle flap, or other type—is the tendency to graft around the elevated area. Thus the nipple itself is a lighter color than the graft. There is nothing wrong with deepithelializing the whole area, performing a "skate worm" or other type advancement, and then grafting over the entire area. Do not use labia minora for the graft, as it tends to get much too dark, and it is an uncomfortable donor sight.

A good general rule is as follows: To create a pink nipple, use skin from behind the ear; it turns pinker with maturity. For a darker areola, use inner thigh skin and close the incision primarily high in the groin. Use a subcuticular closure in two layers with good eversion, resulting in a flat scar without hatch marks. Trim the skin graft and then suture it in place with a stent dressing. Several surgeons have incorporated rubber bands into these tie-over dressings but I prefer the old way: Place half-buried 4-0 silk mattress sutures (so there are no suture marks outside the new areola), and leave them long; gather them up for hemostasis, and then place a Vaseline gauze (e.g., xeroform) and some moist cotton pads inside the area, and tie them down around it. Do not forget to fold some xeroform around the edge of the stent dressing. This reinforcement prevents the ball of the stent dressing from rocking (caused by occasional pressure within the brassiere). Examine the graft at about 1 week and then recover it with elastic tape over a nonsticky substance such as Telfa. To prevent edge disruption, replace this dressing with paper tape around the periphery at about 2 weeks but have the patient wear a pad inside the brassiere for safety.

Inverted Nipples

The most common inverted nipple is a simple cleft in the center of a raised section. You can actually see the two subcutaneous portions.

Although complicated, the method of repair works well. Excise the epithelium along the duct surface so you can see down into the cleft. The tissues on either side are freed, so the central ducts are now completely mobile. Moving them upward is accomplished by placing a series of dissolvable sutures in lateral fashion beginning from below, bringing the sides to the center, and then moving upward. The top two points on these side pedicles are then joined, and the areolar nipple skin is brought upward and anchored to them with a few tacking stitches. Occasionally, a crossing stitch is placed at the base. The advantage of this technique is that the ducts are not transectioned.

An even simpler method involves transection of the ducts and then using crisscross sutures in a square pattern to hold the tissues into the gap. That method works well also. An even simpler method is reported by P.J. Chandler (Richardson, TX). He makes a small stab wound, cuts through the ducts while elevating the nipple with a hook, and inserts a through-and-through rubber drain, tacking it into place. If the drain is left in place for a couple of weeks, the fibrosis forces the nipple to stay in its elevated position.

The fascinating thing about all of these transection techniques is that occasionally patients can still breastfeed!

Richard Schultz (Chicago) suggests this for nipple projection in mastopexy and reduction mammoplasty. The recipient site is simply deepithelialized and folded under to form a "platform." This additional tissue makes up for any defects in infolding from below, so the nipple–areolar complex points forward. His inferior pedicle is then advanced over the platform and anchored into position. The results shown were good.

John Hamilton (St. Petersburg) has the simplest idea for repairing inverted nipples—so simple that we all should have thought about it. He makes a semicircular incision two-thirds around the base of the nipple, elevates it, completely frees it from underlying connections and then closes off the space underneath with heavy sutures. The nipple then lies back on a firm base and must project. It sounds too good to be true, which means it probably works a lot better than all the complicated methods with which we have been struggling.

Another method for creating a projected nipple in mastectomy patients is reported by Ernest Cronin (Houston). In the bed that is being prepared for the full-thickness graft, he outlines an S-shaped incision. Transposing the tissues and bringing them together creates an elevation. The donor area is then closed, pushing the new projection even higher. The full-thickness skin graft is placed over the entire area. The only better method, he says, is a composite graft from the opposite areola. The S-shaped procedure is excellent if the mastectomy scar has been placed directly through the site you want to use. Let the mastectomy incision line be the center part of the S.

Transumbilical Breast Augmentation

Breast augmentation has been done through the umbilicus. We must applaud Gerald Johnson (Houston) for his imagination, but there are problems, real and potential, that are not addressed using this technique. With this technique, expansion of the pocket depends on manual manipulation of a tissue expander, which is introduced with a fiberoptic scope inside a long tube passed upward at a 45 degree angle through a supraumbilical incision.

You have to admire the ingenuity needed to devise an instrument blunt enough and round enough to dissect upward and into the subglandular pocket. The blunt tip of the instrument is withdrawn, and an inflatable prosthesis is rolled up like a cigarette and placed inside the tube. The tube then passes back into the tunnel it has created underneath the breast and is withdrawn. After filling the prosthesis, the filling tube is simply tugged loose. Hence there are no incisions in the breast and no sutures except in the umbilical entry site.

Johnson has noted only one deflation among 100 consecutive cases. Several patients have shown evidence of bleeding, but there is a "safety valve" built into this operation. Any bleeding, unless it is excessive, simply runs down the tunnel and can be easily removed from the mid-abdomen. The current equipment, however, does not have a coagulation tip in the laparoscopic part, and I question whether laparoscopy is necessary at all. Johnson has reported inadvertent submuscular placement on several occasions, but by visually inspecting the tunnel it is easy to see when one is in the wrong spot. Practice should eliminate that difficulty, and the method can probably be effective without the laparoscopic aspect.

There are some problems. First, many breasts are too high, and there is no easy way to lower the inframammary fold without direct scissors dissection, which means dealing with bleeders. How can bleeders be controlled when you are looking at them from the umbilicus? Second, if the inframammary fold is not lowered, you lose the aspect of breast augmentation we call the "illusion mastopexy." Lowering the fold in a moderately ptotic breast allows the nipple to ride upward, and the lower-placed prosthesis then gives a pleasing and natural look, simulating a mastopexy. This effect cannot be attained through the umbilicus.

What are the potential problems? Even though you have obtained permission from the patient to use a periareolar direct approach if there are problems—and Johnson has not had to do it yet—such a step would more likely anger a patient who came to you because she did not want any scars. The second problem is that an inflatable implant is being manually pushed in different directions to create a pocket, placing stress on the filling mechanism. The question is what will happen a year from now, 2 years, even 5 years? Will this extra manual compression that has been necessary to tear the soft tissues loose damage the filling mechanism or the seams? You certainly would not have to worry about inadvertently cutting a sensory nerve because there is no dissection except directly in the midline. (That is one reason many of us abandoned the transaxillary approach for augmentation. Another was not being able to carefully establish a chosen inframammary fold point.) Other potential problems include the inescapable hucksterism that some surgeon will employ to gain patients at the expense of others by promising them a procedure that may not, in our opinion, give as natural or as uncomplicated a result, as established techniques. Even with overexpansion and manual stretching of the pocket in all directions, how can it be better than physically releasing the adherent bands with a sharp scissors to create a full pocket and expansion. Who will pay for the replacement if the stress causes a significant number of mechanical breakdowns and saline leakage during the first few years? The manufacturers will not replace any implant inserted in this manner. With the current highly successful periareolar incisions that are generally undetectable within the first few years, is it a good trade-off to have a 1-cm incision in the umbilicus versus a 3-cm incision at the edge of the areola? Despite these objections, trying new techniques is admirable, and this method is worthy of investigation.

Atypical Mycobacterial Infections in Breast Augmentation Patients

The following material is excerpted from testimony given by Malcolm Foster, Professor of Medicine at the University of Florida at Jacksonville, in a 1982 court case involving a postsurgical infection with atypical mycobacteria. Prior to his testimony, a board-certified plastic surgeon who admittedly had no knowledge of the subject had testified that implants should be removed immediately in the face of these infections, that these infections were a threat to the patient's life, and that hospitals were preferable to office surgical suites because of their lower incidence of infection and greater degree of safety.

Malcolm Foster had been collecting data and performing research into the problems with atypical mycobacteria. This case began when he was "called by Dr. Wilkinson from San Antonio concerning a clinical problem he had where a patient had cultured out this particular organism from the site of augmentation. I told him that there was very little known . . . about the particular sequence of events, that organism, or that infection. This started a whole cascade of investigation that is continuing to this date."

The first break in the investigation came from three cases in Hollywood, Florida. Investigations led to other case reports from several states.

Atypical mycobacteria are similar to tuberculosis bacteria and were usually discussed in the literature on chest diseases. To date, we have no definite source of the infection.

> The organisms are ubiquitous, which means that it is in dust, in the air, in plants, in animals, and can be grown from tap water. A report came from the CDC [Centers for Disease Control] that atypicals had been found in sterile water and in sterile saline for injection.

The surgical literature had also lists infections in other clean wounds, notably after thoracic surgery. Despite knowing that the bacteria were widespread in nature and zeroing in on sterile irrigation solutions, no common denominator has been found. In the initial cases in eight cities by eight surgeons, there were hospital and office surgical procedures. Four manufacturers were involved as well as multiple manufacturers of the steroids or saline.

The organisms involved in these cases were difficult to study in the laboratory. Antibiotics that were considered effective against one strain were ineffective in cultures of others. "In other instances the patient seemed to respond to an appropriate antibiotic, and in several instances we now know that people are responding to some very simple drugs like sulfa and Vibramycin. Patients responded to injectable or topical antibiotics, leading to a conclusion that there is no fixed way of treatment and that many ways seem to be effective."

The conclusion was that implants may be left in place until all other measures for treatment fail and *should be removed only as a last resort.* This practice is particularly applicable in the case of an atypical mycobacterial infection, as the organisms do not pose a systemic threat other than occasional low grade fevers and occasional skin redness. The patients studied showed no signs of toxicity and no instances of spread of the bacteria beyond the breast.

There are reports of silicone shunts in patients with kidney or cardiac disease and successfully treated with antibiotics without removing their prostheses.

Comments and Commentary

1. Simeon Wall (Shreveport) releases the origin of the pectoralis major from the ribs between three and six o'clock for breast augmentation when he is planning to allow inferior displacement of the implant in patients with minor degrees of ptosis. These patients do not have lateral displacement of the implant with contracture of the pectoralis if the lateral fibers are underneath the implant and the medial fibers are released from the ribs. *Technical Forum* had criticized other surgeons who used total submuscular coverage, even in weight lifters and body builders. "I feel that the secret is to have some part of the implant behind the pectoralis even if it only includes the upper fibers from the clavicular head. The upper pull of the implant is behind the muscle and does not allow for the spherical contracture that results when the implant is totally retroglandular." How do you explain the patients with severe capsular contractures after submuscular implantation?) Perhaps we should tailor our operations to the patient and use all of these techniques in flat-chested women. Or perhaps these women are the very ones who require total subglandular release so the tissue can expand to a greater degree.

2. John Bostwick (Atlanta) reminds us that every time we cut into the breast we encounter bacteria, and so it would be logical to think that infection of some type influences capsular contracture. The overall statistics have improved since we adopted Boyd Burkhardt's suggestion of irrigating with Betadine.

Betadine tends to stay in the tissues for weeks and is an effective deterrent to bacterial multiplication.

Bostwick thinks that cautery dissection is probably not a good idea, as fat necrosis with dead tissue should breed bacteria, another argument that he believes favors submuscular implantation. The problem with that argument is that most people who use submuscular implantation today are those who completely separate the pectoralis from its origin. This maneuver must liberate some serum or blood, which pools in the lower portion of the pocket and is in contact with the forming capsule.

3. Quotes one surgeon: "I think people who say that subpectoral implantation is the way, the truth, and the light for the breast augmentation are simply nuts. In my experience the small potential benefits for most patients are more than offset by the extended recovery time and by the cosmetic deformity frequently caused by flexion of the pectoralis muscle. We do have one surgeon in town who tells patients he is using the subpectoral approach and that he is the only one in town who never gets capsule contractures or other problems. I'm happy to have him in business, as he generates a lot of traffic into my office for [release of] contractures."

4. Anthropologist Max Bartels groups breasts into 48 types, depending on whether they are: "(1) highly developed and exuberant; (2) full; (3) moderate; or (4) small and flat. And in each category: (a) firm; (b) soft; and (c) flabby." He continues, with even more complicated divisions: subgroups of "I—bowl-shaped; II—hemispherical; III—conical; or IV—elongated." Maybe he got a government grant.

5. For those of us who believe that submuscular placement adds little if anything to one's success rate, it is good to be able to identify a factor that does make a difference. In many breasts Cooper's ligaments are inelastic and have never been stretched. Imagine tying a rope between two trees. Even though the rope appears to be strong and fibrous, by the time you have swung on it once or twice, it has stretched and becomes longer and less rigid. This principle of ligament stretch is employed in operative expansion. Unfortunately, the muscle does not participate well in this maneuver, so the best results are with subglandular augmentation.

The best method for accomplishing such a stretch is as follows. After you have created an adequate pocket and inserted the prosthesis, place the tip of your finger underneath the areola and push upward. Then press outward in all quadrants with sustained pressure. Tissues can be felt to give way under your finger. The initially tight, round breast is now flattened and softer. Another way to reach this condition is to insert a tissue expander and expand it while you are doing something else. It can be filled with air, deflated after a few minutes, and reused on the other side (and for several other augmentations before you have to buy a new one). The finger technique, however, is effective. Perhaps it is responsible for our seeing fewer early contractures. Once the breast tissue has been stretched it is easier for the patient to do her postoperative maneuvers, particularly if you instilled 20 ml of 0.25% Marcaine before closing the subcutaneous tissue.

6. We sometimes have used the jacuzzi as a therapeutic tool. In postoperative breast augmentation patients it seems to reduce edema and ecchymoses—or at least that is what we thought it did. More important was the secondary advantage—the early and late postoperative patients were in the same exercise class and in the same jacuzzi, where they could trade experiences and discover that their problems were not major or unusual.

A research paper has now identified the reason for the improved healing that accompanies heat therapy. Local application of heat is the most ancient of methods for treating wound infections. Medical science, however, had not traced the reasons for it or why the swelling of noninfected wounds appears to resolve more rapidly after heat is applied. Two surgical investigators looked at the problem and identified increased blood flow and oxygen tension as the two products of heat application that promote benefit. Using a new technique that allowed them to continuously measure tissue oxygen tension in postoperative patients, the investigators found that oxygen tension rose an average of 80% over baseline concomitant with the application of heat. The local rate of blood perfusion increased at least threefold. Heat application can be used prophylactically as well. With increased oxygen tension and blood flow, there is less chance for bacterial invasion to succeed. These same investigators are gathering additional data on the "infectability" of patients and are looking at superoxite and chemiluminescence in white blood cells in wounds after heat therapy. To support the contention that heat is a prophylactic influence, they demonstrated a direct antibiotic effect with the oxygen tension; and other research found a correlation between leukocyte bactericidal capacity and elevated oxygen levels.

Hence it seems like a good idea to have postoperative patients immersed in soothing, heated waters. Remember, though, to coat the incision line with some scalant such as collodion. We found that breast massage is easier to accomplish after a period of soaking, as much of the postsurgical edema has now subsided. It has been true for most patients who have had cosmetic and reconstructive procedures, from abdominoplasty to breast augmentation.

7. In the ongoing discussion of delayed complications after breast augmentation, one disturbing occurrence has become sufficiently common to warrant recalling patients for mammograms. We refer to implant shell breakage. The gel prostheses that replaced collapsing saline prostheses during the early 1970s were designed with thin walls, and the gel interior was distinctly different from that of modern gels. Some contained liquid silicone. There have been reports of free silicone surrounding intact breast prostheses when patients were reoperated to obtain biopsy specimens or because of changes in size or shape.

We originally thought that these "exudates" were innocuous and that the worst that could happen was a decrease in the mobility of the prostheses, with a greater chance of capsular contracture. It was theorized that the capsular contracture was related to implant mobility and the varying stretching pressures exerted during normal daily activities. However there was a consistent contracture rate when gel prostheses were fixed to the chest wall, whether they were Dacron or perforated silicone patches. The Dacron certainly made a difference, but there were also cases of one-sided contracture with silicone patch prostheses. The contracted side was adherent through its silicone patch in every case, whereas the side without contracture had no adherence. If these patched implants did not adhere to the chest wall, the breast was softer 5 to 10 years later. If the only problem was decreased mobility, why worry? The answer is that we are now seeing siliconomas, dense fibrotic reactions, and silicone migration into the shoulder. Moreover, after approximately 10 years, a number of patients have developed sudden capsular contractures. Some have distinct siliconomas.

Three such cases surfaced in our practice in one year. Two had breaks in the prosthesis wall, and one had an intact implant. The gel that escaped after 10 years created havoc. Woe betide the surgeon who would have performed a closed release. The watery gel was forced into the capsular tear and caused an immediate inflammatory response. Pain, fibrosis, siliconoma, or all of these problems resulted. Other surgeons are now reporting similar changes in their patient population.

We suggest that a recall letter be sent to all patients in whom gel prostheses were implanted between the years 1970 and 1984. X-rays, physical examination, or endoscopy can reveal any problems.

We have discovered hidden siliconomas, free gel, or both in patients who reported a sudden onset of pain and contracture during the ninth or tenth postoperative year. On the other hand, about 40 others we examined have had no problem with their prostheses, and their breasts are soft and natural. It is good practice to be careful, however, as in one case the free silicone had migrated into the shoulder soft tissues, and one with migration to the arm, both problems that are difficult to correct.

Did closed contracture play a role? It would be difficult to assess this factor in the first two cases (with breaks in the prosthesis wall) because the breasts of both patients had remained soft and had not required medical attention for at least 6 years. Should a closed capsulotomy be performed on a 1970's gel prostheses patient if she returns to your office today? Probably not. Even a 1984 case. If there is a free silicone that cannot be detected by xerogram, it may be forced into the soft tissues. I have seen two such cases, presumably due to prior closed capsulotomy performed elsewhere.

A reasonable plan of action for avoiding later complications due to the early gel implants is as follows.

1. Send a note that includes information about the safety of breast prostheses to all implant patients. Ask them to make an appointment with your office.
2. When you examine them, if they have a early or late contracture and the implant was of the thin-walled less-than-cohesive gel type, do not

attempt a closed capsulotomy. Advise them that implant replacement is in their best interest.

3. If you see evidence of a broken implant or siliconoma, advise the patient to seek corrective surgery within a reasonable time.

8. Did you know that the patient who had the first Cronin-Gerow breast prostheses in 1962 still has the implants in place and is comfortable and satisfied?

9. How does an implant break? Terry Tubbs surveyed 22 patients with broken prostheses and found no history of trauma in 16. Four of them had no symptoms, but most developed tightness and constriction. Two of the implants were polyurethane. One of the worst contractures I treated this year was in a patient with a 1983 Meme prosthesis. I believe that the implants have been improved dramatically since 1985. We certainly are not seeing these heavy contractures today.

Tubbs says he is not seeing siliconomas as often, and I agree. The 1979–1983 series of thin-walled silicone prostheses are associated with a small percentage of siliconomas in intact or broken prostheses. (We recommend triple-view Xrays. The plastic surgeon may give a better evaluation of the implant with a than can the radiologist, although there are some false positives. In one case, we saw a double shadow, which usually indicates a broken prosthesis with extension outside the original shell. The original surgeon had somehow placed half of the implant under the pectoralis muscle and the other half on top. Needless to say, it was easy to correct.)

10. John Young commented on the subject as follows: "I have been using the double-lumen Heyer-Schulte implants for several years. I have had two spontaneous ruptures, one in 9 months and one at 11 months after surgery. This is admittedly a low percentage, but both of these appeared to be so-called 'stress factors' of the implant. I suspect there may be more of which we are not aware."

By 1989 we saw more women whose breasts had changed after minor-trauma X-rays confirmed an implant rupture, but most had *no* tightness or inflammatory reaction. Siliconomas came later in some cases, so we were wise to advise recalls, reexaminations, and replacement.

11. Does ultrasound therapy have a place in capsule release? Several readers have found a beneficial effect from the use of ultrasound in patients whose capsular contractures after breast augmentation were resistant. Gerald Kakascik (Paducah) found that several patients whose capsules could not be released by other means were easily released with minimal pressure after a period of exposure to ultrasound. Has anyone else had this experience?

12. Richard Toronto (Plano) on periprosthesis infections: "I would like to share with you a small item that been most useful to me. I had an occasion to see a young lady with atypical mycobacteria in both breasts who had been [operated] through inframammary incisions. She was draining freely out of both incisions with a 1 × 2 cm necrotic area under one and about a 2 × 2 cm necrotic area under the other. I took her to the operating room where I applied our usual technique. Through a periareolar incision, I turned down a muscle sling flap based laterally of serratus and pectoralis based inferiorly and laterally. I put complete full thickness of muscle between the prosthesis and the hole. I then took a Limberg flap of skin and closed the hole from the outside of both sides, giving it effectively a two-layer full-thickness closure—the skin and muscle to support the prosthesis. Even with the edema and all one usually sees accompanying the treatment of atypical mycobacteria, she healed uneventfully with a beautiful result. Since that time I have had occasion to use the flap three times, and I have found it to work superbly. It is a really neat trick [to add to our] armamentarium."

13. A suggestion that merits attention: Because the controversy is not resolved about the role of infection in breast augmentation despite some excellent work by our colleagues, it might be wise to follow a suggestion: After dissecting the pocket, irrigate with half-strength Betadine. It should destroy any superficial *Staphylococcus epidermidis* that have been introduced into the wound or may have been living in the adjacent tissue. Half-strength Betadine is innocuous to the tissues and can be washed out with a subsequent rinse of Xylocaine or Marcaine.

14. Can tampons indirectly cause capsular contractures? Reports of capsular contractures with positive cultures are numerous. There are many documented cases of bacteremias in which an augmented breast suddenly became hot and tender and subsequently developed a contracture. We know that tampons are widely used in the United States and in many cases are considered responsible for transient bacteremias.

15. Greg Hetter (Las Vegas) used Keflin in the outer lumen of double-lumen prostheses for a number of years, along with Betadine irrigation of the pocket (started soon after Boyd Burkhardt's study indicated that minimal contamination from the breast bacteria was a potent cause of contracture). Because Kefzol was less expensive, however, Hetter began to use it instead of Keflin. The first time one of the outer-lumen bags broke, the Kefzol was released into the pocket, and the patient experienced rapid contracture of the breast and marked pain. Surgical exploration revealed that the Kefzol had created concretions in the outer lumen, a finding that Hetter had not seen with Keflin. He subsequently saw three similar cases and stopped using Kefzol. There is little doubt in his mind that because Kefzol has a different solubility and different tissue toxicity it can cause problems if used in the pocket or the outer lumen of a double-lumen implant.

Technical Forum has reported that one of the complications of double implants was deflation of the outer lumens due simply to wear and tear and "wearing out." We now add Kefzol irritation as a cause of late contracture, along with bizarre folding over of the collapsed outer lumen. Of the many causes of breast contracture, this is certainly one that can be easily eliminated.

16. Ron Berggren reports four cases of delayed infection around a breast prosthesis. In the first, he removed the prosthesis and then inserted another. The second one was also removed. In the third case, he immediately placed a new prosthesis subpectorally, and in the fourth case he removed the prosthesis. All the results were satisfactory (reinforcing the idea that infections are not overwhelming disasters. Many can be controlled with pocket sterilization or antibiotics alone, sparing the patient a long period of disagreeable recovery between removal and reinsertion).

17. Mary Martin reported a case in which Prostaphlin irrigation controlled periprosthetic infection. Jay Ellenby (North Miami Beach) removes the prosthesis after capsular contracture following infection. He performs an open capsulotomy and then inserts a new prothesis and covers the infection with intravenous and oral antibiotics—with good results.

18. James Rybka (Carmichael) presented a suction-assisted lipectomy patient who developed a localized soft tissue mycobacterial infection some time after the procedure. Fortunately, he did not perform massive debridement, as was suggested by his first consultant. The bacteria generally clear if you leave them alone or use an intravenous medication such as Amikacin. His case responded to simple treatment with oral erythromycin, for example.

19. Atypical bacterial infections usually show up in warm weather areas. They occur naturally in fresh water and, in fact, can be cultured from many normal stomach washings. They do not seem to become aggressive unless there is an abundance of sunshine.

A board-certified plastic surgeon had done a simple closed capsulotomy some years after a breast augmentation. Surprisingly, the patient developed the massive outpouring of fluid, which is typical of intracapsular atypical infection. Another plastic surgeon removed the implant, but he apparently had not read the literature that says because the bacteria are relatively benign and the prosthesis can be retained and the infection treated by simple irrigation with antibiotics. (We know of another case from the 1970s in which the fluid was aspirated simply because the patient refused implant removal. Not surprisingly, the bacteria disappeared and the breast remained soft.) The "expert witness" in the case against the original surgeon stated unequivocally that closed release had caused breast infection. Such ignorance should not be allowed in a court room.

Kel Cohen (Richmond) experienced a delayed periprosthetic breast infection he successfully treated by instillation of antibiotics without removing the prosthesis. His report agreed with numerous others.

20. It seems fairly well established now that the breast prosthesis does not behave as an ordinary foreign body. If it is used to maintain the space and expansion of the breast, antibiotic solutions administered orally, intravenously, intracapsularly, or intraprosthetically have a more than fighting chance to eliminate late developing infections. The greatest successes seem to be with the nonthreatening infections, such as with atypical mycobacteria and *Staphylococcus epidermidis*. There have been a few spectacular successes with the more serious infections as well, such as *Staphylococcus aureus* and *Pseudomonas aeruginosa*. Perhaps someday we will find that failure to attempt to "salvage" the breast with an intact prosthesis would be a cause for a malpractice action, rather than the sorry state of affairs that we have witnessed (i.e., attempting to salvage the prosthesis, leading to a charge of malpractice by a colleague).

In a recent *Technical Forum* survey, more than 35% of the respondents stated that they had encountered delayed infections after breast augmentation. Sixty-nine of the respondents gave detailed information. In most cases the implant was removed arbitrarily with no attempts to sterilize the pocket or replace the prosthesis. There were four successes with inflow-outflow antibiotic irrigations and some form of "salvage" procedure, and nine patients responded to simple antibiotic therapy. Today, infection is quite rare.

An interesting point regarding my personal experience with eight cases is that only two developed capsular contractures despite what initially appeared to be an overwhelmingly threatening and destructive situation. One patient had a *Pseudomonas aeruginosa* infection in the periareolar and periprosthetic areas. She was treated for the infection, and both breasts are now equally soft and completely natural in shape and appearance 1.5 years later.

21. About 5% to 10% of our patients once required minor or major closed capsulotomy, performed as an outpatient office procedure. In our experience, almost all cause only a small, sharp pain, usually during the routine monthly testing within the first 6 months after surgery. When a patient appears with a definite advanced capsular contracture, consider offering them this alternative.

For a small additional medication charge, the patient may choose a brief "twilight" procedure. We have successfully employed this method about 100 times over a 5-year period. It can be safely performed without cardiac monitoring, and it is best done in the office recovery room with a nurse in attendance. An intravenous line is established and 5 mg of diazepam (Valium) is slowly injected. No premedication is employed. Stadol 2 mg is then given slowly. Stadol provides pain control postoperatively but in this low dosage does not inhibit respirations or create mental confusion. Ketamine 20 mg IV is then slowly administered. With the low dose of ketamine and a small amount of Valium, a brief period of painless "twilight" dissociation is obtained. The closed capsulotomies are then completed within approximately 60 seconds. If it takes more pressure or time, you should plan later open capsulotomy instead.

22. Why is aesthetic surgery difficult? "The average patient in an aesthetic practice is a perfectionist. The surgeon has the responsibility of surpassing normal, not simply restoring back to normal" (Millard).

23. Most unusual closed capsulotomy case: John Royer had a patient who told him that her once-hard breast had suddenly become soft. How did it happen? She stepped on a rake, and it flipped up and hit her in the chest.

24. Jerry Nelson (Wichita) reported more than 30,000 closed capsulotomies with only a 1% hematoma rate. There were some ruptured implants with gel migration, but these cases were rare. His record is reassuring to those of us who believe that periodic hard compression is the only way to prevent capsular contracture. On the other hand, if you decide to go ahead with an open capsulotomy, hematomas appear at almost 2.5 times this rate. If a capsule releases easily and you continue to release it weekly until the breast stays soft, there is less risk than if you immediately perform an open capsulectomy. Do not worry about that "30% recurrence rate after closed capsulotomy." Some probably were not done well and had limited follow-up. It is important to recheck the patients at weekly intervals to prevent early reattachment of the capsule. If expansion is maintained for 6 weeks, open capsulotomies are necessary today only 2% to 3% of the time.

25. After presenting a learned review of closed capsulotomy, open capsulotomy, and capsular contracture, Hollis Caffee (Gainsville) summarized the problem well: "We're confused as ever, but we're confused at a higher level and about more important things." To add to the confusion, he rightly pointed out that "firmness" is not an all or nothing quality. "Firmness" is related to the thickness of the breast parenchyma, the size and compressibility of the implant, the thickness and elasticity of the capsule, and so on. It also depends on what you consider "firm" and what the patient thinks is "firm."

26. Capsulectomy sometimes causes a considerable amount of diffuse capillary oozing that cannot be stopped with cautery. Knowing full well that some blood will accumulate even after a section device is removed, we make the following suggestions. Create a small extracapsular pocket at the inferior border. A 1.5-cm opening is created with blunt dissection and a large pocket developed beyond that by spreading the scissors blade. This opening is not large enough to allow the prosthesis to stretch into a "balloon" at the inframammary fold but is sufficient to allow fluid to drain away from the forming capsule. On the second or third day after surgery, one can safely aspirate through the skin without risk of touching the wall of the prosthesis. Repeated aspirations over 2 to 3 days allows us to remove any serosanguineous fluid.

27. Jim Baker (Orlando) on breast scar contractures: Most contractures peak at about 6 months in a bell-shaped curve. In Baker's follow-up study about 92% occurred during the first 12 months. He reemphasizes the use of vitamin E preoperatively and postoperatively. In patients who show evidence of contracture, he increases the dosage of 1000 units of synthetic α-tocopherol per day to 1000 units four times a day. This dosage is continued many months and then decreased to 1000 units twice a day. No bleeding problems have occurred.

28. Ed Melmed restates the general rule concerning breast massage and textured or polyurethane implants. "The whole interface between the cover and the cavity is an active one. The cover must not be torn or secondary capsule contracture may occur." "Leave them alone and they will soften nicely on their own." In view of the late contractures seen with textured and polyurethane implants, which usually begin in the upper inner quadrant, perhaps we should compromise and begin a form of gentle upward pressure at about the third week. This practice may prevent separation of that part of the prosthesis due to gravitational force. Retraction and separation of the attached parts of the implant allow the chest tissue to contact the upper portion of the breast by sealing off a portion of the cavity. It occurs when textured implants become more mobile, at about 12 weeks.

29. In an article in the *Southern Medical Journal*, plastic surgeon Leroy Young discussed calcification of breast implant capsules and would have us believe that it is a rare complication. That may be true if you consider only the fact that few cases are reported in the literature, but most working plastic surgeons see two or three every year. Calcification due to seepage of silicone or catalytic materials in the old type implants is going the way of the dinosaur, much to our satisfaction.

30. Ignorance, denial, neglect, and complacency—not breast augmentation—cause delay in breast cancer diagnosis.

31. We have reported cases in which double-lumen prostheses deflated their outer lumens, resulting in being folded into a cigar shape. This problem plus the thick unyielding feel has led me to discontinue their use in practically all cases.

32. Siliconoma development is definitely time-related. In other words, if you detect a broken gel implant, replace it. It seems that the gel eventually breaks down into smaller bits, similar to a liquid state, that evoke a foreign body reaction as the material is pushed into the tissues.

33. Other than training anesthesia residents, is there any reason to continue the practice of intracostal blocks in wide-awake, pain-feeling augmentation mammoplasty candidates?

34. Are you having trouble getting a textured implant under a breast through a small incision? Dick Jones was struggling with those implants when he realized that lubricants might be useful. Betadine is a good lubricant and it certainly is beneficial. Some surgeons use a sterile tube of K-Y jelly, which is not tissue-friendly, assuming that they can wash this water-soluble lubricant out before closing the skin. (Editor's note: If you do not wash it out, it may cause capsule formation.) Looking at both lubricating possibilities, Jones decided that a new product was needed. He remembered high-molecular-weight dextran, the plasma expander we used during the 1970s as an antithrombolytic agent and immediate volume expander. It is available in any pharmacy and has been cleared by the FDA for use within the body. Best of all, it is slippery. Jones has the pharmacy provide the operating room with sterile Hyskon. He pours it over the implants, and "they become so slippery that I could practically lob them into that incision from across the room." We tried the dextran, and what he said was true. Because this dextrose solution is easily metabolized by the body and does no harm, it seems to be a good choice.

35. Kuros Tabari reemphasizes the need for total capsulectomy when you treat a severe capsular contracture by replacing the original implant with a textured one.

36. Luiz Lamana dos Santos (Brazil) performed 1088 breast reductions over a 4-year interval and lived to tell about the experience. American surgeons in the RAPS audience to whom dos Santos presented his cases agreed that three-fourths of his breast reduction candidates would have undergone simple breast augmentation, with or without an areolar lift "crescent" excision, had they been in the States.

37. Frank Walchak reports a patient who developed a spontaneous postaugmentation venous bleeding episode and decided because of her work schedule to put off evacuation. Walchak used a large suction cannula from a lipolysis set to aspirate 200 ml of old blood clots. He palpated within the cavity and found a small indentation, but the breast was otherwise normal. He implies that the use of the textured implant may have had something to do with the bleeding, citing as a reason another case in which a textured implant's rough surface and attachment to the tissues may have caused irritation and erosion. The problem in the present patient developed 3 months after textured implant augmentation. Two of my polyurethane reconstructure patients developed the same syndrome 6 *years* postop.

38. Peter Linton was asked by a patient if there would be a problem during her cremation because she had had breast implants. Peter asked Dow Corning for the answer. Silicone prostheses burn at 600° to 700°F, forming silicone dioxide. This sandy material mixes well with the ashes.

39. About 3 weeks after every flu epidemic, we see numerous breast augmentation patients with unilateral contractures. Fortunately, all of them release easily and stay released. Next time you see someone with a delayed contracture ask them if they have had a recent febrile episode. Some patients tell you that their breasts became warm and tender, some detected redness, and all tell you that the discomfort in the breast went away fairly quickly. Why does this reaction cause a contracture a week or two later?

40. Shel Rosenthal is satisfied with textured implants, but he warns us to be prepared for more incisional erythema and serous drainage around the incision site. Is it due to the trauma of the insertion or to early motion of the prosthesis within the breast? Seromas are a known complication of textured implants. They are sterile but can certainly become infected. We had such a case last year.

41. Jim Moore has no hesitation about going directly through the breast using a periareolar approach to augmentation mammoplasty. Several prominent plastic surgeons have made a fuss in the literature about the infections that surely must occur after such a dastardly deed, but Moore has not seen them. For the record, he prefers submuscular placement but releases the origin of the muscles so completely that it is almost the same as subglandular placement. He experiences the same 4% contracture rate that is seen with submuscular, subglandular, or foam-covered prostheses.

42. Did you know that some people have an intense allergic reaction to the triglycerides that make up peanut oil? What if one of the proposed peanut oil breast implant leaks?

43. Why do presenters of papers slip in statements that just are not true? Here are two that deserve awards. *1st Place:* "People who develop contractures after implant rupture have a different immunologic response to silicone." *2nd Place:* "Closed capsulotomy has a 70% complication rate." This statement was made in an effort to promote endoscopic sectioning of breast prostheses capsules ("scoping for dollars").

44 Apparently some of our colleagues are using bogus diagnoses to indicate a reason for removing a breast implant in a patient who demands removal for nonmedical reasons. If you list "adjuvant disease" or "autoimmune disease" as a reason for removal, it will eventually backfire. These diagnoses may be politically correct, but they are not medical diagnoses. If you have to put anything down for a diagnosis, put the following: "severe anxiety caused by-self-appointed and uninformed consumer advocates."

45. Charles Vinnik suspects that unhappy patients do not return to their physicians. One of his patients had been operated on in San Francisco by an "expert in subcutaneous mastectomy," who claims a tiny complication rate with polyurethane foam implants. His colleague had had great difficulty removing the material as the pectoralis muscles were "greatly disturbed." I saw a high incidence of this problem with the implants used prior to 1985, but the rock-hard complication factor seem to be diminishing with the newer implants. Vinnick's second patient had a polyurethane submammary implant with which the patient reported a rash, recurrent axillary nodes, and diffuse breast tenderness and pain. Her surgeon's last notes indicated that she was a Baker 1, but Vinnick classified her as having a class III contracture. Dense bands of fibrous tissues were surrounding inflammatory reaction. We now know many such cases were bacterial in origin.

46. Who are you going to believe? One surgeon on the West Coast reported a 40% deflation rate for inflatable breast implants and another on the East Coast reported a 4% deflation rate. Latest surveys show between 2% and 5%. O'Neal Engeron (Houma) noted that he had used three pairs of inflatable implants over the last few years, and two had deflated, one of them 1.5 years after insertion. That is not a satisfactory record. Maybe the answer is to use the top loading design with a textured surface, which allows tissue growth to stabilize the valve. Perhaps the textured implant does not move as freely so there is less trauma.

47. Is it not odd that Norplant, the birth control device in a silicone casing that is inserted into the forearm as a birth control device, was approved the day before Dr. Kessler called for a moratorium on breast implants? "We, as scientists, forgot that Dr. Kessler is a lawyer."

48. Tom Biggs (Houston), on studies of implants in young women: "Why do we not do retrospective studies? There is a gigantic pool of patients in stable communities." The only thing wrong with this totally logical demand is that the government is not willing to accept retrospective studies.

49. At one aesthetic plastic surgery meeting, a flat statement was made that in all patients, except those who are small-breasted, better visualization was obtained with submuscular implants. He might have told his audience that most of his patients had old calcified subglandular implants. This situation certainly affects the ease of mammography as well as totally skewing the statistics. My impression is that the issue is not one of subglandular versus submuscular augmentation. It is an issue of competence of radiologists as new techniques evolve. Excellent evaluations can be obtained with both types of implant. Balanced against the known problems of submuscular augmentation (pain, movement, upward or downward displacement), ease of visualization should be a moot issue.

50. The rheumatologists who were supposed to bring new information to the FDA on autoimmune connections to breast implants turned out to be as fraudulent as the single dog study they cited. One wonders how the distinguished representatives from the American College of Surgeons and the College of Radiology and the immunologists and rheumatologists who were listening to this "new evidence" maintained their equilibrium. The AMA also rejected these and subsequent "studies."

51. Augmentation patients who become pregnant are seen at least once a month in our practice. When such women ask for specific directions to preserve the breast contours, the following points are essential for counseling: (1) Pregnancy can do strange things to the breast. For the patient who has not been wearing a brassiere because of having nonptotic, good quality breasts with no loss of elasticity, the rules change. A support brassiere should be worn all day during the first 3 months and at night as well for the final two trimesters. (2) Skin creams are essential for protecting the breast from the deleterious effect of dryness, which would compound the effect of circulating hormones on the collagen. (3) It is possible to lose breast tissue, so the present implant may have to be replaced with a larger one after the pregnancy. (4) If it is the first pregnancy, the nipple color will probably darken, and the scar may become visible if a periareolar incision was used simply because pigment may appear outside the incision line. Scar touchup may be necessary. (5) When the breast regresses after delivery and cessation of breast-feeding, contractures are likely. In our experience, however, they are easily released by the closed technique. (6) Few patients gain breast tissue with pregnancy. It is conceivable that the fibrocystic content will vary, and the patient may be asked to resume vitamin E orally.

52. I have had a number of cases, even during the 1990s, in which Kenalog placed in an augmentation pocket or a double-lumen implant settled by gravity into the inframammary fold area. Kenalog does that. Aristospan and Solumedrol do not. The worst mistake is to remove the implant when this happens. *Removal of a prosthesis should be a last resort.* Internal repair using flaps of muscle, capsule, or breast tissue with proper knowledge of the dynamics of breast prostheses in relation to breast tissue is essential for restoring these breasts to normal without a prolonged period of deformity. Prolonging the deformity by implant removal makes the reconstruction infinitely more difficult. Implant replacement with internal flap reinforcement can be done immediately, however, if needed.

53. In reference to sudden capsular contracture, an apt phrase was coined by Robert Ersek (Austin). Fortunately rare, "firestorm fibrosis" is the sudden emergence of a dense capsular contracture after a relatively benign cosmetic breast procedure, such as a biopsy following augmentation or replacement with a larger prosthesis. Less commonly, it occurs after a primary breast augmentation. Early massage, intraoperative antiseptics and antibiotics, and other measures make no difference. (I have seen a few such cases diagnosed in the past as *Staphylococcus epidermidis* infections via culture specimens taken from the capsule. Others seemed to be related to changes in oral hormone therapy. Oral vitamin E capsular releases by closed compression and frequent massages can often slowly soften the breast over several months. In others, one must do yet another open surgical capsulectomy.)

Ersek described their experience as follows:

> "We would wait for several months thinking that hope and prayer might deliver us from a fibrotic fate. We did not usually reoperate until 6 or 9 months. With the development of the silicone textured implants, it was thought that no capsule could or would form." [It is true that replacement with a textured implant seems to give less chance of recurrent fibrosis, but it is not a sure alternative.] "After placing these [textured] prostheses in repeated-failure patients, and seeing the patient develop a second contracture, we thought surely there was a hematoma. Because

> we wanted tissue ingrowth into the surface, we decided to reoperate quickly to be sure the hematoma was evacuated. Alas, we found a brand new fat, thick, fibrotic area that had been formed within a week or two! These scar capsules measured more than 0.005 inch in thickness, and there was *no* tissue ingrowth. No frank hematoma was found, although there was bloody fluid."

This case indicates that no implant is perfect, but it is no reason to give up on the textured implants, particularly in the failed implant patients. There are more successes than failures and certainly a few more successes than if one uses a double-lumen prosthesis with antibiotics. Ersek's answer to the problem: He removed all the scar tissue and placed a drain with a vacuum bulb in the pocket. Every 3 or 4 days he injected 40 mg of Solu-Medrol into the drain and instructed the patient to wait 2 to 3 hours before restoring the vacuum. In three cases, the breasts remained soft and comfortable, and the "firestorm" did not recur. The three patients have now been followed for more than 12 months.

54. Surgeons who perform a large volume of breast surgery are hearing questions about nipple discharge with increasing frequency. A survey published in 1988 is still a good reference point: "To be significant, a discharge should be truly spontaneous, persistent, and nonlactational." Remember that water, serous, or serosanguineous discharges are surgically significant even though most are caused by intraductal papillomas or fibrocystic changes. The survey covered 503 patients operated on for nipple discharge: 13.3% had cancer and 7.2% had precancerous changes. More significantly, among 67 patients who were found to have cancer on biopsy, 10 had no palpable masses, 11 had negative cytology on the fluid collection, and 7 had negative mammograms.

The multicolored sticky discharge due to dilated ducts is usually treated medically, except when it becomes purulent and forms an abscess. Even then one should send the abscess wall to the laboratory to make certain there is nothing unusual present. Unless the patient is young, a "complete central duct excision" is advised for those with surgically significant discharges.

Technical point: To be sure if blood is present in the nipple discharge, use Hemostix, which can be obtained from any laboratory. Also remember that nipple discharge can be seen with the syndrome known as "joggers' nipples," due to traumatic erosions and irritation. Another interesting point is that patients taking oral contraceptives, tranquilizers, or rauwolfia compounds and those who have had oophorectomy or are near menopause can usually express a few drops of cloudy, gray, or green discharge by firmly squeezing the nipple. In general, it is no cause for concern. Also, remember that reddish-brown discharges can be easily mistaken for bloody discharges. The reddish-brown ones are simply due to duct ectasia and are most often seen in women who have borne children.

13 Breast Reduction and Mastopexy

In this chapter we discuss the techniques used to avoid the horizontal scar that may plague breast surgery. At times the standard T incision must be used, and some patients require a free nipple transplant, but I do not like to perform this surgery. Following are the major points to consider for mastopexy and reduction.

1. Most of the continuous problems with breast reduction and mastopexy are the horizontal scars, medially and laterally.
2. There is no reason to extend either one past the area that is covered by the breast itself. Use liposuction laterally and leave an extra fold of skin, even a "dog-ear," medially: The weight of the breast and the pressure of the brassiere will flatten it.
3. The new trend is to use liposuction liberally to reduce the breast, particularly in hard-to-reach areas. Gene Courtiss and Alan Matarasso discussed a group of older patients in whom liposuction alone gave them a comfortable and acceptable breast.
4. There is no excuse for hatch marks. Close all T incisions with subcuticular sutures. Any tacking stitches that are needed around the areola should be half-buried mattress sutures tied on the areola itself.

5. Always use drains. The one time you think you do not need them will be the time a small hematoma forms.
6. Spend time counseling young patients. Explain to them they can definitely have the operation, but it must be at a time that suits their life style.
7. If possible, use variations of the donut technique (see later in the chapter). General principles are exactly the same as for mastopexy or reduction, but the entire upper two-thirds of the breast serves as the pedicle, with blood supply and nerve supply left intact. Liposuction is used to reduce the bulk.
8. Instruct patients to wear a good support brassiere for at least 3 weeks and to sleep in a support brassiere for another 4 to 5 weeks to prevent late distortion. Start a program of skin care immediately after surgery so they can tolerate the brassiere. The regimen involves gentle cleansers, surface creams, and topical oils for flattening the incision.
9. Keep incisions covered with paper tape for at least 2 weeks. We use collodion on top of the tape to make it waterproof so patients can get it wet without fear of moisture pulling against the incision. Once the tape is removed, a good massaging oil helps to reduce irritation and flatten the everted skin edges.
10. Be prepared to tattoo (a good technique to know) because some patients lose color in the nipple despite good blood supply. Always tattoo a shade lighter than you think is needed.
11. This rule is obvious: Always examine the breast the night after surgery. There is nothing wrong with taking all the surface stitches out. If you think the nipple is getting dusky, it may indicate impending necrosis. Do not wait until the next day or a week later when you change the dressing for the first time to make this discovery.
12. What you leave behind is more important than what you take away. Preoperatively patients may focus on the weight of the breast, but later they are concerned with how well they fit their clothing and how easy it is to buy a two-piece bathing suit or a brassiere and panty set.
13. Do not hesitate to establish lateral blocks along the ribs with bupivacaine (Marcaine) at the end of a breast reduction. Adding epinephrine to the Marcaine does not significantly change the blood supply. Do not infiltrate around the nipple, however.
14. Make the breast smaller in an older woman who already has permanent changes from strap marks and permanent kyphosis. Advise young patients about the possibility of breast loss following pregnancy. Impart this information when planning the eventual size and shape of the breast.

Choices When Correcting Breast Ptosis

The primary goal of the aesthetic surgeon is to correct physical deformities with minimal detectable surgical sequelae. In cases of ptosis of the breast, certain patients must be resigned to accept a circumareolar and lateral or a T-shaped incision to restore the shape of the breast. In many cases, however, alternatives to standard mastopexy may be employed with long-term correction and decidedly improved appearance due to fewer external scars. Factors of patient selection and technical consideration that we have developed in our aesthetic surgical practice are as follows: If reduction of mass is needed, liposuction is required. The skin, particularly over the inferior half of the breast, must be of fair to good quality. The patient must be willing to accept the chance that correction to the absolute "youthful" idea may not be achieved and must understand that future surgeries, including even standard mastopexy, may be required. The choice of technique depends on the degree of ptosis, the position of the areola, and the need to reduce the breast envelope.

Patients who may be considered candidates for these procedures fall into four distinct categories and must fulfill certain requirements. In the first category are women with mild to moderate ptosis and atrophied breast tissue. Restoration of fullness is the major objective. A 1.5 to 2.0 cm inferior periareolar junction

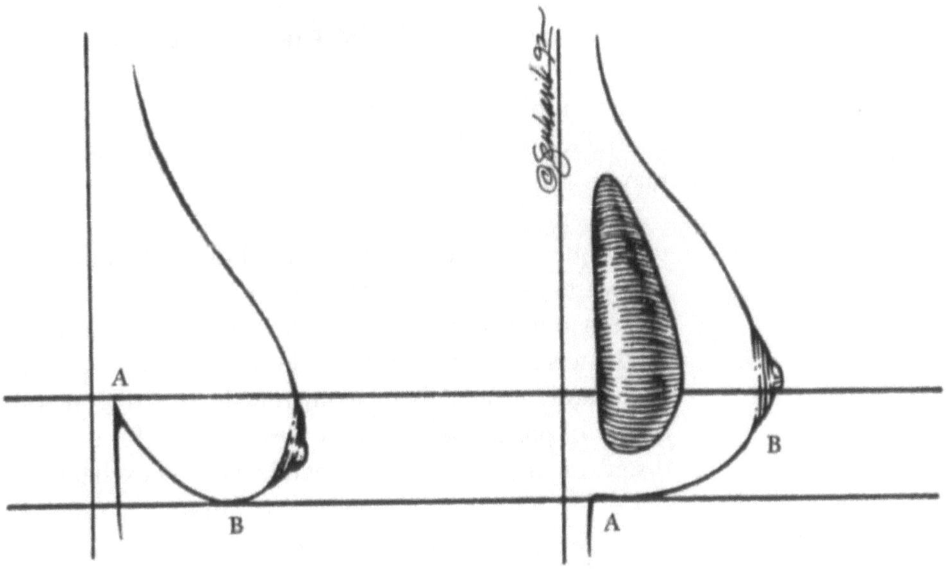

Figure 13-1. Lowering the inframammary fold without elevating the areola gives an illusion of breast lifting. If the fold is lowered only 2 cm, a normal-appearing breast is created. This type of illusion is performed through a short incision at the lower one-third of the areola.

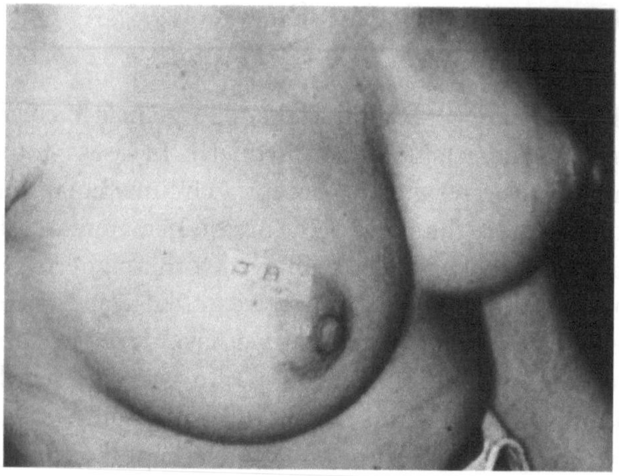

Figure 13-2. See text for explanation.

incision allows repositioning the inframammary fold from within and textured breast prosthetic augmentation. Repositioning the fold aids in concealing the breast descent, and the areola is pushed upward, as in Figure 13-2.

In the second category are women with a similar deformity but with descent of the nipple–areolar complex. Textured gel prosthesis breast augmentation with elevation of the nipple–areolar complex is performed via a single incision, which includes excision of a supraareolar ellipse of skin and soft tissue. Repositioning of the inframammary fold may or may not be required for visual correction.

The third category of women are those in whom stretching of the inframammary breast tissue has progressed to a greater degree. With normally contractile skin, the technique of "internal" mastopexy and areola repositioning may be employed.

A small number of women fall in the fourth category. Here internal repair techniques are used to correct stretching of the infraareolar portion of the breast or breasts years after breast augmentation.

In our experience, most mature or postpartum patients seeking breast aesthetic surgery are not fixated on the "youthful" upturned breast. Their peer group and role models are women with attractive "mature" figures that include a degree of ptosis of the breasts. Restoration of the lost fullness and, to a degree, disguising the ptosis are acceptable goals in exchange for minimal skin scars.

Category I

If moderate ptosis is accompanied by atrophy of the breasts, the first alternative to standard mastopexy may be proposed for approval. Rather than totally reshaping the breast with obligatory external scarring, as with standard mastopexy designs, we illustrate a compromise. An illusion of mastopexy correction can be created by prosthetic augmentation and lowering the inframammary fold from within.

Technical aspects of category I correction are as follows: A curvilinear incision along the junction of areolar and breast skin in the lower third of the areolar circumference is sufficient for developing a submammary pocket. Later, subcuticular closure of this incision rarely leaves a detectable scar. Medial and superior sharp scissors dissection allows choosing a wide-based, low-profile, textured prosthesis of a size consistent with the patients' wishes for superior fullness and cleavage without excessive forward protrusion. Under direct vision, scissors dissection inferiorly lowers the position of the inframammary fold 1 to 2 cm. A solution composed of a local anesthetic (Marcaine) with epinephrine, a cephalosporin antibiotic (Kefsol 500 mg per side), and a steroid (Solu-Medrol 20 mg per side) is instilled by a removable catheter during closure.

More than 200 such patients were reevaluated after 2 to 5 years. Continued ptosis occurred in fewer than 10%. The breasts of only five patients have progressed to the degree of ptosis that requires mastopexy for correction.

Category II

A smaller number of our patients have avoided standard mastopexy because a disguising optical correction may be obtained by the simple technique of elevating the nipple–areolar complex to a higher position on the breast mound, the so-called crescent mastopexy (Fig. 13-3). The new prosthetically augmented breast is normal in all respects except for the semicircular periareolar

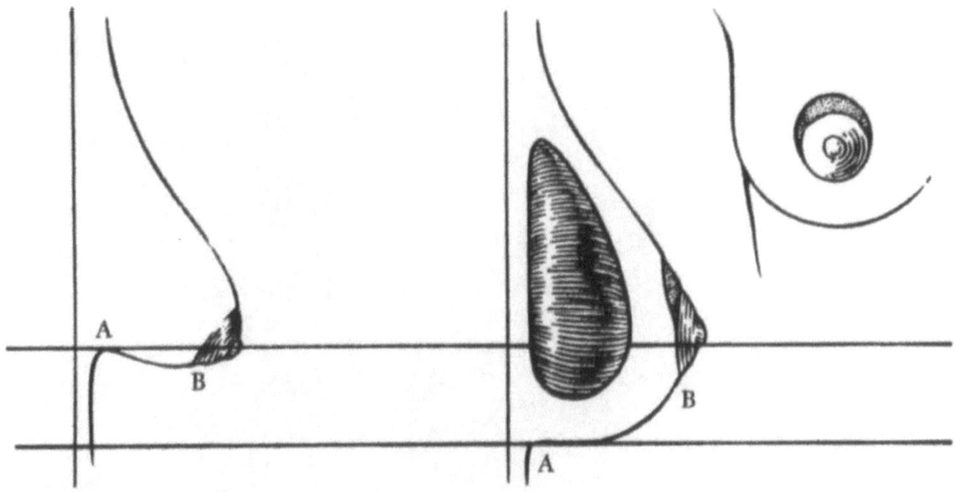

Figure 13-3. See text for explanation.

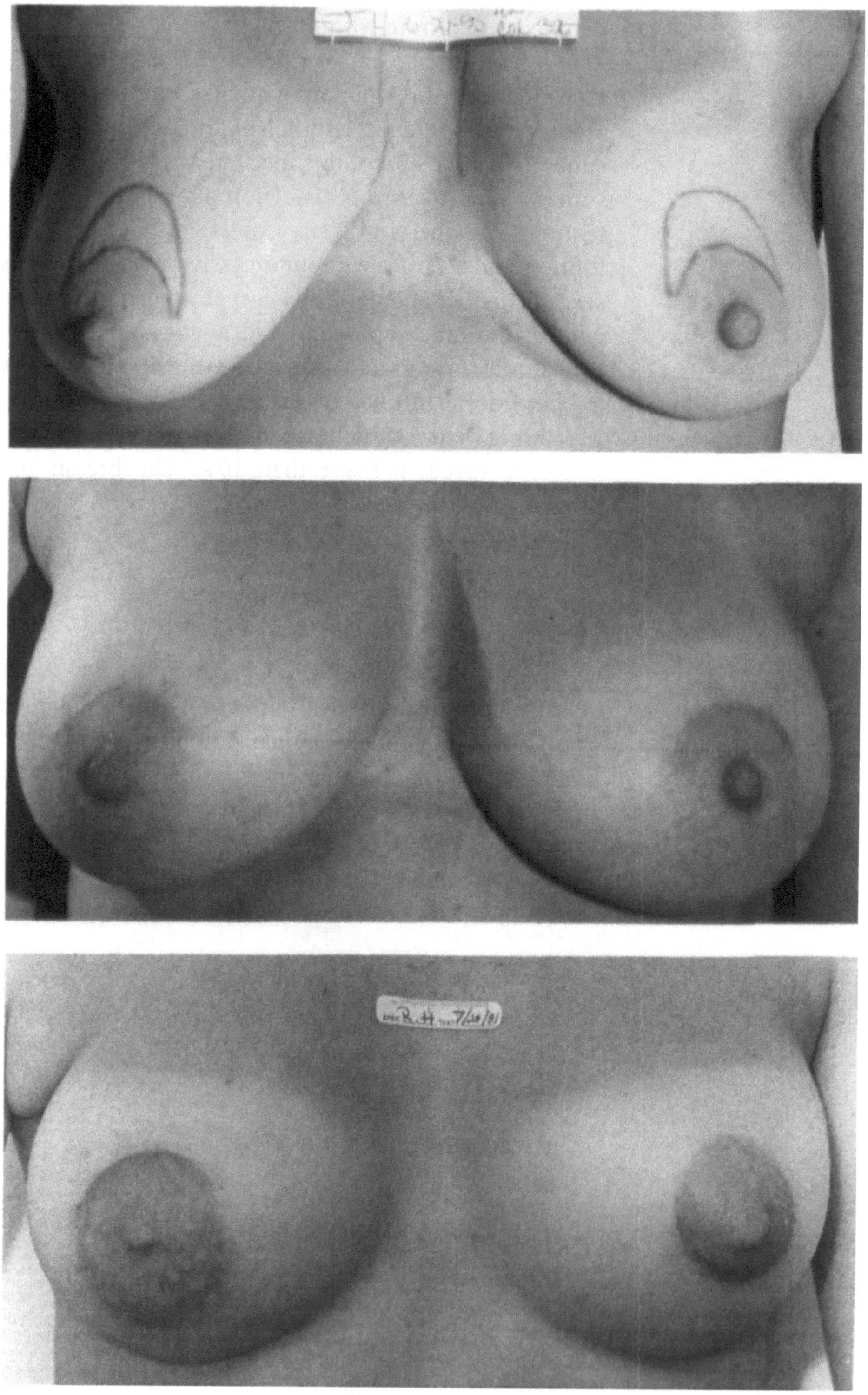

Figure 13-4A

B

C

Figure 13-5A

B

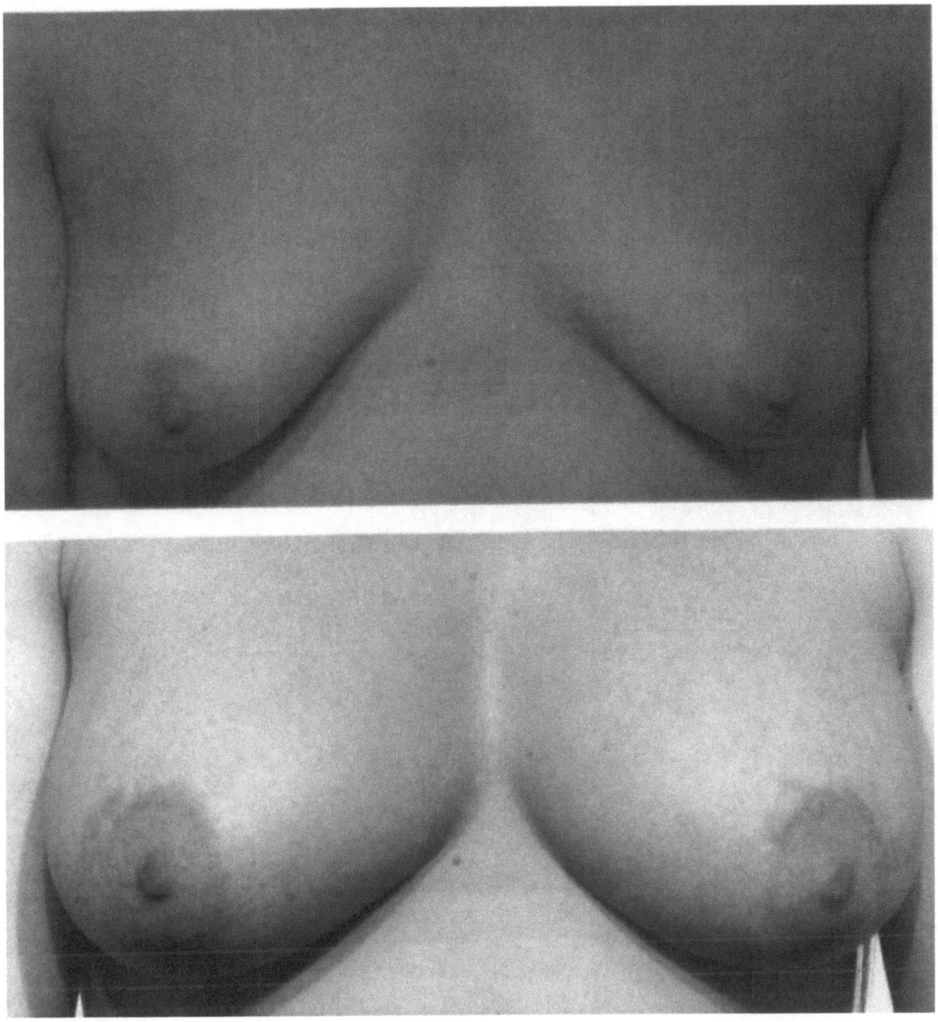

Figures 13-4 and 13-5. Unilateral and bilateral areolar elevation with augmentation. If one does not have to reduce the size of the areola, there are obviously fewer problems with hypertrophic scarring or stretching of the areola.

Figure 13-4. This ptotic right breast was realigned with a crescent excision, and the left breast was simply augmented through a standard short periareolar incision at the lower third junction. Lowering the inframammary fold further contributes to the illusion of mastopexy.

Figure 13-5. Manual stretching of the medial and lateral quadrants of the breast plus the choice of a wider-based prosthesis allowed us to create a normal-appearing breast for this patient without the circumareolar scar or the T scar of mastopexy. Three years later, the patient requested an increase in size because of atrophy due to pregnancy and delivery. At that point, she chose a slightly fuller contour, which was easily obtained by replacing her prosthesis through the original supraareolar incisions.

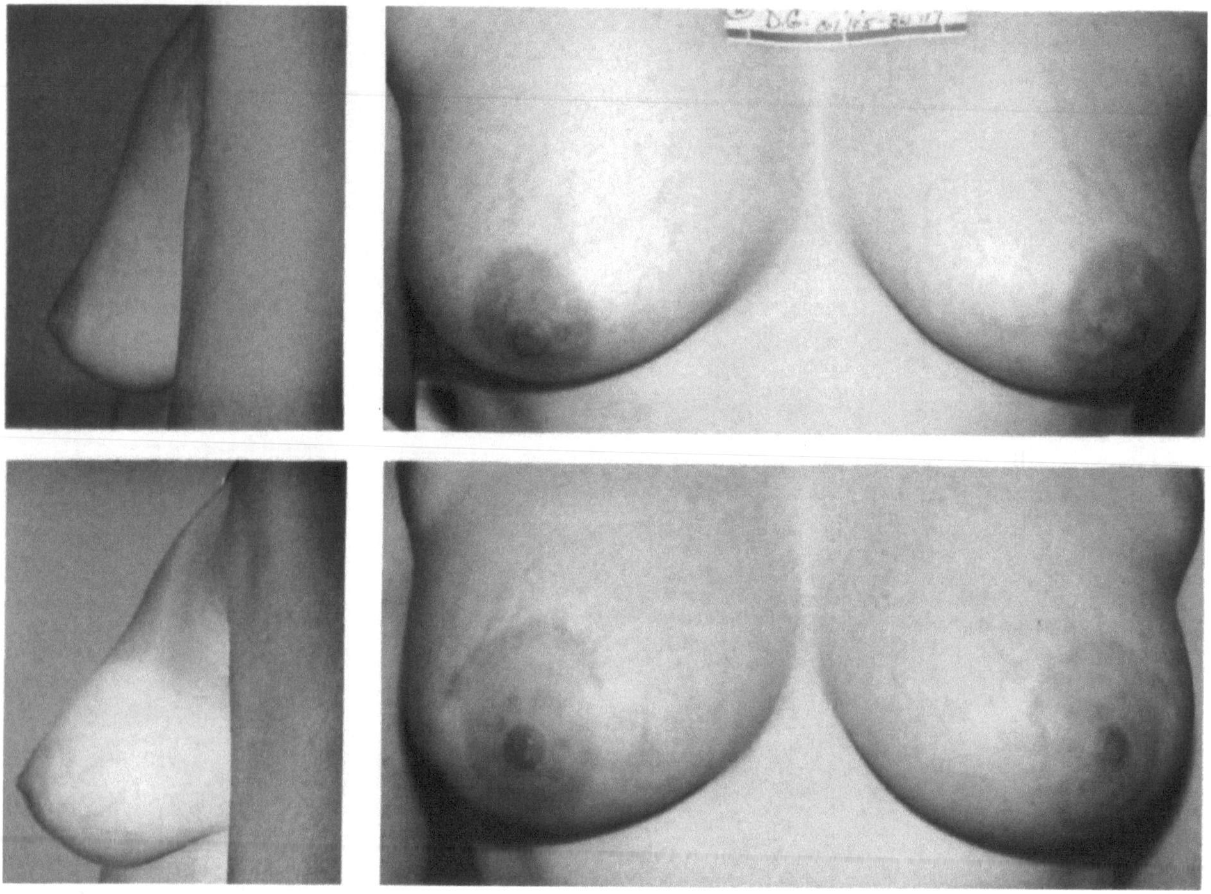

A B C D

Figure 13-6. See text for explanation.

scar above the areola and its relative position on the thorax (Fig. 13-4). Lowering the inframammary fold may or may not be indicated (Figs. 13-5 and 13-6). Insertion of the wide-based gel prosthesis and the sculpting of the submammary space are performed through the supraareolar excision site. With this exception, technical details of the operative procedure are the same as for category I.

A number of patients were reevaluated at 10 years. Only a few exhibited a degree of continued ptosis that required correction by "standard" or "donut" mastopexy and only after many years of satisfactory correction.

Category III

The technique for repairing the stretched parenchymal portions of the breast underneath the skin was developed because of the unpredictability of breast scars. The basic concept, which we have adapted, involves areolar

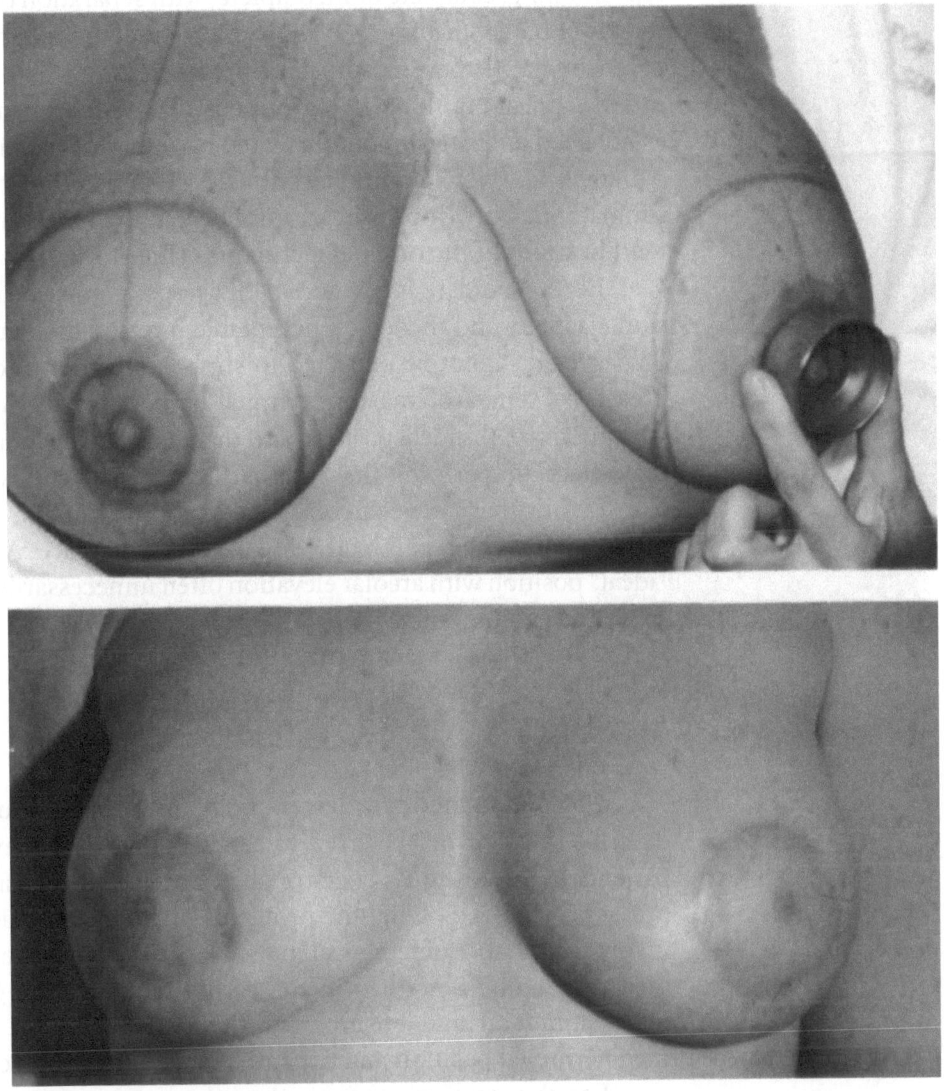

Figure 13-7. For this type of circumareolar repair with retention of the same breast prosthesis, the left-to-right overfolding maneuver is done after the inferior flap of skin and subcutaneous tissue have been reflected. The double Benelli advancement sutures bring the surrounding skin to the base of the areola. Internally, the soft tissues have been repositioned at a higher spot, and left-to-right overfolding has reinforced the breasts between the areola and the inframammary fold.

repositioning, complete or incomplete, with separation of the dermis and skin of the lower half of the breast to allow plication of the redundant underlying breast parenchyma. If there is sufficient breast tissue to give an acceptable mound, internal plication alone is performed. A new inframammary fold position is established and a new mound created by infolding existing tissues. Most of our patients, however, require additional size and fullness (Fig. 13-7). Adding a submammary breast prosthesis complicated the repair and led us to add several modifications of the original techniques (Fig. 13-8).

Each candidate for "internal" mastopexy must be evaluated for adequate skin elasticity and the lowest acceptable limits of areolar position. If the skin is damaged, it cannot be expected to shrink to conform to the new shape of the breast. A "standard" mastopexy must be performed. However, if the areola is within 2 cm of the ideal position and there is relatively normal skin elasticity, one may elect to perform the internal repair with or without areolar lifting. Considering that a lower areola is acceptable for patients past 25 years of age, we often simplify the repair by leaving the areola in place. An attempt to achieve an "ideal" position with areolar elevation often unnecessarily complicates the repair as well as adding visible scars.

Category IV

Obviously, there are fewer problems if ptosis can be disguised by the described maneuvers, referred to as "illusion" mastopexies, or in category III patients by repairing an overstretched breast and repositioning or removing a breast prosthesis. Solving the problems of "internal" mastopexy and reduction involves a number of technical maneuvers to prevent the areolar expansion and breast flattening described in the early literature. The goals are to create the internal mound and ensure that the reduced nipple and areola stay at a predetermined position and expand to an acceptable size.

For the small mastopexy, the inframammary position must be securely sutured at an acceptable level. One problem was solved by anchoring this tissue after completion of the Erol-type infolding. The infolding must be with multiple lattice-like sutures to ensure that stretching does not occur with subsequent flattening of the cone.

Figure 13-8. Internal repair. If areolar elevation is required, the procedure begins with removal of a circle of excess areola, skin, or both. The top point of the circle is the new site of the upper edge of the areola. Undermining the skin of the lower half of the breast helps the skin conform to the new mound shape. (A) With the inferior mantle of skin retracted, a parenchymal splitting incision is made from the new areolar site to the level of the new inframammary fold. A transverse incision is made at this level, and excess tissue at the base is trimmed away. These patients typically have an areolar–mammary fold of 8 to 10 cm. If preoperative evaluation

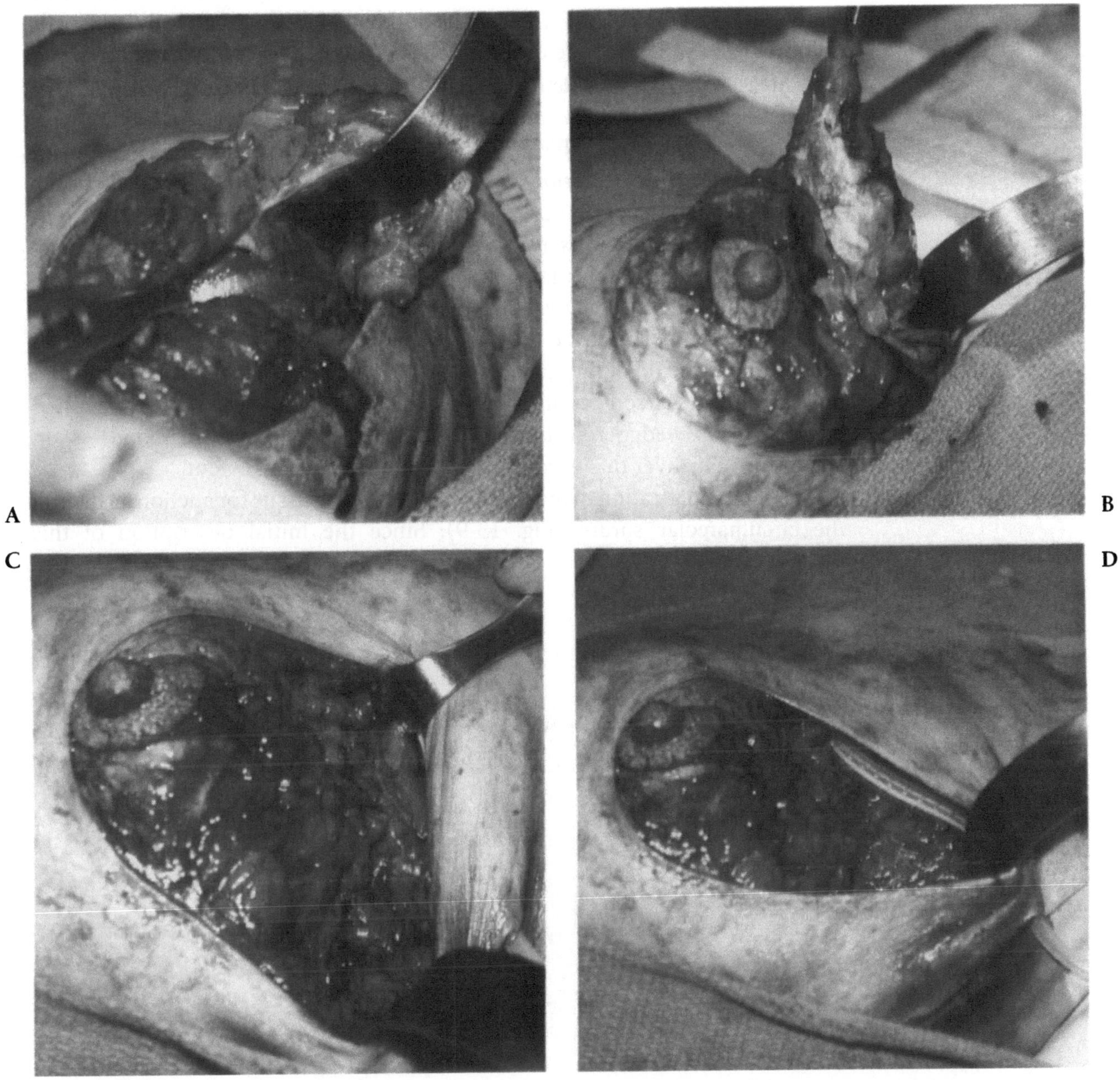

indicated the value of adding a mammary prosthesis, the submammary dissection is carried out at this point and a textured prosthesis inserted.

Two methods of internal repair were evaluated in our series. With the first method the excess tissue was simply excised and the edges joined in the midline with a series of heavy inverted Mersiline sutures. The new inframammary fold was attached to the posterior surface. After following several of these patients and noting that continued stretch became evident within 12 months, we adopted the technique we currently use. **(B)** A crossover multilayered closure is effected by passing the lateral wing of tissue underneath the medial breast and anchoring it to its undersurface. **(C&D)** After the inframammary fold has been established with sutures, the wing of medially based tissue is plicated over the closure. Imbricating sutures are used to obtain a smooth contour.

Adding liposuction, even for small reductions and mastopexies, was popularized by Luis Toledo. It solved the problem of the rounded ball shape with fullness at the superior edge of the areola. Aggressive use of liposuction in the large breast solved the problem of irregular distribution of breast parenchyma, as the major resection is in the inferior quadrant.

Creating the cone in the large and small reductions is no longer a problem if one considers this operation as a "subcutaneous Pitanguy wedge resection." Simply closing the wedge is only the beginning, however. The wedge is removed, the breast coned, and the excessive tissue at the base of the cone trimmed away until the desired shape is obtained.

With the circular removal of skin, the areola tends to remain in the center of the circle rather than at the superior edge, which would give it normal positioning at the tip of the cone. Removing a wedge of subcutaneous tissue and breast prior to the conization allows us to set the nipple at its predetermined position. This wedge resection (Toledo triangle or Texas diamond) is an anchoring maneuver that is completed before skin advancement.

Deepithelialization of the circle provides firmer tissue for anchoring bites of the circumareolar suture (Fig. 13-9). Since the initial description of this

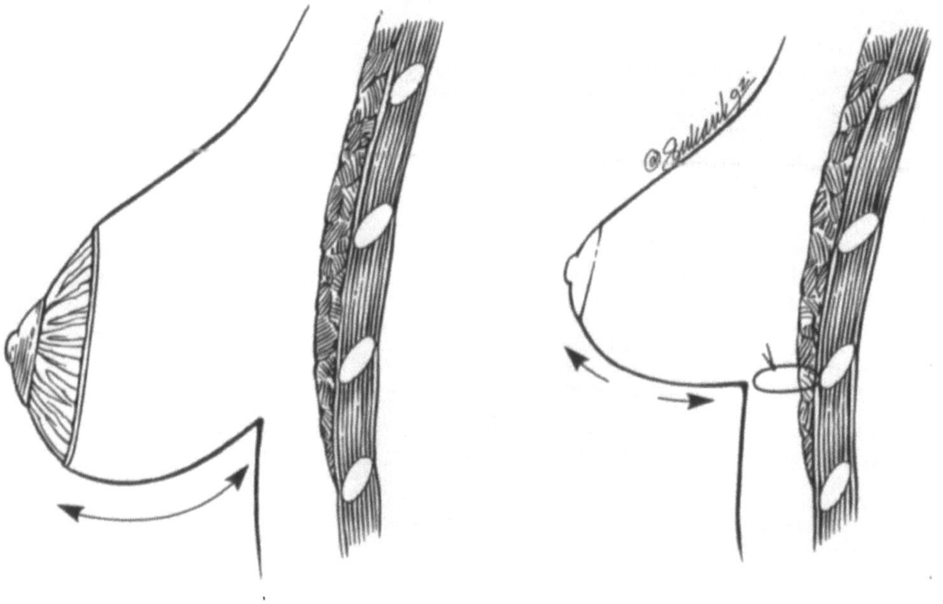

Figure 13-9. When one marks the area to be deepithelialized, the only absolute point is that to which the areola will be raised. Remember that the breast is to be made smaller with liposuction and then elevated. The skin in the lower half then shrinks and falls into the new position. Instead of reducing the length of skin between the deepithelialized zone and the areola to the usual 5 cm, leave an extra 2 cm or more to adapt to the new position. It is important to remember that the smaller the deepithelialized ring, the smoother is the closure. This figure also shows the internal anchors that reset the reduction or mastopexy breast to the desired inframammary fold level.

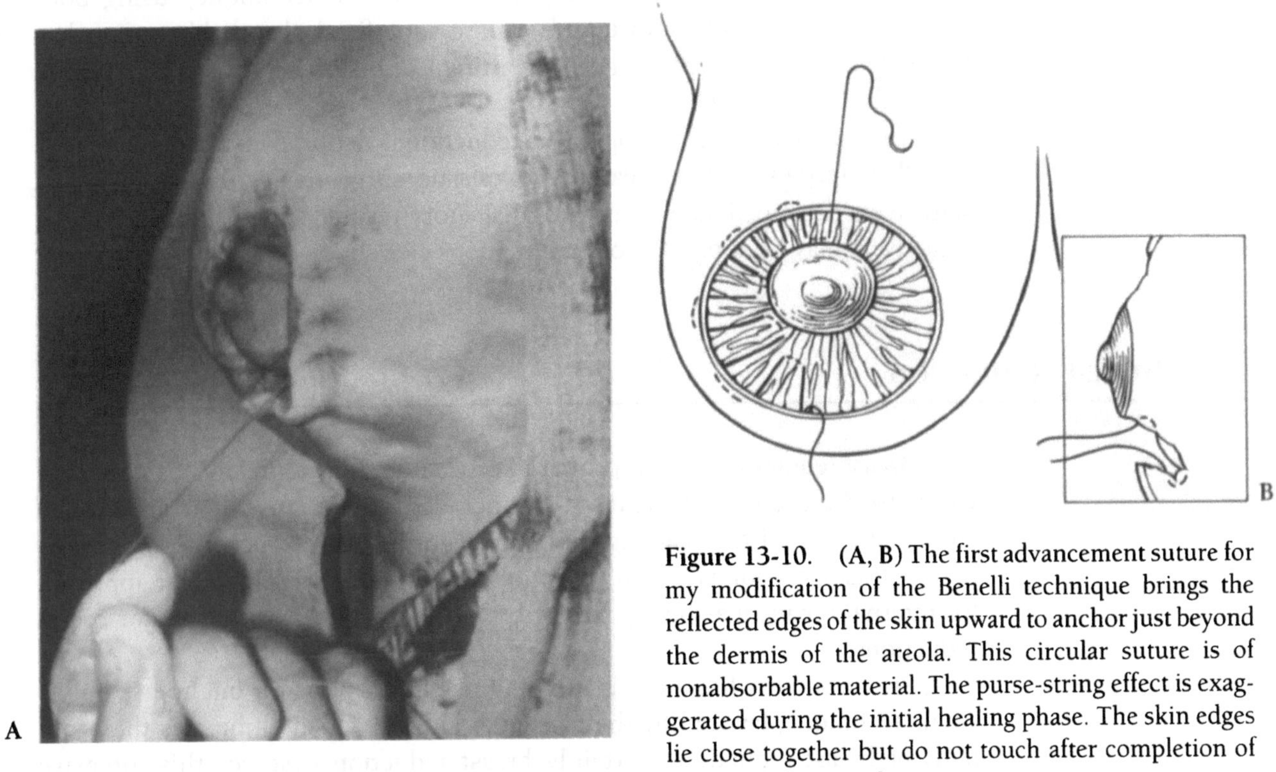

Figure 13-10. (A, B) The first advancement suture for my modification of the Benelli technique brings the reflected edges of the skin upward to anchor just beyond the dermis of the areola. This circular suture is of nonabsorbable material. The purse-string effect is exaggerated during the initial healing phase. The skin edges lie close together but do not touch after completion of the first circumareolar suture.

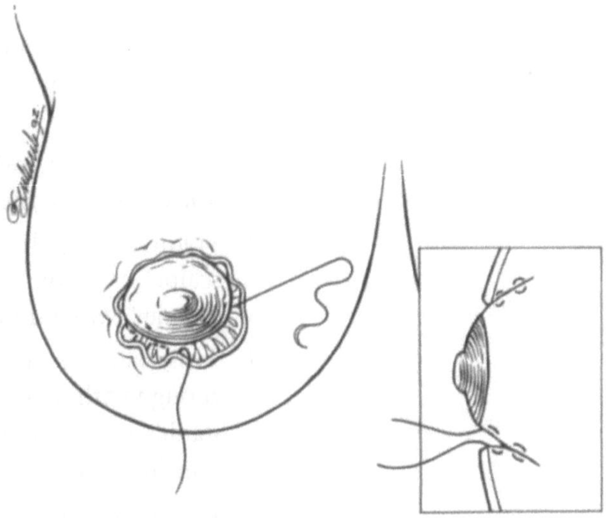

Figure 13-11. After first undercutting the areola so the skin edge can evert, the second circumareolar suture is placed using an absorbable suture, which prevents many of the problems of extrusion. Note that before placing this suture there is still a gap between the advanced breast skin and the areola. After placing the second suture in the subcuticular zone, there is still no tension on the areola. The suture bites are taken below the surface in the everted skin edges. Simply insert a few tacking sutures. A 6-0 nylon suture may be required for excess gapping. Ignore the fact that the areola is not perfectly round; it will return to its natural shape within the next several weeks. Anchoring in two layers, the weight of the breast skin is attached to the deepithelialized dermis, which largely avoids the complication of areolar stretching.

technique, the addition of crossing sutures (Benelli technique) using both Benelli's nonabsorbable suture and a more superficial absorbable suture has eliminated many of the problems of "spitting," or distortion due to knot failure (Figs. 13-10 and 13-11).

The circumareolar mastopexy or reduction is definitely a hands-on operation that appeals to the creativity of plastic surgeons. With the technical maneuvers described later, many unsatisfactory results can be avoided. (These maneuvers may be applied to other situations as well.)

Breast Reduction

Breast reduction is a compromised procedure. It is not really cosmetic, but we are working hard to make it so. It is included here because there are ways to eliminate much of the scarring. In contrast to the other procedures described herein, this operation is still in transition. I refer to the circumareolar approach for internal repair, mastopexy, minor breast reductions, and now major breast reductions.

Plastic surgery literature is full of impassioned pleas for one to use only a single technique, favored by the particular author, which eliminates the problems of breast reduction. Certainly breast reduction deserves this intensive consideration because, frankly, the results are often not optimal. The major points to consider are as follows.

1. Learn one good procedure, whether it is the inferior pedicle, superior pedicle, or (my favorite) the double pedicle McKissick method (Fig. 13-12A).
2. For standard breast reductions, it is important that the pedicle be kept thick to reduce the risk of areolar loss.
3. Traditionally, the lateral flaps were thinned with electrocautery or scalpel excision. Today, much of this step is done in a preliminary manner with a liposuction cannula.
4. Cross hatches are forbidden for breast reductions. The scars are bad enough without cross hatches. The same applies to closure with clamps, staples, or any other metallic device. Make all closures with subcuticular everting sutures.
5. Tacking sutures may be required around the areola. If so, make them half-buried mattress stitches so they are tied loosely on the areolar skin. These sutures evert the two skin edges. If a mark is made, it is a white dot that appears to be a new Montgomery gland.
6. For standard mastopexy, make the inferior incision as short as possible (Fig. 13-12B). Extend it only if absolutely necessary. Use liposuction

under the arm and defat the area directly under the skin beyond the incision. Remember that scars, laterally and medially, are the most troublesome.

7. The vertical scar is the least troublesome, which is why we discuss converting certain other large circumareolar procedures to a "lollipop" skin excision. The only thing wrong with this technique is when the scar extends beyond the new inframammary fold it becomes obvious, irritated, and is unattractive.
8. Always undercorrect. The worst problem in breast reduction is "star gazing." I have had to close the areola site in order to bring the nipple down to an acceptable position in patients who left their original surgeon because of this problem. Remember that ptosis elevates the areola over the next several years.

Circumareolar Approach to Mastopexy and Reduction

By definition, the circumareolar approach allows repositioning the nipple–areolar complex and reshaping the glandular portion of the breast from a subcutaneous approach. In contrast to "skin brassiere" techniques, the skin here does not play a role in maintaining the shape of the breast. The internal conization, reduction, and fixation at the new inframammary fold play the major role. In contrast to these skeletonized pedicles described in the plastic surgery literature, the entire breast serves as a pedicle for the nipple–areolar complex, and the mound itself is repositioned. In theory, this technique would preserve sensation to a greater degree as well as preserve the ductal structures. In the young patient, breast feeding is often impossible; even with the thicker bipedicle McKissock technique. Breast feeding is not compromised when the circumareolar technique is used.

The major advantage of the circumareolar technique is the avoidance of scars on unpredictable breast skin. Scars are a major concern for the young patient. Therefore in all patients except those with severe ptosis and extreme skin damage or those with massive, hypertrophied breasts, the circumareolar technique should be presented as a reasonable alternative. The circumareolar scar itself is no more predictable or controllable than the circumareolar scar that results from standard mastopexies or reductions. The major concern of many patients is clothing choices, irritation of the horizontal scar by brassieres, the probability of loss of sensation, and, most of all, minimizing visible reminders of the prior abnormality.

Our initial experience with the circumareolar technique was not good (Fig. 13-13). It is true that the circumareolar scars required frequent revisions—more so than the circumareolar scar from standard mastopexy-reduction. Moreover,

(Text continued on page 364)

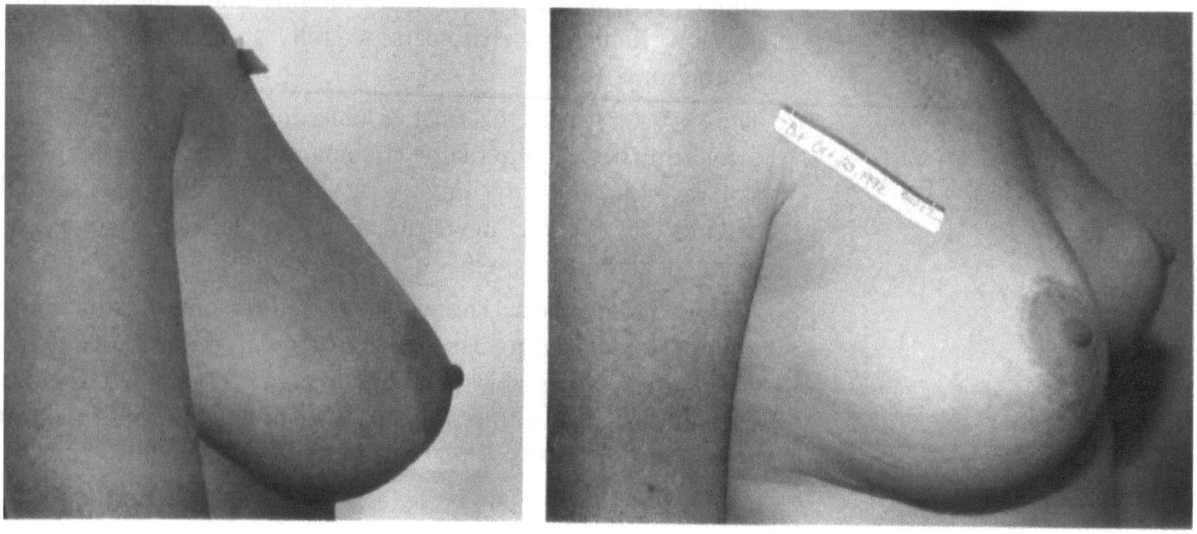

A B

Figure 13-12. McKissock reduction. Because it is as easy to perform a double-pedicle procedure as it is a superiorly based or inferiorly based single pedicle procedure, I prefer the security of the double-pedicle procedure, particularly in patients such as this one. **(A)** At this breast length, a free nipple graft is not the best choice; neither is a circumareolar reduction because of the quality of the skin and the size of the circle that would require deepithelialization, although we are now approaching more patients of this type with the circle procedure.

(B) Note the excellent elevation of the areola. Note also, however, that even with careful multilayered approximation, thick scars are present in the circumareolar area at 2 years. Experiences such as this one have led me to apply the techniques of "internal" reduction with the circumareolar technique in patients with this degree of breast hypertrophy. The question arose: If the best bipedicle reduction still requires touch-up surgery of the periareolar incision, why not avoid incisions elsewhere if one can obtain this degree of projection?

(C, D) Circumareolar surgery is contraindicated in this patient, who has suffered extreme thinning of the breast following pregnancy with descent of what was once an acceptable breast augmentation. The principle of circumareolar surgery is reflection of skin and formation of a stout internal brassiere with autologous tissues. These patients have little internal tissue. The standard mastopexy with the short-limb, lower, inverted T scar is the better choice. A multilayered closure of the dermis for a "skin brassiere" effect provides a longer-lasting result in these individuals.

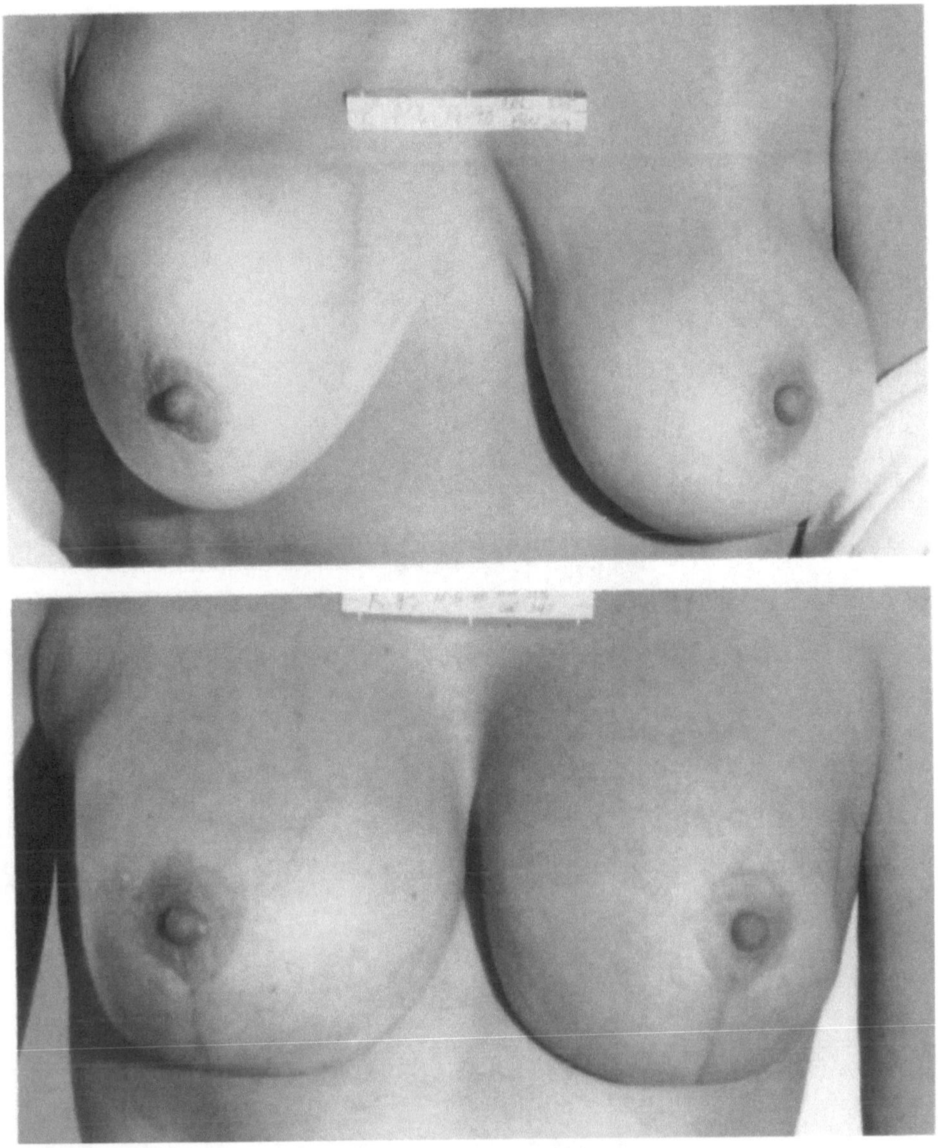

C

D

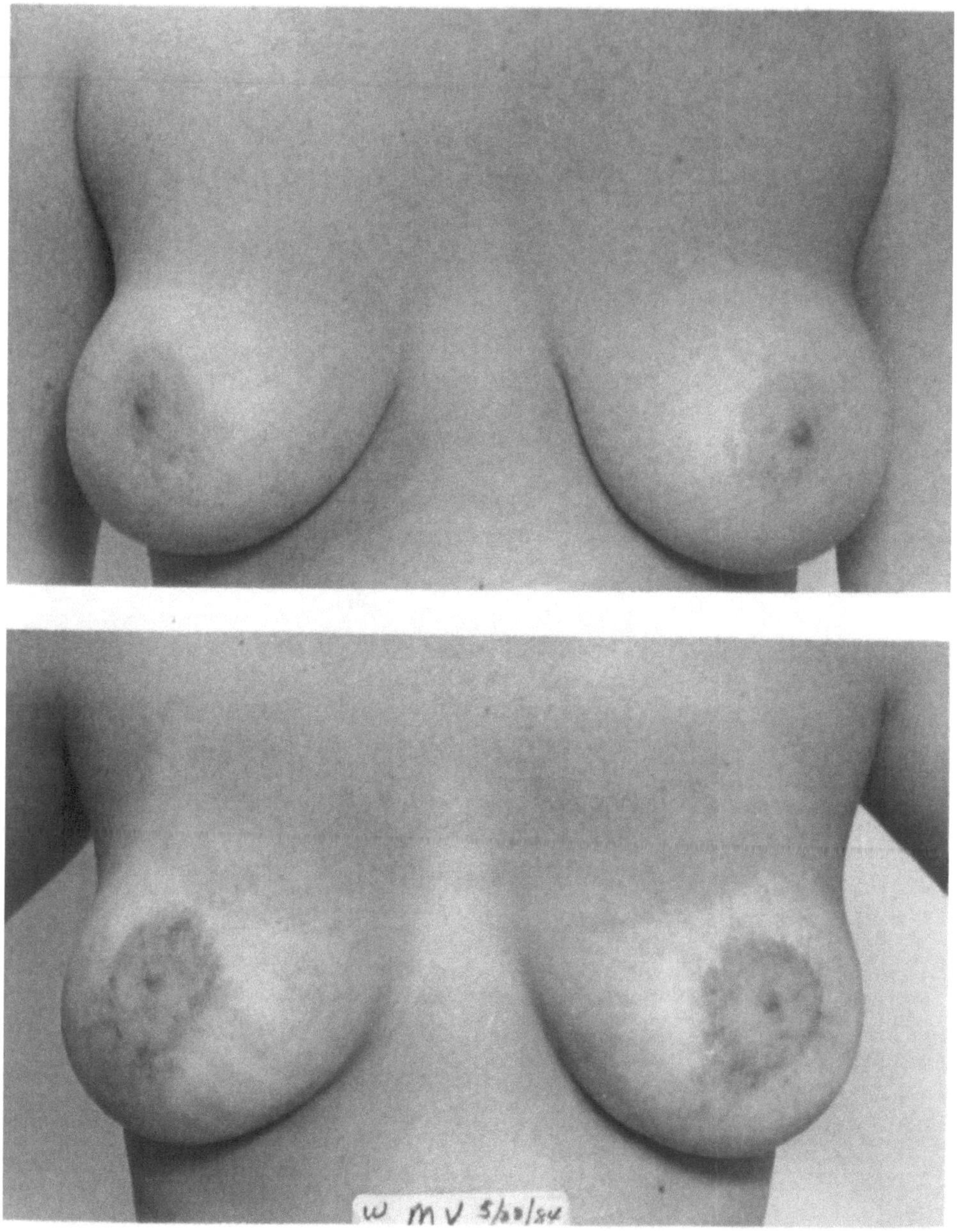

Figure 13-13. Circumareolar reductions in the past. Results such as those shown here indicated that we could at least make a forward-projecting breast; but without liposuction, double-advancement sutures, and multilayered internal coning of the breast, the results were not as satisfactory as those expected today. In this patient today, we would anchor the areola at a higher position by removing the "Texas diamond," perform deeper infolding and/or use liposuction to adjust the size and position, and prevent areola spread by using multilayered circular sutures.

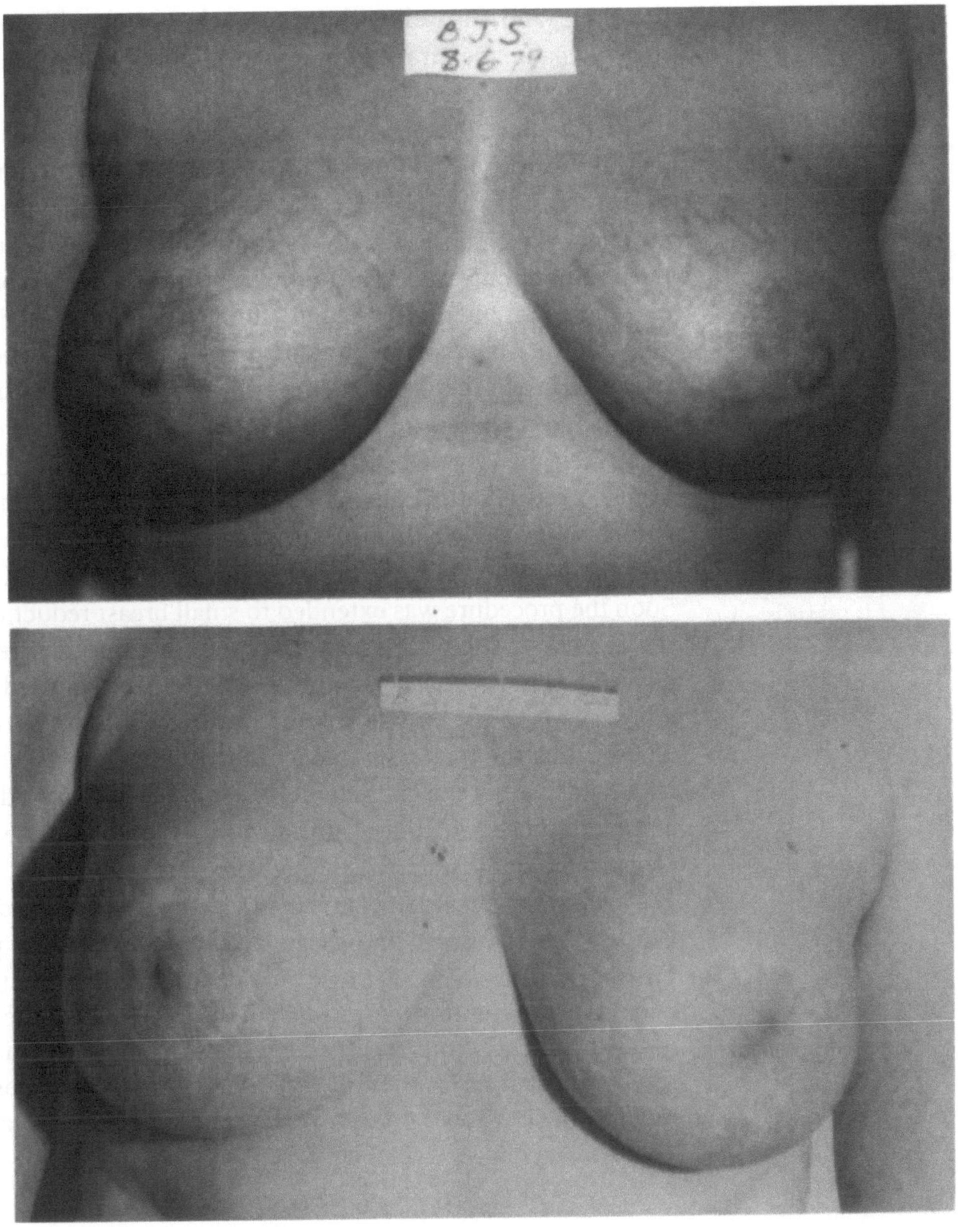
BJS
8.6.79

flattening of the breast, fullness above the areola, areolar descent to the center of the circle, and, most disturbingly, areola stretch with concomitant scar hypertrophy made the procedure less desirable. Many authors had contributed technical innovations and enthusiastically supported the procedure. Recent reports in the literature, however, must be considered as setbacks. The flat pancake breast is no longer an expected trade-off for avoiding vertical or horizontal scars. With increasing familiarity with the procedure and the incorporation of technical maneuvers contributed by many surgeons, it is unfair to refer to the circumareolar technique as unsatisfactory to physicians and patients, or, as one presenter described it, "the Benelli disaster" (Figs. 13-14 and 13-15).

The circumareolar technique became increasingly popular in South America and Europe thanks to the pioneering efforts of Onur Erol, who should be considered the father of the procedure. The techniques of infolding through a small incision provided elevation to small breasts. When the areola was elevated, a small excision of circumareolar skin allowed repositioning the nipple–areolar complex upward. With success in the small breast, measures were adopted to prevent distortion in these breasts by using mammary prosthesis augmentation. Soon the procedure was extended to small breast reductions (Fig. 13-16). With the aggressive use of liposuction, it soon became apparent the "lollipop" skin excision was no longer required. We had often used liposuction for final adjustments of the breast volume during reduction surgery (Figs. 13-17 and 13-18), but the aggressive use of liposuction as a primary tool is now an invaluable part of the circumareolar approach and indeed has been described as a primary procedure for certain categories of individuals who do not require the elegance of breast reshaping along with mass reduction.

Adopting circumareolar principles to repair distorted or stretched breasts is valuable for the practicing surgeon. Due to either low placement of a breast prosthesis or stretching because of gravitational or muscular factors, a number of patients are presenting with stretch of the lower half of the breast without areolar descent. Subcutaneous repair allows the surgeon to recreate the original shape of the breast with restoration of the inframammary fold position; with reinforcement by the crossover procedure, future ptosis of this area may be deterred (Fig. 13-19).

Mastopexy

The trend in traditional mastopexy is to shorten the horizontal limb, but one does not eliminate the vertical limb. With many mastopexies, breast implants are added for fullness and projection. Although mastopexy by the circumareolar technique is still the operation of choice for most of our patients, it is by no means the only approach.

I began to work with the circumareolar mastopexy technique in 1976 after seeing reports from Rossell, Bartels, Erol, and others. I was impressed by Erol's presentations. Onur Erol was first noticed by the American surgeons when he and Mel Spira coauthored an article on circumareolar mastopexy. He emphasized making a cone of tissue by infolding the breast after separating the skin and elevating it. It was not emphasized that a thick pad of subcutaneous fat should be left, nor was it noted that large breasts would require other procedures to prevent the aforementioned problems of areolar spread.

In 1986 I presented an update on a number of patients I had been following and pointed out that scar hypertrophy was still a problem and perhaps more so than with standard mastopexy; moreover it was difficult to maintain a cone shape with the techniques we were using. I also showed a number of patients whose breasts had more of a ball shape with projection above the areola than I had wished and others in whom the areola did not stay at its elevated position. Louis Benelli and Luis Toledo also gave presentations on the circumareolar technique. Each emphasized a different approach, both of which have been incorporated into mastopexy and reduction procedures. Following this 1986 RAPS symposium, a number of us have borrowed from each others' techniques and ideas and have settled on a general approach to reduction of large and small breasts and to mastopexy.

Benelli's contribution was the deepithelialized circle, although we use smaller circles today. The dermis provides a stable bed for attachment of an advancing circumareolar suture.

Various forms of infolding of the breasts with rotation flaps may be employed. In American series, we commonly add a breast implant to give fullness, as large breasts are considered desirable.

Holding the areola at its superior position was a problem, but Toledo suggested removing a triangle, a wedge, of subcutaneous tissue and then anchoring the areola at its new position before beginning the circle advancement. His emphasis on liposuction to maintain the final contour was the last piece in the puzzle.

The goals of circumareolar mastopexy are the same goals as for standard mastopexies. The only difference is that the skin over the lower half of the breast is reflected and the tissue is infolded with or without augmentation.

Internal Repair from an Areolar Approach

The two categories of patients who require repair of the breast parenchyma are those with the "Snoopy nose" deformity and those in whom breast protheses have overly stretched the wall of the breast between the inframammary fold and the areola. The latter is unfortunately common.

The "Snoopy nose," or areolar breast is an underdeveloped breast with a shortage of tissue below the areola and excess tissue directly underneath the areola. As shown in Figure 13-20A, this breast can be adequately corrected through a short periareolar incision. It is not necessary to rotate flaps or to make

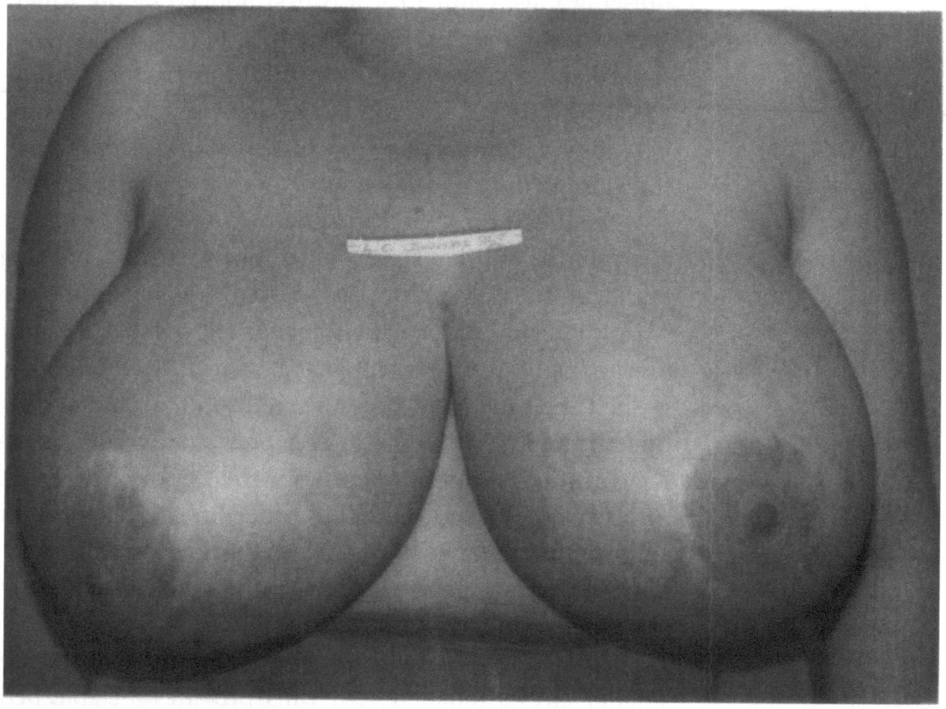

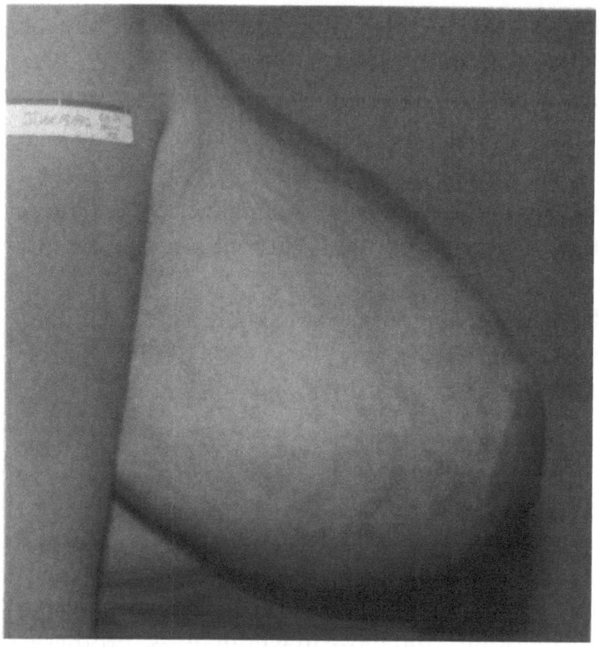

Figure 13-14. When not to use a circumareolar reduction. I am not comfortable with circumareolar reduction for massive breasts, as in this patient or for breasts that have multiple stretch marks (indicating poor-quality skin retraction and poor dermal blood supply). In 1983, at age 23, this patient asked for a premarital breast reduction, as her breasts had reached a size that caused considerable symptomatology. Note the strap marks on her shoulders and the relative symmetry of the breast enlargement. We used a standard McKissock reduction which resulted in her being able to wear a C cup brassiere. However, her breasts continued to enlarge almost from the day of the operation. At 9 years after the

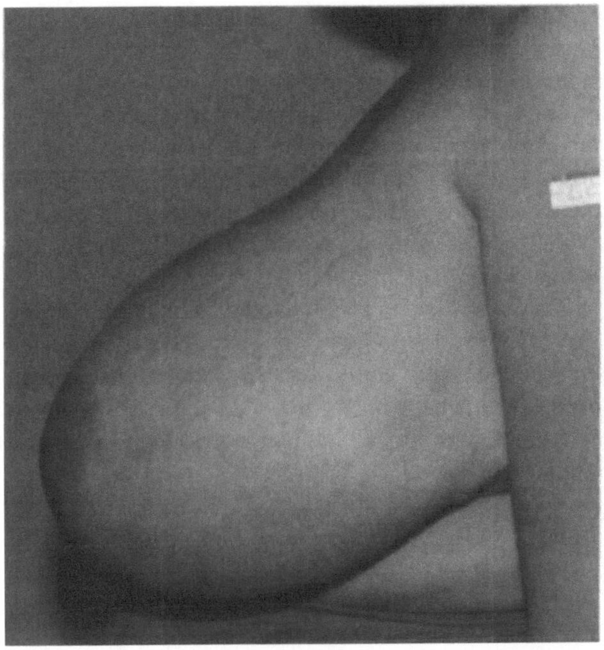

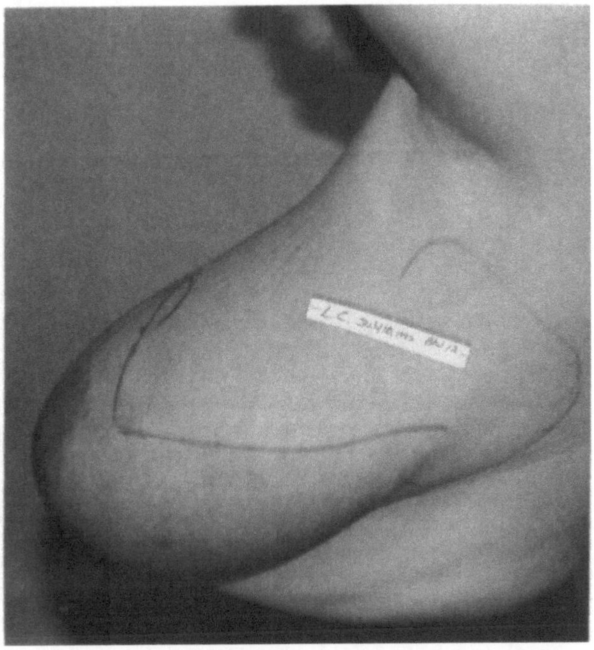

reduction, her breasts were once again troublesome. When this amount of tissue has regenerated, it is advisable to remove the nipple (replacing it later as a free nipple graft) and the entire ductal system at the same time. This method is not a 100% guarantee against recurrence of virginal hypertrophy, but it should reduce the risk. At 6 months her breasts have retained the size and shape we recreated. Note in the preoperative drawings that liposuction will be used in the anterior axillary line area. The long incision is placed to meet the original long incision made in 1983. Today we keep these incisions shorter, even in large-breasted patients, because the "dog-ear" that is located underneath the breast fold flattens with time.

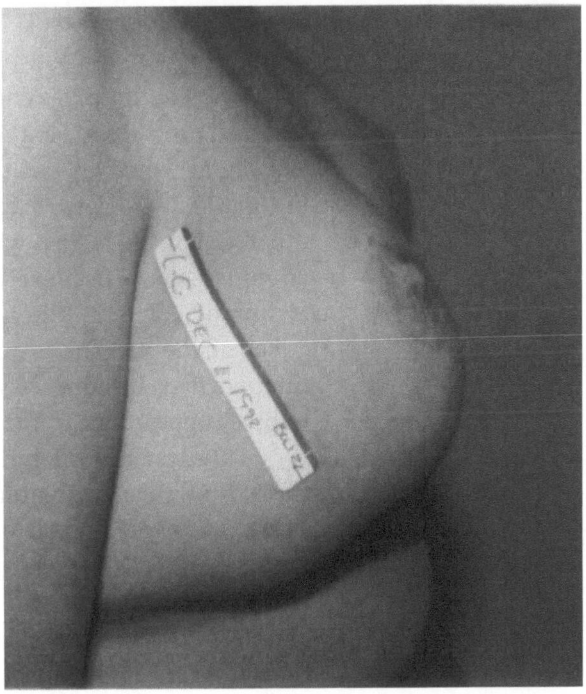

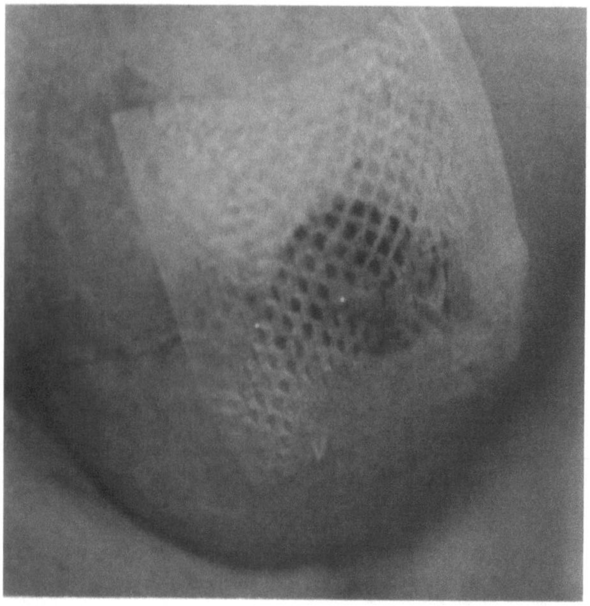

Figure 13-15. For standard reduction mammoplasty, the areola–skin edges are usually tacked with half-buried mattress sutures. It is imperative that these sutures be removed rather quickly to avoid stitch marks on the areolar skin. For the circumareolar mastopexy, the same eversion of the skin edges occurs. Standard Steri-Strip tapes applied following suture removal are often accompanied by pooling of exudate from the everted edges. Mesh tape provides support as well as free drainage.

As a resident in plastic surgery at St. Louis University in 1969, I developed mesh tape as a means of immobilizing skin grafts. A mesh skin graft device had been developed during my general surgery residency in Atlanta, and it was a simple progression to design a similar tape.

any scars on the breast skin itself. The technique involves internal stretching of breast, rotation of a soft tissue flap from underneath the areola to reinforce the depression at the lower edge of the areola, and augmentation of the breast with a textured prosthesis. Textured prostheses are chosen because of their immobility. They hold the newly created space in position. These young women have small but markedly fibrotic breasts, and a soft prosthesis would be distorted by the inherent tension factors within breast parenchyma. When the areola is large, the circumareolar procedure we have described is used as well as the internal flap technique (Fig. 13-20B–E). Long-term results are excellent. The gravitational effect of the prosthesis rounds out the lower portion of the breast; and the internal flap, in concert with the gravitational effect, eliminates the "double bubble" appearance of the original deformity.

I always reset the inframammary fold internally, several centimeters above the old inframammary fold to shorten the areola–inframammary fold distance. This may involve resection of breast parenchyma as well. The typical patient requiring internal *repair* for mastopexy requires reinforcement. The technique of left to right "pants over vest" reinforcement, shown in Figure 13-20F, is extremely useful. I have been following patients with this type of repair for more than 10 years, and their breasts seem to resist the effect of gravity (Fig. 13-21).

The last category of patients are those whose breasts have enlarged to the point that a breast implant can be removed. A rotation of tissue similar to the Benelli "round block" procedure is useful here to fill out the empty space. It is not necessary to resect the capsule, but it is important to move the excess tissue into position underneath the areola to prevent extreme flattening. Fortunately, most of my patients had developed such increases in breast volume over a period of 10 years or more that natural-appearing breasts could be obtained with minimal tissue rotation.

In the "ballooned out" breast, the prosthesis has been placed in a position that is either too low or under a completely divided pectoralis muscle in an active young woman (Fig. 13-22). Over time, a significant number of these patients have shown excessive stretch with a rather bizarre "balloon" deformity of the breast in the space between the areola and the inframammary fold. As distressing as it may be, it would be more distressing to correct this defect with an external mastopexy incision of the inverted T type. Internal reinforcement and repositioning the prosthesis is the answer.

The technique for repairing the areolar breast with a large areola is as follows. A 3.8-cm incision is made around the nipple, leaving a smaller than than normal areola. All other pigmented tissue is deepithelialized as described by Benelli and others. Entry is made into the submammary pocket through the tissue just below the new areola between 3 o'clock and 9 o'clock, and a pocket is prepared using blunt and sharp dissection. Sharp dissection is particularly useful for reestablishing a correct inframammary fold position and dissecting superiorly and medially. Once internal dissection has been completed, the undersurface of the areola is everted for direct visualization. A U-shaped flap is developed with its base at 6 o'clock. Once this tissue has been dissected, the areola is now reduced to one-half its original thickness. A prosthesis of the appropriate size is positioned, and the flap is rotated downward and sutured. This reinforcement brings the tissues between 6 and 9 o'clock up to a normal curvature, repairing the original indentation. It may be necessary to break up circular fibroses between 9, 12, and 3 o'clock as well. Standard subcutaneous subcuticular closure with absorbable suture is then completed. We instill Keflin, Marcaine, and 20 mg Solu-Medrol at the end of the procedure and then withdraw the cannula that had been left in the incision.

After 10 days the patient is allowed to bathe without the brassiere and then to slowly progress to going "braless" as much as possible. Once the textured implant begins to become more mobile, the breast slowly assumes an even more natural shape. Because a number of these young women were originally ptotic, we advised resumption of brassiere-wearing once the shape has been achieved so further stretch would not occur during the years to come. This program has been successful for maintaining a natural and unscarred appearance (Fig. 13-23).

A short periareolar incision is also utilized for the "ballooned-out lower half-breast, even if the patient's original augmentation may have been performed through another approach. As for the circumareolar mastopexy, the skin and subcutaneous tissue is reflected over the lower half until the breast wall is visualized. A vertical split is then made with cutting cautery, and the prosthesis is removed. If the prosthesis was underneath muscle, a new expanded pocket is

(Text continued on page 377)

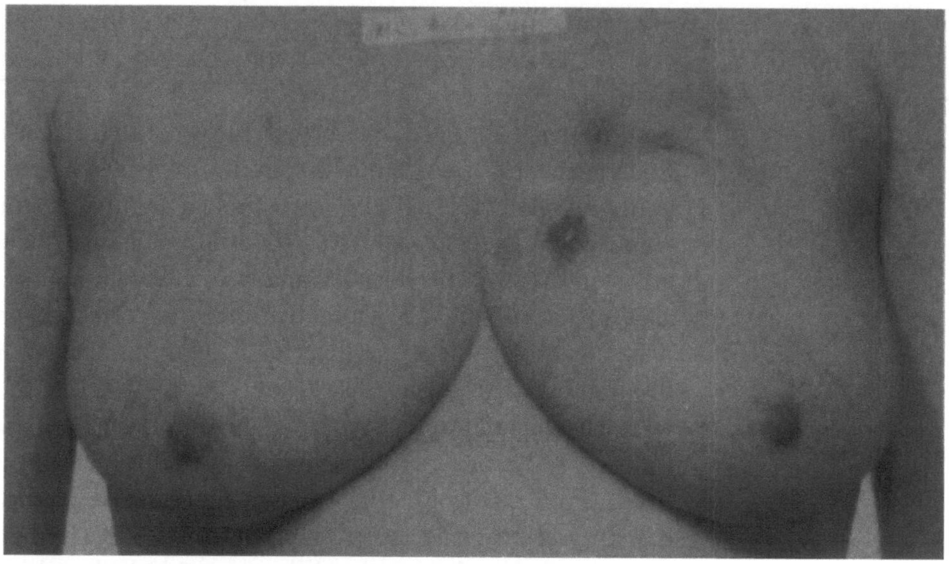

A

B

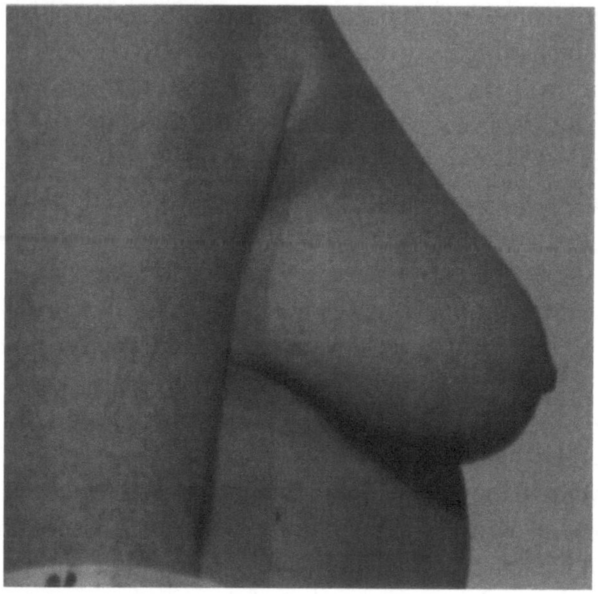

Figure 13-16. Moderate reduction of the opposite breast using the circumareolar technique. **(A)** This patient presented with a biopsy-proved carcinoma of the left breast and underwent immediate reconstruction **(B)**. **(C&D)** At the second-stage surgery, a balancing procedure was performed on the right side. The xerogram was negative, so it was an option to simply reduce the breast volume. For moderate reductions of this type, the circumareolar technique is more predictable. A small wedge is resected after the skin and subcutaneous tissue have been reflected, and a small cone is created using the multiple-suture technique.

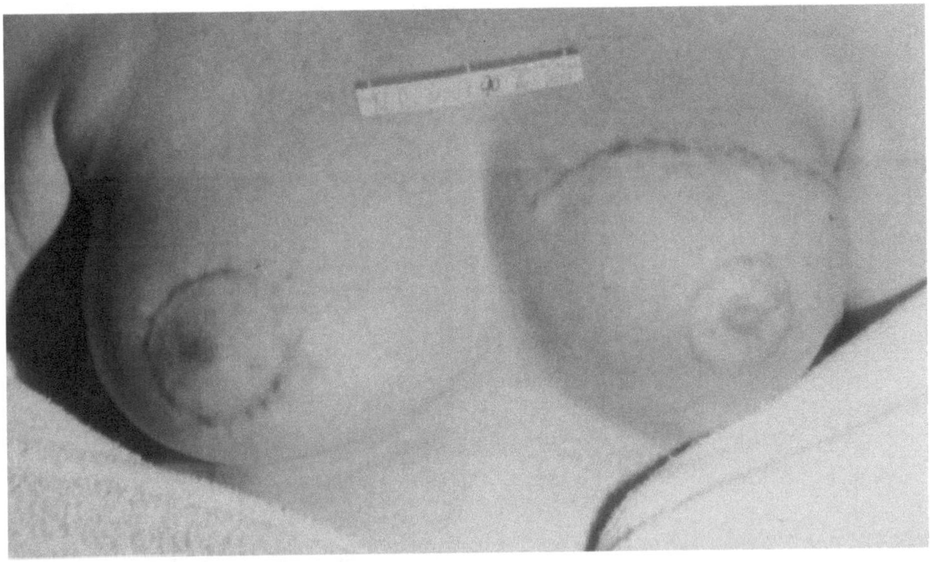

C

D

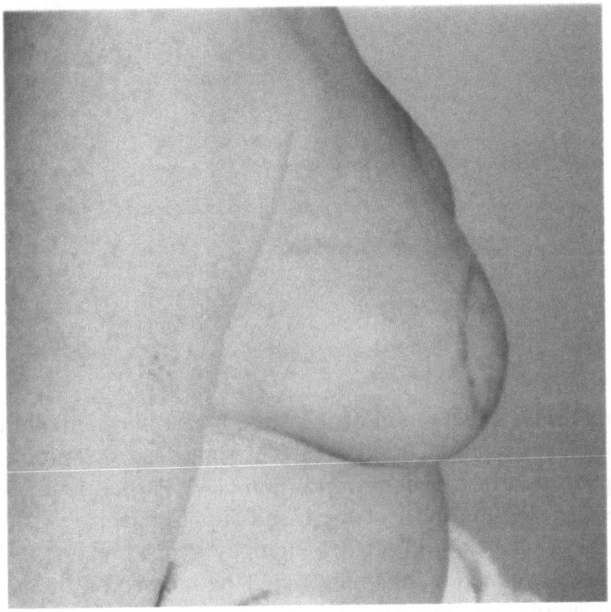

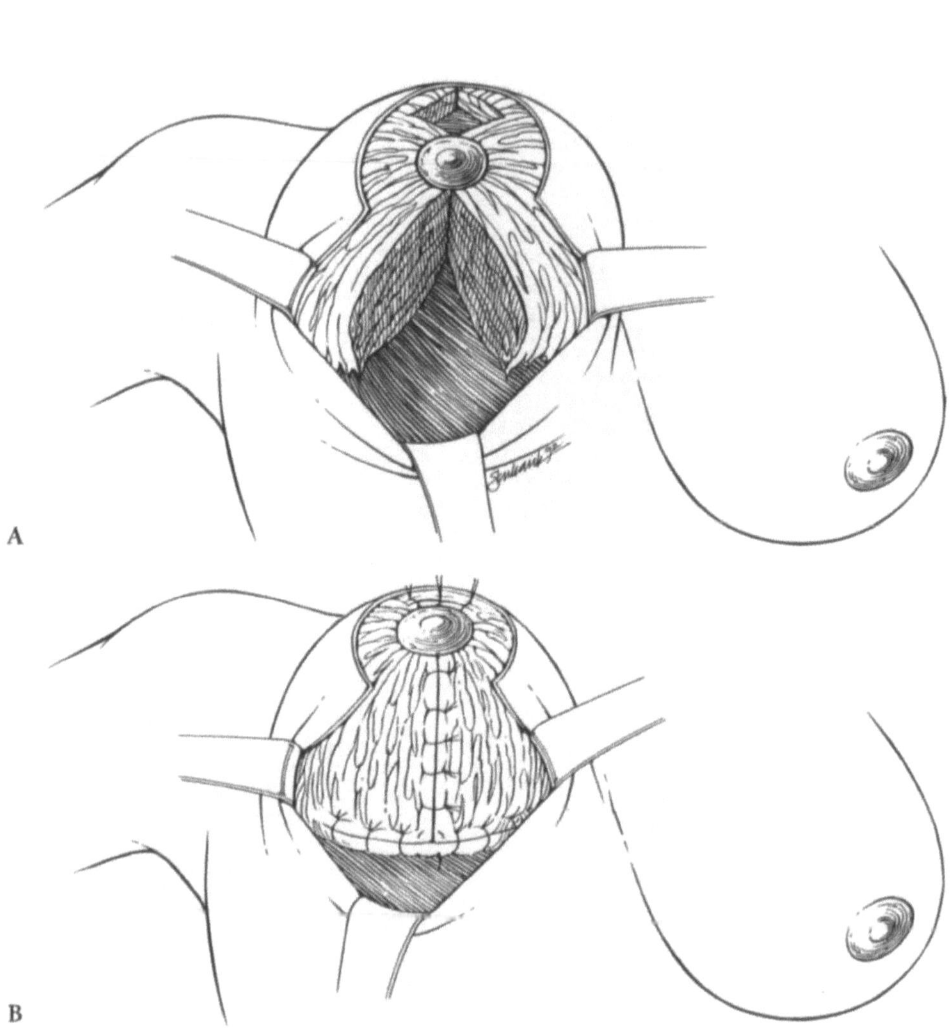

Figure 13-17. Reduction of the large breast is essentially the same as for the small breast. The deepithelialized area is designed so the nipple–areola complex may be brought upward to its new position. **(A)** Partial-thickness soft tissue excision is performed, leaving most of the blood supply intact over the upper two-thirds of the breast. With the skin reflected, a Pitanguy wedge is excised. **(B)** The left and right sides have been trimmed to an appropriate length based on the position of the now secured nipple–areola complex. This distance should measure 5 to 6 cm. Anchoring sutures are then used to secure the lower edges to the pectoralis fascia, and a series of imbricating sutures are used to secure the cone shape underneath the skin.

Our experience with large reductions using the circumareolar technique came as a result of requests from patients who did not want scars that would rub on brassieres or be obvious when changing clothes. The addition of liposuction has made it an even better procedure than in the initial cases. Patients C.J. and A.C. are young women who initially desired only a modest reduction in volume. Because the skin quality was excellent, I decided to try the circumareolar technique with only a moderate amount of liposuction adjustment.

Patient C.J. is shown preoperatively in 1989 and then 5 months postoperatively. The shape conformed exactly to her wishes for a modest reduction. We have received reports that the shape has remained the same and the wrinkling has disappeared

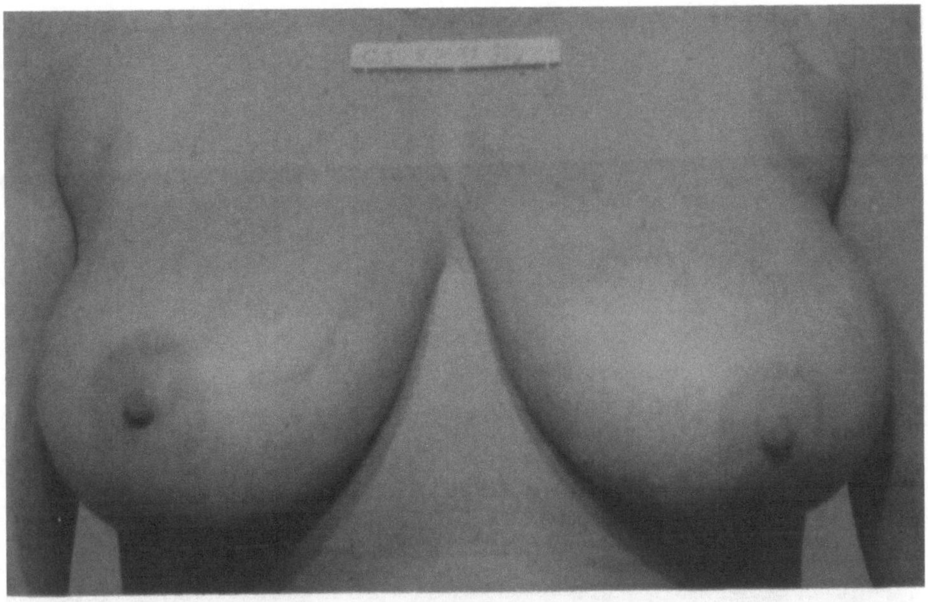

C

D

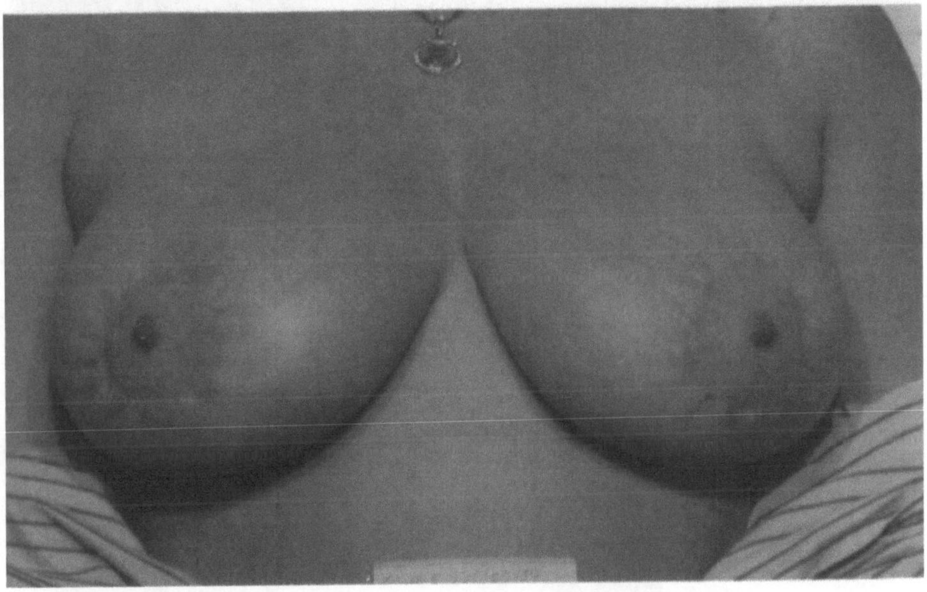

subsequently. Note on the lateral view that the breast retains a cone shape due to the internal wedge resection and cone formation with resetting of the inframammary fold. In this initial group of patients I was concerned with subsequent areolar lifting to an unacceptable position and purposefully placed the areola at a somewhat lower spot.

Patient A.C. underwent reduction in 1990, requesting a moderate reduction. In this patient the single Benelli suture surfaced, leaving an unacceptable scar, as shown in the upper quadrant of the right areola. The scar was still evident at 18 months, so further revision was planned. Six months after the revision a reduction has been performed on both sides and the areola repositioned. Fortunately, the edema that was still evident on the right side at 6 months resolved over the ensuing 6 months, and secondary liposuction was avoided.

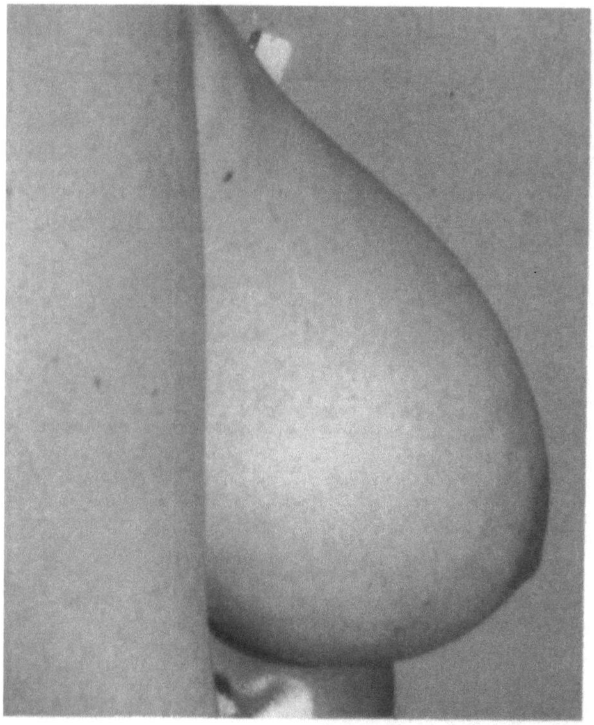

E

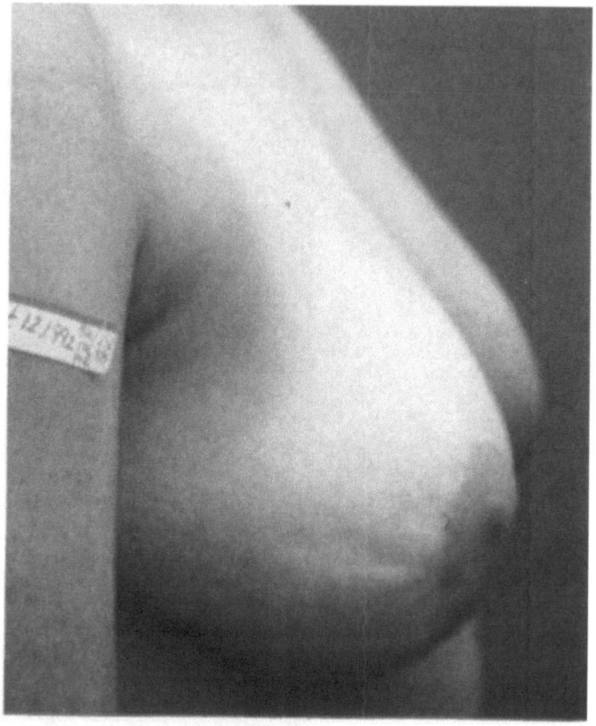

F

G

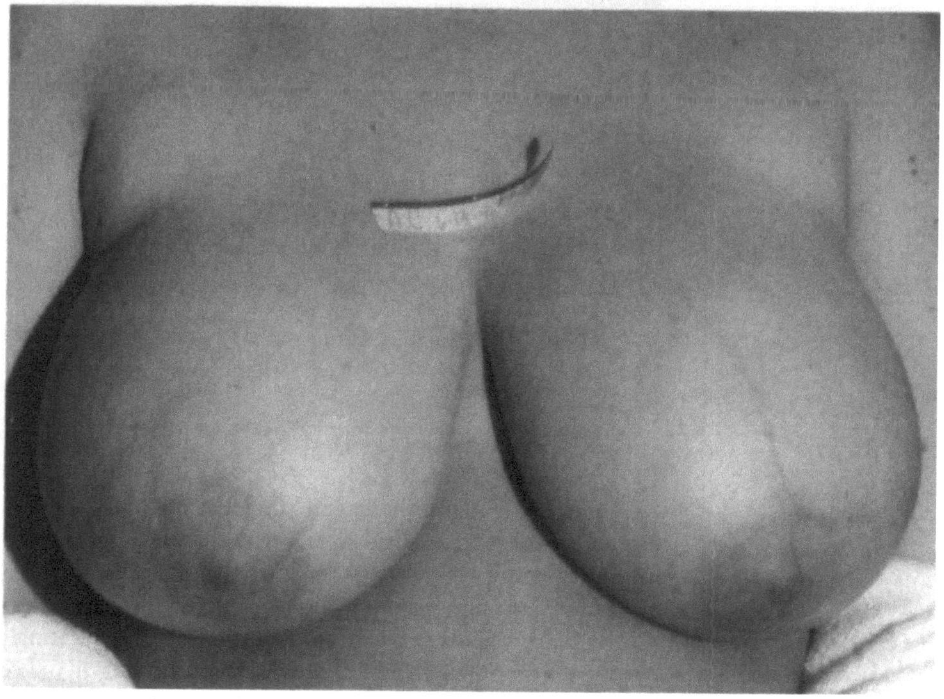

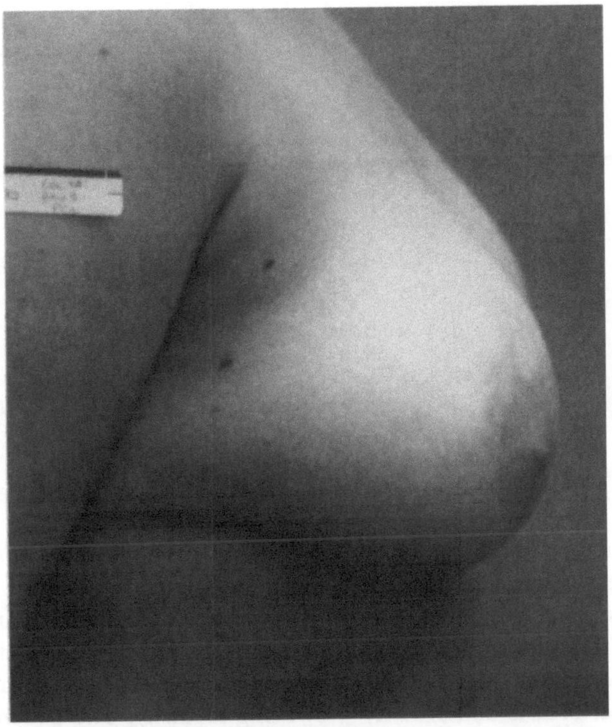

H

I

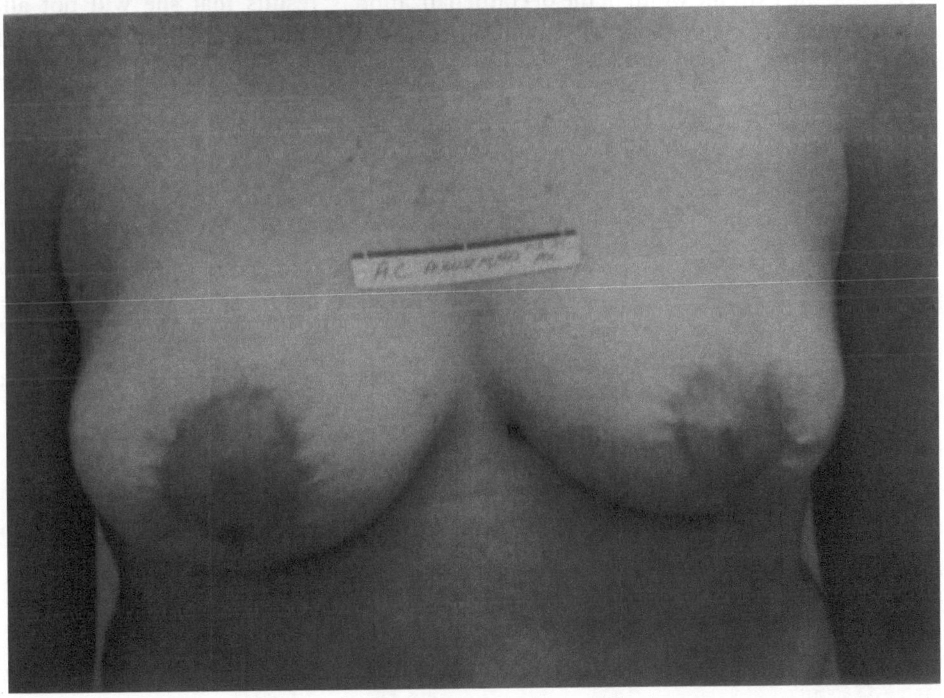

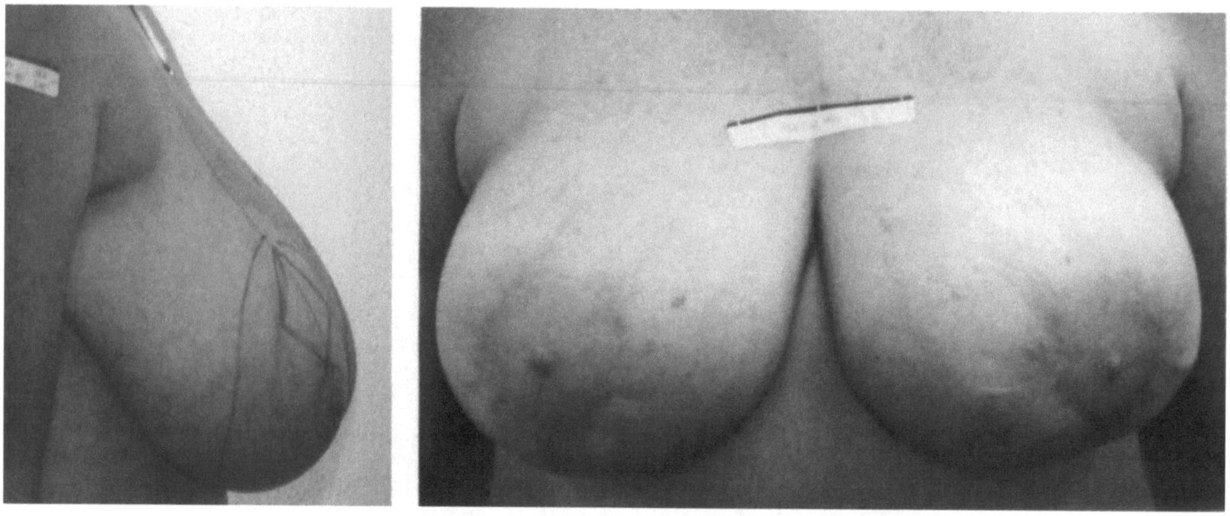

A B

Figure 13-18. Major breast reduction in an older patient. Fortunately, this patient requested that her breasts be reduced only moderately. Because of her large bone structure and perhaps in response to her recent abdominoplasty and major liposuction of the lower body, she had requested that her breasts be left fairly large. Note the extreme width of the deepithelialization and the wide "Texas diamond" that will be removed from each areola.

This patient's reduction was performed under ketamine-Valium anesthesia. One error was made in that we did not use drainage, and a seroma developed 10 days postoperatively on the left side, resulting in extrusion of the Mersiline suture and a moderate amount of swelling medially. The patient is so pleased with the results that she will not allow the final adjustment, which would include minor liposuction and revision of the scar on the left side.

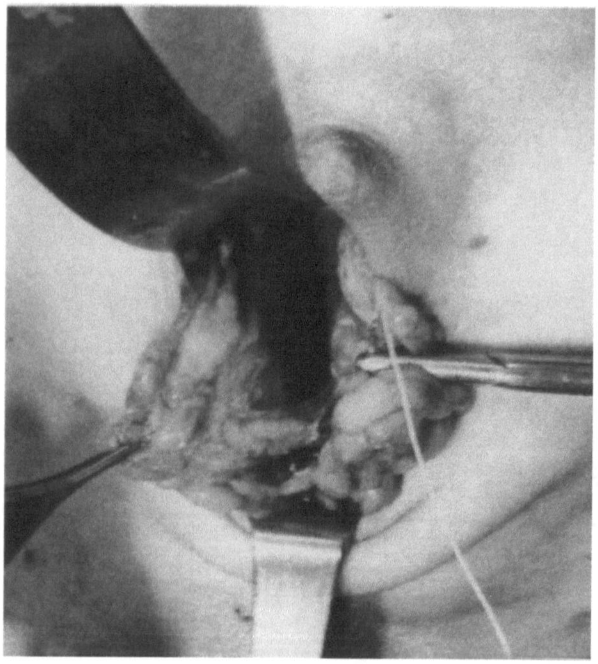

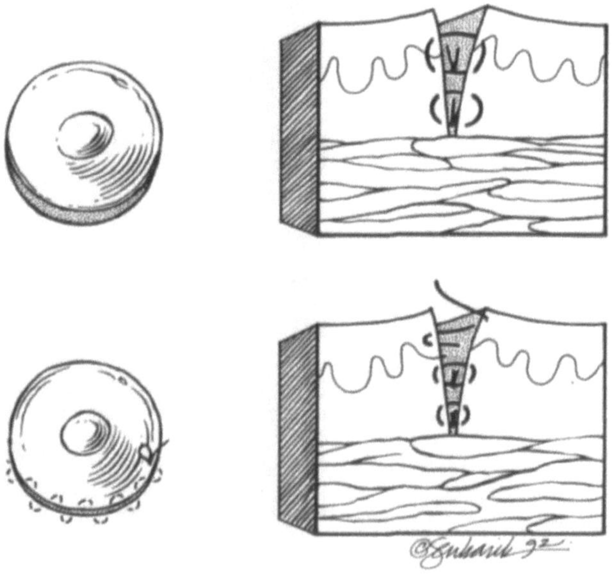

created above the muscle. Textured implants offer the advantage of early immobility, which gives more time for the internal reinforcement to become stable. There is usually excess length between the areola and the inframammary fold. This tissue is excised, and the left side is then brought into position and anchored to both the chest wall and the undersurface of the right flap. By crossing the flaps "pants over vest," double-layered reinforcement in the midline is achieved, as is a new inframammary fold. Drains may or may not be necessary. The surface tissue is then returned to its position and subcutaneous and subcuticular closure of the short periareolar incision is effected.

Although areolar enlargement is not rare, it occurs to a lesser degree in patients whose circumareolar mastopexy does not require an implant. Simply restoring fullness, usually to a larger size than the original, is preferable. These patients are generally scar conscious. Unless the areola is very large, it is better to leave it untouched than to attempt an elevation or reduction of diameter. We show patients counseling books that illustrate early and late appearances of these incisions, as well as before and after pictures of patients who have had the internal repair. For their information, we include a page of photographs from popular men's magazines that show even more bizarre "balloon-outs" than theirs. These individuals should continue to wear a brassiere indefinitely because their tissues are likely to stretch over time. Few have disregarded these instructions, with most maintaining their breast shape and position after the internal repair.

Comments and Commentary

1. Preceding me on the program at the 1991 American Society of Aesthetic Plastic Surgery convention was a good friend who discussed his short-term experience with the Benelli "round block" procedure. Although he admitted that the repaired breast looked acceptable at the beginning, he became disenchanted

Figure 13-19. Stretched-out breast. A common problem of patients after augmentation, particularly submuscular augmentation, is overstretching of the breast from the nipple to the inframammary fold. For most breasts areola repositioning is not required, but it can be accomplished by a variation of the circumareolar technique, as shown here. To avoid external scars, except at the edge of the areola, most of these operations are performed through a lower-half perioareolar incision. After the skin and subcutaneous tissue are reflected, a capsulotomy is performed and the implant is usually replaced with a textured type because it holds a superior and medial position for a longer time and thus protects the reinforcing repair that will be performed. With the implant in position and held out of the way, the tissue at the base of the breast is resected so the inframammary fold can be reestablished. A left-to-right, over-and-under, "pants-over-vest" repair is then performed. After following these patients for many years, it appears that the reinforcement has slowed or prevented ptosis of the breast.

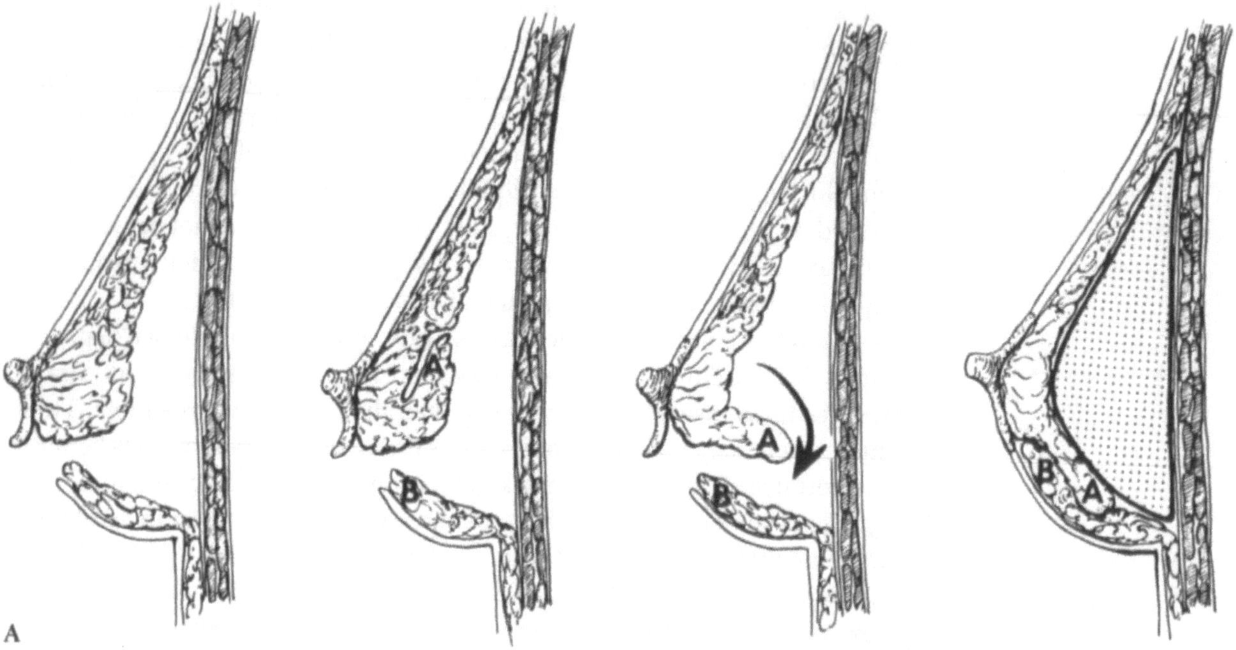

A

Figure 13-20. (B) This patient had a original "Snoopy" deformity with a small, extremely narrow-based projection from the chest wall that was almost entirely areola. (C) Two years later contractures have occurred on both sides. These patients are good candidates for the combination circumareolar mastopexy plus secondary reinforcing rotation flap (A). Full expansion and lowering of the inframammary fold play a role. (D&E) At 3 years postoperatively, the areola scar has not spread, thanks to the double Benelli suture. The breasts are soft, and there has been no further descent during these 18 months.

(F) For the repair of most overstretched breasts, the only access needed is to the lower half of the breast. A fingertip is used to break up the contracted upper half of the breast once the pocket has been reestablished. I use a short periareolar incision. It is not necessary to resect skin if the nipple is of normal size and position, which is usually the case. Wide undermining of the subcutaneous tissue is easily accomplished through this minimal exposure. After the breast parenchyma has been split vertically and the prosthesis removed and replaced (or simply repositioned), the new inframammary fold is established by suturing the freed-up lower edges of the breast parenchyma at a higher position with an overlap. A textured implant, chosen primarily for its width and stability, is then positioned. A left-to-right "pants-over-vest" closure of the breast parenchyma not only reestablishes the normal curvature but reinforces that area as well. Skin closure should be in several layers ending with an everting Vicryl subcuticular suture, as shown. After one additional pass, the end of the suture is brought out through the areolar skin and tied in a loop knot, exteriorizing the end of the subcuticular suture. (These knots frequently migrate superiorly over time.) After 3 to 4 days it is safe to elevate the exteriorized knot and clip it flush with the skin surface.

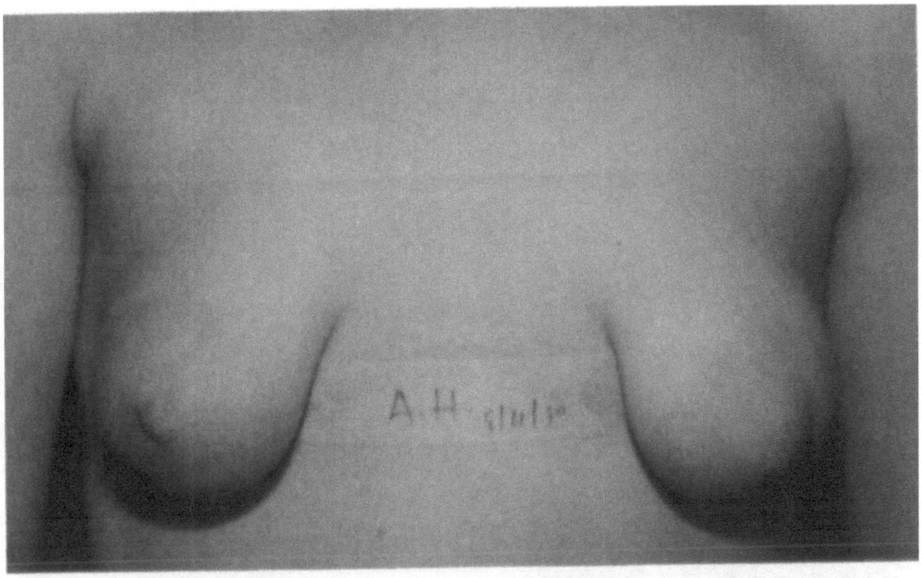

B

C

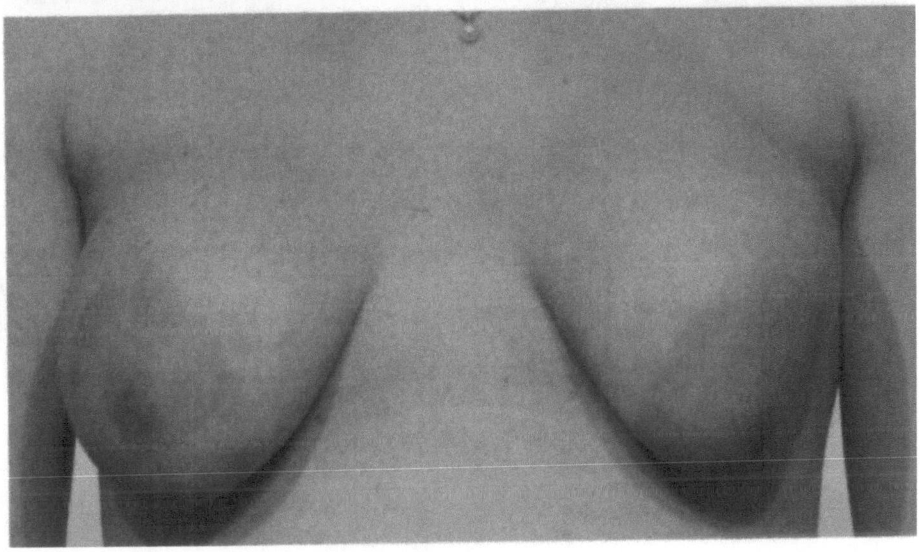

D
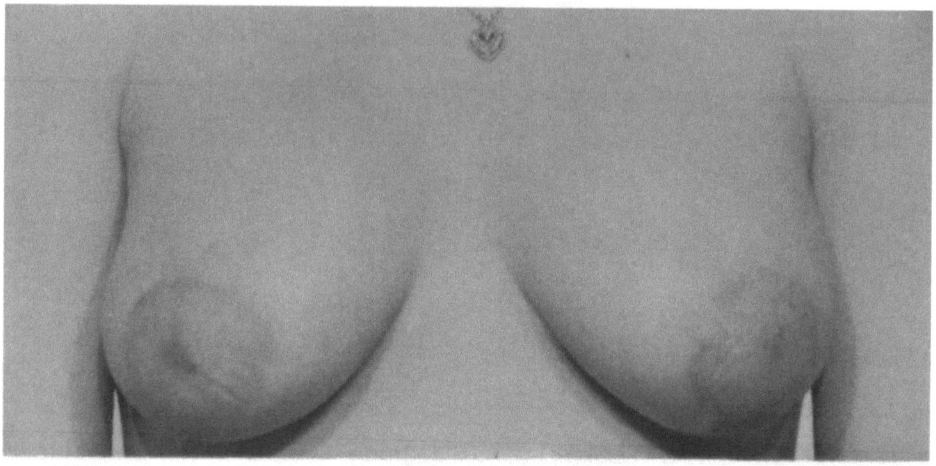

E
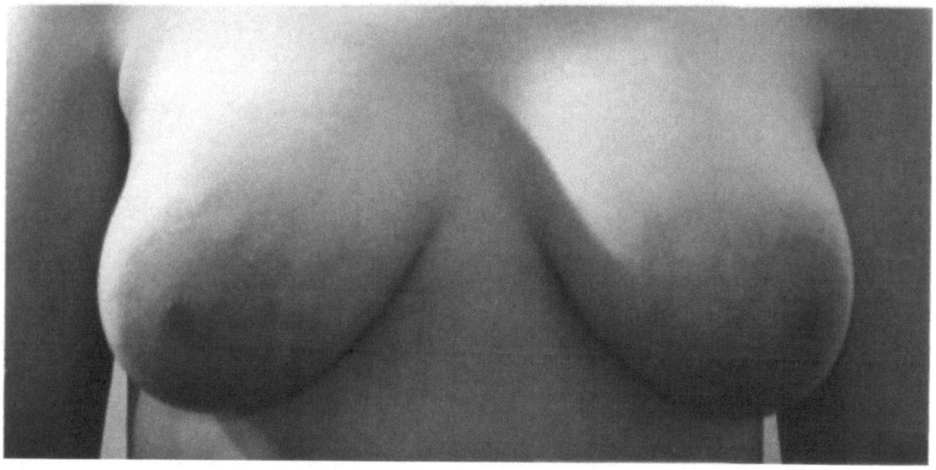

F
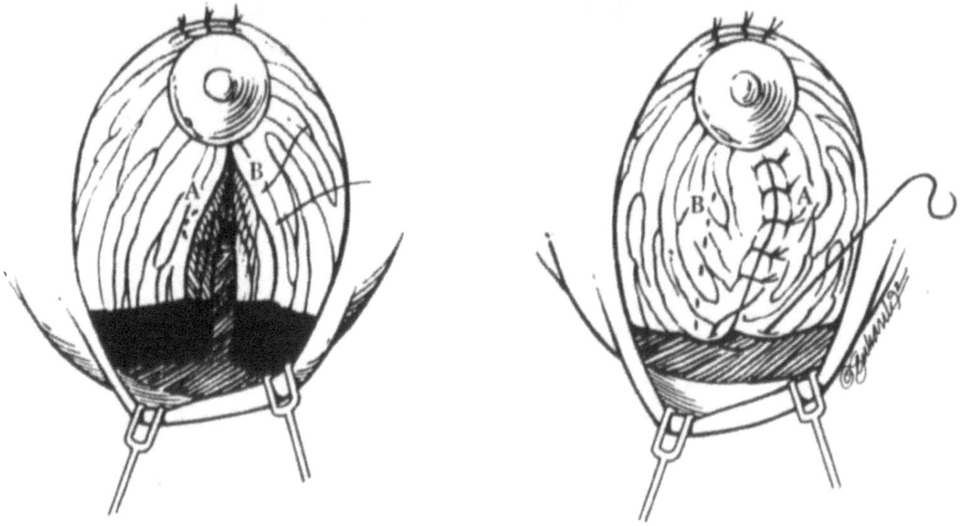

with the operation. Other American surgeons have been equally vocal in their disapproval.

When it was my turn I stressed the technical changes that have been made and emphasized that a firm, well attached mound must be created underneath the skin envelope. I also showed the techniques for anchoring the areola at its new position and our addition of a second "Benelli circumareolar stitch" to reduce tension upon the areola. I believe my presentation of 4- and 5-year follow-ups was impressive enough to counter the negative impression.

My opening slide referred to the circumareolar approach as the "Erol procedure" giving due credit to the surgeon I consider to be the leading expert and most erstwhile proponent of circumareolar surgeries. He has improved the technique and reported many excellent results, although, admittedly, all were in small breasts.

2. No one has a magic formula for perfect breast reduction. I conducted a survey that showed the rising popularity of inferior pedicle techniques. Some disagreed. We are constantly alert for new concepts and eager to understand the technical maneuvers that make the next result a little better. John Silverton (Stockton, CA) commonly uses a standard McKissock approach. His second most common technique is the superior pedicle method, and the third is the free nipple graft technique. He considers the inferior pedicle method a last choice. His preoperative design varies with the consistency of the breast as well as its original shape. Breast consistency includes denseness, firmness, and degree of fullness. Silverton disagrees with the plastic surgeons who limit the width of the inferior incision. He plans the medial and lateral ends wide to produce the most conical result. Technical point: Be sure the inframammary crease is no further than 4.5 to 5.0 cm in the low point of the areola.

Others also have had difficulty with inferiorly based dermal pedicles. James Diller (Toledo) decided there might be intradermal residual bacteria in the skin appendages that could not be cleansed by the preoperative preparation. Quantitative bacteriologic studies were done on several deepithelization areas, and *Staphylococcus epidermidis* was present in every deepithelialized zone. If the colony count was below 1000 per gram of tissue, there were no problems, but if it increased to 3000 colonies per gram and diphtheroids or *Klebsiella* species were present, the pedicles seemed to be in trouble. Technical point: In addition to a Hemovac, Diller places a small Silastic tube inside, under the nipple. If dermal viability seems threatened, he injects kanamycin daily through the tubing. Cefamandole can also be used intravenously if true infection surfaces. In a further effort to reduce infection, topical Sulfamylon cream was tried preoperatively but has been abandoned. The only truly effective technique was to deliver antibiotics to the embedded dermal pedicle and the bacteria that were still growing in the reconstructed breast.

3. Gerhard Schmidt (Bakersfield, CA) uses the Ribeiro technique. He prefers this technique for medium to large areas of hypertrophy and has noted fewer problems with healing and areolar survival than with other methods.

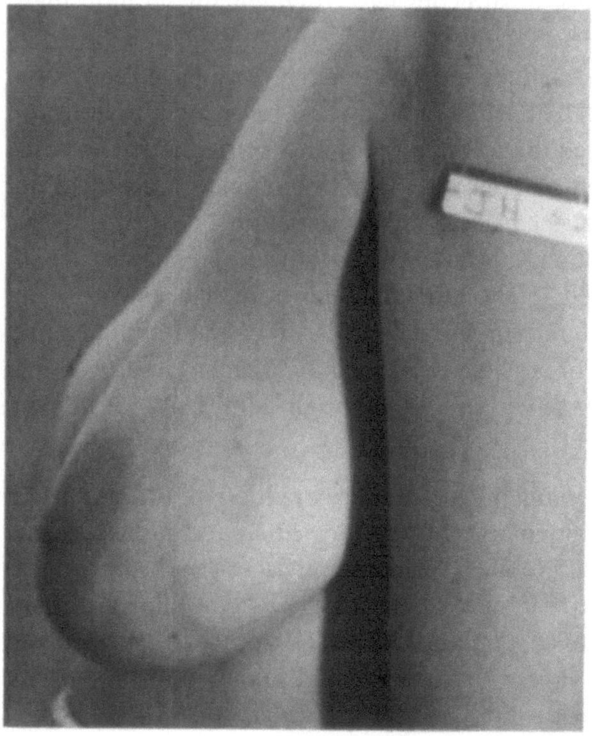

A

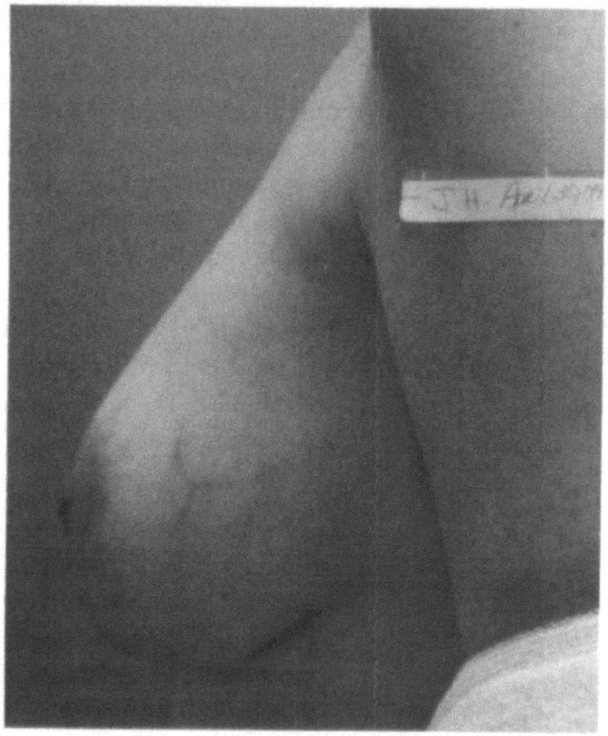

B

C

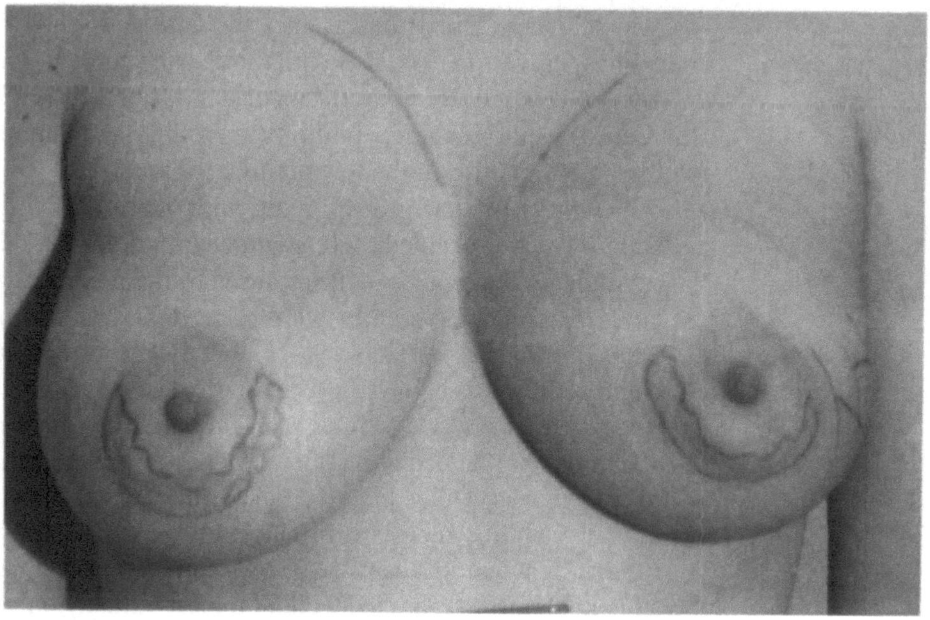

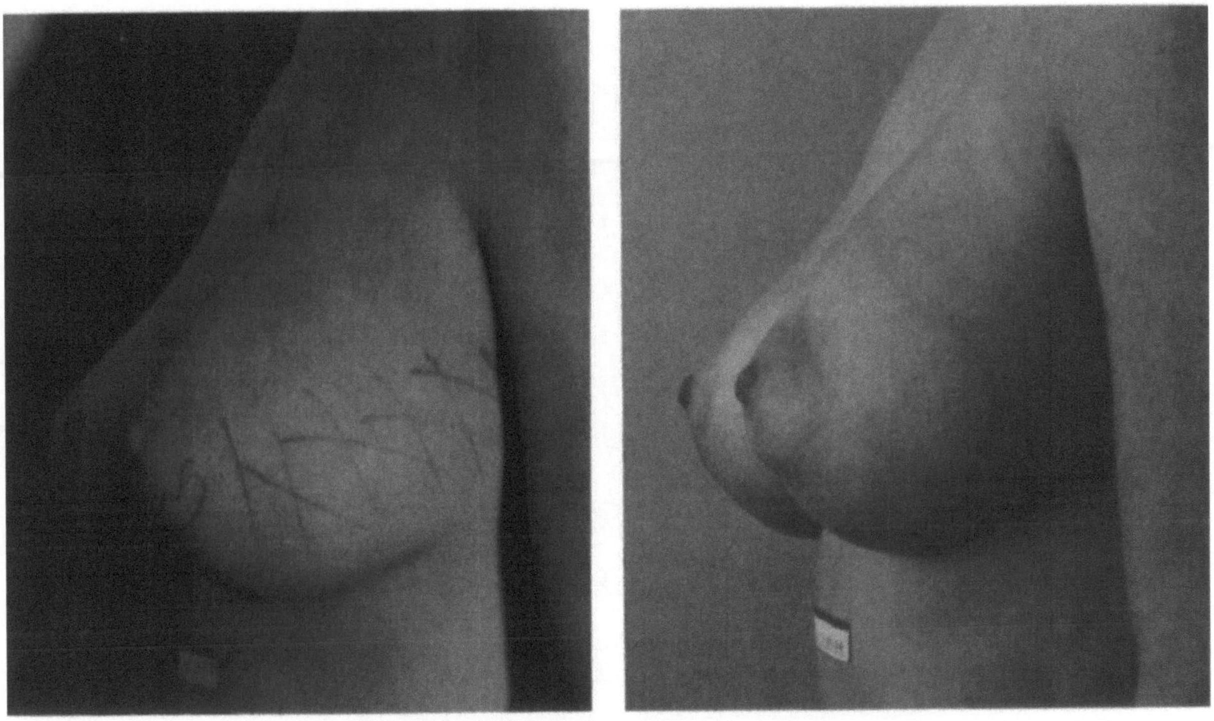

D E

Figure 13-21. The greatest application of the internal mastopexy procedure is in the patient with postpartum or non-support-induced breast stretch following breast augmentation. These patients fall into two categories. The most common is the patient with "stretch out" from the areola to the inframammary fold without areolar descent. Correction involves detaching the skin and subcutaneous tissue from the lower half of the breast through a short periareolar incision, which also allows access to the overstretched zone. Vertical splitting of the breast is followed by resection of the excessive length at the inframammary fold level. Left and right flaps of breast tissue are designed and then folded one upon the other; and a new, higher inframammary fold is established using absorbable polyglycolic sutures. Compression brassieres hasten realignment of the overly stretched skin in the lower half of the breast.

A&B show a patient with postaugmentation ptosis, more exagerrated on the left side. A circumareolar repositioning with internal repair reset the nipple/areolar to match the opposite side, and corrected the bowing of the breast between the nipple and old inframammary fold.

The patient shown in (**C**) not only had amateurishly cross hatched wide scars around ⅔ of each areola, but bilateral breast descent and dense fibrosis distorting the left breast (**D**). Since the areolar position was acceptable, the correction (**E**) was performed with a scar revision incision.

A

B

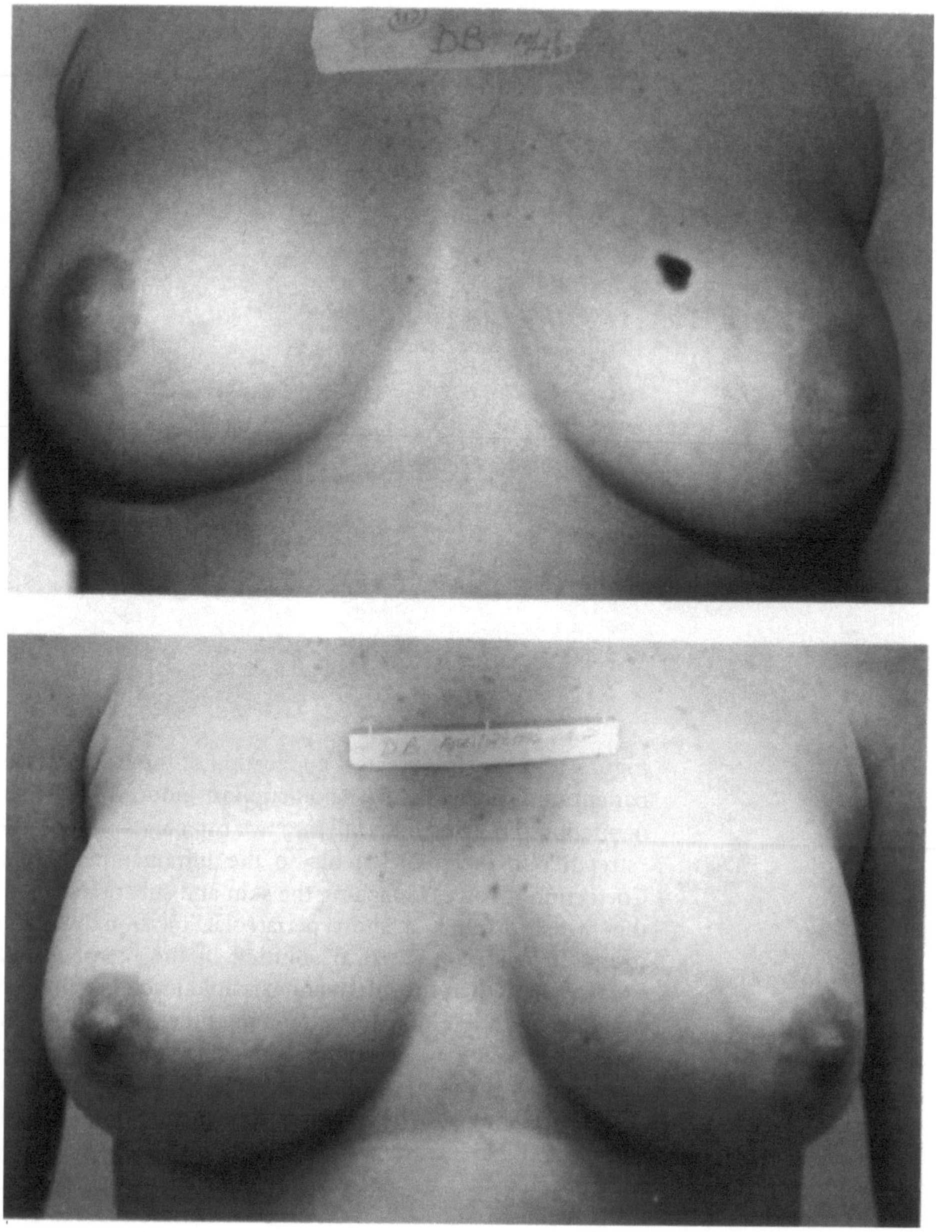

Figure 13-22. Unilateral ptosis. **(A)** Patient D.B. several years after bilateral breast augmentation. She presented here (1984) with a left breast that had been dropping for approximately 3 years. Note the degree of asymmetry. Bilateral implant replacement to correct width and volume was performed, with concomitant internal overlapping and repair on the left side. **(B)** The results (1985) indicate that the overstretch of the lower portion has been corrected. Six years later, there is still some stretching and asymmetry bilaterally but to a relatively minor degree.

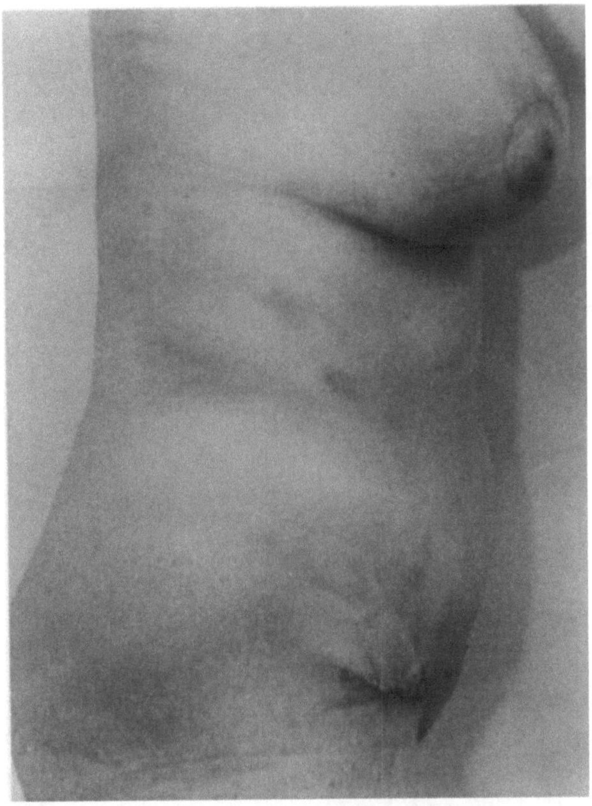

Figure 13-23. Mastopexy augmentation using a circumareolar technique in conjunction with abdominoplasty. An acceptable circumareolar scar has been obtained, even though the patient underwent augmentation of the ptotic breasts at the same time. The difference is that a smaller circle was deepithelialized and advanced to the base of the areola. Note also that the tissue between the areola and the inframammary fold is overcorrected. It was done purposefully using a crossover double-reinforced closure after the breast prosthesis has been positioned because the breasts of these patients inevitably stretch.

Schmidt uses this technique in large breasts for subcutaneous mastectomy, folding the inferior flap for bulk without the use of a prosthesis.

4. Alberto Sanchez and Jose Iglesis (San Juan) have a breast reduction practice that rivals even those of the "great uncharted Midwest." After working with a number of techniques, Sanchez and Iglesis concentrated on the basics but have always been willing to try new techniques that might improve the contour and reduce the complications. During the early 1980s they used a basic triangle inferior pedicle, but instead of correcting one problem they found more. The small triangle tended to become necrotic because the pull at its base strangled the rest of the breast. If a large amount of skin was added at the triangle base, the base appeared more square or almost bilobed. The other problem they found with the inferior pedicle technique is the tendency to make the vertical scar too long. We are all familiar with the "star-gazing" effect of gravity on a long inferior incision line. Sanchez keeps the inferior pedicle between 4.5 and 5.5 cm because of the difficulty they found when correcting elevated nipples.

When they used the Stromback or McKissock technique, they rarely saw skin necrosis at the junction of the inverted T. After having used the inferior

A

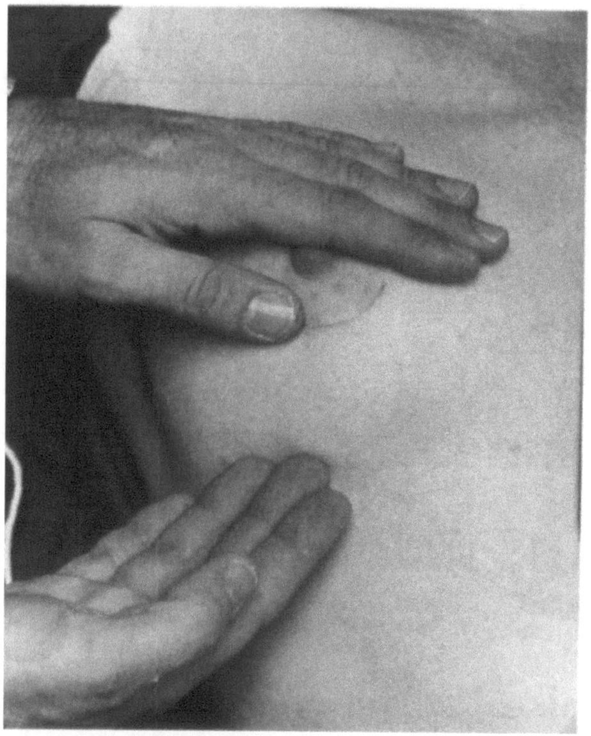

B

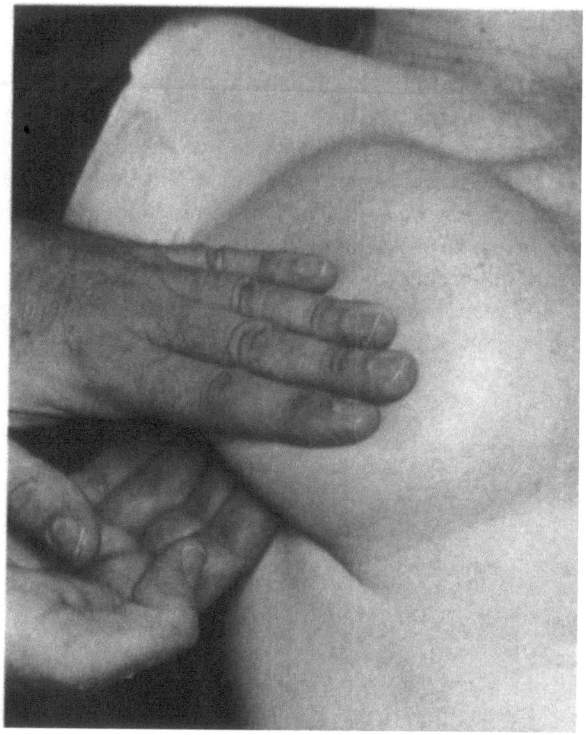

C

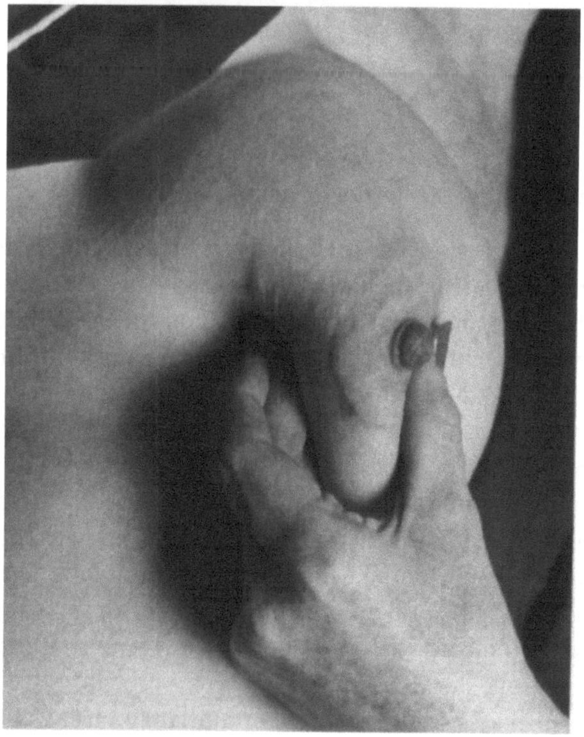

Figure 13-24. One advantage of adding a breast prosthesis rather than infolding is the obvious fullness and contour preferred by North American women. The second advantage is the ease of self-examination. It is well known that the presence of a breast prosthesis does not increase the incidence of breast cancer, but it does not decrease it either. Small tumors are pushed upward by the prosthesis and are more easily detected and still small when found by fingertip palpation. **(A&B)** The patient is being shown how to examine the posterior surface of the breast. With one hand in position above the areola, the other fingertips are curved upward and the implant is displaced. A stroking maneuver then can detect new growths. Patients may prefer to do this with two hands as illustrated or with the finger and thumb **(C)**. Three of my patients have detected malignant growths on the undersurface of the breast that were not detected on multiple-view xeromammograms.

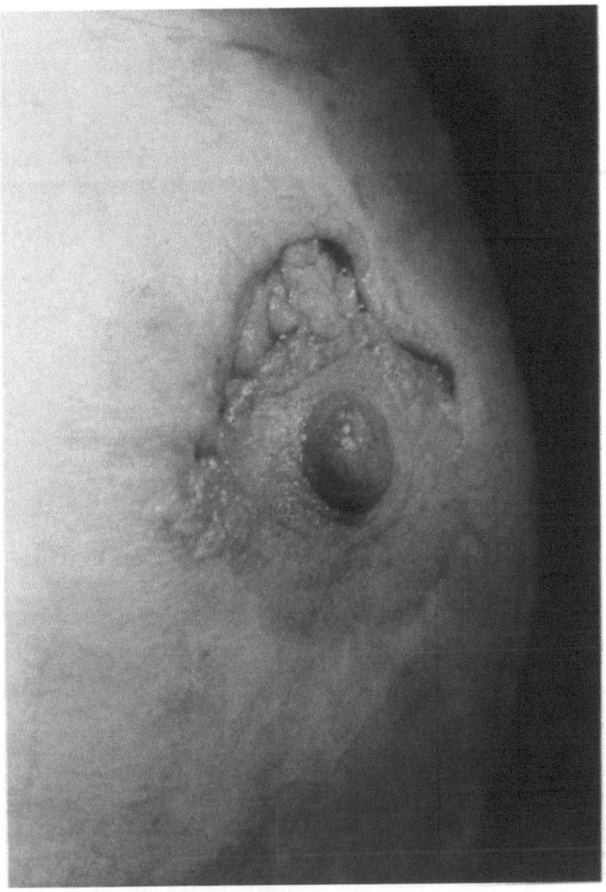

Figure 13-25. Closure of the short skin incision for the Erol type infolding mastopexy or crossover internal repair mastopexy is a multilayered everting procedure that reduces the chance of scar widening. The first two layers bring the soft tissue together with inverted knots of absorbable suture. The final subcuticular and everting suture is exteriorized at its end and tied as a one-loop knot on the pigmented areolar skin. These knots too often "spit" if they are buried. Five days after surgery, the loop is lifted and clipped off flush with the skin.

pedicle technique for 2 years (100 cases), they have not seen a single case of nipple necrosis, and the breasts have recovered most of their sensation even though there is more necrosis at the junction of the inverted T.

In an effort to convince insurance carriers that reduction mammoplasty is not a cosmetic procedure (a battle already won in most states), Sanchez and Iglesis prepared a questionnaire for 54 patients. Preoperatively, 83% of these patients said that they hoped the surgery would help them improve their posture; 80% stated that they were ashamed of their figure; and 90.7% described tiredness and pressure on their chest due to the breasts. As expected, more than 90% complained of brassiere strap pain as well as chest, back, and neck pain. Postoperatively, 98% said that their breast pains were completely gone or "improved" (22% were in the "improved" group). The "proof of the pudding" regarding the procedure was that 98% recommended the surgery to friends. The important point is that many of the patients who described complete or almost complete relief of symptoms had less than 250 g of breast tissue removed.

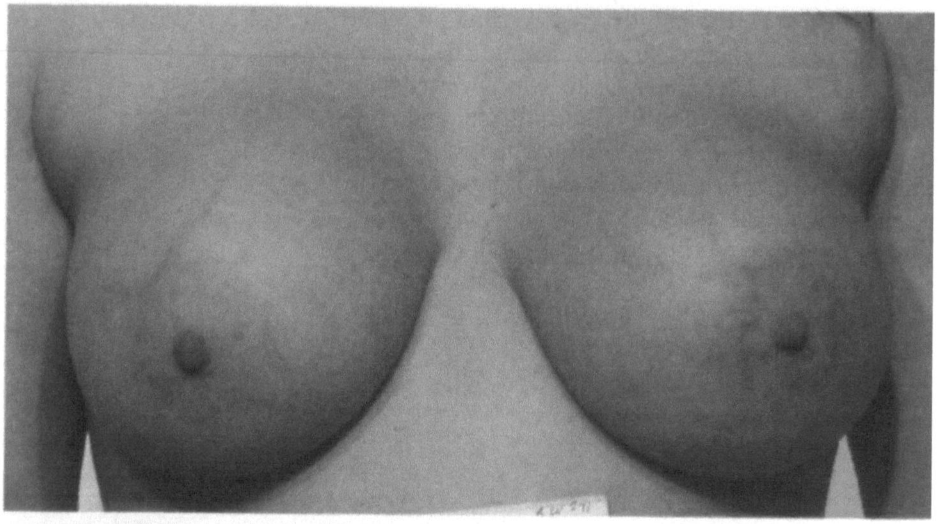

A

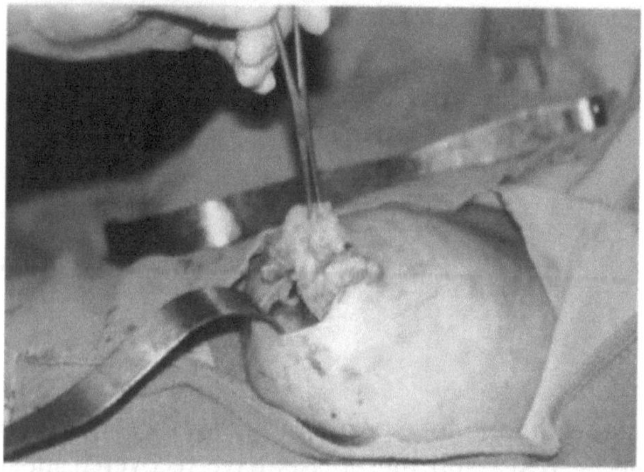

B

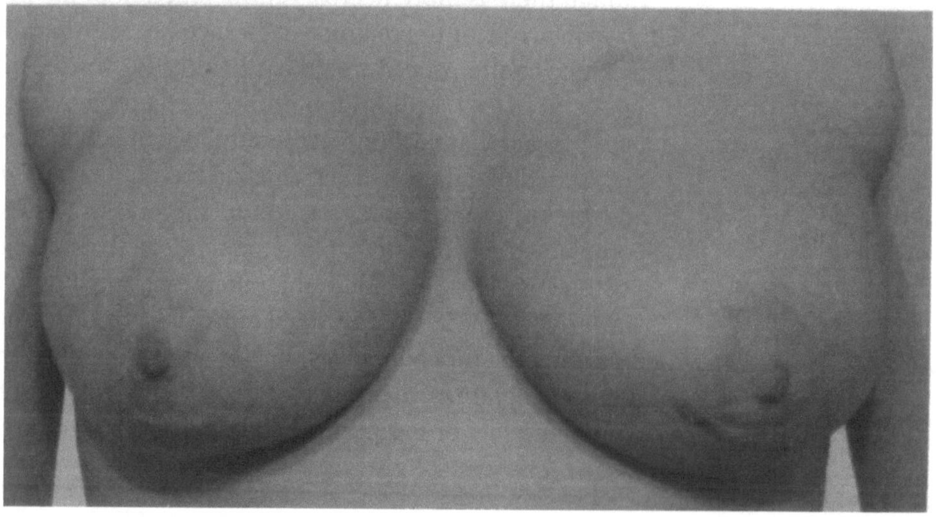

C

5. The volume of breast tissue does not necessarily correspond to its weight. It is unrealistic for an insurance company to base compensation on the weight of tissue removed. Dense, fibrotic breasts obviously weigh more than the relatively lighter fatty breasts, but the volume could be equal or greater in the lighter-weight breast.

6. After reading my account of the circumareolar incision for internal mastopexy, Enrique Rossell cried "foul." He had presented a paper in 1973 on this same subject and had submitted it for publication but it was rejected. Rossell's original paper was based on his experience with 18 patients. Since then he has used the procedure often and "every time I am more enthusiastic."

7. According to Rossell, small breast reductions can be performed in many patients without the need for a T scar. The augmented breast that sags too soon can also be treated this way. Now we use the technique for larger breasts.

Figure 13-26. Internal repair of a vertical split using "internal mastopexy" techniques. This patient presented as a dilemma. She had severe capsular contractures after saline prostheses had been implanted elsewhere through fairly large inframammary incisions (**A**). During a closed release, she had suffered rupture of the left breast internally so the prosthesis was palpable in a defect extending from the inferior margin of the areola halfway to her shoulder. The defect measured two fingerbreadths.

She adamantly refused visible incisions, so correction was performed using bilateral implant replacement through periareolar incisions (**B**), which allowed us to expose the entire overstretched portion of the left breast so a reinforcing closure could be effected. A modification of the circumareolar technique was employed. The central zone from the edge of the areola to the inframammary fold was incised as a superiorly based flap. The flap was turned on itself and sutured into the defect of the breast, filling it completely. Once the new prosthesis was in place, anterior wall repair was carried out and the inframammary fold repositioned to match the right side.

Hence with a minimal incision we were able to achieve relative symmetry of her dissimilar breasts, to repair the defect in the upper portion of the left breast, and to repair the overstretch on the left and right sides with internal reinforcement (**C**).

14 Abdominoplasty

At one time abdominoplasty was a rarely performed procedure, reserved for huge, waddling people. Today abdominoplasty is a relatively common procedure and is used in its limited, mini, and modified varieties for a large group of individuals, male and female.[6] As cosmetic surgery has become more acceptable and bathing suits more revealing, requests for abdominoplasty are coming from women who have had a single low pregnancy or a rapid weight gain that has damaged the lower abdominal skin and musculature. When the muscles are stretched—whether the entire length of the rectus abdominis (requiring complete abdominoplasty repair) or simply from the umbilicus down, one does the patient a disservice by not making a repair at the time of fat removal and skin excision.

We review here the technical points of patient selection as well as unusual maneuvers such as elevation or fixation of the mons, advancement of new or old incisions medially to fit under "French-line" bathing suits, and conversely methods used to prevent an incision from drifting outward.

The most important factor when selecting the surgical procedure is the length, quality, and excess skin *above* the umbilicus. This evaluation leads to one's operative choice: whether to "float" the umbilicus, to "float" the umbilicus and lower the mons to give an effective symmetry between the upper and lower skin areas, or to simply close the original umbilical site as a vertical slit. The latter maneuver is the one I most commonly employ. It retains extra flap length there, so the closure is without tension but with minimal deformity. It allows the surgeon to proceed but through a shorter incision than the "classic abdominoplasty" incision.

In past years incisions were made from iliac crest to iliac crest with a bizarre V in the center and curlicues in the ascending limbs. Suction was unheard of. Today we make the incision shorter and attack the "dog-ear" problem aggressively by defatting underneath the lateral limbs and suctioning the flanks. Carefully performed, this method provides a better waistline. In the past we also flirted with the idea of crossover muscle flaps and other complexities. As one surgeon remarked, "If you plicate laterally in patients who need it, it won't show. If you plicate laterally in patients who don't need it, it still doesn't show." In other words, a good anterior plication of the rectus sheath is all that one needs.

I prefer a two-layer fascial closure that can be accomplished in a short time by using the buried figure-of-eight suture technique. Handling the umbilicus was once a major part of the procedure. Turnover flaps, tuck-under flaps, and other variations have had their advocates. I discuss the simplest procedure, the "four-stitch anchor," which is less complicated and gives a natural appearance to the new umbilicus without the risk of stretching or close-off. Lastly, I discuss the role of liposuction in the new abdominoplasties and why it can be safely employed today.

Rather than discuss at great length the techniques of full abdominoplasty, I concentrate on efforts to reduce the scope of the operation while obtaining the goals of a shorter, less obtrusive scar and a full, tight contour without deformity. My first article on limiting the abdominoplasty to short incisions in 1986[1] reflected an 11-year experience. I was aware of the limited incision procedures

---

Figures 14-1 to 14-4. Liposuction technique.

Figure 14-1. Note that the umbilicus has already been separated and left attached to the abdominal fascia. We have completed the plication and elevated the mons veneris to its desired position. At this point, one measures the patient in an only slightly flexed position. We remove the panniculus to the point where the edge simply touches the new mons position without tension.

Figure 14-2. An incision has been made to a depth of 1.5 cm, and the scalpel is then turned horizontally to complete the dissection. This direct scalpel excision is carried up to the point where the excess tissue begins to thin.

Figure 14-3. In a similar case, note that the thin panniculus is touching the midline. It is before the French-line advancement and before the new umbilical position has been chosen.

Figure 14-4. The new umbilical site has been opened, and the old umbilical site has been closed as a vertical midline slit. The suction cannulas are now being introduced to create the midline and lateral rectus groove and to suction the area marked by the circle, which has not been undermined. Note also that the lateral edges of the incision have been advanced upward and anchored to the deep fascia to bring the scar well within the French-line position. Overcompensation is required.

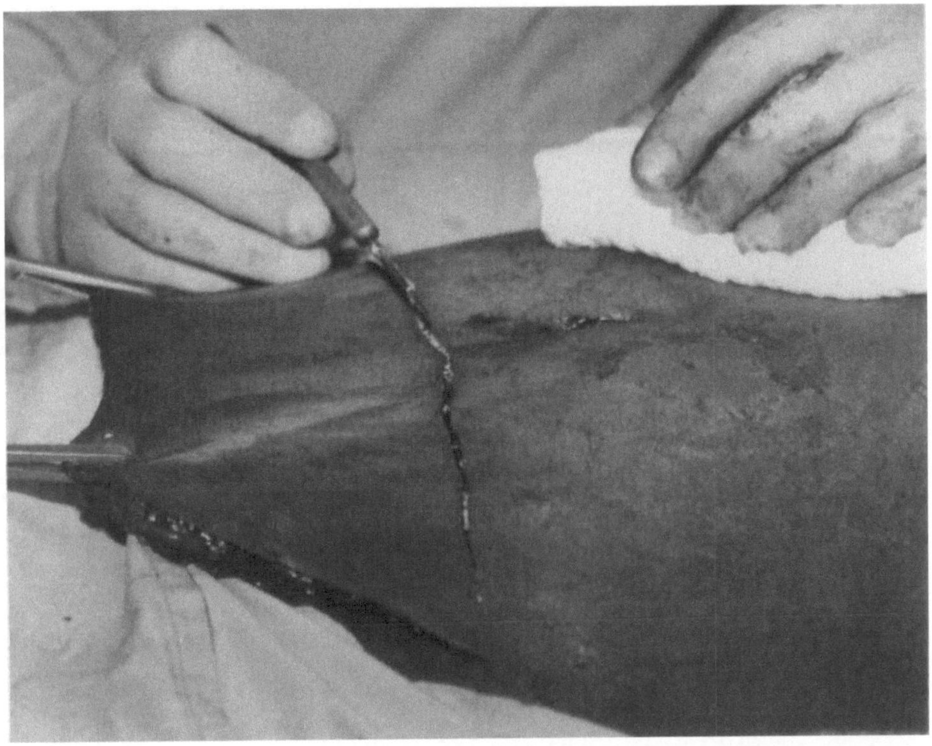
Figure 14-1

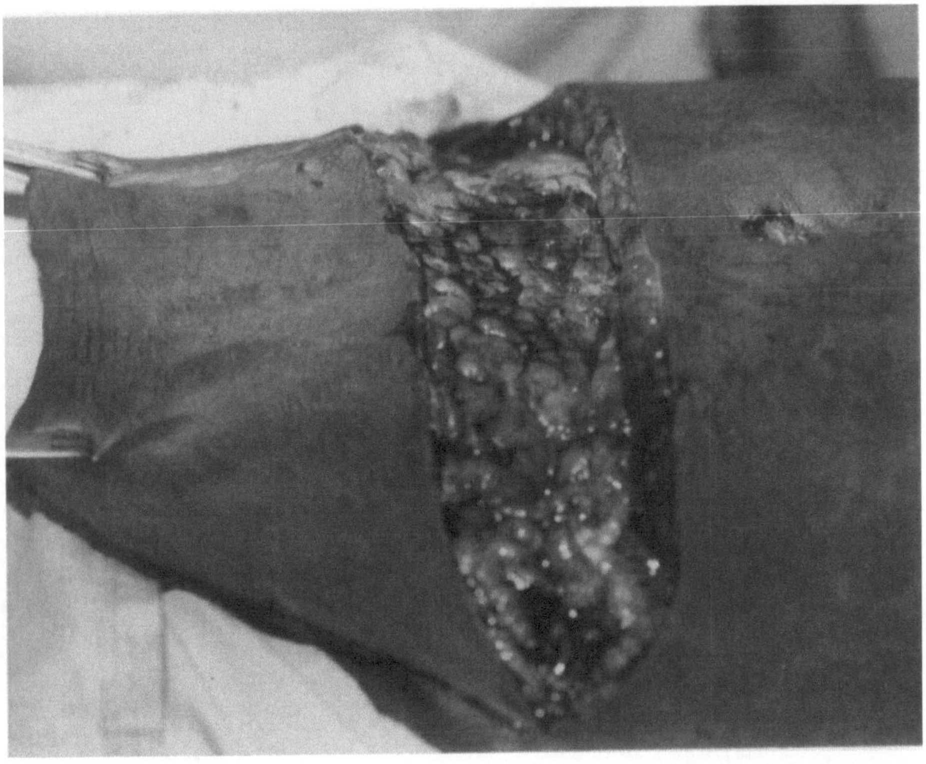
Figure 14-2

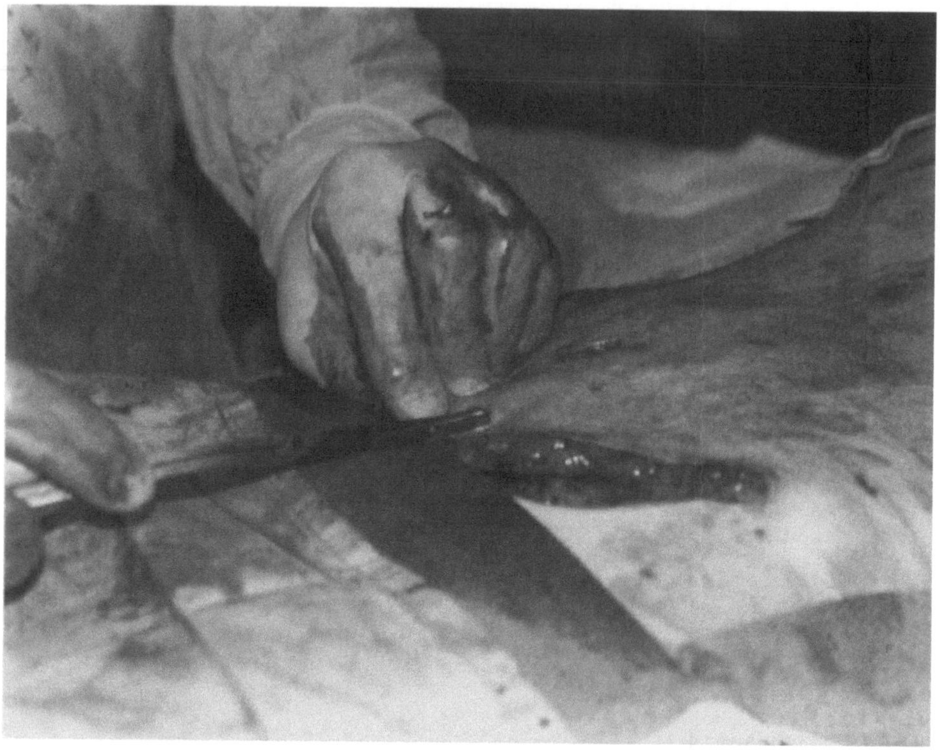

Figure 14-3

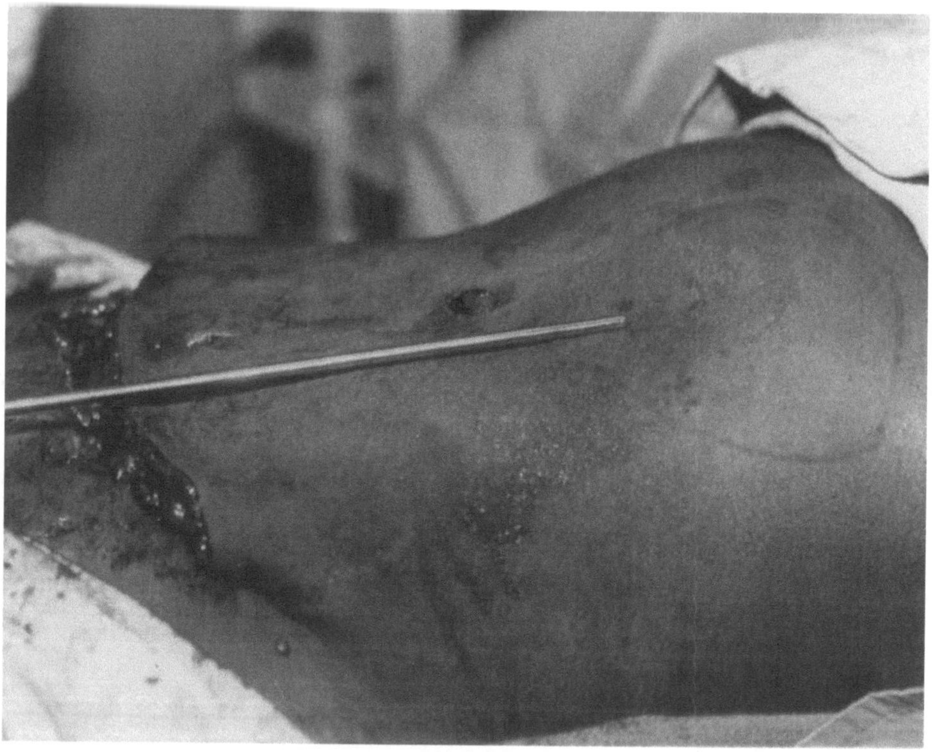

Figure 14-4

described in the European literature by Elbaz and Gleicinstein, but these authors did not address the problem of fascial plication, the distance between the mons veneris and umbilicus, or other factors. My results with W-shaped incisions, which were popular at that time, were abysmal: The scar was too high, the mons was in an unnatural position, lateral scars were too visible, and scars hypertrophied because they transversed the natural body lines.

Therefore I designed a "smile" incision for full abdominoplasty, and it was from that point I began to work to shorten incisions for the new group of patients who required or requested this procedure—largely women who had had low pregnancies. The upper abdomen was not "broken" so we did not "fix" it. With the advent of liposuction, "limited abdominoplasty" became an even better procedure. Most of these patients did not have excess fat in the upper abdomen, so our results prior to 1983 were impressive. These basic principles are now applied to the patient who requires a full abdominal plication with or without separation of the umbilicus.

Separation of the umbilicus to gain exposure for upper abdominal plication is an old procedure. We found that certain individuals with long abdomens and wrinkling above the umbilicus were best treated by separation and by what we call the "umbilical float" procedure. The umbilicus was allowed to drop a distance of up to 2 cm.

One may wish to excise skin above the umbilicus in certain instances to make the umbilicus appear to be in a natural position. We added the idea of reducing the bulk of the mons veneris and removing hair-bearing skin to create a greater expanse of smooth skin between the new umbilical site and the hairline. "Mons reduction" allowed us to center the umbilicus and still drop it down enough to unfold the upper abdomen and yet keep a normal bare area above the hairline of the new, lower mons veneris. This maneuver was also helpful for redoing abdominoplasties that had intruded on the visual areas.

In 1975 no one wore French-line bathing suits, and bikinis were not popular. Today we have changed the operations to fit the current demands of patients. This challenge involves the techniques we discus in this chapter. The same techniques are applied to the full abdominoplasty as well.

In my opinion, there are few patients who benefit from the French version of the "miniabdominoplasty" or Illouz's suggestion of a small skin excision after liposuction. After all, if the abdomen is to be opened, repair it. It is not difficult to do a plication through a small incision. Patients who have not been pregnant, who have good skin quality, and who are young do not need plication. They require only abdominal liposuction, which is discussed in Chapter 15.

Superficial liposculpture can play a role in the intermediate abdomen because it induces more shrinkage and causes less wrinkling. The method is useful in older patients who do not desire the flat contour and do not plan to wear a two-piece bathing suit. For most patients, the goal, of course, is the natural looking abdomen with only a short incision that is angled upward to stay within the "French line." Shorter incisions mean shorter healing times.

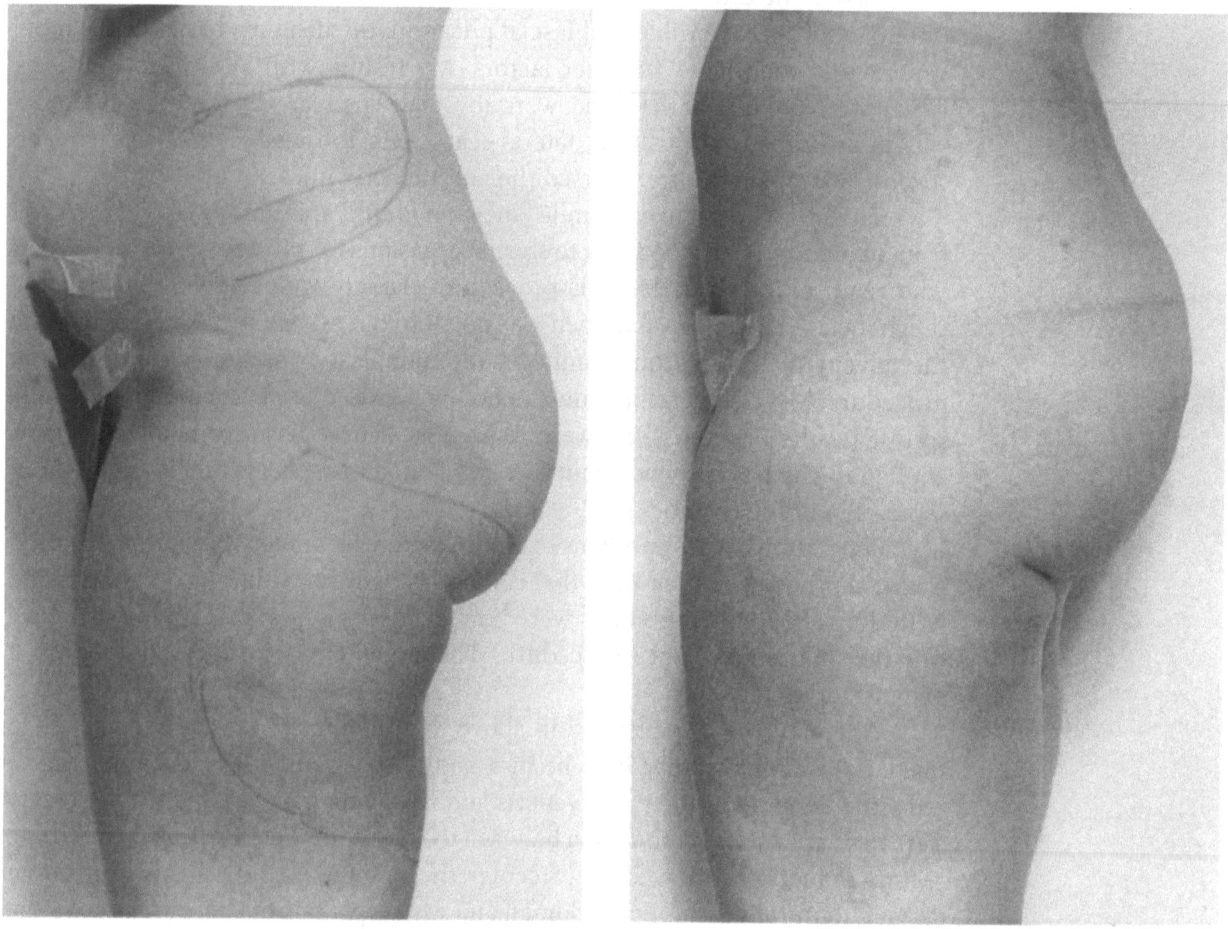

Figure 14-5. In 1983 we did not aggressively attack the "banana roll" underneath the buttock; nevertheless, one can see the excellent infolding of skin after liposuction in this zone. This patient also underwent limited abdominoplasty with flank suction. The important technical point is to avoid a grid pattern in the flank so as not to interrupt blood supply but to approach the hip and thigh zones with multiple entry points so complete grid functioning is effected. Today, we would attack the "banana roll" area with an open Becker-type cannula, which would curet the undersurface of the skin to ensure maximum contracture.

The second major change was our insistence that the skin flap meet the mons without tension, a total departure from what I had been trained to do. Remember how we were taught to tie the abdomen so tightly you could bounce a coin on it? It led to hypertrophic scars, wide scars, elevation of the mons, and skin necrosis. Now that we can decrease closure tension with the techniques in use, we can also be more liberal in our use of liposculpture to create the natural folds of the abdomen.

The procedure usually involves closing the umbilical site as a short, vertical slit. It is then almost invisible in most patients, even those who are wearing their

French-line bikinis. This simple maneuver saves additional flap skin, so closure is completed without tension. Preventing upward migration of the mons means anchoring the mons to its new position. This step is also important in the large patient because the mons has drifted downward. The fixation maneuver also removes tension. Next is the French-line advancement of the lateral wings of the incision. Overcorrection and fixation to fascia are the keys to keeping the scar under the French-line bikini. Liposculpture, direct excision, and tapering up the abdominal flap laterally are also important for preventing persistent edema above the incision line.

Basic Principles

The basic principles of abdominoplasty—whether complete, modified, or mini—are the same. Keep the incision short, and anchor the ends upward. Suction parallel to blood vessels, and suction the entire area above the umbilicus if you can get away with it and the musculature is still tight. (If only the lower abdomen is tightened and you have misjudged the upper abdomen, a balloon effect results that is bizarre.) Even if you think you can remove all of the skin between the umbilicus and the mons, do not. Leave an extra 3 to 4 cm after separating the umbilicus. Defat the lower half of the abdomen directly—a more controlled and less traumatic procedure than liposuction. After the muscle repair is completed, fix the mons in its new position by anchoring it to the deep fascia. Advance the lateral incisions upward and anchor them so they do not drift downward. Trim the flap last. Flex the patient only 15 to 20 degrees, and make sure the skin edges touch without tension.

The absence of tension reduces the risk of unsightly or hypertrophic scarring, the most frequent complaint of patients. They soon forget how unsightly the original condition had become. On the other hand, I have seen a half-dozen patients whose skin continued to stretch! Removing the extra skin and occasionally re-setting the umbilicus is required.

Technique

The patients we see in private practice today are rarely the large patients who require major hospital surgeries. Most of my patients undergo repair by variations of the "limited" abdominoplasty. Because most of the deformity is below the umbilicus, it can be safely and efficiently corrected in an office setting. The principles of limited abdominoplasty may also be applied to any individual who requires a neoumbilicoplasty.

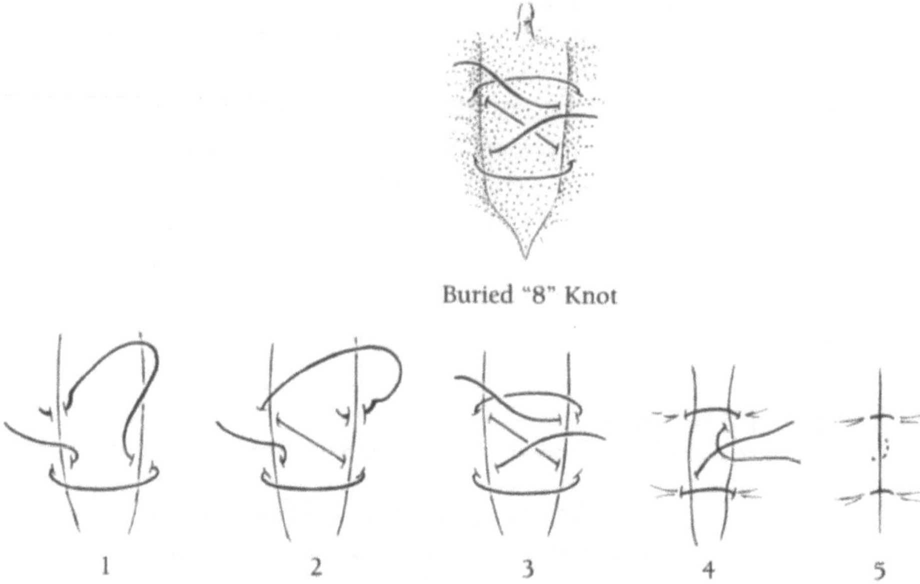

Figure 14-6. Closure. Everything from nylon to wire has been used to close the fascia. No one opens the fascia anymore, and plication causes the least morbidity. How can you plicate with the least chance of dehiscence? One way is using 40 to 50 closely spaced silk or Mersilene sutures, but it is time-consuming. I use the figure-of-eight closure. Mersilene is strong, easy to tie, and green (in case stitch extrusion occurs, it is easy to spot). The problem is the size of the knot. In thin women a large knot can be felt through the skin and fat. The technique illustrated here buries the knot and allows full closure with fewer knots—and saved time.[8] I started with a Mersiline retention suture on a long "swaged" needle. The second layer (for insurance) is No. 1 Vicryl. Mersilene lasts forever but may untie if the patient coughs repeatedly.

1. Keep the initial incision short and angle it upward for any type abdominoplasty. You can always extend the incision if you need to take care of a "dog-ear."
2. Most "dog-ears" can be prevented by manually defatting just past the distal end of the incision. Taper the flap, leaving its thickest part in the center and its narrowest part at the ends of the incision. The bulges that occur after an abdominoplasty are usually in that zone or laterally. Scissors defatting is more efficient than liposuction.
3. Once the initial incision has been made, it is easy to raise the flap with cutting cautery, which allows you to stop the small blood vessels before they retract into the fascia.
4. If the patient's deformity is limited to the lower abdomen, stop the dissection when you reach the umbilicus. If not, there are two choices: (1) separate the umbilicus from its attachment to the fascia and

proceed; or (2) dissect around the stalk so there is room enough to place a figure-of-eight stitch above the umbilicus.

5. Base the preoperative decision regarding the choice of abdominoplasty procedure largely on the amount of loose skin above the umbilicus and its position. If the umbilicus is high, it can be separated and allowed to "float" down 2 cm. It will still be centered. This step unfolds the upper abdomen.
6. If the umbilicus is central or low, do not use the "umbilical float" maneuver. Either leave the umbilicus alone or detach it from the skin and create a new umbilical site. If there is extra skin above the umbilicus, a new site is the best choice. Close the original site as a vertical midline slit; it leaves a negligible scar and provides a longer flap with less tension. The umbilicus can serve as a tether to fix the upper flap under moderate tension & stretch.
7. Avoid undermining in the upper abdomen as much as possible. After the plication is completed, use your fingertips to spread the lateral tissues below the rib cage until everything lies flat. Do not cut bands if you can avoid it, as that blood supply is needed.
8. With most limited abdominoplasties there is a pouch of fat in the midline above the umbilicus. Remove it using a small liposuction cannula. Do the same for fat just under or over the rib cage and in the flanks.
9. If the flanks are to be suctioned, use a single entry point and fan in the direction of the blood vessels coming in—at a 45-degree angle. Do not try to remove every ounce fat, as blood vessels may be damaged.
10. After every abdominoplasty, no matter how moderate, drains are required. Leave the drains in 3 to 4 days even though the wound looks dry the next morning. Drainage reduces the incidence of seroma. Moreover, the suction helps the flap attach to the fascia.
11. The drains should exit through the end of the incision. Close with a subcuticular 4-0 Dexon suture, bringing it out beyond the drain. Three days later, when the drain is removed, tie the Dexon suture down with a loop knot to close the incision, leaving the knot outside the skin where it can be easily clipped off 4 to 5 days later.
12. Aftercare is important. Gently massaging the flap downward helps to move the edema out. Oils applied with pressure to the incision line flatten the incision quickly and hasten resolution of the redness. Start this scar massage the second or third week. Until then, use protective taping to avoid any shifting or pulling due to sudden movements. Coat the tape with collodion so the patient can shower. Protect the wound, as patients sometimes pull at it when they are asleep.

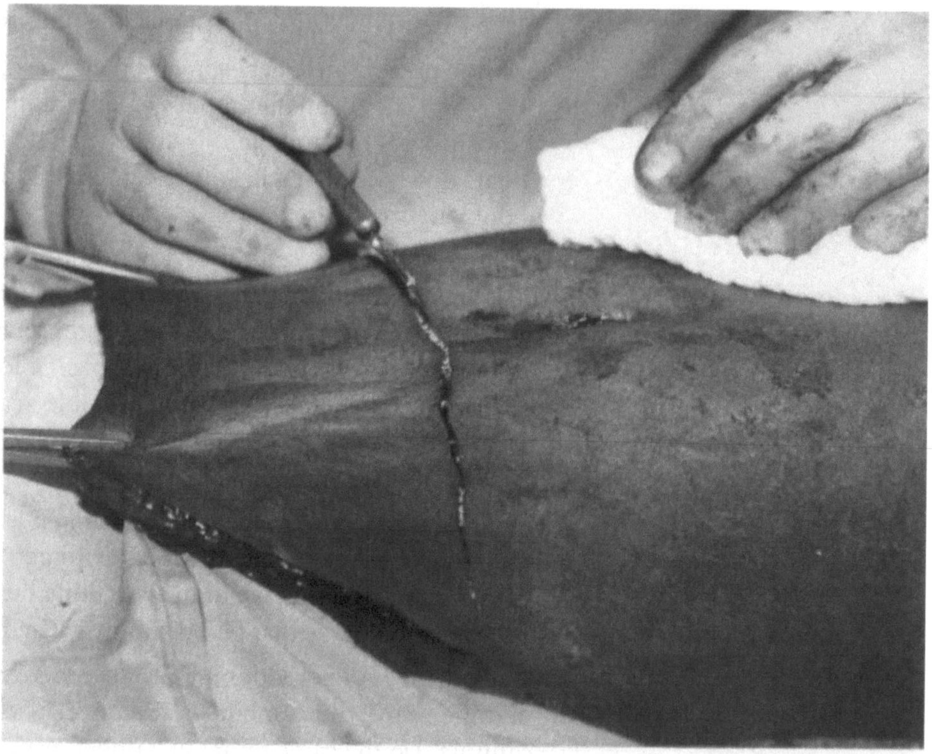

A

B

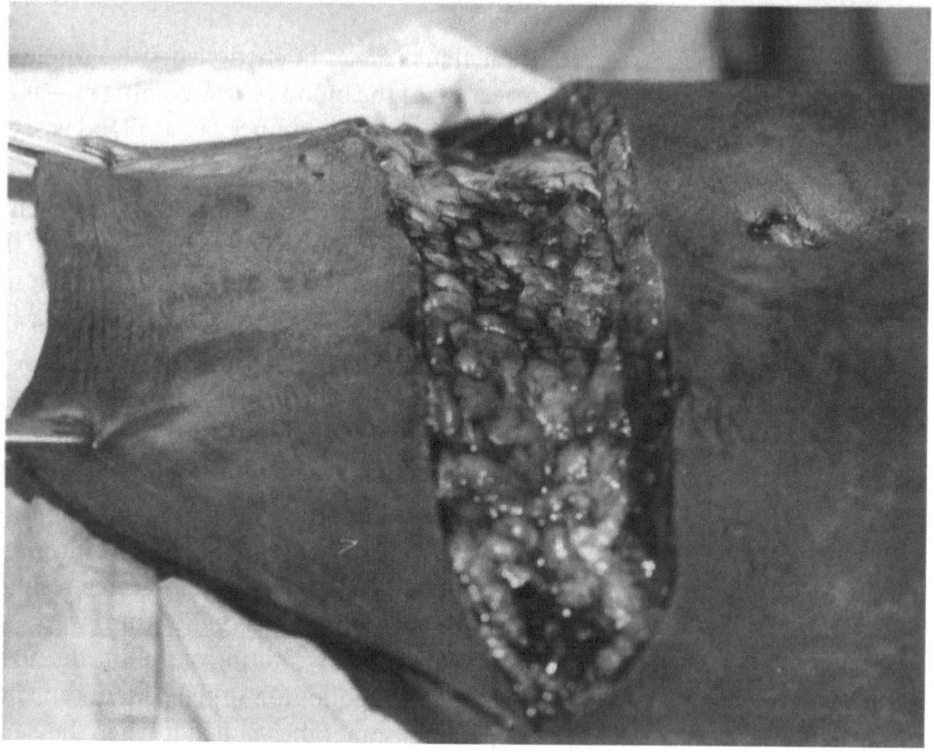

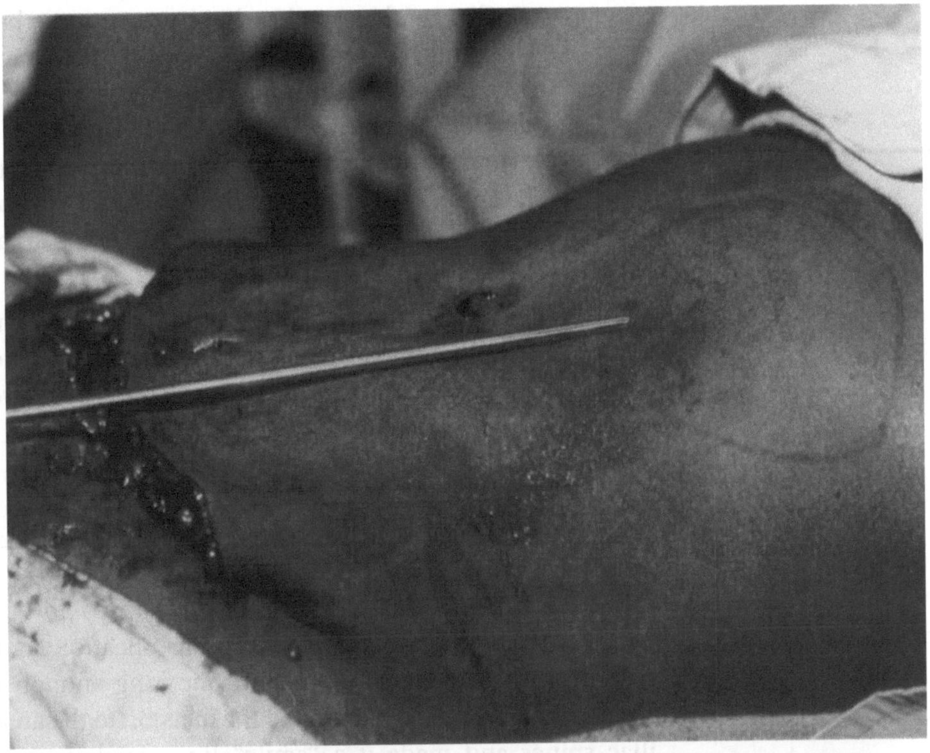

C

D

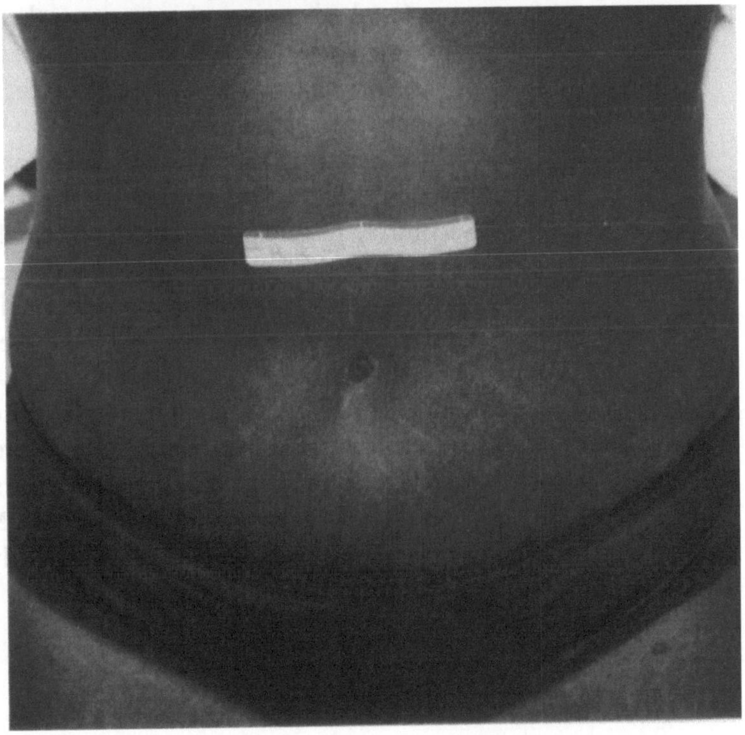

Figure 14-7. Abdominoplasty in African Americans. It is extremely important in these patients that there be no tension on the skin closure. (A) Rapid, efficient technique for defatting the panniculus. The incision has been made in a limited abdominoplasty fashion, stopping short of the amount to be removed. Our initial cut leaves extra skin below the umbilicus, which has now been separated from the overlying skin. After deepening this incision, traction is placed on the area to be removed, and a broad scalpel blade (No. 20) is used to separate the superficial fat from the deeper layers. This method is much faster than liposuction. (C) French-line advancement has been performed so the lateral wings are anchored in an overcorrected position and the mons veneris has been anchored with No. 1 Vicryl sutures into its restored position in the midline. This is the point at which we use liposuction to avoid undermining the upper zones of the abdomen marked by the circle. Small (No. 6 and No. 4) cannulas are used for spray-type suction. (D) End result. The four-suture umbilicoplasty has anchored the scar below the surface, and the lower incision is well hidden within a French-line garment. Visible above this garment is the midline closure site of the old umbilicus.

13. Advise the patient not to wear a girdle immediately postoperatively. Girdles tend to bend and put pressure on the incision line, usually in the center where the blood supply is the most tenuous. Prescribe an abdominal binder and have the patient loosen it three or four times a day for 30 minutes each time. (Plaster casts are no longer used. The heat they generate can be harmful and their rigidity even more harmful.) Choose a binder that has a soft undersurface all the way around. Use enough padding so there is an added layer of protective cover for the panniculus.
14. The patient should start leg lifts in bed during the second week and situps by the third or fourth week. If some exercise is not undertaken, the muscles stretch, as does the tight fascial repair.

Types of Abdominoplasty

As early as 1983 I discussed alternatives to standard abdominoplasty. Because abdominoplasty entails muscle plication in the "crumpled tummy" patient, a short skin excision—but one long enough to allow plication—was needed. With my design, I limited the incision to the area well within the anterior iliac spines and made it a "smile" line. At that point I had recognized the occasional advantage of separating the umbilicus from the fascia to facilitate plication above the midline. Experience convinced me that most patients needed at least one or two figure-of-eight stitches placed above the umbilicus to prevent postoperative ballooning.

Plication of the midline rectus fascia sometimes creates a dimpling effect laterally, so the flap should not be freed laterally any more than necessary. Secondary fingertip movements or careful cautery to separate the skin is then done to avoid a "pinched" upper abdomen. A pad of fat is left in the midline just above the mons, and the mons is defatted. Liposculpture facilitates this step. The fatpad is left in place to make sure there is not a midline dropoff above the incision due to the plication. It is easy to trim that pad just prior to closure if too much fat has been left, whereas it is difficult to elevate a depression.

Shortly after we published our first national paper Richard Greminger[2] reported a similar technique but with a shorter version of the W incision. The terminology is still confusing because Matarasso,[3,4] I,[5] and others published articles on these procedures subsequently.

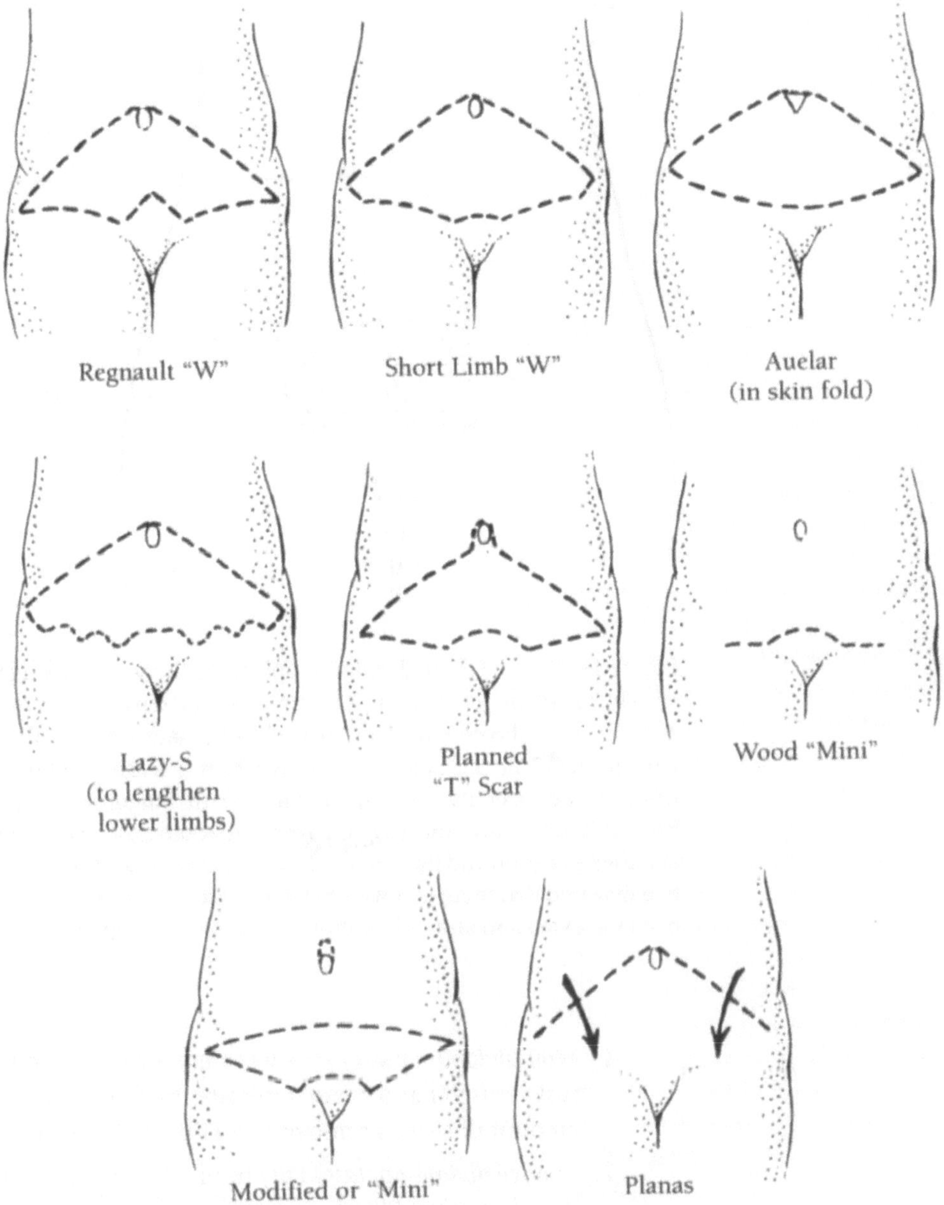

Figure 14-8. In 1978 I described the problem of abdominoplasty incisions in a discussion of what is now known as limited abdominoplasty.[9] Note that most of the incisions then in use crossed the natural skin lines or left an unnatural scar line. We changed from the Regnault W to a short-limb W with the ends angled upward, then to the "smile" incision placed in the skin fold. I also suggested making a lazy S on the lower incision to make the limbs more equal in length. The Wood mini incision was a too small, similar to French mini excisions. None of these incisions addressed the real problems. In fact, few patients with this tiny amount of excess skin needed surgery.

My original description of the modified incision shown in the bottom row had more of a V than the one we later adopted. We also moved the limbs higher than the skin fold and made them more curved, eliminating the V.

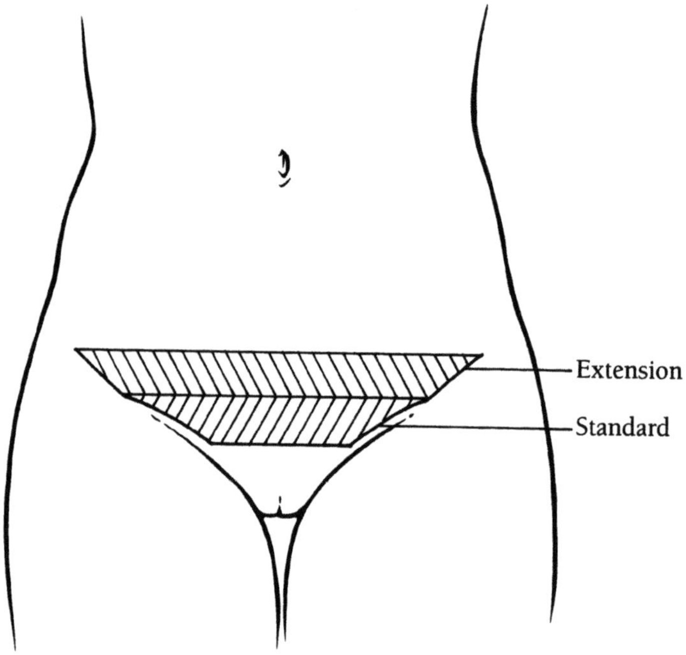

Figure 14-9. The limited abdominoplasty as shown has a longer incision than the mini variety, in which one is doing a lower abdomen repair. For a modified abdominoplasty, the extension shown would be incised in the midst of the procedure if there are extra stretch marks in the area or excessive lateral folding. Note that the extension goes upward and laterally, staying parallel to the inguinal crease and well within the French-line bathing suit design. I advise that only the least amount of skin be resected and then plication and liposuction be performed. Once the patient is flexed at 30 degrees you may find that there is still extra lateral skin to be removed. More often, I find I did not need the extension after all. A shorter incision is a happier incision.

1. *Mini abdominoplasty* requires only a short, curved incision that allows just enough hand room to plicate the fascia up to the umbilicus. A small amount of skin is removed and liposuction can be freely employed.
2. *Limited abdominoplasty* may be of several types, including the "umbilical detachment and float" procedure or a dissection above the umbilicus for one or two figure-of-eight sutures. Again, liposuction may be employed freely because of the extensive blood supply.
3. *Modified abdominoplasty* is a term now used to distinguish the incorporation of limited abdominoplasty techniques in patients who require complete mons-to-xiphoid plication and a large amount of skin removal. The most common type is closure of the umbilical site in the midline to provide a greater length of panniculus so closure may be effected without flap tension.

Choosing the Abdominoplasty Procedure

There have been many developments in the operation once called "limited" abdominoplasty. As with other surgical procedures, enterprising surgeons have continued to refine and tailor the operation according to individual patient requirements.

For each of the three variations—mini, limited, modified (see above)—follow these rules: (1) make a short incision with upward curves at the end; (2) avoid any transgression across the inguinal ligament; (3) avoid V incisions in the midline; and (4) vary the length or angle of the lateral limbs according to bathing suit preferences. For example, in patients who prefer French-line swim suits, angle the incision to roughly parallel an old diagonal appendectomy incision.

New technical point: *In the operating room*, the surgeon decides whether to separate the umbilicus and allow it to "float" downward. If there is still laxity in the upper abdominal skin following limited abdominal resection and fascial repair, detach the umbilicus from the fascia. The other common variation in technique is detaching the umbilicus from the skin, repositioning it, and closing the umbilical site as a vertical midline slit. This operation is indicated for patients in whom a standard abdominoplasty resection would result in a long scar and tight midline closure. "Vertical slit closure lessens the risk of midline necrosis."

There are other variations, each being a legitimate variation of "limited" abdominoplasty. The "beer barrel belly" midline excision and repair has been discussed by Jon Sattler (Columbia). Repairs in his male patients are performed through a circumumbilical incision. Suction and direct excision of fat is employed, and undermining is done only to provide exposure of the midline fascia for plication. Because these men have obviously never been pregnant, the skin should shrink well. Sattler reports good results with negligible scars. I have not had much success with it.

Next is the mid-abdominal repair of Ewaldo De Souza-Pinto (Brazil). He uses a supraumbilical skin incision that can be extended to resect those crumpled areas that occur in the supraumbilical zone. My criticism is that he uses a percutaneous plication when one could easily do a direct plication using Sattler's method of elevating the surrounding panniculus.

My colleagues Gus Colon, Robert Wood, Richard Greminger, Maxwell Cooper, Barrett Noone, Brian Murphy, David Reath, and others will be interested in the following comments from one of our British colleagues regarding the limited or mini abdominoplasty.

According to our London expert, who voiced these opinions as an authority in a malpractice suit to be heard in an American court, this operation was "not an acceptably used procedure" in 1982.

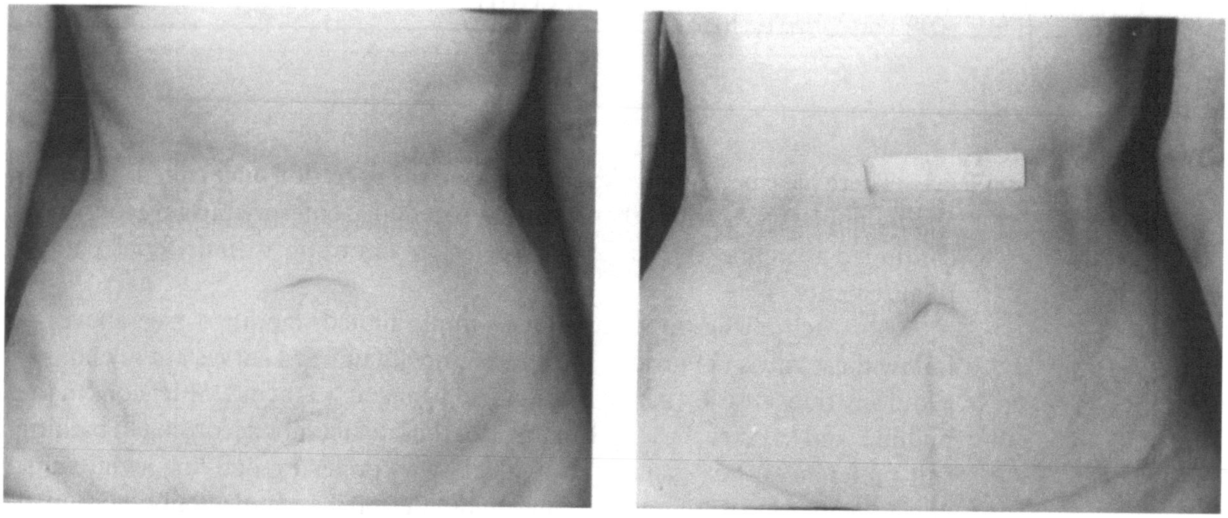

A B

Figure 14-10. The procedure we described as limited abdominoplasty is applied primarily to patients such as those who have little or no abdominal wall stretching above the umbilicus but a fairly extensive diastasis below. The incision is a smile line. In patients who have bold scarring in the midline, it is advantageous to try to remove as much as possible even though the umbilicus now has a down curve. In this patient, we have maintained the natural folding of the abdomen with selective liposuction above the umbilicus, plication from the pubis to the umbilicus, and resection of 4 cm of skin, which included much of her old scar and stretch marks.

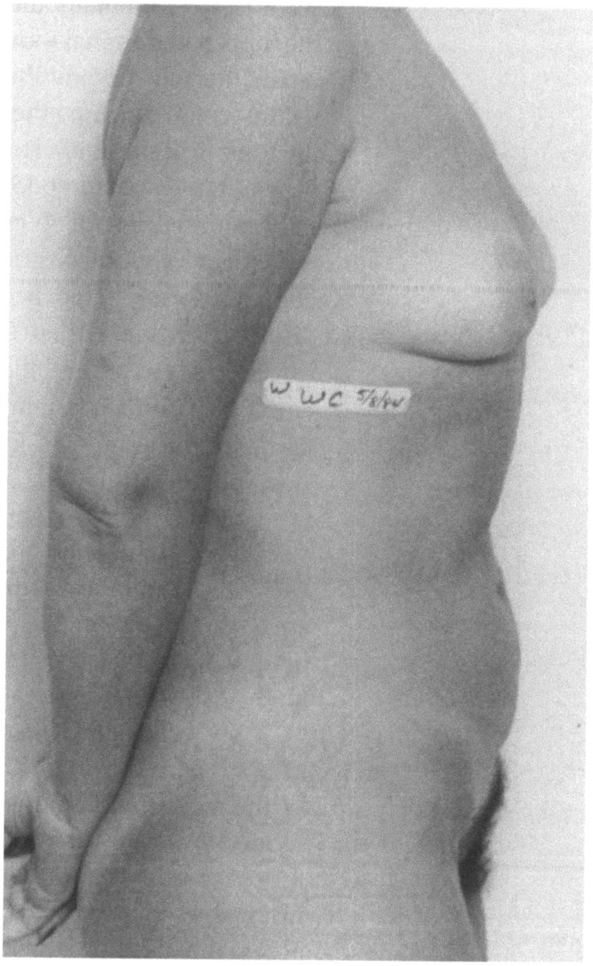

Figure 14-11. By 1984, we had established a criterion for evaluating patients for limited abdominoplasty. This patient is typical of those who fit the requirement. Note that the upper abdomen is taut and relatively fat-free. The stretching of the fascia begins just above the umbilicus, but there is little excess skin. A short incision, plication up to and above the umbilicus, and moderate skin removal with lateral flank suction was a revolutionary idea in 1983.

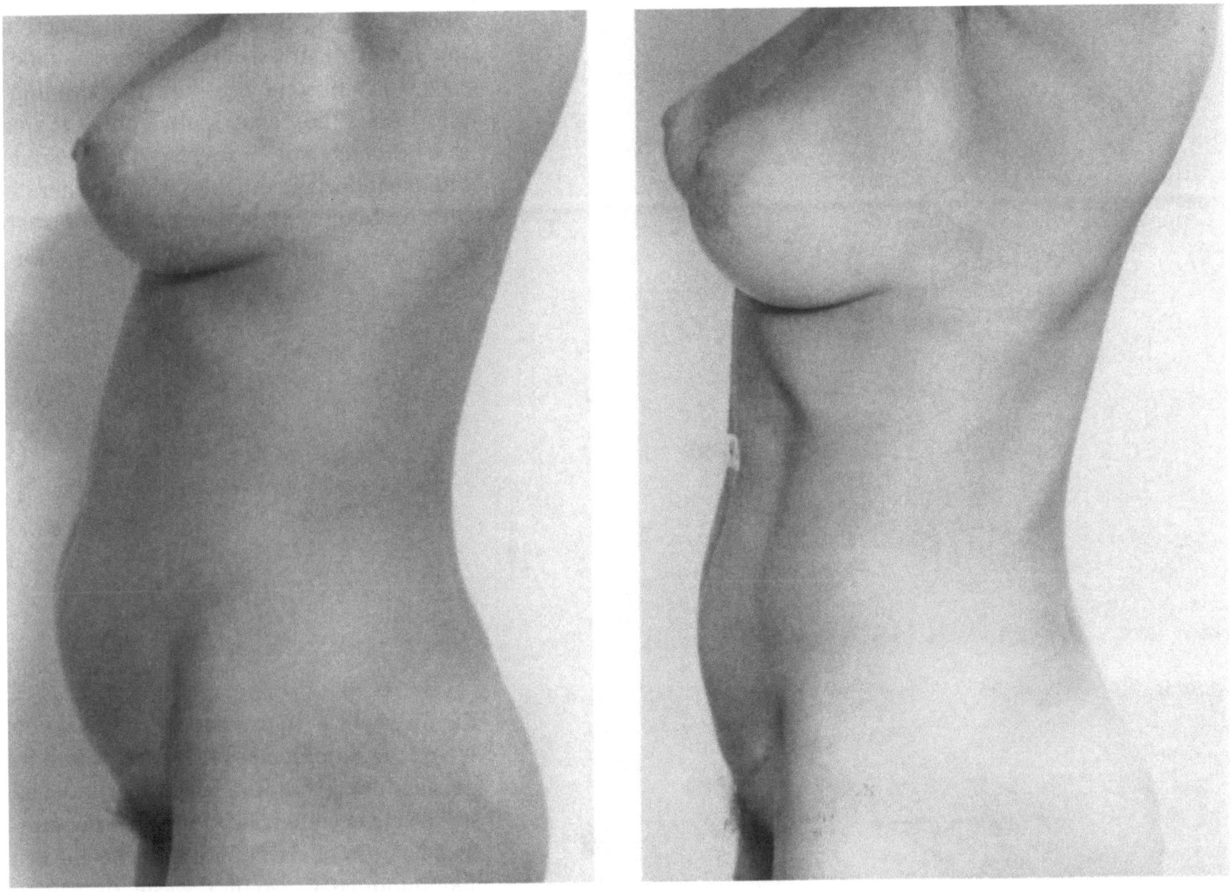

Figure 14-12. This patient had previously had breast augmentation and now requested abdominal repair. Note on the side view that I have repaired the fascia to just above the umbilicus via an old cesarean section scar. I extended it only minimally and upward so she could still wear a French-line bikini.

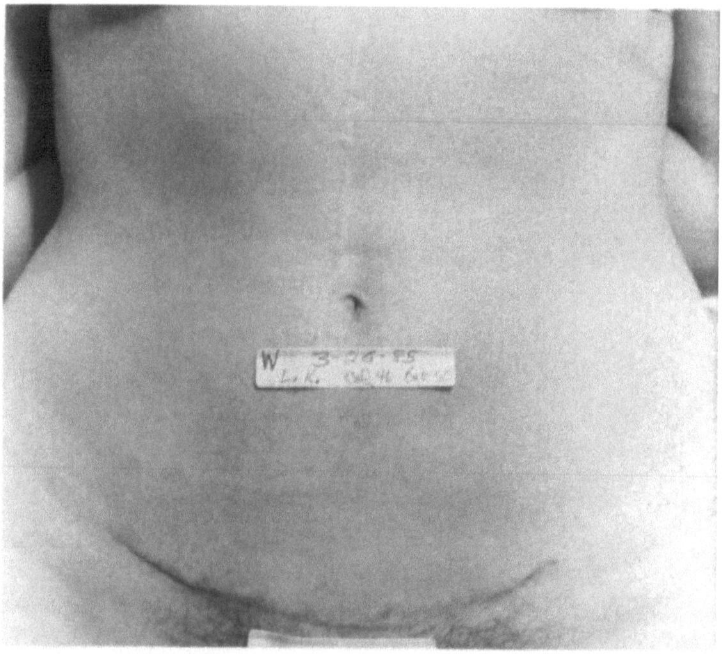

Figure 14-13. By 1985 I was using suction much more aggressively in the upper abdomen but still kept the limited abdominoplasty scars short and repaired only the area that needed repair. Scars placed in the smile line position fade quickly. Because there is little or no tension, hypertrophy is unusual.

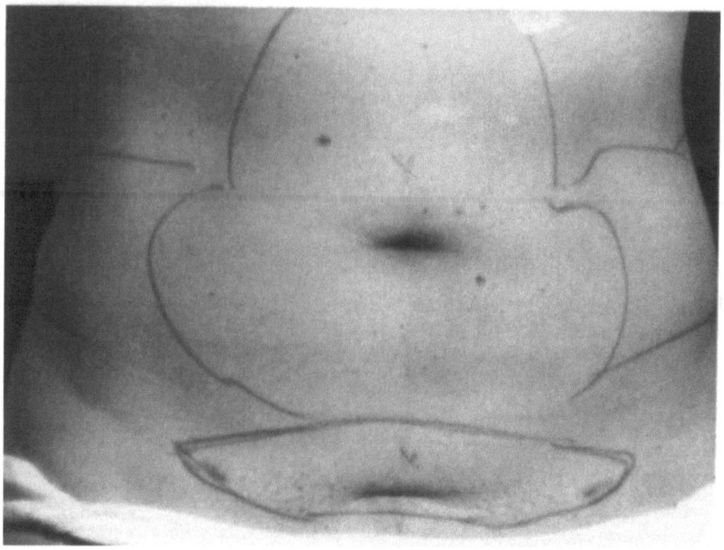

Figure 14-14. In this patient the marks on the upper abdomen show areas that will be liposuctioned, but the lower portion will still be elevated for plication. Note the minimal amount of skin removal in this limited abdominoplasty. Do not waste time with liposuction below the umbilicus. It is easier to trim fat under direct vision. With the limited abdominoplasty one can be more aggressive with liposuction because of the minimal disturbance of blood supply.

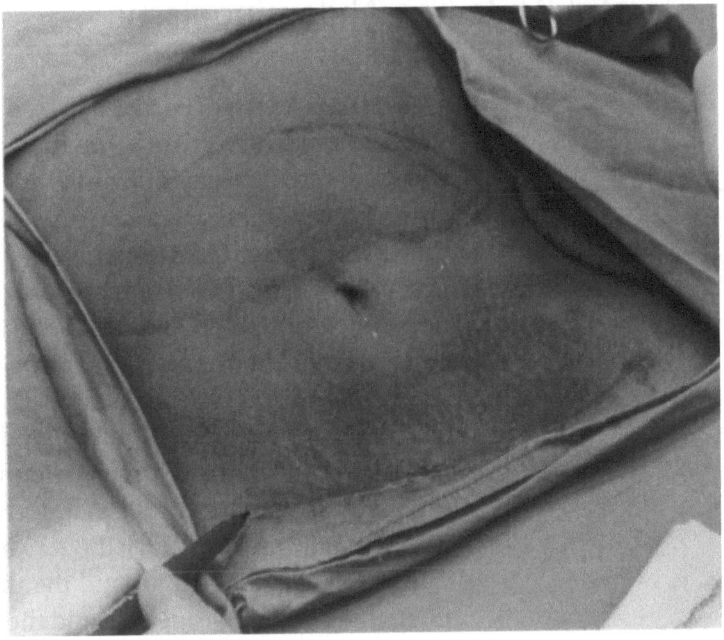

Figure 14-15. When limited abdominoplasty patients gain weight, it is typically in the upper abdomen. Prior to the availability of liposuction we generally left this area alone. In this patient, secondary liposuction is required, as fat has recurred in this area. The small amount of fat around the umbilicus will not be removed because it gives a more natural appearance.

WARP Procedure

The wide abdominal rectus plication (WARP) of Richard Toronto (Plano) is a waist-cinching maneuver to obtain more lateral pull on the oblique and rectus muscles.[7] These muscles then distract the vertebrae so certain types of back pain are relieved. Imagine a triangle. Pulling in both lateral points to the center elevates the tip of the triangle. Lateral-to-lateral plication pull translates into longitudinal lift (i.e., separation of vertebrae compressed by muscle tension). The oblique and transversalis muscles are brought up to the lateral rectus sheath, and the rectus is plicated in the midline. Toronto reported that a series of patients did obtain relief from their refractory low back pain. Could it have been simply from repositioning the weight of the infraabdominal contents?

Tom Biggs (Houston) has observed that abdominoplasty does reduce lordosis. Maybe intervertebral distraction is a factor. Many of my patients who have undergone the WARP procedure have been pleasantly surprised to find that they may resume normal activity without their accustomed backache. Thus our version of the WARP procedure must have an effect beyond the abdominal wall, as Toronto described.[7]

Mid-Abdomen Abdominoplasty

Marcus Melvin (Portland) asked if anyone has had experience with patients who have extensive tissue breakdown only in the mid-abdomen. His solution was to excise directly horizontally across the mid-abdomen and do the repair through this approach rather than the traditional low abdominal incision. "If there is significant scarring from old surgery or from extreme stretching during pregnancy in the mid-abdomen it might be unsafe to work from below." At that point one must accept the fact the scar will be more visible than the others and certainly more unpredictable. I have not used this method and prefer not to deal with a mid-abdomen horizontal scar.

Melvin's repair is somewhat different from the de Souza-Pinto type mid-abdomen repair. With the latter method a circle of skin is removed around the umbilicus and drawn in as a purse-string after some type of mid-abdomen fascial repair has been carried out. This technique is said to work well in men. The problem is the scar around the umbilicus. "Men seem to accept this better than a long bikini line incision and the longer recovery [the latter] would entail."

Effect of Smoking on Abdominoplasty

Does smoking cause complications in abdominoplasty patients? The answer is a resounding "yes." I was initially skeptical of the first reports linking decreased blood flow to resumption of smoking after surgery. Subsequent reports in the literature, however, as well as laboratory data and personal communications with other surgeons, have convinced me that smoking can play a part in creating complications after abdominoplasty, face lifts, breast reconstructions, breast reductions, and so on. At one time we would have attributed these complications to acts of God rather than to acts of nicotine. We now know that nicotine can effect large changes in the circulation in some people, especially if it is already compromised.

Touch-Up Surgery in the Postabdominoplasty Patient

Surgeons who have performed aesthetic or reconstructive abdominoplasties since the mid to late 1970s are well aware that a small percentage of these patient do not maintain their original (postsurgical) appearance. There may be descent of soft tissues with some stretching, usually in the lateral folds. In some individuals it is simply due to weight gain, and in others this skin has stretched to the point that touch-up surgery is complicated. Suction-assisted lipectomy can be a useful tool in these individuals.

The usual patient has one area of scar widening or hypertrophy. After a few years it is easy to remove the scar and perform the repair with standard multilayer techniques. We prefer two deep layers of Vicryl, which completely evert the skin edges, and a final subcuticular 4-0 Vicryl suture to hold the edges. A few patients require lateral extension of the scar, but often I find that "dog-ears" can be smoothed out without the need for skin removal. Simply making a small opening in the lateral incision or even taking out 1 cm of skin allows insertion of a Becker curette suction cannula to reduce the bulk laterally. Abdominal skin is tough. It more often than not shrinks to an acceptable contour if the undersurface fat is removed.

The same is true in the upper abdomen. For some reason a number of women have added fat or a fibrofatty deposit due to suture breakage in the midline. Technical point: Use 4-mm, short suction cannulas to debulk. These instruments are much easier to control than the long ones. Make the opening inside the umbilicus. If the old periumbilical scar is visible, as was the case in some of my abdominoplasties, it is a good time to use a turnover flap technique to hide the incision and create a skin fold across the upper border.

Do not forget the "pinch technique." After you have suctioned with a 6-mm cannula and then criss-crossed with a small facial cannula, you can identify remaining areas of thickness with the pinch technique: Lift the area and pass the deepest retractor through the base of the pinch. Let the patient relax and then crisscross above this area using the small suction cannula. No drains are necessary, and if a panty girdle or abdominal binder is applied immediately there is little bruising. Try the flat-end cannula in the superficial plane to break up subdermal adhesions.

Role of Liposuction in Defatting

Direct defatting of the panniculus is not only faster, but easier on the surgeon's arms and shoulders. Moreover the end result is a much more uniform thickness. Liposuction has been used to make the midline and lateral rectus grooves and to suction the areas above the panniculus that have not been dissected. By not dissecting these areas near the lower rib cage, one preserves more of the blood supply.

See Figures 14-1 through 14-5 for descriptions of liposuction techniques.

Open Abdominoplasty

With tongue in cheek, I published a letter to the editor in *Plastic and Reconstructive Surgery* in November 1990 which detailed some of the technical points we had used in addressing abdominal wall problems in patients who had

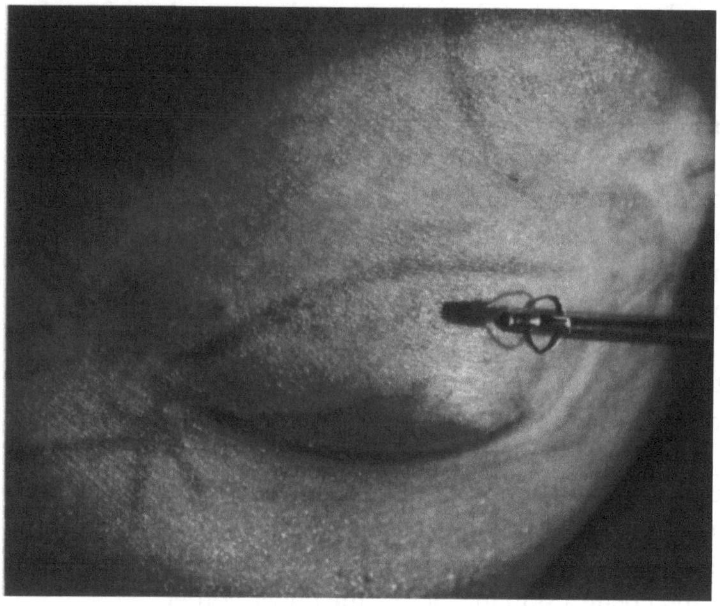

Figure 14-16. Liposuction can play a role in the direction of "dog-ears." I use this Becker curet cannula to scrape the undersurface of the skin beyond the incision in order to enhance shrinkage—then I do not have to extend the scar. Standard liposuction cannulas are used above and below for tapering. If in such cases this triangle is defatted aggressively during the original limited abdominoplasty and the upper flap tapered, the problem seen here will become a rarity.

previously undergone major abdominal surgery and must be approached in a different manner because of the previous undermining and damage. Such individuals have wide hypertrophic scars from the xiphoid to the pubis. The only way to control scar hypertrophy in this unfavorable orientation is to create a series of W-plasties and leave a section of old scar intact, preferably in, above, or below the umbilicus. This area is simply undermined and the fat trimmed under direct vision from the midline scar excision. Leaving the intact area creates two scars that respond favorably to the W-plasty closure technique.

Liposuction, of course, plays a major role in attacking the flanks and areas beyond the direct excision. Direct excision of subcutaneous fat 4 to 5 cm past the midline to the left and right is a quicker way to remove the fat. Furthermore, this area can be advanced by the plication sutures.

Once the fat has been removed, the plication brings the soft tissues together so the resulting W-plasty closure is already everted. A multilayered subcuticular and subcutaneous closure with running Vicryl sutures brings the tissue together.

In certain individuals, it has been necessary to resect loose skin just above the "smile line," as for the limited abdominoplasty. A half-buried nylon suture tied on the hair-bearing surface of the mons brings this T scar together without tension. Only a few 6-0 nylon tacking stitches are required to keep the ends of the W-plasties from drifting.

The umbilicus may be detached, as in the "abdominal float" procedure, or left intact, depending on the particular requirements. The umbilicus may also be allowed to float downward, and an ellipse of skin can removed in exactly the same manner described earlier in this chapter for limited abdominoplasty because scars are more problematic around the umbilicus and the umbilicus may easily distort. Even though the original surgery, scar crosses the umbilecus it is advisable to leave this area untouched on the surface as a zone free of incisions.

Hence when faced with a vertically scarred abdomen, the open abdominoplasty approach is a quick and easy way to obtain good contouring, waist plication, safe liposuction, and more predictable contouring of the abdominal fatpads.

Comments and Commentary

1. Current taboos for plastic surgery

   1. Plaster of paris casts after abdominoplasty
   2. "Elastoplast" tape after augmentations
   3. Incisions 2 to 3 mm below the eyelid margin "to reduce the danger of skin necrosis"
   4. General anesthesia for limited abdominoplasty and for breast augmentations because "you can't make a large enough pocket with a local"

2. Shape of the umbilicus: It is reported that 63% of all umbilical shapes are oval in the horizontal direction, and about 12% are oval but vertical. Those with round belly buttons (25%) are in a distinct minority.

3. Bob Wiemer (Houston) incises each new umbilical site as a U and then sutures this flap to itself, rather than suturing the flap directly to the fascia. Turning the flap on itself creates a shelf that effectively hides the suture line. It also recreates the superior fold frequently seen in the normal umbilicus.

4. Occasionally one reaches the point of umbilical placement and discovers that the midline markers have been lost. There is then a fear that the umbilicus might have been pulled to one side or the other by differences in muscle suturing. It would be reassuring to see a reliable mark to indicate that you are indeed on target. One suggestion is to mark the undersurface of a steridrape. Simply slide the marking pen underneath and twirl it a few times. This maneuver leaves an indelible mark that does not wash away no matter how wet the field or how well it is cleansed.

5. One of the good points in Jose Guerros-Santos' article about patients with absent umbilicuses who require a new abdominoplasty is as follows: Measure the spot for the new umbilicus, cut out a round spot of skin still attached below, and anchor it to the fascia for the base of the new umbilicus.

6. The recurrence of fluid underneath a flap is not limited to plastic surgery patients. General surgeons tell us that a seroma under a radical mastectomy flap

(Text continued on page 421)

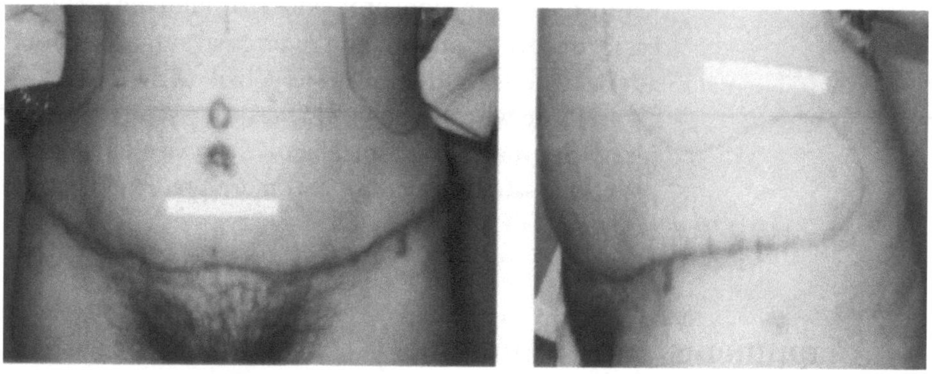

A B

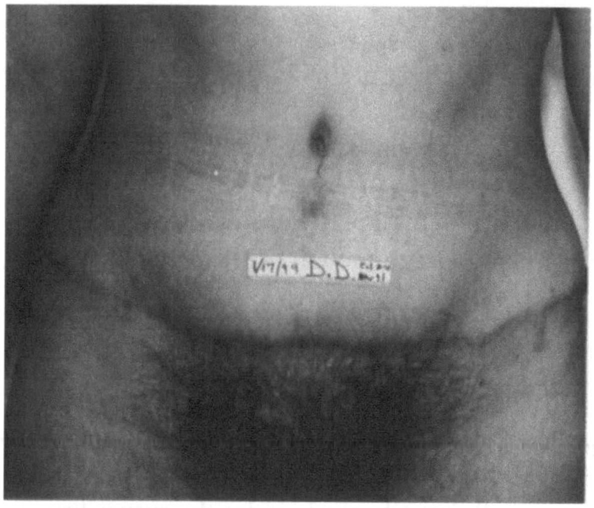

C

Figure 14-17. (A–C) What is wrong with this picture? First, the other surgeon left the mons far too high. The umbilicus has hatch marks, and it is too low. It will be relocated to the marked area and the old umbilioplasty closed vertically. Her internal repair was intact, and liposuction corrected the rest of her problems. Long scars such as this one should be avoided at all costs. We only can improve them. Adding mons reduction and mons fixation gave a balanced shape and appearance.

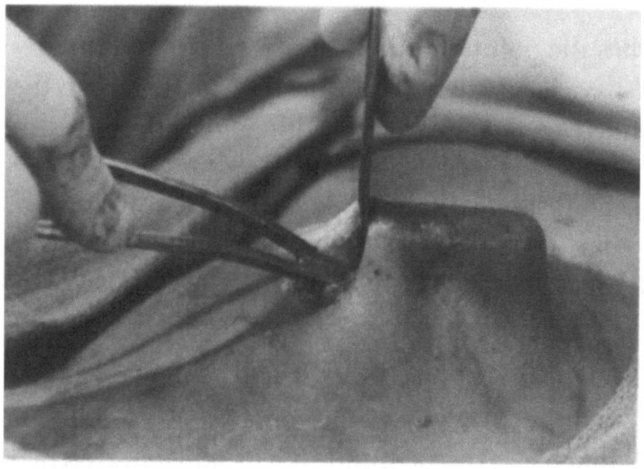

Figure 14-18. Occasionally men have stretching of the mid-abdomen fascia and little excess skin. After liposuction, one can elevate the flap easily from a supraumbilical approach for plication sutures. I use a short needle and heavy material such as No. 1 Vicryl to make it easier. For most men, however, a standard limited abdominoplasty is a better choice. The average patient has so much excess skin they must be treated exactly the same as the postpartum woman.

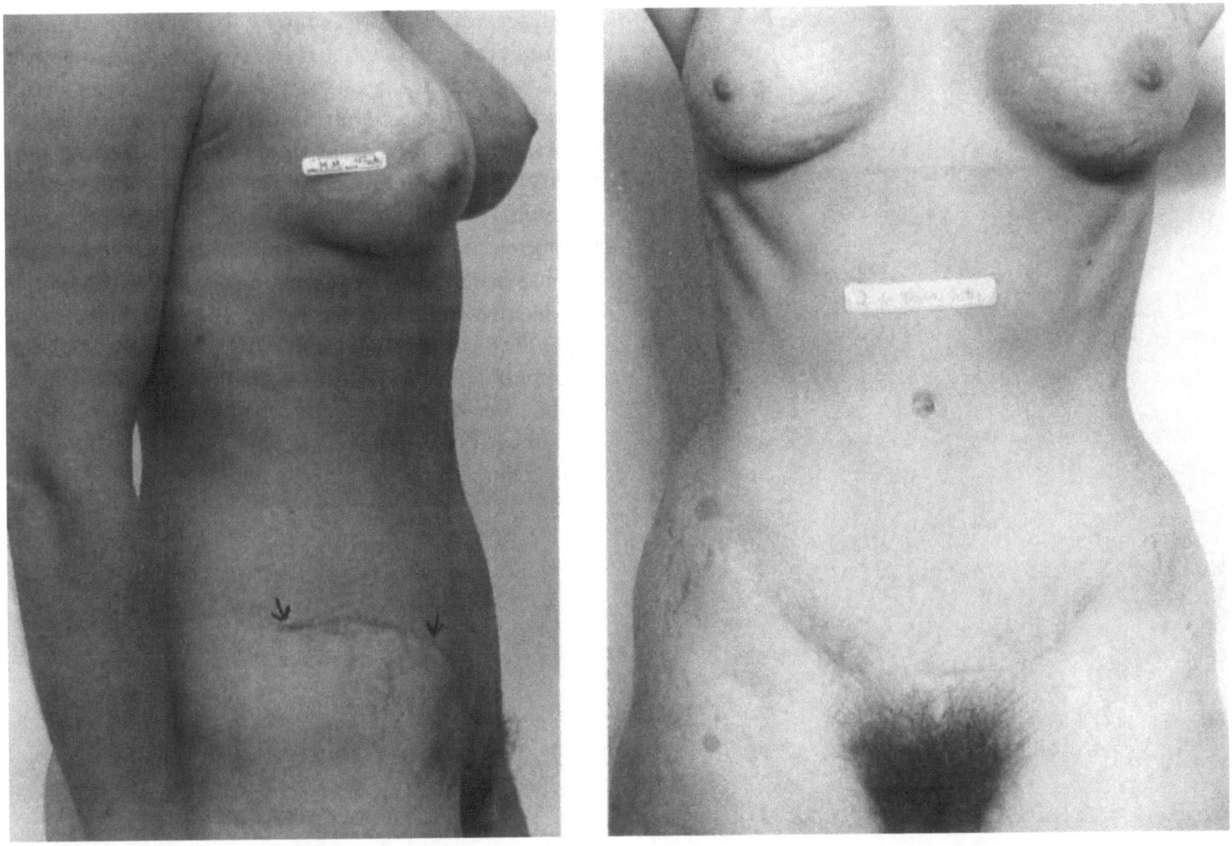

Figure 14-19. A few patients do require an extended excision. If it is necessary, at least place it within the bikini line, as in the "gull wing" procedure described by Fred Grazer. These individuals have loose, damaged skin laterally. In 1980, at 2 years after operation, this patient's incisions are just beginning to fade, and she can now wear a French line bikini. Today we would make every effort to induce shrinkage in this lateral zone (marked by the arrows) by suctioning and subdermal curettage. There are cases in which the skin simply must be removed as a primary procedure.

Note the good results of the breast augmentation performed from within the abdomen. There are only a few technical points for augmentation: I make a wide incision under the mammary fold to expose the surface of the pectoralis major for good lateral dissection and stretching. Today, I use textured breast implants because they do not move. The brassiere keeps the new inframammary fold sealed. I tack the undersurface together with just a few sutures to keep the implant in place but leave space for it to drain. There may be undetected bleeding, so it is wise to leave enough space for any blood or fluid to flow down into the abdomen, where it will not cause problems.

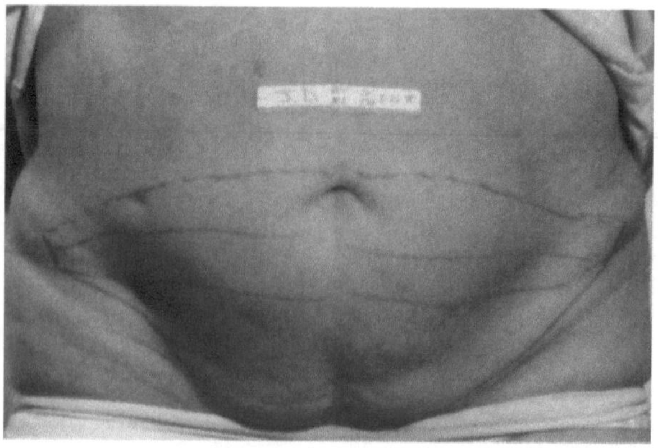

Figure 14-20. In patients with gallbladder incisions, I may use either line (as drawn). I excise the minimal amount of skin first. Once I have fixed the mons upward and advanced the lateral tissue forward, I can decide if I need to resect more skin. In this patient, applying the principles of limited abdominoplasty will decrease tension on the closure. Blood supply will be compromised somewhat by the previous gallbladder incision. Once the abdominal plication is complete and the abdominal flap has been raised by separating the umbilical stalk, I can decide whether to resect more or less of the skin flap depending on the new position of the mons and the amount of laxity above the original umbilicus. When in doubt, I leave the flap long. In this case, I chose the "umbilical float" procedure. She has a long abdomen and lax skin *above* the umbilicus.

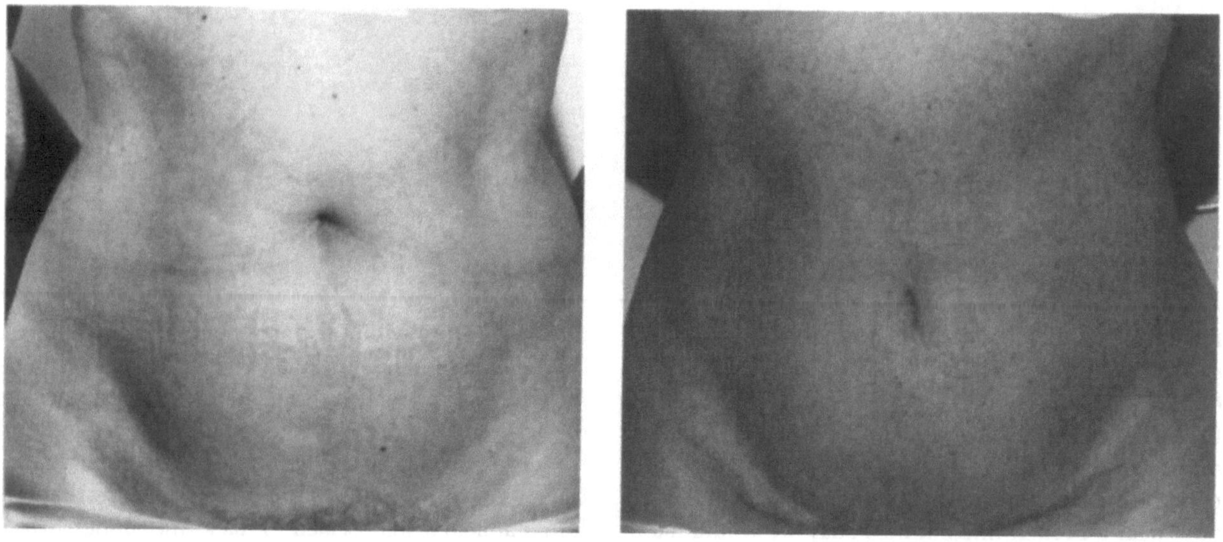

Figure 14-21. Freeing the umbilicus from the fascia and allowing it to float to a still natural position allows correction of the entire area.

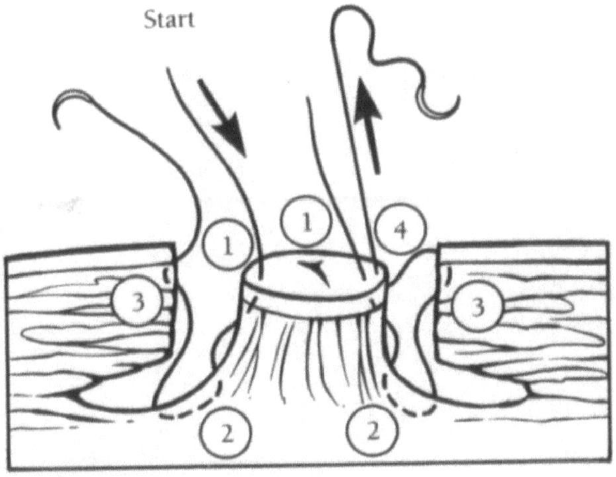

Figure 14-22. Four-suture umbilicoplasty saves time during "full" abdominal repair or modifications of that repair where the umbilical site is closed at the central slit to allow a longer panniculus flap. With the abdominal flap elevated, pass a 2-0 nylon suture through the umbilical skin and into the deep fascia at 12 o'clock. Then come upward and take a bite of subdermal tissue below the skin margin, then back down for another bite of fascia. The suture ends with an exit on the umbilical skin. Before tying this one, place the second suture at 6 o'clock (steps 1–4). After the abdominal fascia repair is completed, tie these two sutures down to secure the umbilical stalk to the fascia. With only two sutures, there is no problem with tangled sutures. The other sutures do not go to the fascia. They start on the umbilical stalk skin, pass subcuticularly into the new umbilical site, and end on umbilical skin. When all four sutures are tied, there are no hatch marks on the surrounding skin.

A 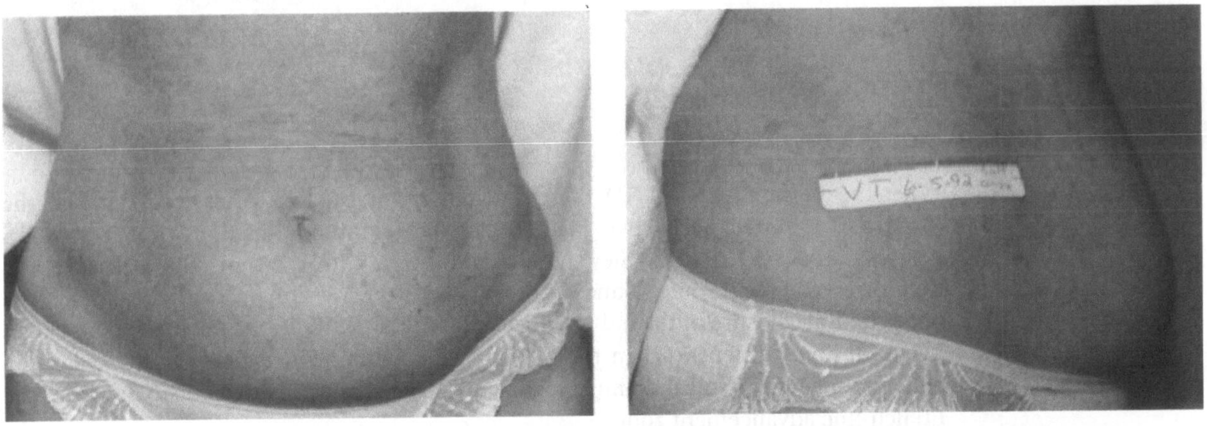 B

Figure 14-23. Two defects are apparent in this patient. The umbilicus sits at a low position, and there is excess wrinkling in the skin above. The umbilical float procedure would make this situation worse, yet she does not have enough loose skin to warrant removal from the umbilicus to the mons. **(A)** Her main deformity on the lateral view is in the lower abdomen, but there is still muscle separation and laxity above. **(B)** We planned to use liposuction in the corners beyond the incision and across the upper abdomen, and to free the upper abdomen so we could plicate from xiphoid to pubis. In figure **(C)**, the umbilical site has been closed and sutures are placed for the "4 suture umbilicoplasty".

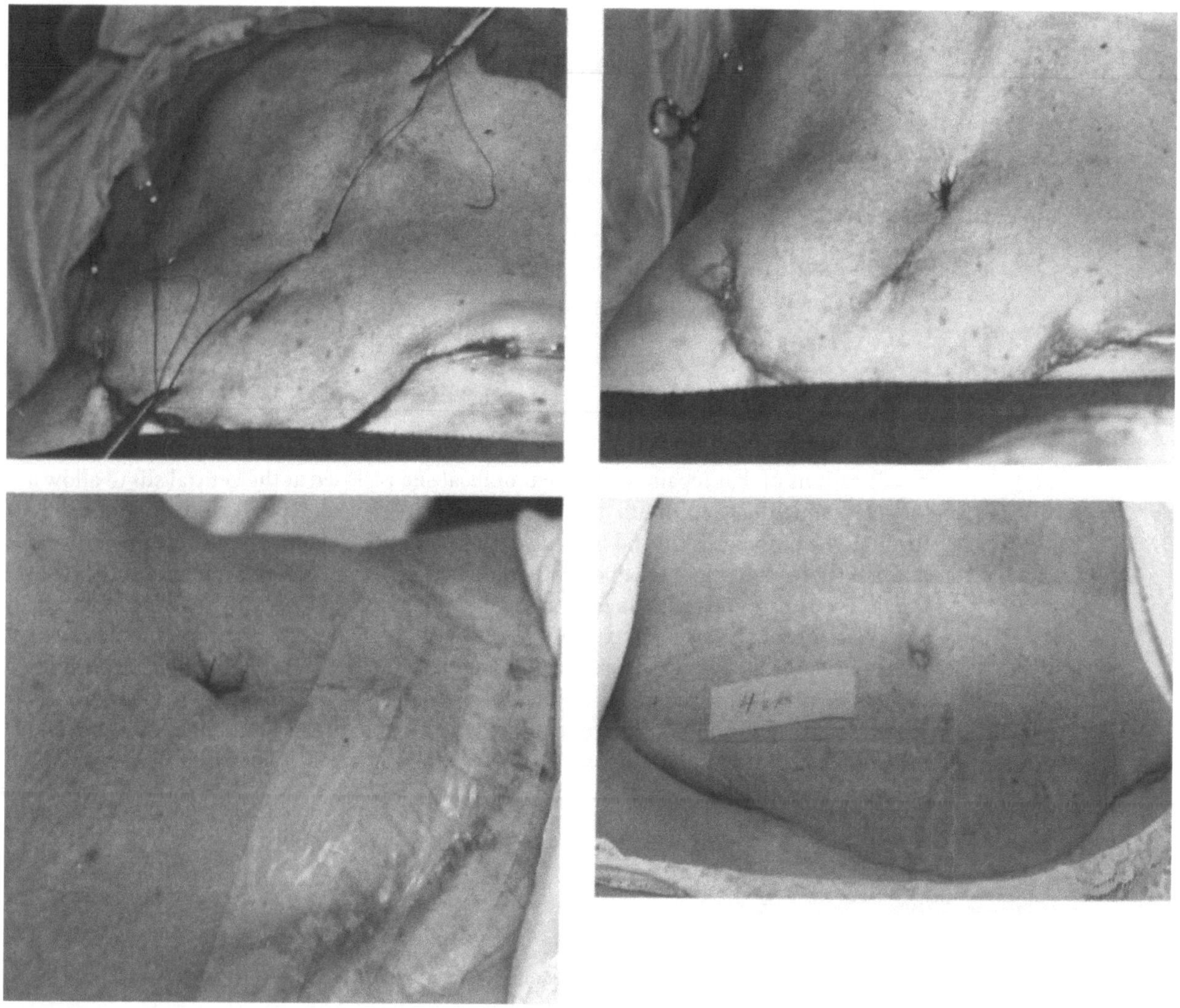

C D E F

When the incision is closed (D), there is no tension on the flap. After drain removal, the lower flap is protected by two inch paper tape for immobilization. (E) At 4 weeks postoperatively (F) note the new umbilical position with the four-suture closure, the overcorrected French-line advancement that leaves the incision protruding, and the area of the midline closure of the old umbilical site. All of the incisions are easily covered by a French-line garment. (G) In this patient we have applied the principles of limited abdominoplasty to a full abdominal repair and have adjusted her incision to fit within the French-line advancement zone.

Figure 14-23. Continued.

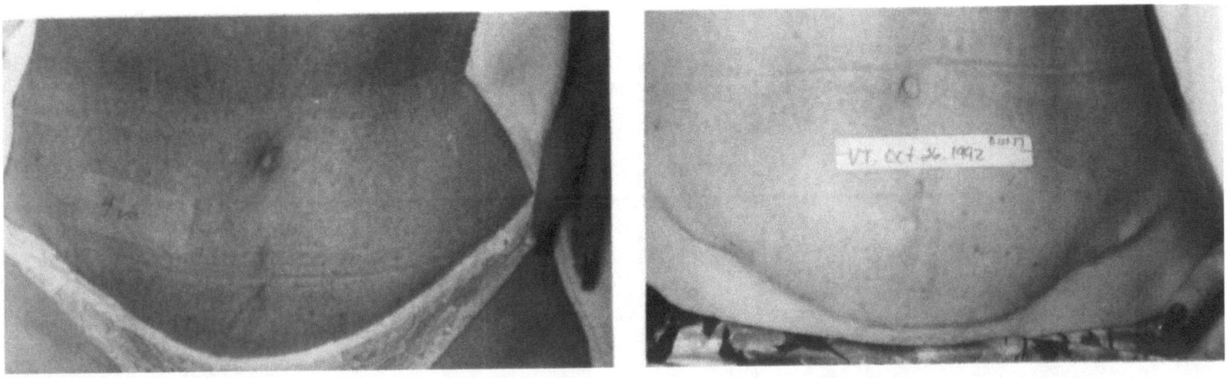

G H

Figure 14-23. Continued.

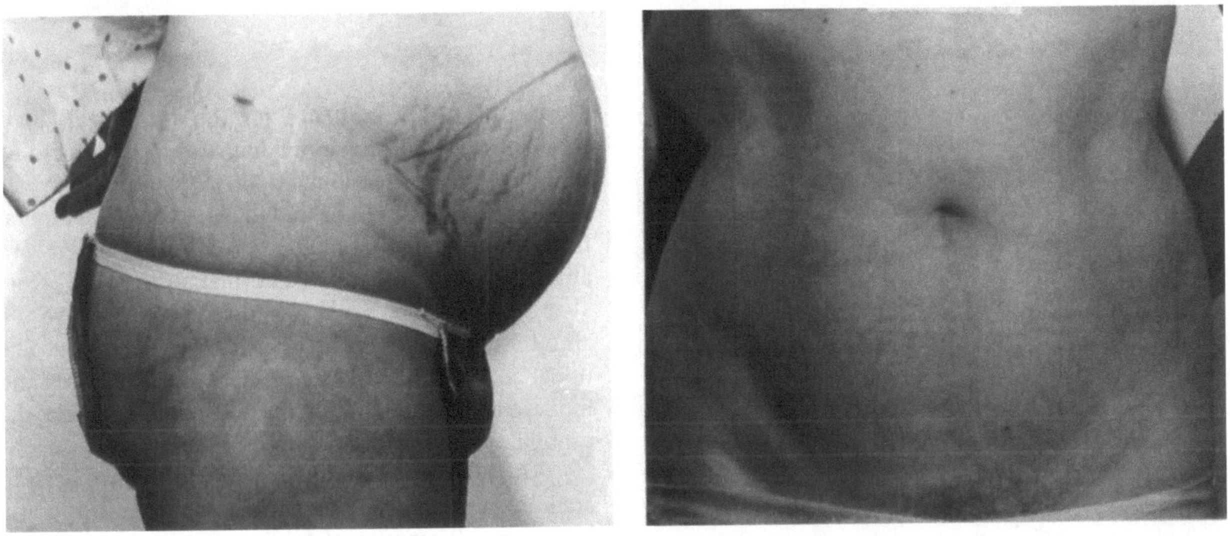

Figure 14-24. *Complete abdominoplasty variation.* For this category of patient, I prefer to remove as much of the distorted skin as possible. With a full panniculus stretch, there will be no difficulty moving the umbilical skin to the mons veneris incision line. The lateral incision curve will be widened during surgery and extended more laterally to trim out more damaged skin. The incision is kept within the "smile" curvature. Her mons veneris has dropped 2 to 3 cm. Anchoring it in a corrected position also reduces tension and allows removal of more stretch mark marred skin.

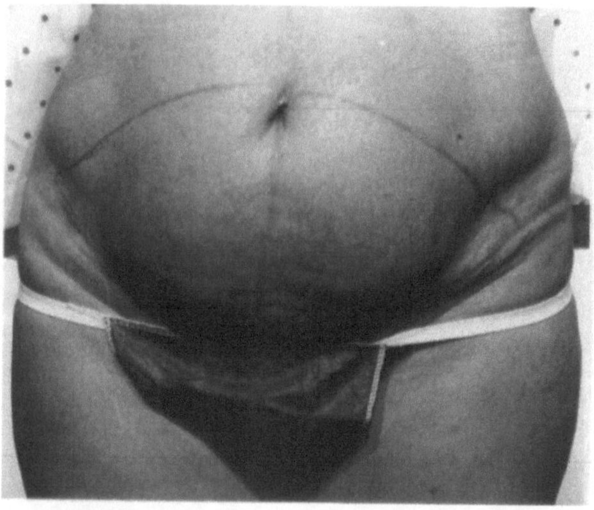

A

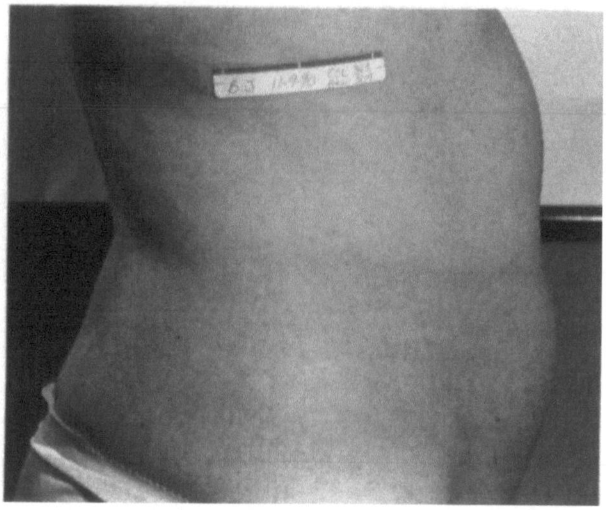

B

C

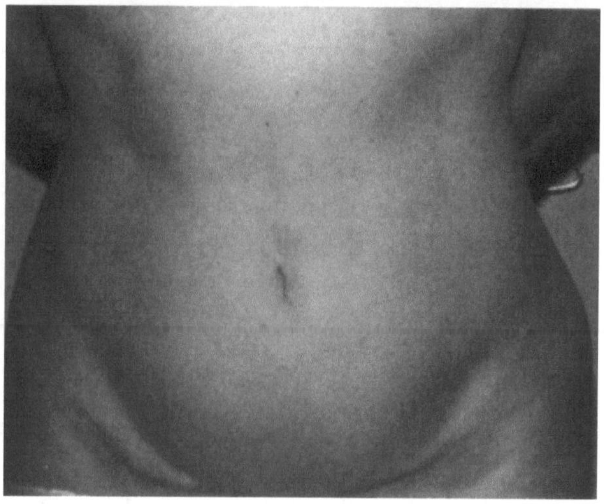

Figure 14-25. Candidates for the "umbilical float" procedure are ideally individuals with a high-riding umbilicus, a long abdomen, and a generous distance between the hairline and umbilicus. **(A&B)** Postoperatively, note that the umbilicus has floated downward almost too far but is still in a normal position. **(C)** Note also the short incision that allowed us to remove the amount of skin and soft tissue that was necessary. The upper abdomen was treated primarily by suctioning and moderate plication up to the midpoint between the umbilicus and the xiphoid process.

An alternative in this patient would have been to anchor the umbilicus at a slightly higher position and leave a small amount of folding, or to resect a small ellipse of skin just above the umbilicus and stretch it upward another 0.5 cm.

is one of their biggest difficulties despite drains and frequent aspiration. I once reported the antiseroma effect of Terramycin and asked if anyone had experienced complications with injecting it into a seroma. Some general surgeons had published a series in which they had injected Terramycin for sarcomas in their mastectomy patients, but they discontinued the practice because patients complained of continued pain. The solution: mixing the Terramycin, Achromycin, or Tetracycline with a long-acting local anesthetic such as Marcaine. The mixture helps distribute the antibiotic and provides long-lasting analgesia.

7. Theodore Dodenhoff (Phoenix) says: "The patient is responsible for his or her epigastrium." After liposuction or abdominoplasty, the patient may reaccumulate fat and distort that area again. Inactivity and obesity then stretch the skin, making a secondary revision necessary.

8. Weight loss patients undergoing body plastic surgery have an increase in self-esteem. However, they do not show any improvement in their weight gain and loss patterns.

9. Most American surgeons do not heparinize or give intravenous alcohol to abdominoplasty patients. After discussing this subject in *Technical Forum*, the following correspondence was received from Leo Rozner (Victoria, Australia).

> We in our practice do approximately 150 cases a year. This has gradually built up from about 20 cases a year. We first went into practice in 1965, and in the early days venous thrombosis and pulmonary embolism was virtually unknown. However, in about 1973–1974 we had an "epidemic" of thrombosis and embolism—about four and five [cases], respectively. Only one fatality ensued, and this was in a patient who was grossly overweight and very sluggish. She also had peripheral venous disease.
>
> As a result of discussion with colleagues, the following regimen has been instituted, and to date no further episodes of significant venous thrombosis have occurred in the legs and certainly no pulmonary embolisms. The patient is given Calciperin 5000 units intramuscularly 1 hour before going to theatre. In theatre, the patient is positioned with the heels on a soft sponge pad, and calf stimulator electrodes are fastened to the legs and set to work about once every 30 to 40 seconds. The operation is carried out with the patient horizontal. Postoperatively, the patient is encouraged to move in bed [and is] allowed to sit out of bed the next morning and walk in the stooped position. Calciperin is continued for 3 days, by which time good spontaneous activity has been restored.
>
> The only other technical assistance we have is to support the area of surgery with a fairly broad piece of tubi-grip around the body. This adds considerable support, reducing the discomfort and thus encouraging movement.

10. One would certainly not praise the general practitioner or other untutored "plastic surgeon" who uses a long midline vertical incision in a patient with the type of abdominal distortion we see in 99.9% of cases. However, there is always room for innovation and changing of principles according to the problems presented. Such variation is the "open" abdominoplasty, in which one

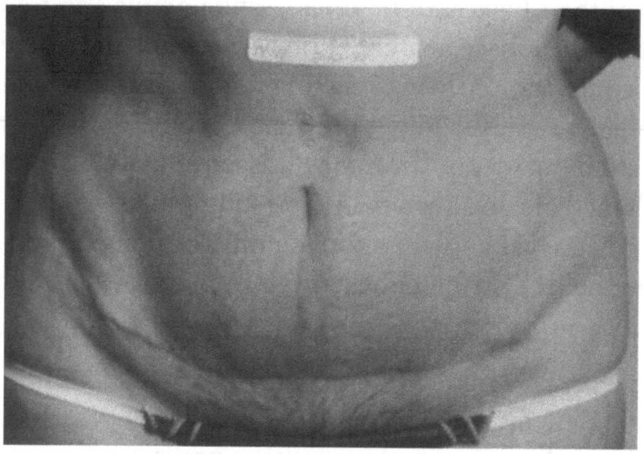

Figure 14-26. Better planning would have prevented the significant problem shown in this patient. The umbilicus has floated down too far. Rather than attempting simply to attach it at a higher position during the procedure, it would have been wiser to have removed a small ellipse of skin above the original umbilicus and anchored it to the fascia to avoid stretching. The umbilicus will be slightly longer, but the position will be good. Second, reduction of the mons veneris would have given the required 13+ cm of non-hair-bearing skin between the umbilical site and the mons. It also would have allowed us to bring the skin in more smoothly. It must be noted that such minor variations disappear with time. It is not necessary to extend the incision to prevent this type of "dog-ear." Subcutaneous fat removal and angling of the incision allow the tissues to fall into place rather easily.

Figure 14-27. Making abdominoplasty choices in the operating room. Ideally, one would like to remove all of the damaged skin that extends from the mons to several centimeters above the umbilicus, but it is neither practical nor risk-free. In these cases, the short incision is outlined with a scenario of varying degrees of skin resection. It is apparent preoperatively that the umbilicus must be relocated, but the good quality of the skin above indicates that little stretching can be obtained; therefore the option of closing the umbilical site in the midline becomes the procedure of choice when the flap has been elevated (**A–C**).

In the operating room photograph (**D**), the flap has been laid in position without tension. After full fascial plication, the decision is made whether to resect a moderate or a full amount, judging by the tension in the 30-degree flexed position. Had we resected the entire panniculus as far as the umbilicus, rather than preserving 4 cm, the tension would likely have resulted in a midline skin slough. Angling the incision upward laterally and advancing the flanks allows us to remove more of the lateral stretch marks, yet keep the midline closure without tension (**E**). The postoperative photographs at 7 years (**F**) show that the contour, scar position, and general appearance of the abdomen are acceptable.

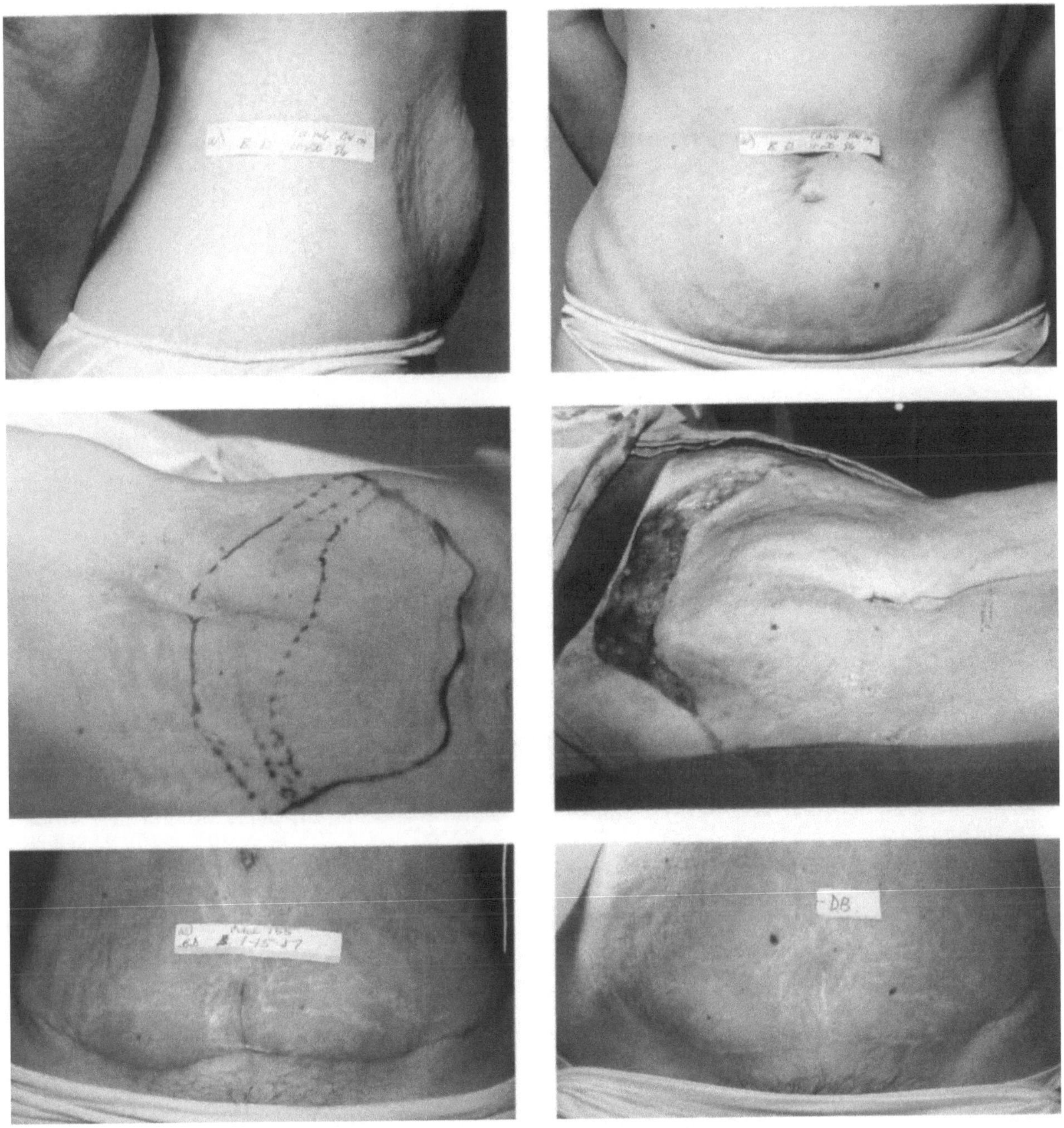

A B C D E F

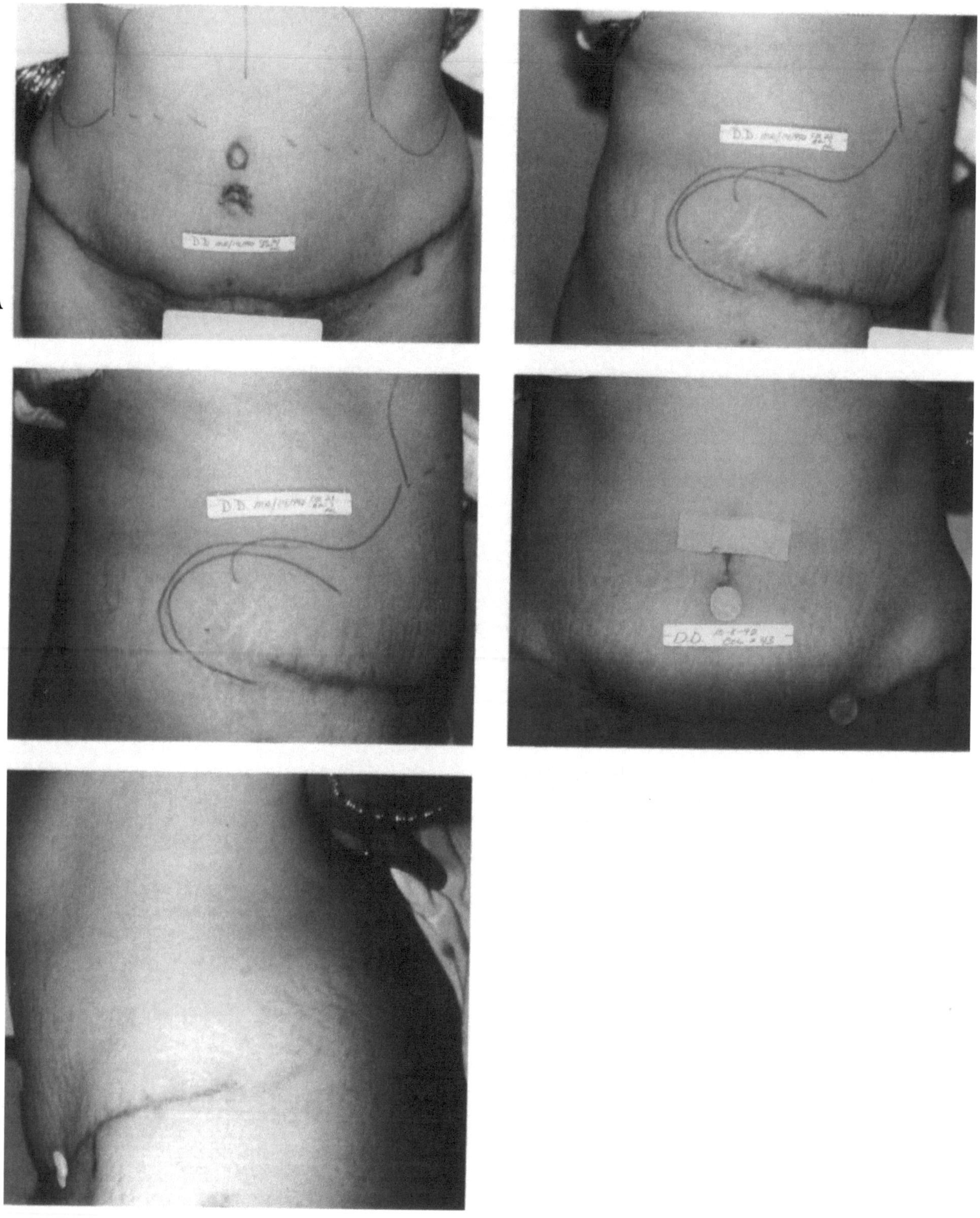

A B C D E

has more than adequate access through a prior long vertical incision. In these cases hypertrophic scars can be improved by **W**- or **Z**-plasties.

11. Why do some experts in abdominoplasty still use those exceptionally long scars that curl down over the hips? Haven't they learned that suction can reduce the need for a long scar? Why do they still make separate drain holes through the skin when a drain can easily be brought through an incision?

12. There are surgeons who still perform reverse abdominoplasties. That is, they create a scar that reaches from one mammary fold to another mammary fold straight across the midline, *as well as* a low abdominal scar so they can tug in both directions. Most of us recognize that both upper midline scars are going to be highly unattractive, unacceptable, and ultimately more trouble than the original condition.

REFERENCES

1. Wilkinson TS, Swartz BE: Individual modifications in body contour surgery: the limited abdominoplasty. Plast Reconstr Surg 77:779, 1986.
2. Greminger RF: The mini-abdominoplasty. Plast Reconstr Surg 79:356, 1987.
3. Matarasso A: Abdominoplasty. Clin Plast Surg 16:289, 1989.
4. Matarasso A: Abdominoplasty: a system of classification and treatment for combined abdominoplasty and suction-assisted lipectomy. Aesth Plast Surg 15:111, 1991.
5. Wilkinson TS: Limited abdominoplasty techniques as applied to complete abdominal repair. (in press).
6. Wilkinson TS: Mini abdominoplasty. Plast Reconstr Surg 82:917, 1988.
7. Toronto IR: The relief of low back pain with the WARP abdominoplasty: a preliminary report. Plast Reconstr Surg 85:545, 1990.
8. Wilkinson, TS: Abdominoplasty and figure 8 closure. Technical Forum 3(4), 1979.
9. Wilkinson TS: Survey on techniques in abdominoplasty. Technical Forum 2(5), 1978.

Figure 14-28. Secondary abdominoplasty. This patient was rightly concerned with her results from an abdominoplasty performed elsewhere. The incision is long; the distance between the umbilicus and the mons is short; and the umbilicus is at an unnaturally low position (**A–C**). In these cases, liposuction is used on the premarked area, and the umbilical site is simply closed vertically. The umbilicus is brought out at a new position. The soft tissue below the midline is resected so the mons can be lowered; liposuction completes the remaining contour. The postoperative photographs (**D&E**) show the only complication of this secondary procedure, extrusion of a suture from the subcutaneous closure of the old umbilical site. The positions of the scars have been improved by moving them upward. The thickness of the waist has been reduced by liposuction. The new umbilicus is now in a satisfactory and natural position, and the distance between the umbilicus and the mons has been lengthened. Although complex, this type of revision surgery is easily accomplished on an outpatient basis in our office surgery center under ketamine/Valium anesthesia.

15 Suction Lipectomy

OUR FIRST ACQUAINTANCE WITH SUCTION-ASSISTED LIPECTOMY (or, using the politically correct term today, liposculpture) was in 1979 when reports filtered in from Europe. Predictably, the results that were acclaimed were not those one would wish to see in Main Street, America. The operation has developed dramatically, however, and has become safe and technically improved. We concentrate here on the philosophy behind the procedure, the technical innovations, and the current controversies and applications.

Liposuction itself is no longer controversial. There have been impressive changes in the equipment used and our understanding of fluid shifts and blood loss. Unfortunately, a number of practitioners in the United States with little surgical experience have undertaken liposuction with questionable results. They (and we) should heed the standards for this procedure.

1. The maximum safe limits for removal are 2000 to 2500 cc of fat at a single procedure, unless one uses saline infusion.
2. Robert Ersek's concept of serial liposuction is a wise one. With it, the patients are subjected to relatively minor procedures on separate operating days spaced several months apart so transfusions are not necessary and the skin has a better chance to shrink during the 4 to 6 weeks between sessions.

3. Liposuction combined with fat grafting has helped us to erase many of the unwanted stigmata of aging in the body.
4. Liposuction has not replaced traditional surgical approaches, such as submental platysma repair, but it has become a useful adjunct to many procedures.
5. Liposuction plays an essential role in the nasolabial fold, the jowls, and the lower neck during face lifting, in breast reduction surgery, and for body contouring.
6. Suction pumps have become less cumbersome and less noisy. The question of aerosolization of AIDS viruses and bacteria is perhaps overblown, as liposuction is performed in well ventilated rooms. Nevertheless, a number of expensive and inexpensive filters are proposed. Cannulas are much smaller now, leaving few instances of ridging or overresection.
7. We approach each area for multiple ports with a crisscrossing maneuver of small cannulas at multiple levels.
8. The syringe suction technique in my hands has been useful for small procedures, but it is too tiring and labor-intensive for major procedures.
9. A number of fat traps have been perfected, as have other means of preserving fat for reinjection into superficial layers or in the face.
10. Superficial liposculpture may be a "buzz word," but the concept of using small cannulas close to the surface is a valid one. Hilton Becker's idea of curetting the undersurface of the skin may be risky in the neck, but it certainly is useful in the upper flank, just below the arms, and in the "banana" area just below the buttock fold where maximum retraction is important and fine wrinkling is not visible.
11. Circumferential suctioning of arms, legs, calves, and ankles is now acceptable. Conservatism is the key, of course, particularly in the calf and ankle.
12. The inner thigh has always been a problem because the skin does not shrink well. The choice between conservative reduction of some of the fat so the patient does not look bow-legged versus suction with a thigh lift should be considered for each individual.
13. Double- and triple-hole cannulas may be useful for certain areas, such as the thick tissue of the nasolabial bulge, but they are associated with a greater degree of risk. The fat may be removed too rapidly, and a superficial defect could easily be created. Most surgeons are not convinced that the three holes are better than one large hole, but the consensus is that a blunt tip is preferable, except in fibrotic areas, and that the suction hole should be away from the skin for safety reasons. Sharp open tips, such as those used by some Italian colleagues, are not

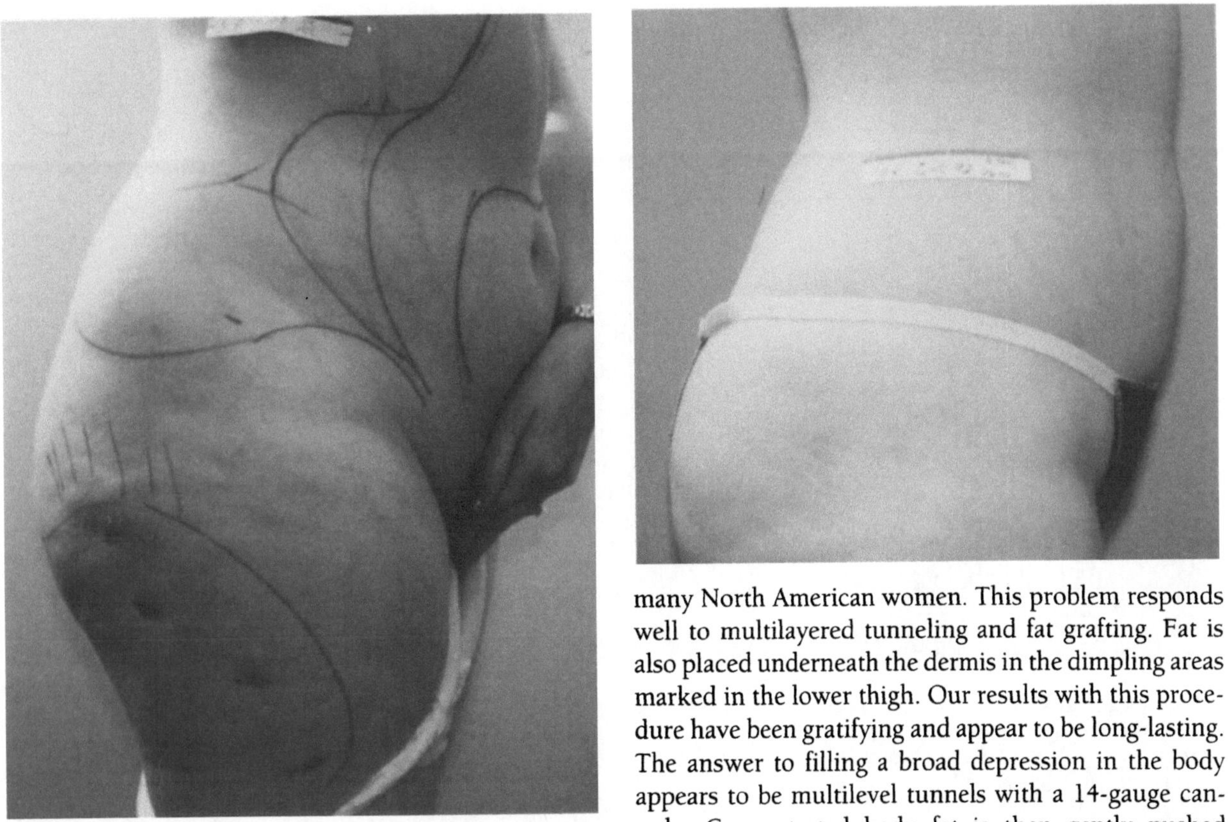

Figure 15-1. Liposuction and reinjection in the "Brazil Zone." Patients who have taut abdominal muscles and good quality abdominal skin usually do not have much distortion. Liposuction, as outlined, is used to reduce the bulk in the hips, flanks, and anterior abdomen. The drawings are to show the topical map of elevations of the fatty panniculus. We also marked with vertical lines the depressed zone that is common in many North American women. This problem responds well to multilayered tunneling and fat grafting. Fat is also placed underneath the dermis in the dimpling areas marked in the lower thigh. Our results with this procedure have been gratifying and appear to be long-lasting. The answer to filling a broad depression in the body appears to be multilevel tunnels with a 14-gauge cannula. Concentrated body fat is then gently pushed through the cannula as it is withdrawn, thus filling the tunnels to prevent their collapse. This principle is the same as that used successfully for chin and lip augmentations. With the "new" liposuction, small radially placed incisions are required for introducing the Toledo fork injector that elevates the dermis in the cellulite dimpling and provides entry for the tunneling for fat grafting.

a good idea except for gynecomastia. Once you have created a surface defect and surgical rippling, it is almost impossible to correct.

14. Separating surface rippling and surface defects from the deep dermis with autologous fat grafting is useful in the patient who has surgical deformities following poorly performed liposuction.
15. An aggressive postoperative skin care program is essential. It involves professional masseuses, patient massage, skin care, and compression.

The "operation that came out of the cold" has sparked more heated air in plastic surgery circles than it deserves. In the history of the procedure, the

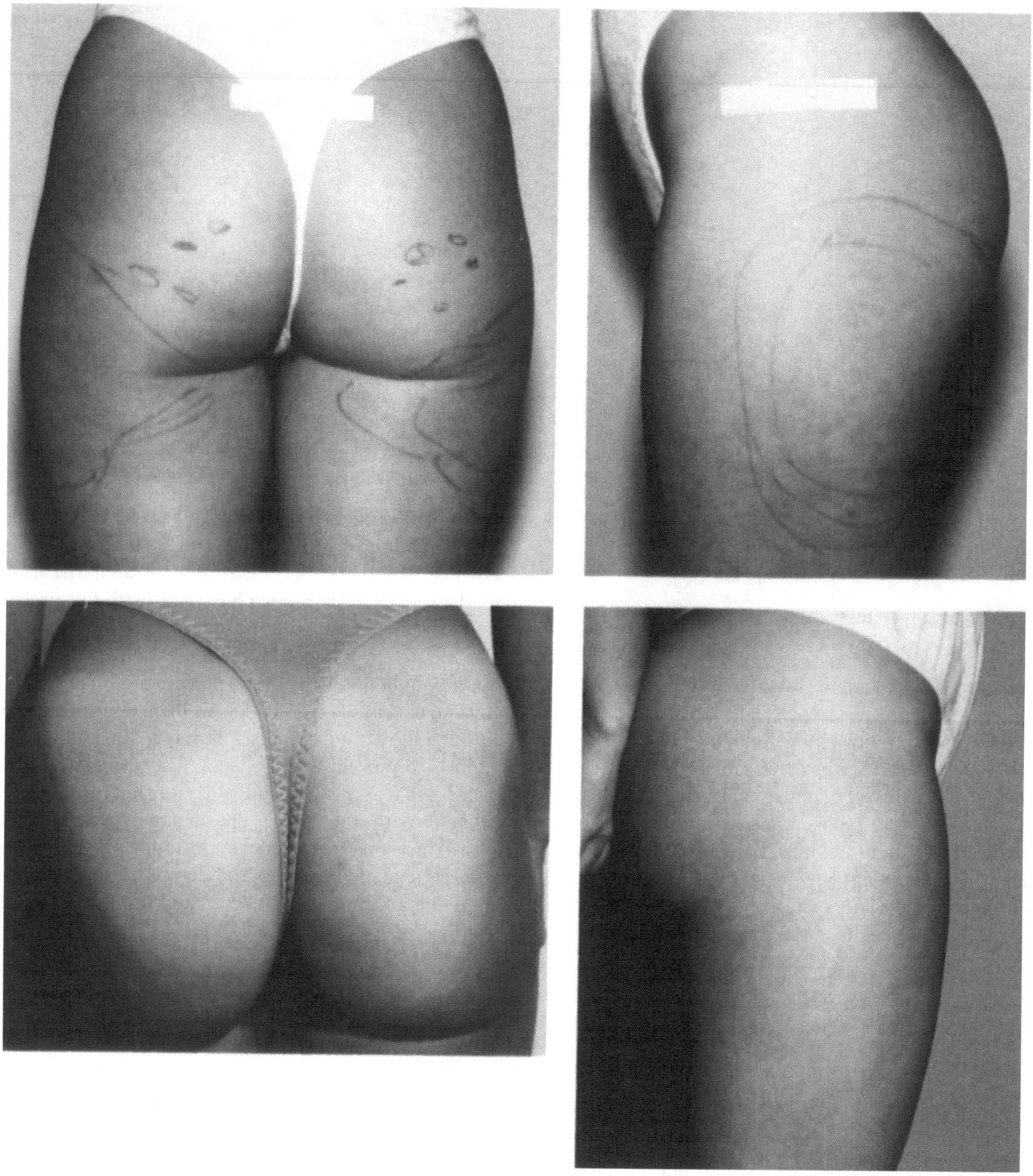

A B C D

pendulum swung toward using suction for everything we could possibly dream of. Now the pendulum has swung back to the realization that suction is a useful *adjunct* to sound surgical treatment of various disorders. Our reconstructive surgery colleagues use it for defatting flaps. People with silicone injection problems can benefit from judicious suction. However, lipolysis should not be used alone for a multifaceted problem. Refusing to admit that certain procedures such as abdominoplasty and submental repair look better if one attacks skin and muscle as well as fat is self-deluding.

Sometimes a patient says, "Doctor, I don't have the time to recover from having muscles repaired in my abdomen. Can't you do something that will make me look better, and I promise I'll be back next year?" There is certainly an argument for acceding to her wishes. She probably never will do exercises, and her several pregnancies have stretched the rectus abdominis to such a degree that exercise would not help anyway. She is in the middle of business deal and yet would like her suits and cocktail attire to fit better during the fall social season. What do you do? You explain the procedure and then suction the abdomen. The postoperative results show a decided improvement, but you must remind yourself that you corrected only part of the problem.

Are we wrong in acceding to these marginal requests? We certainly would be if we did not point out that a short incision and partial skin incision plus muscle repair would give a definitely more youthful, longer-lasting result.

Saline Infusion Technique

There is definite merit in sometimes injecting moderately large volumes of sterile saline mixed with small percentages of lidocaine (Xylocaine) and epinephrine in patients who are to undergo suctioning. In the proper setting it makes sense. The injection guns and long dispersal needles make it an easier

Figure 15-2. Liposuction with fat grafting in buttock dimples. Some years ago, it seemed a good idea to take concentrated body fat and inject it to elevate buttock dimples with a sweeping motion of a 16-gauge needle. It was a more complicated procedure than the one we use today, but it certainly worked in this patient. In the preoperative photographs **(A&B)**, each dimple is outlined. The postoperative photographs **(C&D)** show the shaping of the buttock fold and the thinning of the thighs from multi-entry-point crisscrossing liposuction. Until I recognized her, I had forgotten that we had tried the "new" approach of lipografting 5 years earlier. Once I had ascertained that she was indeed the same patient, comparison between the Polaroids, the black and white photographs shown here, and the color photographs left no doubt that the procedure had been a success.

procedure than injecting with a standard 20-gauge spinal needle. Whether it is more efficient is undecided.

In my experience, those who claim blood loss is diminished have not made their case. The initial blood loss may be less, but thorough suctioning still produces a bloody aspirate, particularly if one uses superficial suction.

The other problem with this entire concept is that it was immediately seized on by the nonplastic surgeons with little surgical experience as a means of performing liposuction in their offices. In a proper operating room, with ketamine, diazepam (Valium), general anesthesia, or at least fentanyl, the initial infiltration phase can be carried out easily. That is not the case in the office setting. From this point on we refer to this procedure not as the "tumescent technique," with its unsavory connotations, but properly as a "saline infusion technique."

Gerald Pitman and Luis Toledo, (their books on this subject are excellent) have used different combinations of infusions, but it basically comes down to adding 30 or 45 ml of 1% lidocaine (Xylocaine) with epinephrine to each 500 ml of saline. Various pumps and syringes make it easier because the surgeon can continue to move back and forth during injection without refilling a syringe. At these dilute concentrations, volume is not a problem. We only fear that someone who is unused to these techniques might employ them with undiluted 1% Xylocaine.

Small stab wounds are made outside the areas marked for suctioning or reinjection. The stab wound must be large enough to introduce a Toledo or other type fork dissector to free up dimples in the buttocks or thighs and allow you to reinject these areas with a long needle or a Toledo dissector. These stab wounds must be large enough to insert No. 4 and No. 6 cannulas. (Byron Medical makes a long injection needle with multiple ports.) By passing the instrument superficially and deeply through all areas, good anesthesia results. The only drawback is that the 20-gauge spinal needle may penetrate the fascia and deposit Xylocaine in the deeper tissues. It is helpful for patients who are operated on under twilight anesthesia, and flooding an area with 500 to 1000 ml is a helpful adjunct to liposuction.

Infiltration Liposculpture

An important reason trained surgeons are leery of the hype about "the tumescent technique" was its sources. One dermatologist claimed that he had "refined" the procedure and had had "no complications." According to an interview in a lay magazine, he claimed, without scientific facts, that "the diluted anesthetic enables fluids to permeate fat cells causing them to constrict. This, in turn, helps prevent the usual accelerated bleeding." We know that epinephrine diluted beyond 1:400,000 has a blood vessel constricting effect, but the rest of his statement does not make sense. He said that liposuction should be a "walk in and walk out" procedure even though he has "suctioned up to an amazing 6000 cc of fat during one operation." This doctor was also quoted as saying, "Dermatologists and cosmetologists generally perform the new procedure, which is regarded by plastic surgeons as too experimental because of the large amounts of body fat being removed." I rest my case.

The shifts in fluids after liposuction and the massive trauma we induce by this technique are an ongoing concern for plastic surgeons. Therefore, the claim that one can remove greater amounts of fat with the "tumescent" technique makes no sense. Furthermore, few patients are willing to lie in a dermatologist's office while someone inserts the large needles required into their subcutaneous tissue followed by liposuction with no anesthesia, or suffer the debilitation and prolonged recovery of massive fat removal in a single procedure.

Laser Liposuction

The ASPRS finally went public and criticised those who claimed that lasers offer great but unspecified benefits to cosmetic surgery. *Technical Forum* dissected the claims of those who used laser for blepharoplasty and contrasted them with reports from pragmatic and practical surgeons. Needless to say, the laser is simply a hot knife and an inadequate and impractical substitute for the cold knife that opens the skin. Damage to the cells surrounding the laser incision and the potential for damage to underlying structures makes the procedure unwelcome.

Reports of laser liposuction have recently been featured on national television. Fortunately, David Apfelberg was interviewed in the press and rightly pointed out that only a few such procedures had been carried and that it is too soon to know if it reduces bruising or facilitates the procedure in any way. "Laser liposuction is just regular liposuction with a laser in the tube, and it is there in hopes of preventing bleeding." Maybe that makes sense and in some way compensates for the additional costs of the new gadgetry, which of course are passed on to the patients. Bruising certainly is not a major deterrent to liposuction. The same argument applies to the purchase of a laser to treat capillary spider veins when one can use a 30-gauge disposable needle and various injectables with good results at reduced cost.

Some advocate biostimulation by laser. They claim that passing a laser over the skin causes cells to constrict and "lessen in volume," which sounds like old scar tissue to me.

The bottom line is that laser liposuction is expensive, unwieldy, and inconvenient for the surgeon. Its possible important advantage lies in the fact that it can be used in the large, bulky, poor-risk patient who should not or cannot afford multiple procedures.

White Fat Suctioning

Some physicians are claiming that liposuction can be done without blood loss. They must be surgeons who can spend all day with a syringe in their hands to "very gently tease our globules of fat" under general anesthesia. The rest of us have schedules to meet and other operations to perform. Theoretically, a method whereby one would not have to replace blood during extensive liposuction procedures would be advantageous. Even with autotransfusion, it is inconvenient to have a patient go through the donation process and pay the extra fee. Nevertheless, "white fat suctioning" is not practical, nor is it conceivable for ordinary application of the technique.

The idea was to suction one "tunnel" until the fat shows color tinges (blood) and then move on. Kesselring does not agree with this method. Frequently, he reminds us, one encounters blood on the first passage, which is not sufficient reason to abandon that area and create a new tunnel elsewhere just to maintain white fat suctioning. Moreover, we no longer create isolated tunnels, and with the "parallel tunnel" technique parallel grooves appeared in the skin. It is for those reasons that many of us waited until someone came up with the idea of *cross-suctioning* to eliminate the deformities and break up the fibrosis.

It is disconcerting to hear the totally different estimates of how much blood is contained in suction specimens. Illouz estimated a 7% blood loss. Others more realistically estimated that 20% of the aspirate measured in the bottle was blood with at least 10% more in the tissues, giving about a 30% blood loss. In other words, for every 1000 cc of fat, the patient has lost 300 ml of blood from the circulating volume. We do agree with Kesselring that these figures vary depending on the individual patient: In some you see little blood with an ordinary suction technique, and in others it seems that every move brings red tinges. I can support the idea of suctioning an area until one encounters bleeding, but it is more important to know exactly what you have taken and what is left behind.

Facial Palsy After Liposuction

Facial palsy after liposuction, in terms of our dissatisfaction, ranks on an equal basis with the oversuctioned cheek that leaves grooves and ripples. (For the latter, liposuction only the J area unless the cheek is extremely fatty. Do not turn on the liposuction until well past the corner of the mandible.)

Transient paresis was known but was not reported until it was discussed in *Technical Form* in February 1989. Paresis has occurred after both open suctioning (direct application of a suction tip to the exposed cheek when the flap is elevated) and closed suctioning. In most cases, nerve function returned within 3 to 6 months. The nerve injury probably did not occur because the entry point was made in front of the lobule of the ear, although one surgeon is certain that that was a factor in his case. It is possible that the injury is to point at which the mandible crosses near the oral commissure. A heavy hand in this area with full-bore suction attached to a rigid cannula with an open suction point could easily traumatize the nerves. The marginal mandibula does cross the mandible near the commissure, and nature has probably designed a few aberrant branches just to keep us on our toes. Overinjecting this area with local anesthesia to balloon the skin is a valuable suggestion. Cross-suctioning is not necessary in this "no man's land." Most faces have a deficiency anterior to the jowl, and it is in these areas that we routinely inject autologous fat. It is possible that in some cases the platysma was accidentally penetrated or the depressors damaged. After consulting with Dick Mladick, Peter Fodor, and a number of other surgeons, I suspect that "rough suctioning" may have been the cause of the facial palsies.

It has been noted by competent surgeons that the fat just under the jaw in the depressor area is adherent and resistant to suction. This condition may have led the surgeon to "try too hard" to remove it with cannula suction. Several respondents to our survey mentioned that they were "overly enthusiastic."

How, then, should damage to the mandibular branch or its fibrils be avoided? Our recommendations follow.

1. It is safer, and indeed easier, to trim the adherent subdepressor fat under direct vision with a curved scissors. In this way you can control the amount removed and be certain that damage will not occur to underlying tissue by either direct trauma or transmitted trauma due to suctioning.
2. If a cannula is used, penetrate the area in front of the ear and in the depressor area slowly. Prior spreading of the skin with a fine-point scissors can establish a safe entry port. Suction should start only when the cannula tip has safely passed that zone. Remember, the fat that is unsightly is in the true "jowl zone," which lies more laterally.
3. Pre-mark the area to be suctioned above and below the mandible. When the edge of the jowl pad is inspected during a face lift procedure, I am always surprised by how much fat has been left after I thought it had been removed by cannula suction. Perhaps it is best to be less aggressive with the cannula.
4. Do not mistake perioral muscle hypertrophy for fat. Pinch the jowl fat that was marked before the injections and lift it away from the cheek before suctioning.
5. Cross-suction the area; but when penetrating from two directions, be certain that the suction tip is just underneath the skin so it does not inadvertently pass too low or penetrate the fascia. Make the motions slow and steady, rather than rapid and "enthusiastic."

One of the survey respondents wrote that he thinks these rare complications are due to a "cavalier approach in criss-crossing across the mandible." Because most of the jowl fat deposits appear just beyond the area where the nerve crosses the mandible to the lip, one is safe in penetrating to that area without suction and then working the cannula in a radial fashion with the power turned on. In our hands, vacuuming with a 3-mm cannula has improved the results of our face lifts. Also, in certain young patients simple vacuuming in the midcheek and jowl can change a chubby, unattractive face to a more natural contour that accents the malar highlight area.

Someone suggested that we look to mandibular intraoral implants to correct aging features of bone absorption and fat loss rather than rely on fat sculpturing. This suggestion is a good one, and many older patients also benefit from a malar or submalar augmentation using prosthetic materials. One precaution: be certain the patient is not one who values a "hollow cheek look." You can offer a choice between a "classic malar face" and an "apple cheek." Structuring the procedure to the patient's wishes is fine so long as you are cautious with the cannula. Most of my current face lifts include malar extended chin prostheses in addition to jowl suction and fat reinjection.

Lawrence LeWinn (Palm Springs) has noted transient unilateral weakness of the lower lip that resolves about 4 weeks after facial suctioning. His three cases appeared after open suction during a face lift. "It is my distinct impression that when you attempt to suction the area just over the depressors, and just under the jaw in the mental region, the fat is adherent and resistant to suction. I found that when I tried too hard . . . I saw weakness after surgery." LeWinn goes on to say that he has learned not to be aggressive in that area and has confirmed that it can be a problem by discussing it with other plastic surgeons. The experience from those who were actually visualizing the area are, of course, directly related to the incidence of temporary paralysis during closed suction of that zone.

Arthur Ship (New York) also has had cases of temporary lower lip weakness following facial liposuction. "My suction is always open, with No. 7 and No. 8 Busse plastic cannulas. This means that suction is done under direct vision and is always above the platysma." Ship was mystified as to the etiology of the muscle weakness because he knows that he did not tear the platysma. He does recall being "overly enthusiastic" when suctioning jowl fat.

It may be that the fat suctioning should be done only when the opening is directly over the area to be suctioned. Moreover, one should be conservative rather than aggressive. Fortunately, most of the fat to be removed is not directly in the area of the nerve but is located more posteriorly. If a submental repair is being done, perhaps it is better to visualize the area directly and remove the fat with a scissors technique. This method seems to be safer, as there is no tugging or pulling on the underlying tissue, and the fat to be sculptured is in plain view, away from underlying musculature.

Syringe Liposculpture

Syringe liposculpture can be either easy or difficult. Having three or four assistants to empty syringes and hand them to the operating surgeon is helpful. Each time a syringe is refilled, however, you have to stop and reinsert it. There is also the annoying problem of having air slip into the syringe when you get close to the opening on the backstroke. I do not use this technique for suctioning large areas because it is just too much trouble. For small areas and for harvesting fat for minor regrafting, it is a good procedure. There is the same amount of bruising but less blood in the aspirate, and smoother skin than with other methods. When resuctioning an area—which should be done to make sure it is smooth—during the second passage of the grid pattern bloody fat is always encountered. It is inevitable because cannulas went through there once before, and it occurs whether you are using the syringe or the suction pump. The concern about aspirating AIDS viruses and bacteria is not valid. Operating in an office surgical suite with good ventilation is a protection against anything that might emerge from the back of your machine.

Syringe liposculpture is a quiet procedure, whereas machine-controlled liposuction is not. I have concluded that each method has its advantages and disadvantages. The machine is noisy and is attached to a hose, which is somewhat inconvenient. On the other hand, with the machine method you can continue suctioning an entire area without having to stop, regroup, and put in another syringe. The fat traps work well for collecting fat, although they are somewhat cumbersome for the larger cases. How do I decide which method to use? If a single area, such as the abdomen, requires liposculpture and the patient is of "normal" size, I use a syringe. If two or three areas are to be suctioned I always choose the machine.

A "mini poll" has asked readers' opinions about syringe lipoplasty. Luis Toledo (Brazil) is an advocate of the technique and indicates that his patients have less bruising than those operated with a suction machine. Carson Lewis (La Jolla) compared two sides on the same patient and reached a similar conclusion. Both men thought that syringe lipoplasty was far easier than traditional suction.

Many surgeons polled disagreed with them, pointing out that a busy surgeon does not have time to spend exchanging syringes. The method is slower simply because of the nature of the technical requirements. I also pointed out that bruising occurs with both methods and disappears at approximately the same rate.

Most of the responses to the poll were negative. Some like syringe suction for touch-up procedures, and some prefer it to fat trapping for obtaining graft material to use in the face or thighs and for use under dimples that are released with the cutting tool that separates the "cellulite" attachments to the deep fascia. Other readers were not as critical but generally tended to agree that syringe lipoplasty has a place but not for the usual patient undergoing first-time suction-assisted lipectomy.

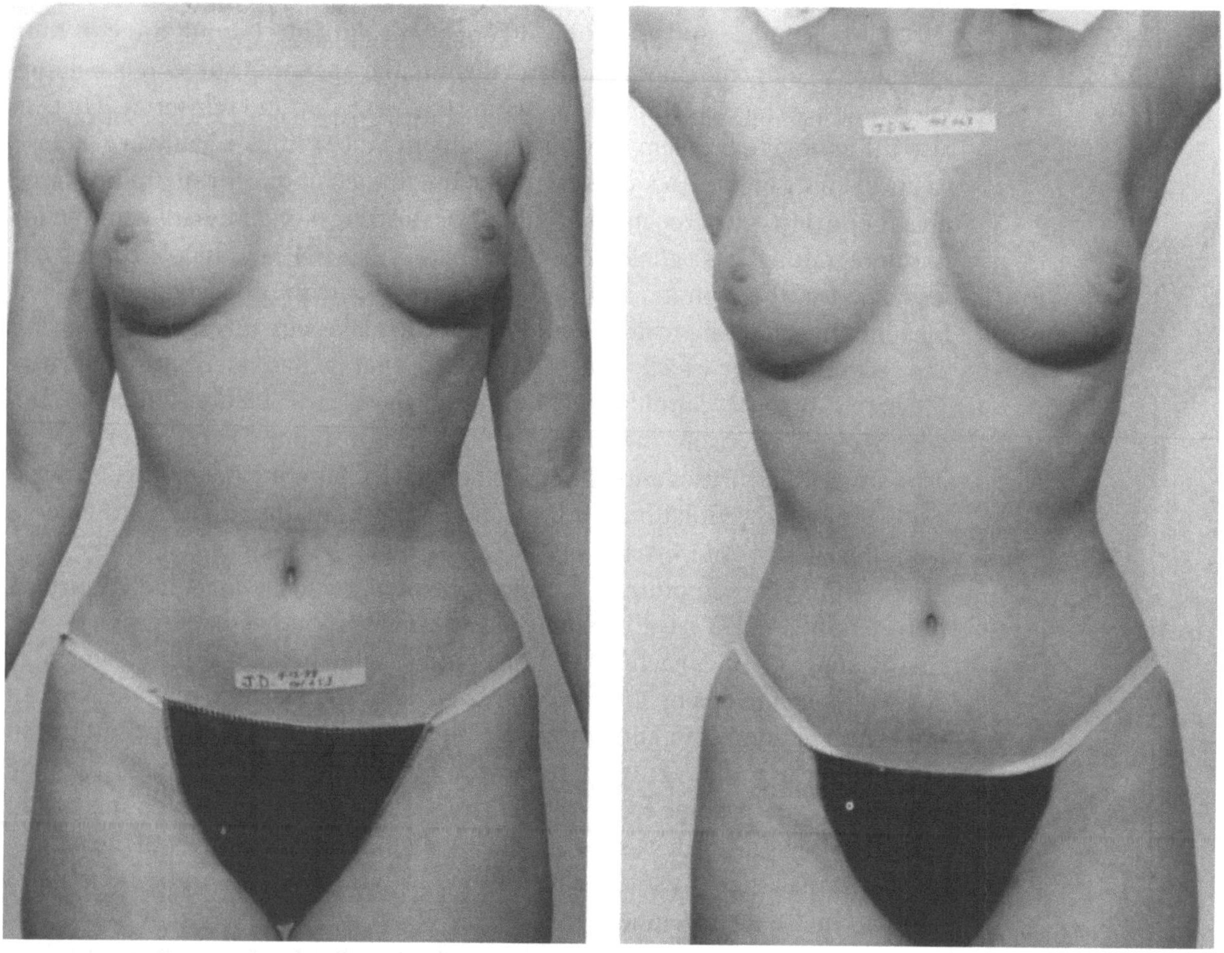

A

B

Figure 15-3. Liposuction of the abdomen, flanks, and thighs with breast implant replacement. One of the advantages of an office surgery center that utilizes ketamine/Valium "twilight" anesthesia is that multiple procedures can be performed safely and efficiently without additional cost to the individual. **(A)** This young woman had good muscle tone and good skin tone. In the postoperative photograph **(B)**, with arms raised one can see that her original inframammary scars were utilized. The implant replacement was with a wider-diameter, full-volume prosthesis, and the dissection was below the original scar site so the scar would rest on the undersurface of the breast in the hands-down position. A change in body contour without rippling or distortion is a credit to those plastic surgeons who pioneered the use of smaller cannulas and crisscrossing, multiapproach liposuction. The evolution of breast prostheses has given us the advantage of creating a more natural cleavage without appreciable increase in breast volume.

Brazilian Bottoms

Much of our interest in regrafting the hip and thigh area came from travelogues that pictured Brazilian women. The plastic surgeons in Brazil (notably Luis Toledo and Ewaldo D'Souza-Pinto) were the first to describe success with multilevel tunnel grafting in the hip and thigh. We American surgeons were skeptical. We also know that most American women like smaller, rather than larger, bottoms; however, there is an increasing demand in my practice for regrafting. A number of the hip and thigh suction patients have large fat deposits in the flank and upper thigh extending to the lower buttock, with a valley in between. It is this area that is often regrafted.

The technique is not difficult. Following the lead of the Brazilians, we concentrate the fat and then use a dissector-tipped 14-gauge long needle to create tunnels subcutaneously and in the deeper fatty tissue. Just as for lip fat grafting, concentrated fat is laid into these tunnels during withdrawal. As in the lip, the secret is multiple parallel tunnels at several depths. Fat placed in these small areas does not migrate, and there is no necrosis. The deepest layer, in the gluteus, is perhaps the most effective one. No one knows yet whether the multiple-tunnel technique is "more effective" than the vascular subcutaneous tissue or the relatively avascular fatty layer (which is practically nonexistent in these people), but it certainly works well for me.

I now have follow-up for patients 3 to 4 years after this type of grafting. The patients are pleased with the rounding effect that we achieved by lowering the "hilltops" and elevating the "valleys"; and I can see the difference in the pre- and postoperative photographs. Because the material is free and the procedure takes only a few minutes, it is another valuable addition to our technical portfolio.

Comments and Commentary

1. An Iranian surgeon fat-suctions his patients standing up. He claims it gives him a better idea of what he is doing. Consultants at the recent ISCPS panel reported good results whether the patient is prone or supine. Once you are used to the supine position and can turn the patient on his or her side, it is an easy position with which to work. Helpful hint: Keep patients awake during the preparation phase so they can lift their own leg; then start the intravenous (or other) sedation.

2. Dick Mladick (Virginia Beach) "Remember, with the tremendous increase in lipoplasty procedures being done by many different specialists other than plastic surgeons, we are going to see more complications. Percentage-wise, though, there is no question in my mind that the complication rate for lipoplasty

(Text continued on page 444)

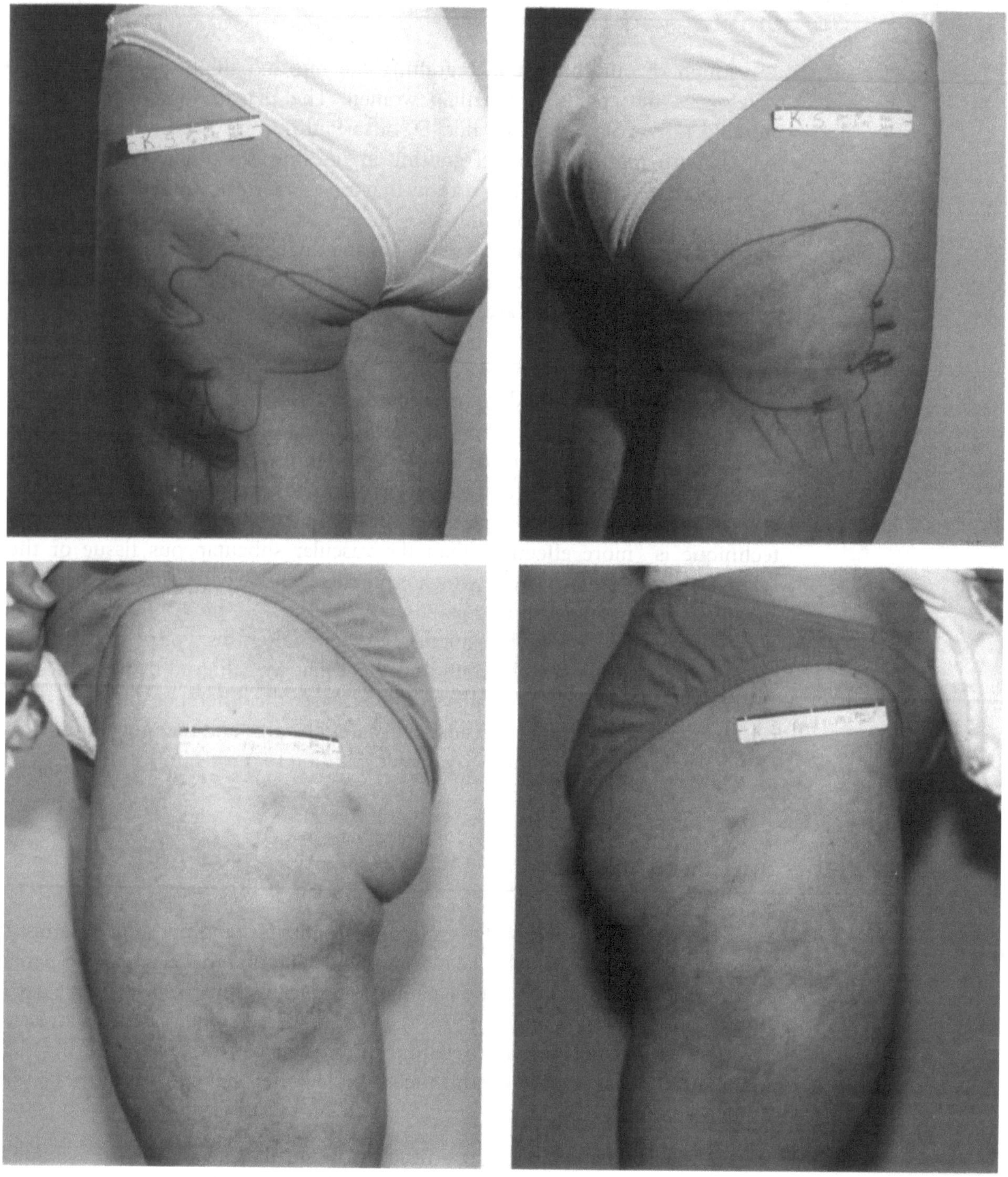

A B
C D

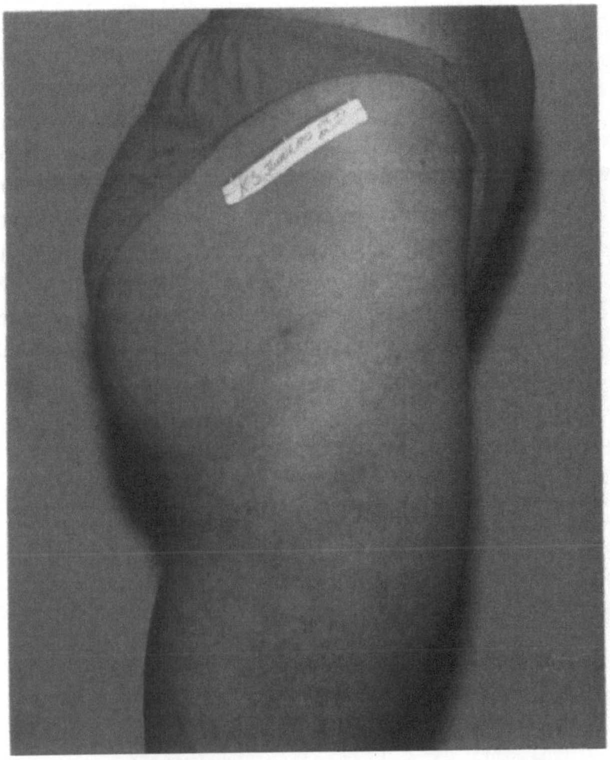
E

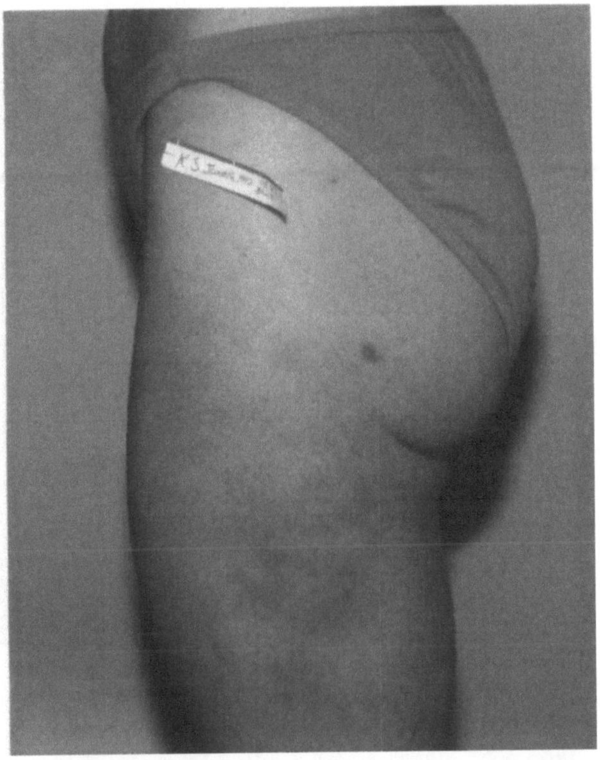
F

Figure 15-4. For Secondary liposuction patients one must use fat regrafting, separation of depressed zones, a multiple-port small cannula, and superficial and deep suction. In my opinion, it is immaterial if suction is performed using the syringe or the machine technique. **(A&B)** In this patient three liposuctions had left her with an obvious deformity. Using multiple approaches, including those unfortunately chosen by her original surgeon, we were able to liposuction the area outlined with the solid lines. Fat was then collected from both sides, concentrated, and reinjected underneath the dark spots and the dimples (marked by parallel lines). **(C& D)** At 10 months, a moderate amount of improvement has been effected. At this point, we decided to undertake minor suctioning and use abdominal fat to further fill the areas that were depressed, particularly on the left side. **(E&F)** These two photographs show the patient 2 months later with considerable improvement after minor secondary, "treatment room" lipoinjection. Note that there is evidence of smoothing following the secondary superficial suctioning with 3-mm cannulas and the additional fat grafting. The latter procedure was performed in our "minor operating room" using the Medi-Frid spray to ease the discomfort of local anesthesia. We also use the "Cryoglobe," which is easy for the patient to hold. Because it comes straight from the freezer and can be held by the plastic handle, the patient becomes actively involved in the procedure by administering his or her own hypothermic anesthesia. One entry point is sufficient to infiltrate the suction and reinjection zones. Use a 10-ml syringe with 0.5% Xylocaine with epinephrine, buffered or not, and a 20-gauge spinal needle. The same applies to the donor site in the abdomen. These minor touch-ups cost you practically nothing, and it is a good thing to do for someone who has had so many surgeries. The best collecting mechanism for this procedure is a tulip-type syringe. We simply pour the collected fat onto a sterile 4 × 4 gauze to soak up the Xylocaine and oil and then scoop it back into the injection syringes, using the gun to control the amount delivered. A total of 30 cc of fat was reinjected to effect the final smoothing in this patient.

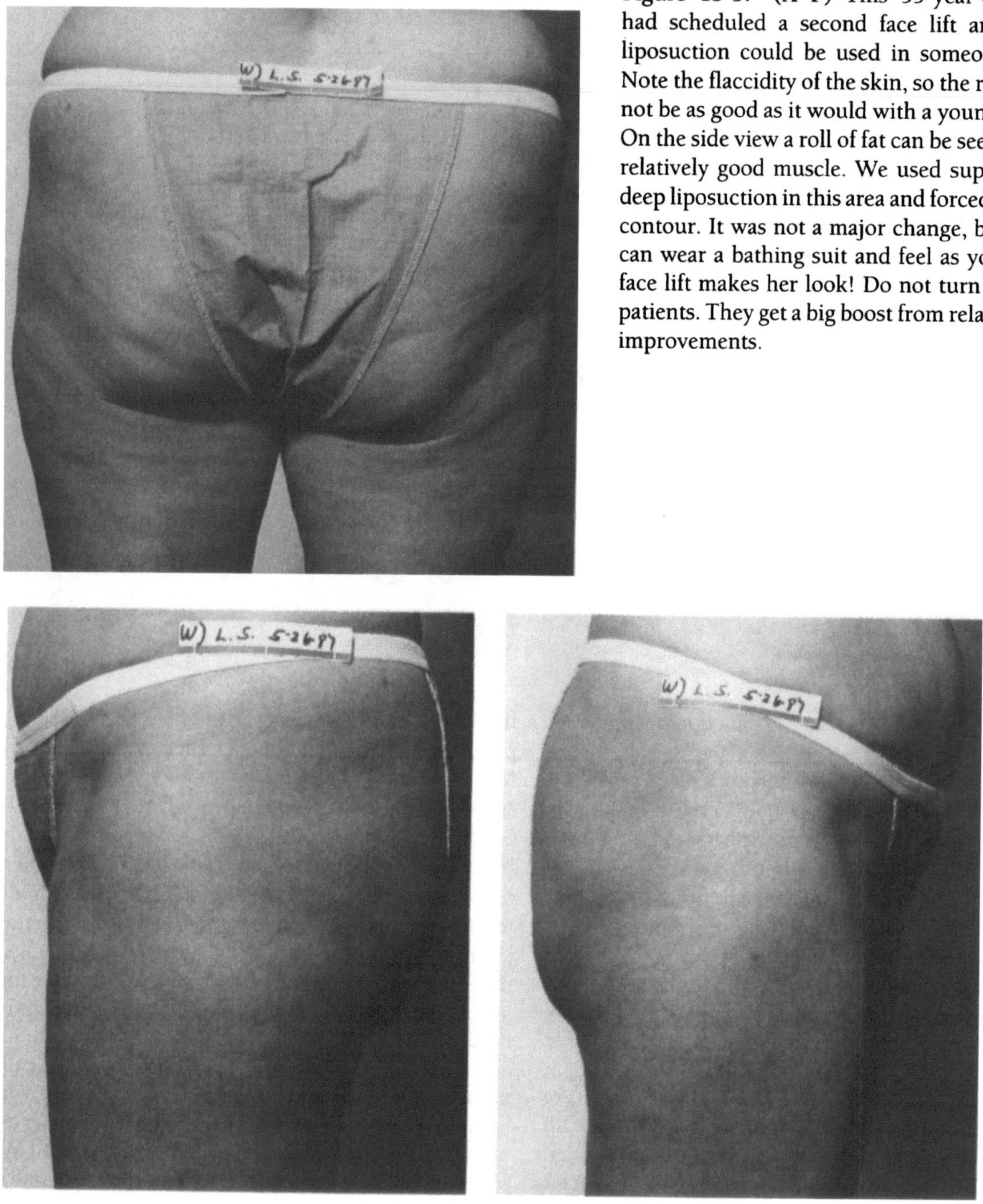

Figure 15-5. (A–F) This 55-year-old woman had scheduled a second face lift and asked if liposuction could be used in someone her age. Note the flaccidity of the skin, so the result would not be as good as it would with a younger patient. On the side view a roll of fat can be seen overlying relatively good muscle. We used superficial and deep liposuction in this area and forced the skin to contour. It was not a major change, but now she can wear a bathing suit and feel as young as her face lift makes her look! Do not turn away older patients. They get a big boost from relatively small improvements.

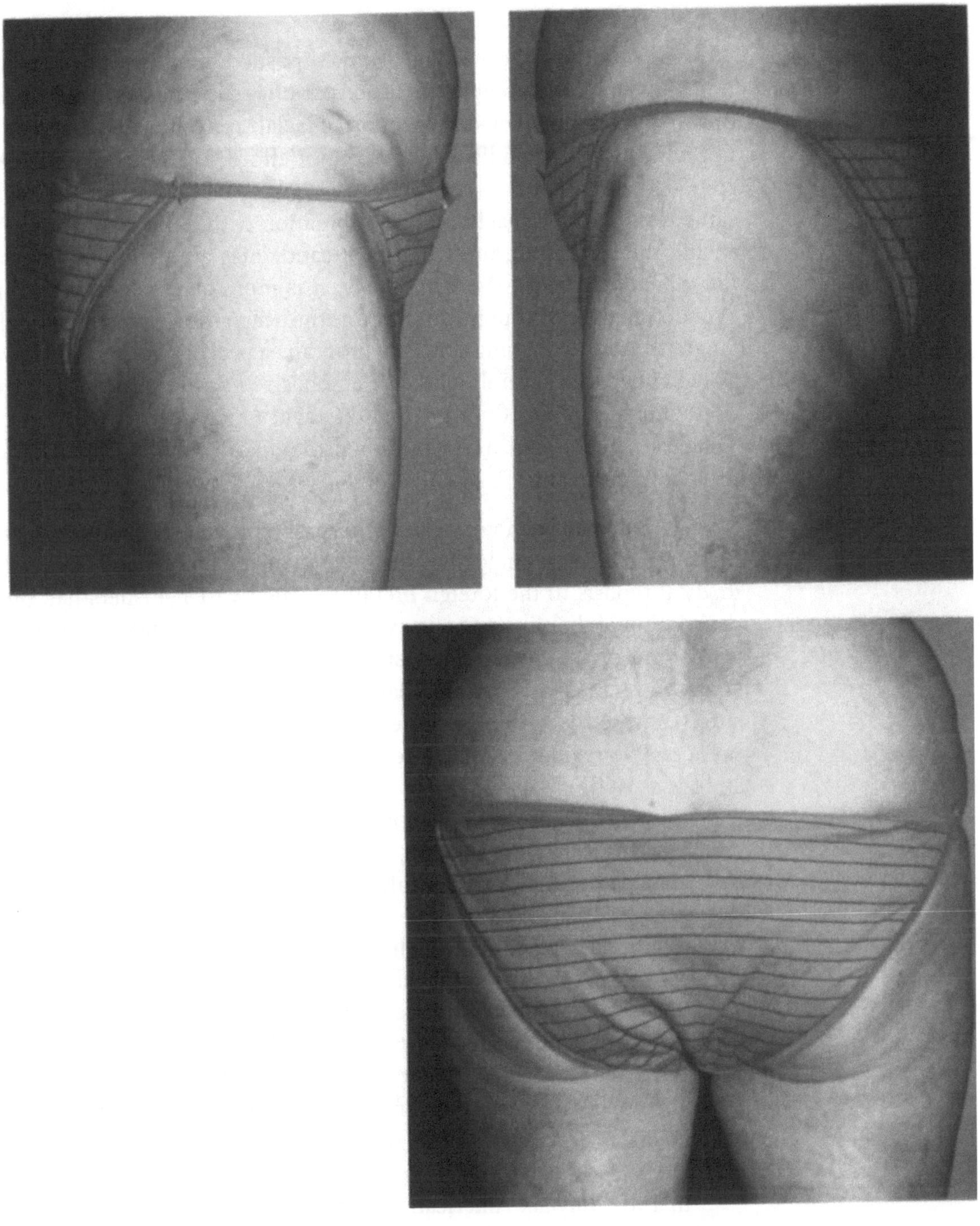

D E F

is extremely low, more so than for virtually any other type of plastic procedure I can think of."

3. You know the warning against liposuctioning the face with the exception of the jowl and nasal fold. The exception is superficial syringe liposculpture of young faces. Luis Toledo has reported facial "refreshing" in this group who do not wish to have a midface lift or cannot afford it. One may disagree that the source of the vacuum (syringe versus machine) is important, as I achieve the same results with a machine. In combination with Retin-A and "light" peels to shrink the facial skin, these marginal candidates are definitely improved with *fine-cannula suction-assisted lipectomy*. It is more of a "maintenance" program. We suction the early bulges, undermine the deep grooves, and then fill them with fat grafts. Add an ongoing skin care program, a peel or two, and you have helped. Toledo injects fat several times. We emphasize rhytid elevation and overcorrection. Our group introduced α-hydroxy acid (AHA) peels and AHA creams to Toledo's regimen and have continued to advise him about medical covering/protective/concealing cosmetic programs.

4. Bahman Teimourian and others who predicted the future usefulness of liposuction were not helped by the inflated media reports and obviously slanted medical reports in the foreign literature. The two Dr. Fishers had published a description of their instruments, which "chewed" away fat with a biting forceps at the end of a cannula. Their statement that "220 of 245 cases had natural smoothness thanks to minimal layers of fat left for this precise purpose" was surely untrue based on our present knowledge of the procedure. Promoting a preoperative regimen of six to ten injections of vitamin K before surgery was strange as well.

By 1979 Teimourian had reported a modified fascial stripper that he connected to a suction machine. In his initial series, he used it only for small saddlebag deformities but rightfully noted the problems with the sharp edge of the fascial stripper. Once again, seromas were a major problem. During the 1980s it was common to place drains in liposuction patients. Today, it is not considered necessary owing to the multilevel, small-cannula, multidirectional approach.

Shrudde developed an effective curettage technique to remove what we now call lipodystrophy deposits. Once again, seromas formed from the curetting procedure. We rationalized that it was better than direct excision, particularly for fat in the upper abdomen or when only a "limited" abdominoplasty was needed to remove flank fat deposits that would ruin the effect of a standard abdominoplasty.

In 1982 only six American surgeons were performing the procedure that would soon be called liposculpture. By 1983 there were more than 800, including myself. Despite the rise in the learning curve, unqualified individuals have leaped into the arena, and there are good surgeons who simply do not take the time or do not have the patients to give the operation its due attention. The techniques of fat grafting and elevation of wrinkles and dimples are now applied when salvaging the results of poorly executed or planned liposuctions.

In the typical secondary liposuction patient, there are ridges of fat due to skin contracture and valleys where the dermis adheres to the underlying muscle or fascia. Some areas can be simply loosened and massaged down, achieving smoothness. In 1985 a young woman asked if there was something we could do about the dimples in her bottom while we were performing thigh liposuction. Not knowing any better, we used a long needle to sweep the area under each dimple to create a pocket and then injected fat and overcorrected. (Today, this procedure is done more precisely with the "mini-fork" procedure and needle dissectors.) On a follow-up visit 5 years later for an unrelated reason, the dimples had fortunately disappeared.

5. Facial suction and nerve damage: Gerald Pitman (New York) says it is unreasonable not to expect some patients to experience a nerve injury.

6. The best summary of the role of facial suction came from Norm Cole (Louisville). He strongly emphasized that suction is not a substitute for standard procedures but a useful refinement. It may make the flaps more physiologic by reducing the area that requires undermining. That might be the one factor in preventing problems in the heavy smoker who just cannot give it up.

7. A prominent gerontologist said: "Surprisingly, large studies show that human beings who are 10% to 30% overweight live longer! According to one of the theories of aging, mutation of intracellular enzymes creates free radicals, which are eventually destructive. Enzyme scavenger systems protect us from premature aging."

Can suctioning fat reduce the life-span? In one rat study, rats that were alternately starved on a daily basis lived the equivalent of many years longer than their compatriots who were fed regular diets. The only problem was that their puberty was delayed for the equivalent of 10 human years! This means we could have started starvation diets when we were children and not have had to shave until we were 30!

8. The Byron Medical self-filling injection syringe is helpful. One would not over inject saline (as with the motorized pumps) because of the number of hand squeezes needed!

9. David Lavine (Fort Worth) does not like the term "tumescent" because it was coined for the lay media. He believes injecting *iced* saline creates the turgidity that prevents him from resecting too much fat. He also thinks it reduces bruising and cuts blood loss. Others believe volume is more important than temperature.

10. There has been much discussion of α and β fat and the reason that cellulite fat appears to be practically permanent. One easy way to explain this phenomenon to patients comes from a magazine article discussing the difference

in fat type as "female" versus "male." "Female" fat cells around the hips and thighs are "more stable." They resist dieting, and the cell is less likely to break down and release its fat. Moreover, "this type of fat is less of a health hazard." "Male" fat cells are more flexible and easily break down and release fat. Why? It is less of a problem to diet away abdominal fat deposits they say and claim that the risk of coronary heart disease increases because this fat is adjacent to the liver and more fat directly enters the liver and causes metabolic changes. "Sex hormones probably influence the characteristics of the developing fat cell," which would explain the difference in the distribution. Doubtful!

Although many readers may be surprised by the lack of sophistication of this discussion, the article makes important points for the lay public. "Remember though, that no one is obese unless they overeat. You control your fat cells; they do not control you." In many families, eating is considered an act of love, and food is pushed on children to reward good behavior. Children and adolescents, however, are vulnerable to fat cell growth stimulated by excess calories. The body's metabolism apparently adjusts to encourage a certain fat cell size that is a precursor to new fat cell development. (It sounds like wishful thinking, but maybe it will give some encouragement to people having trouble with diets.)

11. If it were not for a few quirks in Western culture, certain plastic surgeons could still be languishing in obscurity and we would not have had the pleasure of watching the biggest fight in the annals of plastic surgery. We are referring to suction-assisted lipectomy and the concept of fat people as deformed, ugly, and gross. Why is it that psychological surveys of healthy people of normal weight, particularly women, reveal that most fear getting fat and are always on diets? Why is bulimia, in which people gorge themselves and then forcefully emit the food, strictly a phenomenon of Western culture? Is it because of the pressures our culture exerts on women to be slender? "You cannot be too rich or too thin" the saying goes. It was not always this way in the United States. During the 1900s thin women were thought to be less desirable. The great suprano, Lillian Russell, in 1890 was considered the absolute ideal of womanhood, and she weighed 186 pounds! Today in non-Western cultures, fat people are thought to possess power and fertility. In Nigeria, one tribe once forced its young women to enter "fattening houses" when they reach puberty. There they were prohibited from working and emerged later as "mountains of flesh" ready for marriage.

So without the aberrations from these ideas in our Western culture, the entire suction-assisted lipectomy movement would have never been born, much less have provoked the intense interest inside and outside our profession. It is interesting how many of our colleagues instantly proclaimed themselves experts in suction-assisted lipectomy once the concept was dignified by American approval. One must admit that the end results today are far superior to those that gave us pause 10 years ago. From the way our culture is evolving, it looks like we are going to be busy for many years to come.

12. In the overall concept of a service-oriented plastic surgery facility, it is commonplace to provide support garments and other essentials to patients. We were amazed to hear a supposedly learned consultant at a recent marketing panel advise plastic surgeons to locate department stores to which their patients could go to try on girdles and brassieres. Whether you take Buck Teimourian's approach of giving each patient three commercial girdles or you stock the girdles in the office, it makes more sense to use commercially available girdles than the overpriced "surgical" variety.

When our patients leave the operating room after liposuction they are in a zippered, snapped, locked, Velcro-closed commercial "surgical" garment. The next morning this garment is removed and washed for reuse (they do get softer after having been washed a few times). We buy commercial brassieres and girdles (wholesale) through Medical Cosmetic Services and stock a variety of sizes, shapes, and colors. Whether you give the patient one and allow them to purchase two or three more or you give them all to the patient, you cut your overhead by buying wholesale. In our office, the patients purchase as many brassieres or girdles as they wish at a private fitting. No matter how you handle it in your practice, do not send people out for fittings. Patients prefer the convenience and privacy of having their girdle fittings in your office, knowing they can get extras of the same type and style without inconvenience.

13. A warning about African American patients contemplating suction lipectomy: Examine the patient in different positions, with the legs extended, standing, and so on. A "false saddle-bag" may be apparent on casual examination, and overresection could result. Joe Nemetz (Encino) has another suggestion. He prepares his patients standing up before they undergo general anesthesia. He also advises the use of antibiotics and plasma expanders, a practice not generally used.

14. Robert Ersek (Austin) prefers the 3-mm suction lipectomy device for facial suction. If you look carefully you can find some with the opening close to the end. Note that it is easier to manipulate the tip into "squirrel pouches" or nasolabial overhangs if it is curved instead of straight.

15. Bucking the trend, Illouz and others continue to see little difference between the pump and syringe methods. My advice is to use both techniques and see which one you like for which situation.

16. A German surgeon talked about suctioning in the neck and was proud of the fact that he suctioned down to the sternal notch. *Only one* of his patients had a clean jaw line. Why did he not plicate or resect the platysma?

17. Hard facts: Among more than 100,000 suction-assisted lipectomies, there have been 11 deaths and 9 major complications. Pulmonary embolism does not seem to be intrinsic to the procedure. It is, however, related to decreased body fluid, blood sludging, and other factors.

18. To suction or to excise? If you attend enough meetings you'll have testimonials on both sides of the issue. Should you use an axillary approach to flatten a gynecomastia, or should you make a small periareolar incision and remove the glandular tissue? There are rights and wrongs on both sides. Many experienced surgeons believe that you cannot remove adequate amounts of glandular tissue by suction. It is good to avoid any scar, but at least you can place that scar in an almost invisible area by weaving it in a wiggle fashion along the areolar edge and closing it in multiple layers. Frank Herhahn likes to excise and then use suction along the periphery. Using suction eliminates the need for drains. Those of you who have attacked large gynecomastias directly know how much of a problem it can be, particularly in active men. We prefer the Becker cannula, a combination curet-suction cannula, and a sharp end Brazillian cannula.

19. Intravenous alcohol is no longer considered useful for abdominoplasty or suction patients by a majority of surgeons. Experts polled were surprised that plastic surgeons still use the "archaic and discredited" technique. The subject came up while discussing a respiratory distress case in which fat emboli occurred after suction-assisted lipectomy. Whether the patient had true fat emboli is difficult to decide. Because urine fat tests can be positive owing to soft tissue trauma, a serum lipase assay can help, but the test shows a late peak at 5 to 7 days—little help for immediate action. The sputum fat assay may be helpful, but it also is not a quick test. An autopsy is the only definitive way to differentiate emboli due to suction lipectomy. What can you do if you even suspect this problem? Give intravenous steroids and provide respiratory support.

20. Suction for hyperhidrosis? John Simons (Paradise Valley) thought it was worth a try. He used the "hole up" technique in addition to thoroughly suctioning the area. Surprisingly, two patients showed a marked decrease in axillary sweating. Someone else has reported similar experiences but that the sweating returned after a time.

21. Have you heard stories about exploding liposuction collection jars? Turning up the pressure does not help you to extract more fat. Some of the liposuction plastic cannula jars, however, have literally "imploded," probably scaring the operating room staff and creating a messy situation.

22. Tim Miller's (Los Angeles) laboratory studies showed that the pressure of injections with a lipoinjection gun can rupture fat cells. This possibility is another reason to pass the needle into area and then inject slowly without pressure as the needle is withdrawn.

23. Peter Fodor (New York) commented on "neuropraxia" of the mandibular nerve after facial suctioning. Among the first 20 cases of facial suctioning, he reported an incidence of 30%. These cases were all done using a retroauricular approach. Fodor thinks that the sternomastoid fibers that joined the skin are thin, and so it is easy for a suction cannula to penetrate underneath the fibers and damage the nerve as it emerges. If one stays above the platysma (it is easy to do this with a preauricular stab wound incision), there is less likelihood of injury. Fodor has used this technique for 6 years and has not seen a single case of temporary nerve paralysis.

24. Jim Carraway (Norfolk) is delighted with his results after fat injection in most people, particularly when he uses a concentration technique. He suctions fat with a syringe and 14-gauge needle and then places the fat in a medicine glass. A Neuro cotton tip is put into the glass to act as a wick to suck out free lipid. The concentrated fat is then replaced with a 16-gauge needle. It appears to work better than nonconcentrated fat. (Editor's note: most surgeons today agree that there's only so much room to place fat in an area underneath a skin depression or wrinkle, and that concentrated fat works better, for whatever reason.) Carraway thinks that removing the fat directly through a syringe produces less maceration than when one uses a side-hole suction cannula. Others disagree, saying that a greater volume can be obtained in a shorter time; and with the traps that are being used, the extra macerated portions are simply disposed of before you are ready to "inject" what is left.

25. Reconsidering laser liposuction: The fat in the suction tubing after laser liposuction looks exactly the same as the fat in suction tubing after using a liposuction machine (without a laser to cauterize the tissue). There is the usual progression from clear fat to blood-tinged fat. When patients who had had both methods used—one on one side and the other method on the other side—were asked which side of the body had had the laser liposuction most were certain of their answers but only half were correct. In other words, patients who were sure they had less bruising and less trauma on one side chose the standard liposuction side as often as they chose the side that had had laser liposuction!

26. Dr. Cohen (South Africa) recently reported his experiences and his recommendations. He agrees that autologous blood transfusion is a good idea and gives 1 unit of autologous blood for every 1000 cc of fat removed. He hospitalizes patients overnight and then, somewhat surprisingly, has them stay in bed for 1 complete day after that. (Editor's note: This practice is in direct contrast to that of most American surgeons, who believe in early ambulation within the protected custody of compression garments.) Cohen's patients wear a girdle for 8 days and then begin massage and physiotherapy. At 8 days the swelling is just starting to go down. He has them wear a girdle off and on for 6 weeks. (Would it not make more sense to keep the girdle on constantly a few extra weeks?) His results are good. When you realize that conscientious surgeons on all sides of the globe have arrived at roughly the same ideas of patient selection, care, and therapy, it is almost amazing. We tend to use autologous blood less now.

27. Another surgeon advocated storing suctioned fat in the freezer and reinjecting it after 2 and 6 months. As *Technical Forum* stated before, "Dead fat is dead fat." Perhaps the dead collagen that is left may be of some help, but would it not be better to leave an area unsuctioned and use living fat for the pre-prepared area at a second sitting? Now that good 5-year results are being reported, one cannot dismiss primary and secondary fat injection techniques.

28. Greg Hetter (Las Vegas) on suction-assisted lipectomy (SAL) fluid replacement: When you measure the amount of fat removed during a routine SAL, 31% of the fluid is blood if you are using general anesthesia. If you have blocked with 0.5% Xylocaine with epinephrine, only about 20% of the fluid is blood. This fact is not a valid reason to give up general anesthesia. Either method does not interfere with evaluation of the amount of fat remaining or the contour if injections are carefully performed. Hetter has transfused only four patients during his extensive experience, and they had had suctions of more than 2000 cc in conjunction with major procedures. One final point: You can get better results by crisscrossing than you can from single-entry suction. There are many places on the body to hide the second incision site, and it is worth the extra effort if a better contour can be obtained. Obviously, large areas that are suctioned have more transudate with immediate fluid and colloid loss. Hetter adds that it is easy to estimate the change in hematocrit, which could be useful when accepting patients for extensive procedures. For every 125 cc you remove by suction, there is a 1% drop in the hematocrit after 48 hours.

If patients are serious about their problem, they do not object to giving a unit of blood for autotransfusion 2 to 3 weeks beforehand. It helps the surgeon sleep better, and it certainly speeds recovery if needed. Remember that it takes several weeks for the bone marrow to resume all production at full capacity. Donating the autounits ahead of time means that the patient is in good shape on the day of surgery and so can replace blood losses more quickly, resulting in quicker restoration of the feeling of good health.

29. Fred Grazer (Newport Beach) was asked about intravenous fluid requirements for suction patients. He recommends lactated Ringer's solution 10 to 12 ml/kg for patients whose suctioned fat adds up to less than 1000 cc. If you have removed more than 1000 cc, he recommends giving blood or colloid. He still prefers intravenous alcohol for large procedures; 500 ml of 5% dextrose with 5% alcohol certainly has a theoretic advantage, although many of our consultants do not use the technique and believe it has little to offer.

30. "Do not turn down obese patients." Fred Grazer and Gil Gradinger are comfortable with using combined suction and abdominoplasty in fat patients. Fat folks are more difficult to manage, but they need your help.

31. How long do you wait before you redo a suction patient? Some patients have residual small spots, and the approach to them varies from surgeon to surgeon. Larry Schlesinger (Maui) repairs these patients in the office under local anesthesia with the patient standing up to better delineate the area for suctioning. Some colleagues agree that this method is a good idea, whereas others would pre-mark the areas and use a more conventional approach in the prone or supine position. If you resuction less than 3 months after the initial procedure, there is more bleeding and more distortion. Four months is the usual minimum wait and certain resolution changes may occur even 6 months after the initial surgery. The advice of our consultants: Do not rush in.

32. There is a question about outpatient versus inpatient therapy for suction patients. Some plastic surgeons send face lift patients home, and others restrict overnight stays to rhinoplasties. Some of us are lucky enough to have overnight stay facilities in our offices so we do not have to worry about face lift or rhinoplasty patients being at home without skilled personnel in attendance. The same applies to suctioned patients. The only firm rule is that you must draw the line somewhere about hospitalization. Anyone requiring more than 2000 cc of fat removal should be hospitalized and watched closely. Some of our colleagues allow patients who have had less suction to leave the office or hospital the same day.

33. A word of advice on suction lipectomy during abdominoplasty: In most cases, suction the area only lateral to the elevated area and make the passages parallel to the incoming blood supply. I firmly believe that tension kills abdominoplasty flaps, not suction. Remember the variations of limited abdominoplasty that preserve extra skin length between the umbilicus and the horizontal incision.

34. Dick Mladick (Virginia Beach) and his group pretunnel for suctioning. They pass a blunt probe in the plane they wish to establish first. Apparently this maneuver prevents one from removing fat too close to the surface by an inadvertent slip of the wrist. Others believe that this move is not necessary once you have gained experience. When I use the saline infusion blunt needle, it is a form of pretunneling.

35. One vote against the triple-lumen cannula comes from Gerald Pitman (New York), who warns us of the risk of using triple-lumen cannulas particularly in the face. "It's just too easy to get grooving." He also says it is easy to remove too much fat around the access sight. There is hope, however. I have seen a number of patients who have had this grooving after aggressive facial suction, and they have done well with a series of small fat injections. The fat tends to stay alive in a rich vascular bed such as the cheek, or at least remains long enough to be replaced by something that appears "permanent."

36. For anyone who might have been taken aback by Hilton Becker's scraping of the underside of the dermis to make tissues "conform" in the neck, consider the gluteal fold. His radical approach to liposuctioning certainly helps the skin conform to the buttock, and the excess slack from the "banana area" shrinks better this way.

37. An early, but appropriate, plastic surgery quote: "In order to achieve true brilliance in plastic surgery, you must walk on the brink of disaster."

38. Arm suction: skin excision first or not at all? During the discussion of case presentations on suction-assisted lipectomy (SAL) for underarm fat deposits, several surgeons discussed cases in which planned excision of skin underneath the arm proved unnecessary. If you are fairly certain you must remove skin, it is better to do the suctioning first; then you can remove the fat without damaging the blood supply to the edge of the flaps. When you do remove the skin, you will note a fine network underneath that ensures quick healing. Be sure the patient knows just how bad these scars can be. With SAL they may be better than you expect.

39. In a presentation on liposuction, Dr. Gasperoni stated that the subdermal layer of the skin must be treated to avoid waves. He uses small cannulas to breech the "arch phenomenon." Dissecting each dimple subcutaneously and adding a fat graft is a better idea.

40. Allen Matarasso refers to the "BLT" suction patient: buttocks, love handles, and thighs. He instructs his patients to do sit-ups preoperatively to tighten the muscles so the end result looks its best.

41. After suffering through a DeQuervain's problem in his hand, Mark Mandel (Beverly Hills) made this statement: "Now that I am older, I wonder if a procedure is good for the surgeon as well as for the patient."

42. Ed Melmed said: "I continue to wonder how anyone can take out 7 liters of fat without questioning either their judgment or their motive (or both). I always thought liposuction was to trim areas, not to make fat girls slightly thinner."

43. Val Lambros (Santa Ana, CA) comments on the difference in the quantity of sharply resected fat and aspirated fat during neck contouring. He has a series of photographs showing "mounds of fat" sitting on patient's necks after sharp excision and similar patients with one to two tablespoons of aspirated fat. The patients look the same, but the patient with sharply removed fat had immediate improvement. This point leads Lambros to believe that much of liposuction is "lipocide." We may not remove everything we want to, but the fat that remains generally dies. "This is why as aspirated neck seems to have so much left-over fat when you open and visually observe it even though the long-term result is good."

44. The most novel use of suction-assisted lipectomy? Hands down, this award does to surgeons who use suction to reduce fatty earlobes.

45. Commenting further on the incidence of seventh nerve paralysis following neck suction, Greg Hetter (Las Vegas) agrees that passing a blunt instrument along the course of the submandibular branch is asking for trouble.

"No one would approach the subplatysmal fat that is highly localized in or near the midline with a lateral approach unless they totally misunderstand the anatomy of the subplatysmal fat." There are those, however, who not only remove the fat they see directly but tell us that it is acceptable to suction under the platysma. Hetter says that the subplatysmal fat can be largely removed through a single submental incision with suction in most young women—and safely so.

46. Ely Lybeer (Brussels) sterilizes Reston foam packs and applies them to liposuction areas. Fred Grazer has demonstrated the antibruising effect of foam pads, but there is an added expense to consider.

47. Another fiction: Fascia lata can "trap" fat and make a lateral thigh suction area irregular.

48. In case you suspected that fat cells injected into soft tissue do not survive: Rat studies of fat cell injections into areas of good blood supply showed a total absence of living cells after 6 months. The fibrosis and microlipid cysts provided the "correction." We do not "inject" fat. It is a free graft in a vascular bed.

49. Dick Mladick (Virginia Beach) no longer places the patient prone for suction-assisted lipectomy. In addition to the difficulty of turning a patient, there is less ventilation in this position, and in some ways it is more difficult to perform thigh or buttock suctioning. Mladick advocates use of the "supine lateral decubitus" position; that is, turn the patient on his or her side and flex or extend the leg as needed. Such positioning eliminates the need for muscle relaxants and intubation, a sizable advantage.

50. Greg Hetter (Las Vegas) on suction in patients who are nearing the indications for face lift: "Don't let yourself get boxed in to the point that you end up paying for their later dermal excision face lift." The point being made was that one must carefully evaluate patients who simply have excess fatty tissue in the nasolabial lines or under the chin versus those who require skin excision, muscle tightening, and so on. If you leave the impression that fat excision is going to give them a truly youthful look, you will have saggy, angry patients. Hetter advises that you make it clear to them what the process of aging will do and that a formal face lift is probably inevitable, whether liposuction is employed this year or at the later date.

51. Carson Lewis (La Jolla) has completed a study on the use of injectable Wydase in suction lipectomy patients. We are aware that there is decreased blood and fluid loss in patients who have local injection of Xylocaine, but was the initial recommendation for using an enzymatic agent worth our consideration? Lewis thinks it is. For some unknown reason, there was less bleeding in the suction specimens when Wydase was added to the Xylocaine. It does not make sense, but Lewis suctioned a series of patients in whom one area, such as the thigh, was injected with the Wydase-containing solution and the results measured against those from a comparable area on the opposite side. The next question for your consideration is this: Is the cost and trouble of adding Wydase worth the minimal savings in blood loss or bruising? Right now most of us do not think so.

52. One point gleaned from a recent panel on suction-assisted lipectomy (SAL): Everyone who does SAL in the calf and ankle considers it difficult. Those who still use this procedure employ bilateral incisions, one on either side of the Achilles tendon, and use a size 6 or 7 long aspirator. Useful hint: Have the patient stand on his or her toes; you can mark exactly where the fatty tissues are. Afterward, use TED stockings, *not* tape. Lastly, ask yourself the most important question: "Can I afford to have a slough in this patient?" The calves and ankles have poor blood supply.

16 Miscellaneous Plastic Surgery Topics

Psychological Impact of Physical Features

Studies published in the *American Journal of Psychiatry* are of interest to plastic surgeons. The following is an excerpt of my communications with Kenneth Nakdimen of New York, who summarized many of the current concepts of sexual stereotyping and their relation to physical features and clothing.

A traditional theory dating back to Aristotle holds that physical features are a true representation of character. Although modern physicians do not accept this theory, one does get a feeling of knowing something about a person's personality by their appearance, including not only their facial features but their body habitus, way of walking, and choice of makeup, the colors they choose, their clothing, even their neck ties. This psychological face is reflected in our speech ("an honest face").

Who would have thought that eyebrows are one of the most important features in personal appearance? Nakdimen reminds us of the famous Mona Lisa, who is considered to have an enigmatic expression. One of the most obvious things that Leonardo DaVinci did was to omit her eyebrows! Another powerful factor in varying the expression of the eyes is the way one positions eyebrows. Low and medial eyebrows express anger or analytic attention, oblique eyebrows express anguish or puzzlement, and so on. Studies show that eyebrow position influences the perception of status in both nonhuman primates and humans.

Low-eyebrowed individuals are said to appear more dominant and high-eyebrowed ones more submissive. Makeup experts note that high, arched eyebrows are associated with credulity, a lack of initiative, and a preference for following other people's ideas; they are inconsistent with firmness and forcefulness. Men's eyebrows are heavy, straight, and close to the eyes. Even unplucked, a woman's eyebrows are more arched.

Eyebrows are not the only "sexual anatomic feature" involved in communication of personality. That most celebrated feature of beautiful women, the high cheek bone, is like a "built-in smile." I agree with the statement that high cheek bones in men are usually severe and bony, at least in models chosen for men's clothing. Photographers' preferences tend to run toward lean faces with high, bony arches. A more universal distinction, however, is that the beauty in women is frequently related to a fullness over the malar eminence. The zygomatic bone itself is proportionately smaller and the soft tissue overlying it extends closer to the nasolabial fold. With masculine high cheek bones, the most prominent point is over the zygomatic bone itself, whereas with feminine high cheek bones it is somewhat lower on the face, at a point somewhere on a line between the zygoma and the corner of the mouth. Feminine high cheek bones are said to mimic the essential contour of smiling. Stereotypically, women are supposed to take a smiling attitude. Arched eyebrows and high cheek bones are considered attractive features for a woman perhaps for that reason. Is this a connection between attractiveness and the communication of personality traits that we expect in women? Perhaps.

Clothing and one's choices of clothing are voluntary expressions of personality. To the psychiatrist, there is more to it than we think. The accepted fact that a suit and tie indicated authority may not be related to the fact that we are living in a "man's world" but that the suit jacket covers the waist, "replacing it visually with the lower edge of the jacket and increasing the apparent waist or shoulder proportion." This appearance is said to mimic a posture of dominance. Jackets are thought to be more authoritative when the shoulders are raised with pads or epaulets. High heels, in contrast, increase the proportion from the waist down. Even tall women wear them when they must look their best. It indicates to our psychiatric colleagues that the proportion of the waist to heel is important in femininity, with the opposite for masculinity. In contrast to men, women also dress to lengthen the line of their necks. Men wearing ties literally protect their necks and enhance the appearance of strength and invulnerability.

It would be simpler to state the obvious! If people take an interest in their appearance—reflected in makeup, grooming, trimming of a mustache, clothing, posture—in today's world it also is indicated by the physiognomy of the face or the contour of the body. Why else would liposuction, rhinoplasty, breast augmentation, and other non-aging-related surgical procedures be so popular? It is interesting and a bit quaint perhaps to hear our colleagues discuss this behavior in terms of Freudian theory and other psychiatric contexts, though.

Recovering from Aesthetic Surgery

According to Steve Hoefflin, the early postoperative phase may be characterized in one of two ways. It may be uneventful, or it may be marked by transient psychological disturbances, usually anxiety. Depression sometimes develops after 2 or 3 days. These [periods of depression] are related, to a large extent, to the uncertainty of the outcome, the patient's personality structure, and the attitudes of those with whom the patient comes in contact during this period. This is one of the difficulties with the current vogue of outpatient surgery in which the patient effectively loses contact with the surgeon and his staff for a number of days following the operation.

There is no doubt that unqualified approval by close contacts is the most important factor in ensuring patient acceptance of the result of aesthetic plastic surgery, irrespective of the degree of excellence of the result.

In the later postoperative phase, the tissue reaction has settled and the patient is able to assess the results in the mirror, as well as the reaction of others to the change in his appearance.

Hair Transplants

In 1981 I wrote about converting the extra scalp that is resected during face lifts in men into square plugs that could be used as donor hair. There is a better way to perform hair transplants today. Donors still have a place, but tissue expansion of the immediate type and scalp reduction are far better ways to attack the problem. Changing this hair into micrografts is probably the best method: That is, a small amount of hair that is resected can be placed into slits made with a No. 15 blade. The technique is to trim away the hair and the skin, leaving only the deep dermis and the hair roots. These micrografts can be inserted into the slits in groups of three or four, and they produce hair growth. Do not place them low enough that the skin seals over and makes the hair curl underneath the dermis.

With another technique, shown in Figure 16-1, plugs are removed from the area to be resected during the face lift. Such plugs still have a place in the partially balding patient. They can be placed well within the existing hairline and the area that is already beginning to thin out. Mention this possibility to your male face lift patients, and they will certainly be grateful for the suggestion. Whether you should charge extra for this service is up to you, but it certainly makes sense not to throw away good permanent-type hair.

A technique that immediately expands the skin during scalp reduction is shown in Figure 16-2. We have achieved 15% to 20% more resection by waiting 30 minutes to let the expander stretch the scalp.

There is another source for hair grafts. When performing a face lift on a

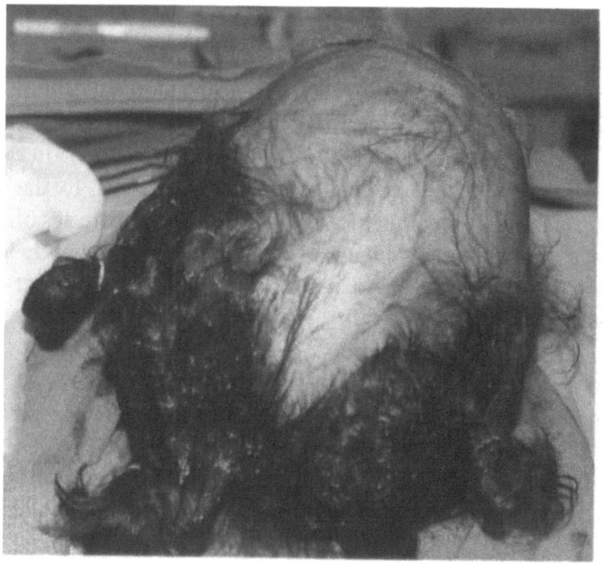

Figure 16-1. See text for explanation.

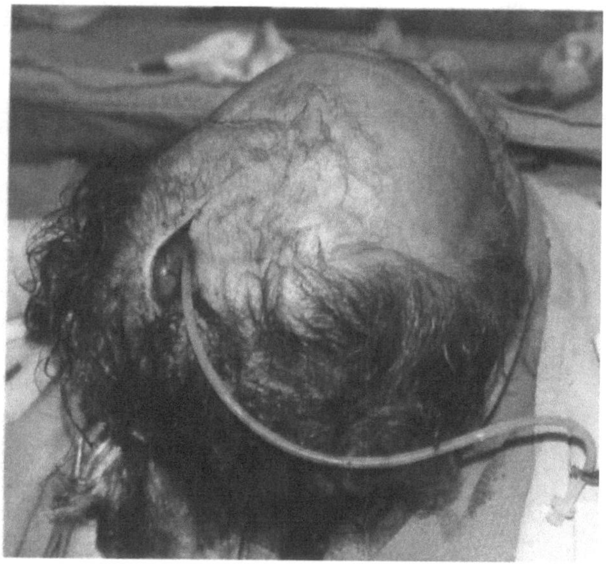

Figure 16-2. See text for explanation.

male patient do not discard the extra hair. As shown in Figure 16-3, we have already marked the area we expect to resect when we advance the neck skin upward. Before making this incision, you may wish to take plugs from it, as shown, and save a portion for slit grafts. Once the excision is completed, proceed with the face lift.

In the patient who is not having a face lift, it is far kinder and gentler to close the donor site rather than leaving it open. Use the same technique but then resect the "swiss cheese" portion that is left and place a few large sutures. You do not need to undermine. The scar is practically invisible. The tissue between the plugs can be prepared for slit grafts as well. This procedure makes hair grafting an easy procedure. Do not forget to reblock the area with bupivacaine (Marcaine) at the end of the operation so the patient can have an uneventful and restful night.

Scalp Reduction

Scalp reduction is effective. The only problem is the scar, which requires a wig to cover it. Do you remember the ads in the major newspapers a few years back asking for people who wanted to sue surgeons who had left scars on their head? There was a crude but effective drawing showing some poor soul with what looked like a tomahawk cut down the middle of the head. We of course have learned not to overresect, to bring the edges together with as little tension as possible by using a few deep undersurface tension-relaxing absorbable sutures and surface tackers, and so on.

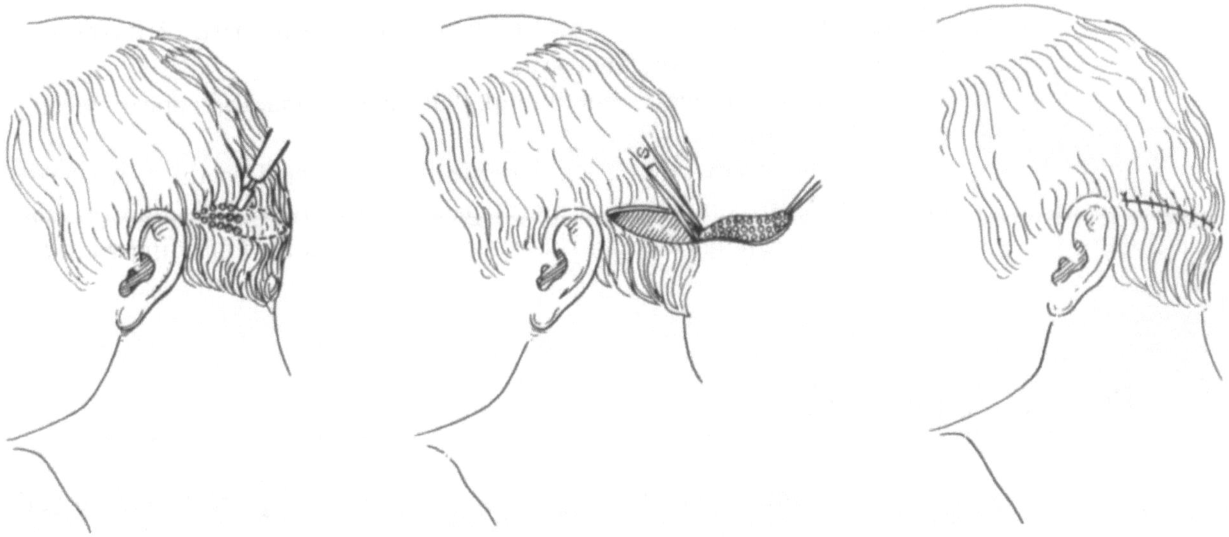

1) Removal of round plugs with electric cutter.
2) Excise "Swiss Cheese" scalp.
3) Close in a single layer.

Figure 16-3. See text for explanation.

No one except perhaps children is willing to undergo long-term expansion. It is just too socially difficult to walk around with a balloon on each side of the skull. Temporary expansion provides an alternative method. An incision is made in the area that we expect to resect, and balloons are place on the left and right sides after full undermining and some cross-cutting of the galea. Full expansion is then done for 30 minutes. It is surprising how much scalp can then be easily excised.

Be sure to advise these patients that second excisions are required and that you may want to make a few small three-hair "slit grafts" with some of the good hairs that would otherwise be thrown away. These one to three hair "micro" or "slit" grafts have largely replaced "plug" hairgrafts, at least in the anterior scalp.

Calf Augmentation

I am not including a section herein on calf augmentation because I am just not trying this procedure. Having seen a number of them, however, and discussed them with Adrien Aiche, Julius Gleicenstein, and Canadian colleagues, I can offer a few points.

The original dual hard "cigar" implants have been replaced by a softer version that is one piece. A second smaller version may be added in a medial pocket. The incisions behind the knee have been shortened, and it would certainly behoove those who use them to spend a little more time on their subcuticular closure. The patients I have seen were not concerned about the harness of their calves, the discomfort, or the possible risk of future skin breakdown: They disliked their scars.

Conversely, athletes seem to think that a hard, unnatural-appearing calf is a desirable feature.

It is obvious that dissection underneath the muscle fascia is the preferred approach. Most complications are in patients who have had polio or other congenital or acquired defects. There is a risk of infection, or bleeding leading to skin loss.

Pectoral Augmentation

The change from hard, cigar-shaped implants is a current trend in both pectoral and calf implant surgery. These implants do not have the textured surface that might prevent migration. They are made of a soft material that can be folded upon itself and inserted through a relatively small incision in the axilla. Several presentations by Adrien Aiache and others have kept us aware of the progress in this area. I myself do not get requests for this procedure.

The smaller implants would be used in someone who has suffered a pectoralis tear. These individuals are left with a true deformity. The others apparently are used to create a more masculine pectoral position. As I understand it, the procedure is no more difficult in these individuals than it is in those with Poland's syndrome, who did not develop part or all of the pectoral muscle on one side.

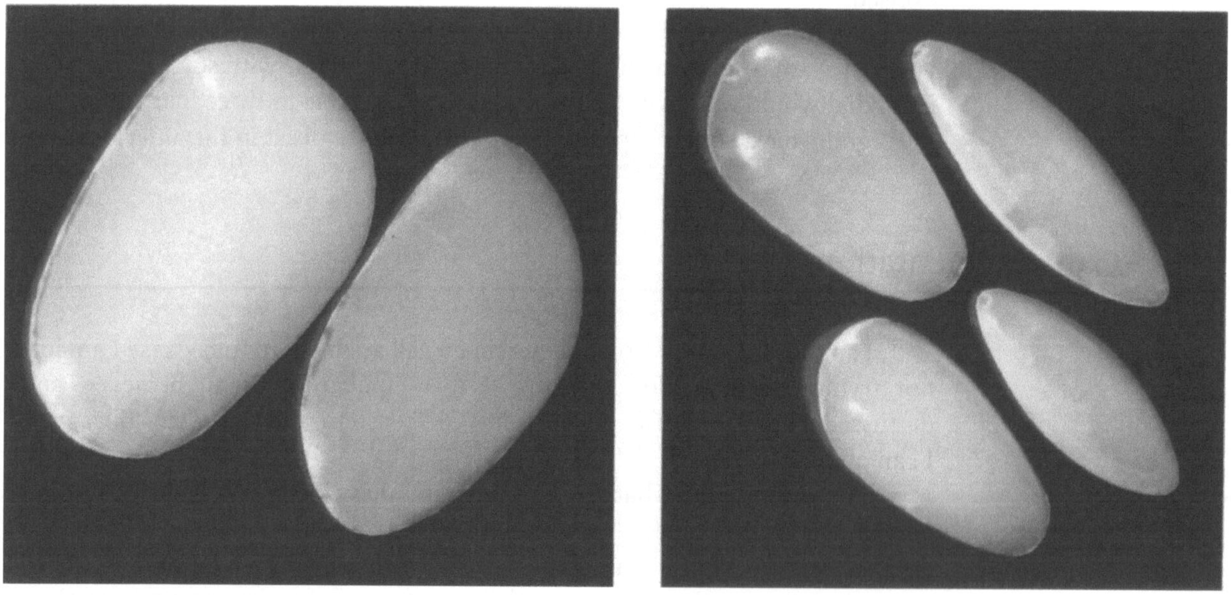

Figure 16-4. See text for explanation.

The wider, softer design should eliminate the reported problem of migration. The story is told of the actor who called in a panic from Bangkok because his hard pectoral implant had migrated into his axilla in the middle of the night and was compressing his brachial plexus. The implants pictured in Figure 16-4 were designed by A.B.T. Corporation.

Tissue Expansion and Tattoos

Until the final problems are eliminated from the laser technique, scarring will result from laser treatment of tattoos. In truth, scarring occurs with practically every method; you just have to choose the method you can live with. Unfortunately, the heat of the laser creates a distinct tissue reaction, and this heat trauma can generate extensive scarring. More recent improvements are promising.

Our best results have been with the light shaving or dermabrasion and soaking technique. Many patients do not require a second dermabrasion because the tissue reaction to the initial dermabrasion is exudative: The serum that pours out from the healing dermabrasion allows macrophages to carry some of the tattoo material into the wet gauze. We do these procedures under local anesthesia, either with a wire brush or a diamond burr in the hand-held instrument. The trick is to dermabrade lightly, so there is little discoloration or full-thickness skin loss. Have the patient change the dressing every 2 hours and saturate each new dressing with sterile saline. (They see the outline of the tattoo on the dressing as it is removed.) Wait 6 months to see if a second dermabrasion is needed. In many patients, the healing process continues and the tattoo is blurred to the point that it is acceptable.

Direct excision is the best choice, but only in areas with extra skin, such as the back of the hand or the wrist. In areas such as the forearm, you must use another technique.

Certain areas of the body form heavy scars. The shoulder, the area in the midsternum, and others are notorious for scarring.

In the individual shown in Figure 16-5, we used a temporary tissue expander on either side of his forearm leopard tattoo. Once we had undermined widely, the expander was positioned and tacking sutures were used to close the incision, which had been made down the middle of the tattoo. Thirty minutes of expansion is usually enough, after which you can excise a much greater margin. Deepithelializing the central part is another useful technique because it gives a firmer base on which to place a series of absorbable advancement sutures. Place one bite into the central area and one bite far underneath the skin. When you tie them, the surface comes together with little or no tension. Six months after the last photograph (C) we did a minor revision to remove the last bits of the leopard paw that were left in the center. Postoperatively, it is important that the patient

A B C

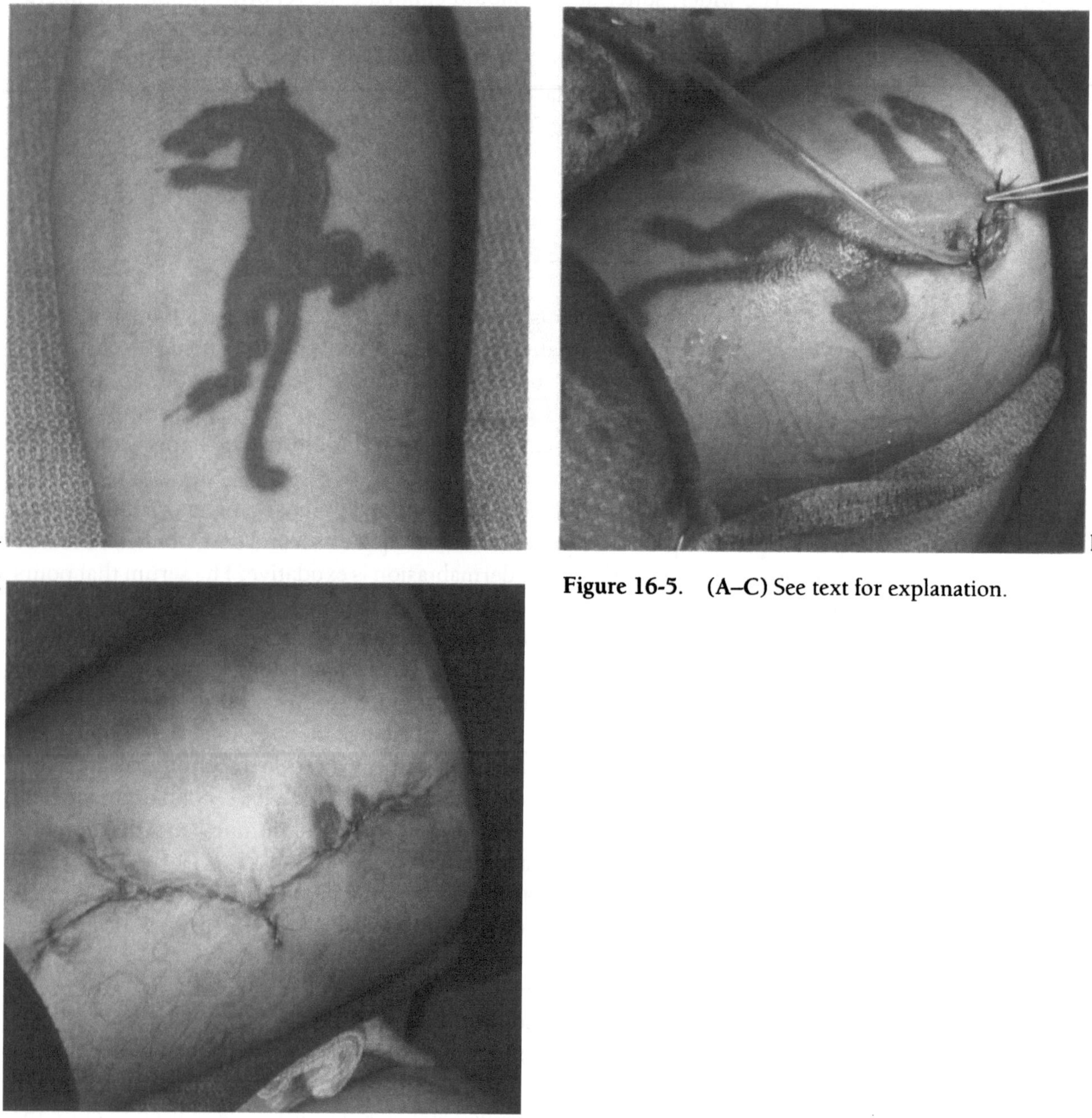

Figure 16-5. (A–C) See text for explanation.

wear a pressure device to prevent scar hypertrophy and that manual massaging of the scar with an aloe vera-based oil is continued for at least 2 to 3 months. Such massage flattens the scar and seems to prevent hypertrophy.

Cardiology "Pearls" for the Office Operating Room

1. Bundle branch block (BBB) is generally a benign condition; 89% of left BBBs occur in normal people, and 97% of right BBBs are not clinically important.
2. Meperidine (Demerol), the least expensive narcotic for office surgery, but it increases the risk of atrial fibrillation and is responsible for 25% of postoperative nausea.
3. Certain brands of implanted pacemakers currently in use turn off when electrocautery units are turned on.
4. Current advice for hypertensive patients: Do not discontinue antihypertensive medication before surgery.
5. For hypertension during surgery, several drugs are more predictable than thorazine: nitroprusside as an intravenous infusion or Nitrocase or a transderm nitro patch rubbed into the skin. Venous dilation drops the pressure. Or, try oral Procardia (Pfizer) under the tongue. Cut into the gel capsule, and squeeze it into the space beside the tongue.
6. More than half of patients with dangerous coronary disease have normal electrocardiograms, but be alert if a report shows "strain," left ventricular hypertrophy, ST or T changes, or an old myocardial infarction.
7. Bupivacaine (Marcaine) overdosage is reflected in seizures, but they may not begin until 15 to 20 minutes later.
8. Systolic elevations, such as minor atrial tachycardias, are not of great concern, but a diastolic rise definitely requires attention.

Office Anesthesia

Most of the abdominoplasties and rhinoplasties performed in our clinic are done with ketamine/Valium "twilight" anesthesia supplemented by intravenous Stadol or Nubain. Each patient is premedicated. My choice is two 30-mg Dalmane tablets, but any sedation can be used effectively. We are warned that phenothiazines should not have a role in premedication because they do not potentiate the analgesia and can present some problems. Valium has the advantage of alleviating anxiety with less sedation. Whether you choose to use Valium, Versed, or Dalmane, the results are similar. Vistaril is still a good premedication drug because it potentiates the analgesia of narcotics. It seems to work as well orally as intramuscularly. Most of us prefer not to use any intramuscular injections. Therefore I have embraced the use of oral Toradol 20 mg and in a short series found good long-lasting analgesia postoperatively. Several surgeons have incorporated Toradol as an intramuscular medication given toward the end of a general anesthesia procedure. That regimen would not help the patient with ketamine/Valium anesthesia because ketamine is effective in the low dose only for the period required for local anesthesia.

What are the problems with ketamine? Large doses (75 mg or more) cause salivation and perhaps hallucination. Our technique has been to use low-dose ketamine in conjunction with Valium or Versed plus a synthetic narcotic. The ketamine is given slowly intravenously over a 1-minute period. After another minute, proceed with Xylocaine infiltration and nerve blocks. An occasional patient still experiences pain, in which case we wait another 30 seconds while the nurse gives an additional 10 to 15 mg of ketamine; that dose usually takes care of the problem. Intravenous ketamine in these low doses can be repeated at intervals as short as 20 minutes without risk of accumulative action.

My patients are sedated for at least 24 hours so I generally choose Valium over Versed. That choice keeps them out of trouble, and they tolerate the ice packs without resistance.

Anesthesiologists unfamiliar with ketamine frequently cite a single literature reference to a problem involving a rhinoplasty. They ignore the fact that the patient received a multitude of other medications. They seem also not to be aware that ketamine/Valium has been used in hundreds of thousands of aesthetic surgery procedures with a marvelous track record. It is particularly effective for rhinoplasty. Clonidine is also a good premedication because it diminishes high blood pressure. A warning is in order, however. If a patient has been taking Clonidine for hypertension or for a neurologic problem and then omits it for several days, there is a strong possibility of a rebound elevation in blood pressure.

Use of a pulse oximeter is not debatable. Even for the experienced surgeon, it is difficult to distinguish between anxiety and hypoxia. The pulse oximeter eliminates the confusion. Our patients do not have to remove nail polish or artificial nails!

A number of adjunctive drugs can be used with local anesthesia. Several surgeons have suggested the use of Stadol infusions, whereas others object to its use. There was no argument from the latter about Stadol itself, just a suggestion that an intravenous infusion could be mishandled by the office nursing staff.

One publication blamed Stadol for "unexpected" hypertension in local anesthesia patients. We asked consultants whether they thought the drug itself was at fault or it was a combination of the following factors. (1) Undiluted local anesthetic. There is a greater chance of inducing hypertension with undiluted anesthetic than if one dilutes the epinephrine in the prepared solutions. A dilution of 1:200,000 works well in combination with 0.25% Xylocaine. (2) Inadequate sedation. If the patient is not adequately sedated and feels pain, the blood pressure rises. Those of us who use ketamine/Valium and augment these intravenous medications with Stadol or Nubain (neither of which depresses respirations) we still occasionally witness hypertensive episodes. Our consultants thought that Stadol was not to blame.

If Stadol did induce hypertension in a significant number of individuals, would we not see it more often? One of our consultants also mentioned that barbiturates used as premedications antagonize local anesthetics. Premedications such as Valium or Valium derivatives (Dalmane) may provide an advantage: prolonged relaxation. Once again we repeat the warning about Versed: Proceed cautiously with this drug. A small dose, less then 2.5 mg, can induce apnea in older patients. It is still a good drug because its duration is much shorter than that of Valium, but perhaps its use should be reserved for young patients who are undergoing short procedures.

Lastly, one must disagree with the philosophy of "pump the Valium so they forget the pain." Those who operate with local anesthesia should consider the humanitarian effects of Brevitol, ketamine, and other medications that eliminate the pain of local anesthetic injection.

Office Surgery Suggestions

One idea for controlling hypertension during office surgical procedures is to use dermal nitroglycerine. It not only improves cardiac function but decreases blood pressure and may even reduce the incidence of tachycardias. There is now a way to deliver the nitroglycerine that is relatively foolproof. Transderm-Nitro-15 is a tape product that covers a pad soaked in 15 mg of nitroglycerine. The drug representatives to whom we spoke said that one or two tapes of 15 mg applied to the arm ensure steady absorption, and this dose is sufficient for most operating room problems.

Another useful drug preparation is the "Monostat Dual-Pak." Many plastic surgeons believe in prophylactic antibiotics when one is placing a large inert prostheses in the female body, particularly when traversing breast tissue, which is likely to be contaminated with intraductal organisms. A short course of oral antibiotics is sufficient, but we still see patients who develop vaginal moniliasis. This annoying complication usually responds to one of the mycostatin preparations. The Dual-Pak is composed of miconazole nitrate (supplied as a dermatologic topical cream) and three longacting suppositories. The dual action usually eliminates the irritation and discomfort more quickly.

Another single prescription item is acyclovir (Zovirax) capsules in 25 or 50 tablet bottles. If a chemical peel patient develops lip herpes after sunburns, it is wise to start oral Zovirax the day prior to the peel and continue it for at least 5 to 10 days afterward. The annoying complication of oral herpes sores can be prevented, or at least ameliorated, although the intermittent 5-day treatment is expensive. Even if it does not stop the emergence of the virus, Zovirax should shorten the duration of the episode.

Monitoring Cocaine Usage in an Office Operating Room

Many plastic surgeons have been through the trials and tribulations of drug control in their offices and office surgical suites. Even the best intentioned employee can be tainted by cocaine abuse. When the only product available was cocaine flakes, which were mixed in the operating room it was next to impossible to keep track of its usage, much less of the total volume and dosage. Roxane Laboratory (Columbus, Ohio 43216) has a product on the market that is sensible. They package unit-dose capsules of cocaine premixed solution. The capsules are double, so if any of the fluid is missing it can be detected. After much trial and error, we settled on the 4-ml 4% capsule and find that it is sufficient for most rhinoplasties. It is available also in stronger concentrations and in glass bottles.

No system, of course, is fool-proof. In our own practice we discovered one day that all of the unit dose capsules were missing. The nurse we had hired 2 weeks earlier with impeccable credentials was ultimately discovered to be a mainliner. For some reason known only to her, she had chosen to inject herself directly with the cocaine. At least it was easy for us to determine exactly how much was gone and to discover the disappearance before she could get approval to reorder in volume—which brings up another point. With the unit capsules, you can order a small package and reduce the overhead as well as the liability. When you are down to the last two capsules, you call the manufacturer for a replacement of six capsules. They deliver promptly.

Xylocaine Versus Marcaine for Initial Infiltration

When reaching the decision as to which agent to use for initial infiltration, the following points should be kept in mind.

1. Marcaine tends to elicit a greater tissue reaction with direct infiltration and is said to be more painful.
2. Marcaine is longer-lasting, but it is roughly twice as toxic as Xylocaine. Xylocaine diluted from its 1:1000 epinephrine strength to 0.25% with 1:400,000 is as much as is needed for the initial 2 to 3 hours of any procedure.
3. Marcaine works well as an instillate to dilute steroids or other drugs flushed into face lift or breast cavities.

4. Marcaine is more effective as a spot nerve block when used at the end of a procedure, particularly if the area is already anesthetized with Xylocaine.
5. Marcaine used with Valium carries an additional risk: According to Howard Gordon (Miami), it is easy to overdose because Marcaine is a protein-bound compound, as is Valium. If the patient becomes restless owing to Marcaine toxicity, it is easy to misinterpret this reaction as emergence from the Valium-induced relaxation. Giving more Valium ties up more receptors and thus causes more problems with the Marcaine.

Marcaine Spray to Control Postoperative Pain

For large open wounds, particularly those seen with face lifts, breast reductions, breast reconstructions, and abdominal lipectomies, after wound irrigation, spraying 0.25% Marcaine with epinephrine 10 to 20 ml (in a 20-ml syringe with a 25 gauge needle) in a fine mist to cover the entire wound at the end of the case provides excellent postoperative analgesia.

Modifying the Pain of Injection with Local Anesthetics

Opinions differ about whether to add bicarbonate to lidocaine with epinephrine to keep the patient from experiencing pain. Val Lambros agrees that the pain varies with the site, the size of the needle, and the amount of material injected. (Slow injection, allowing the local anesthetic to diffuse, is more humane.) Lambros points out that lidocaine with epinephrine is at about pH 4.5, and this low pH is responsible for much of the burning. He adds sodium bicarbonate to buffer each solution to about pH 7.0 to 7.4, at a ratio of 1 mEq of bicarbonate for each 10 ml of lidocaine. The result is less pain but a shorter duration of anesthesia. Diluting the Xylocaine also reduces injection pain.

John Strausser (Sarasota) disagrees with this method. The technique of adding bicarbonate was suggested at a meeting several years ago, prompting Strausser to conduct a brief randomized double-blind experiment. His patients were asked to rate their degree of discomfort on a scale of 1 to 10. After 20 cases he broke the code and found no significant difference in the two groups. Although his was not a formal trial, he abandoned the use of bicarbonate.

My advice is to use Ketamine and Valium to induce the "twilight" state. At the end of the procedure create a nerve block with Marcaine or instill the Marcaine into a breast cavity. Patients appreciate the freedom from pain. For hospitalized patients who are undergoing more serious operations, such as subcutaneous mastectomy, the established technique of leaving a small instillation catheter in the top of the pocket is still a good one. The nurse injects 15 to 20 ml of 0.5% Marcaine with epinephrine every 4 hours and then clamps the Jackson Pratt drains. When they are reopened, old blood or debris that has accumulated is flushed out. Our patients who have undergone such procedures recall the immediate relief from discomfort that followed the flushing maneuver. Marcaine is more irritating to inject, but topically it is painless and seems to work well.

Can you overdose a patient with local anesthetic? It is unlikely if the anesthetic is not injected directly into a blood vessel. Richard Mladick reports that many plastic surgeons use much greater volumes of local anesthetic than is recommended. It was pointed out that Marcaine can be toxic and has an affinity to bind to heart muscle. For this reason, diluted Xylocaine (0.25%) is preferred or (0.125% Xylocaine for the modified saline infusion technique used for liposuction).

Spider Veins

Current thinking on spider vein injections is as follows. All plastic surgeons eventually receive a request for vein injections. Spider vein injection is one of the service items we tolerate. In terms of financial reward, the procedure cannot be justified.

Use a magnifying light and your best magnifying glasses, a 1-ml syringe, and a 30-gauge needle. Dilute one or more vials of Sotredecol solution, & draw it up in 1.0 cc syringes. Ask the patient to bring in pantyhose (it is not necessary to wrap the legs or use TED hose unless you are injecting into the wall of another varix). Always take care of the larger veins first and come back later for the tiny ones. Doppler identification for tiny veins is unnecessary. Just look at the veins and inject the ones that are easy to identify. The patient can return for further injection later if necessary.

Hassle Indexes

Some psychiatrists and psychologists are now studying physician-patient relationships and working out some rather sophisticated "hassle indexes" for our social relationships with our patients. They found that the doctors who were most unhappy in their practices were those who as medical students were the "least guarded, most self-derogating, and least extroverted." These physicians also scored lower on their information sections of their MEDCAT. Doctors who had "low self-esteem" were much more likely to be annoyed by patients with "trivial or undiagnosable complaints and by patients whose problems fail to respond to treatment." The same applied, of course, to doctors in general.

According to the researchers, physicians tend to put diseases and disorders into "likeable" and "unlikable" categories. For example, for the internist hypertension is generally rated "likeable" and obesity "unlikable." Interestingly, "liberal" faculty members are just as likely to discriminate against undesirable patients as "conservative" physicians in private practice.

Perhaps the researcher should ask: Is it fair to refer some of the undesirable, irritating, complaining patients to the physician in the next office whom you do not particularly like either? We propose that being blessed with the ability and talent to flourish in a field that does not involve dying cancer patients calls for us to accept, with good will, irritating, hypercritical, questioning patients whom we do occasionally see. We like to think of ourselves as some of the least prejudiced human beings, as we receive much of our training with minority group patients who reveal their personalities to us as perhaps they had never before to an outsider.

Subcuticular Closures and Steri-Strips

Plastic surgeons should never leave hatch marks and wide scars. I can understand cross-hatching and scar-widening if a patient was sutured in a major emergency room—but not if done by someone in our specialty.

Basic plastic surgery rules do not have to be repeated here, but there are a few suggestions. First, when excising a scar, leave a good shelf of deep tissue for the sutures and a skin overhang of 1 to 2 mm, which allows eversion at the final closure. Be sure to do a good back-cut underneath the skin so the skin does not retract. Bury the knots in deep suture layers. For abdominoplasties, we place a series of No 1 Vicryl sutures, then 2-0 Vicryl sutures, and finally a subcuticular 4-0 Dexon suture. Why change to Dexon? Vicryl tends to split after some months, and Dexon does too, but to a lesser degree. Another suggestion: Always exteriorize the end of the stitch. It is easy to bury the initial starting knot and back-track at a more superficial plane, but the distal knot cannot be buried with any assurance that it will not pop up a few weeks or months later. We exteriorize the suture end and apply a Steri-Strip to hold it down. After 5 to 6 days, the stitch can be lifted and clipped at the skin level with impunity.

How you apply the Steri-Strips is important also. Do not use long strips around the breast, where some edema is expected after augmentation. Cut them in half and place them horizontally. Otherwise, blistering often develops from the stretching effect around the upper areola. I often replace Steri-Strips on the second or third day just to be sure there is no accumulation of fluid underneath them.

By the fourth or fifth day, it is acceptable to cover the entire Steri-Stripped area with a strip of unsterile 2-inch paper tape. We use collodion on top of the tape to seal it. The patient can then get the area wet during a shower or a tub bath without danger of water soaking into the incision. By the eighth or ninth day, this collodionized tape peels away and the patient can begin direct scar massage. We provide each surgical patient with a small bottle of an aloe vera/vitamin E-based oil that we obtain from Medical Cosmetic Services. Whether it is the pressure of the massaging or the oil itself, with this regimen the incisions lose their redness quickly and flatten ahead of schedule.

We once had only one choice in skin closures, the classic Steri-Strip. Every reader is familiar with its advantages and disadvantages. Despite porosity, a certain amount of thick fluid is trapped underneath the strips. With expansion or motion, blistering at the end of the strip can create difficulty. To avoid this problem, several companies are investigating stretch material for skin closure tapes. There is also an "everting" strip that has a plastic circle in the center.

Choose 0.25 or 0.125 inch widths to cross the incision lines, particularly if there is a chance there may be some oozing (as in the corner of a blepharoplasty incision or a periareolar breast augmentation incision). Flesh colored tapes may or may not be an advantage: Once you remove blepharoplasty surface sutures or clip off the subcuticular closures in other areas, a tape becomes a surface protector and an additional safety closure for the incision.

Celestone Injections for Keloids

After a few bad experiences with Kenalog injections for scar tissue, plastic surgeons are looking for the ideal injectable to reduce hypertrophic or keloidal scars. Suggestions have ranged from topical Synalar with Saran Wrap, Cordran tape, and repeated injections of higher and higher concentrations of Celestone or Aristospan.

Irradiation of keloids incurs the risk of thyroid malignancy, problems with growth disturbance in children, and dermal atrophy. Simple excision is associated with at least a 60% recurrence rate in children. Multiple steroid injections are certainly effective, but in children this treatment can be traumatic. Children do have a greater tendency to form and re-form keloids than adults. The subtotal excision & intraoperative steroid injection combined with compression earrings and elastic garments may be the best combination.

Autotransfusion

Patients frightened by the headlines that "over 100 units" of donated blood in the Washington, D.C. Red Cross system were found to be contaminated with HIV (AIDS) virus can relax. The fact is that the units were labeled "positive" for the virus when they were actually negative. That is the good news. The bad news is that Chagas disease, which is endemic in Salvadorian and Nicaraguan immigrants, can be transmitted by blood transfusion. Apparently the blood is treated with methylene blue in South America to destroy the parasite but not here. There have only been two cases of blood-transmitted Chagas disease reported in the United States.

According to a National Institutes of Health conference, we overtransfuse patients if we give them blood for a hematocrit of 30%. These investigators say that patients become hypoxic only when their hematocrit falls below 20%. Mark Mandel, a pragmatic plastic surgeon, rebutted this argument. I agree with his conclusion that patients recover quicker and are able to return to work and normal activities faster if they do not go home with anemia.

Patients do better with autotransfusion if they donate 4 weeks ahead of time instead of 2 weeks. It takes about 2 weeks for the reticulocytes to resume full production. Blood bank experts say they have no problem storing blood for 30 days. They also have no problem freezing the patient's blood and can point to the great advantages of storing this blood for 20 years. (The down side of such storage is the excessive cost of the preparation.)

Autotransfusion is safe, relatively inexpensive, and helps people feel well enough to resume activities. The fact that they have already started manufacturing red cells is helpful as well.

Ultrasound Therapy—Any Benefit to a Liposuction Patient?

The question of ultrasound therapy in liposuction patients has been discussed repeatedly regarding its use for breast capsules and to resolve the edema of suction lipectomy. The only conclusion to date is that it does no harm. Ultrasound therapy became popular after one surgeon promoted its use in suction lipectomy patients. His girlfriend was the ultrasound operator and since then double-blind studies have refuted its value. Most say that ultrasound offers no benefit except that of "laying on of hands," which can be better handled by a skilled masseuse. Fred Grazer (New Port) disagrees. He believes it is beneficial and prescribes it for all his patients. At the least, ultrasound therapy, at no additional cost, is another indication that the surgeon cares about the patient's recovery—and it does no harm.

Achievement-Driven Psychopaths

According to one psychologist, industry trouble-shooters, like plastic surgeons, are achievement-driven (AD) psychopaths, but "in the best possible sense." Many plastic surgeons fall into this category. They cannot endure being dominated. They feel compelled to exert control over their immediate environment and associates. Sometimes this drive is appropriate, and sometimes it is not. According to the psychologist mentioned above, "Without AD psychopaths we would have virtually no consultants, lawyers, producers, politicians, surgeons, or underwriters. These are all professionals who in the course of their daily lives introduce change and influence others. These people give ulcers; they don't get them."

Does that sound familiar? The typical AD individual is extroverted but not particularly sociable. Some plastic surgeons also seem to be hooked on crisis. Nothing can equal the "high" derived from single-handedly resolving problems, meeting impossible deadlines, fighting lost causes, or putting out fires in business and medical endeavors. You know the type. "They are very confident, and they can do just about anything, except follow conventional rules. They rarely listen to higher authorities or allow their staff people free reign."

One AD individual, when asked what other profession he would choose, said that he would like to be a conductor of a symphony orchestra. "When you wave the baton, the entire orchestra comes to life at your command, and you have the power to create something special and an audience to appreciate your performance." Is that not to what we plastic surgeons aspire? It would not be fair to say that most of us are achievement driven, but there are certainly many of our respected colleagues who fit the mold.

Comments and Commentary

1. How do you handle an overreactive steroid injection? Everyone who has injected a scar with steroids has occasionally been appalled by the subsequent atrophy of fat and soft tissue. Saline injections into the atrophic area may reverse the atrophy. Irrigation and withdrawal of the saline puts the steroid back in the solution so it can be removed. Some of the steroid-atrophied fat cells can then regain their "fatness," restoring a normal skin appearance.

2. A few years ago medical use of leeches was a novelty. In 1988 Dennis Lynch (Temple) reimplanted a finger on an infant and was troubled by postoperative venous insufficiency; he promptly air-freighted in a supply of leeches. The continuous removal of venous blood and the anticoagulants injected by the leeches saved the finger during the period of microcirculation reestablishment. Unfortunately, so much blood was lost transfusions were necessary. The finger was saved, and another surgical milestone was established. Technical point: Because the leech's intestinal tract contains bacteria, put the patient on tobramycin. Also be sure you are dealing with venous congestion, not arterial insufficiency.

3. We understand that there is no benefit whatsoever from heat-coagulated fibrin injected into wrinkles, despite some extravagant claims.

4. Surgeons who use tissue expanders to reduce hairless scalp areas cosmetically or for posttraumatic situations are causing a surge in the stock market for the Abe Lincoln stove pipe hat company. We have heard from reliable sources that patients like the stove pipe hat for its perfect fit over the tissue expander. Beards are not required.

5. Lasers (even the tunable-dye variety) were not as effective or problem-free as in a comparative study on spider and feeder small variceal veins on the legs.

6. Once the sotreclecol has been injected into a vein, milk it into connecting smaller veins.

7. David Lavine, who has performed eyebrow tattoos, reports that all of the tattoos have faded, and the brown pigment faded more after 3 years than did the black pigment. He is now having to retattoo these individuals. It seems that eyebrow pigmentation has become a losing proposition. The tattoo dye manufacturers now tell us *not* to use black because the iron oxide fades to gray. Technical point: Use brown-black so the gray does not show.

8. Marcus Melvin (Portland) concurred with warnings about "spitting" Vicryl and PDS sutures. PDS is a stiffer suture and seems to work its way up through the skin more easily; moreover, it takes 6 months to dissolve. Patients who have individual sutures in the deep dermis, even with knots down, are unhappy when the PDS suture comes to the surface. Most of our serious problems recently, though, have been with Vicryl sutures. A stitch that surfaces 30 days after surgery can lead to a full infection of the suture line. Melvin originally performed all cosmetic surgery in his office operating room. Because of a lack of personnel he moved to the surgicenter, and the change involved a switch from Dexon to Vicryl sutures. For the first time he began to witness "spitting" sutures from subcuticular closures. It led to his first and only infection in a breast augmentation patient. As soon as he restocked the surgicenter with Dexon to use for subcuticular closures, the "spitting" problems stopped.

9. In defense of ketamine/Valium sedation for local anesthesia, Charles Vinnik and Howard Gordon point out that critics of the technique are critical simply because of their inexperience. No other combination has a similar safety record.

10. David Wood (Long Beach) uses the blend tone Epilator, normally used for hair electrolysis, to eliminate tiny red capillaries in the nose, face, and legs. He admits that it takes a good deal of experience, but he prefers this technique to direct vein injection.

11. John Kelleher (Amarillo) purchased the AN-74 Anprolene (gas sterilizers) and has used it extensively for 3 years. He finds that he rarely needs to

heat-sterilize any of the instruments except those that require rapid turnaround. He adds one note of caution: Despite the ventilation hood, the Occupation Safety and Health Administration (OSHA) requires ventilation of the gas and is not satisfied if there is no mechanism to remove the gas from your office. "Incidentally, the cost of sterilizing one pack in the large gas unit is about $2.13 and perhaps another dollar or so for the bags." For anyone doing a large amount of office surgery, Kelleher recommends the AN-74 over the AN-72 because of its versatility and the ability to sterilize a large amount of material at the end of the day.

12. Clonidine, usually administered at 0.1 mg PO preoperatively, has many benefits. It stabilizes blood pressure, which is particularly important during face lifts and chemical peels. It has some sedative properties and decreases shivering postoperatively. Use in hypertensive patients, even if they claim that their hypertension is under control.

13. El Melmed (Dallas) likes a product called Coveroll, a stretchy, nonwoven bandage. Because it is in a roll, Melmed cuts off what he needs and uses it on all curves such as fingers and breasts. Exudates can come through, but the tape does not come off in the shower. It can be sterilized, but Melmed uses it directly on surgical wounds and has done so for years with no ill effects and no infections. After augmentation he simply cuts off a square, notches it for the nipple, and applies it for 4 to 5 days. He prefers it to Steri-Strips.

14. David Lavine says there are three stages of learning: First is not knowing enough to stay out of trouble. Second is knowing just enough to get into trouble. Third is knowing enough to stay out of trouble.

15. Weirdest case? Luis Vasconez noted that one of his patients looked so obese *after* abdominoplasty a pregnancy test was done. The "enlargement" was a huge Marlex mesh cyst.

16. True story: A female jogger was using minoxidil to restore thickness to her hair. When she sweated, the minoxidil ran down onto her ears and she unfortunately developed hairy ears. If you use a placebo, 0.4% of patients experience a dense regrowth of hair. The figure with minoxidil is 0.7%. At last report, 7.5% of patients had a moderate regrowth, but the regrowth tended to plateau after a year. Moreover, when the minoxidil is stopped, the regrowth is lost. There is some evidence that using Retin-A with minoxidil might help.

17. There are many ways to treat ear keloids. Injecting them is not the best way because the keloids of patients who are seen in your clinic have usually progressed beyond the point at which injection would help. Several surgeons, including Leon Block, believe that standard simple excision and closure is still the best way to do it. He does not use steroids or pressure devices, and he reports only one recurrence in 18 years. Those of us who are not as bold ask the patients to wear pressure earrings, which are readily available. Pressure plus topical steroids underneath the earring covers is an effective adjunct. The new pressure earrings are attractive enough that your patients will wear them (even men).

18. Plastic surgeons do receive requests for buttock implants, and many have tried to find a way to do it safely and successfully. Silicone prostheses, similar to mammary implants, may be used. Technical point: Placement is now high and well away from the sitting surfaces. The problem is that many of our colleagues still use large incisions with large stitch marks. No drains are used, but one patient in a recently presented series developed what was described as a "fistula," although it looked surprisingly like an extruding implant. Capsular contracture was not reported. (I have seen only a few of these cases, and *all* the implants were rock hard.) Maybe the answer is to use gel textured or solid prostheses, which tend to stay in place, and, if possible, use submuscular placement. Now we know it is possible to dissect a space under the gluteus.

The last word on a buttock augmentation involved a Brazilian colleague who places a breast-type prosthesis between the gluteus maximus and the gluteus medius. The usual volume is 200 or 220 cc. Immediate expansion prior to placement has been helpful. Where do they place the incision? After seeing Brazilian bathing suits, there can be only one place: vertically, between the buttocks. This incision is also preferred by Jorge Hidalgo (Miami) & Jose Robles (Argentina)

> The incision is vertical starting at the very tip of the coccyx, then cephalad on the midline for about 5 to 7 cm. "The incision heals so well that the scar is hardly visible."
>
> The first submuscular augmentation gluteoplasties were in 1988 with good patient satisfaction and minimal complications. An important technical point: As it is in breast augmentation, the location, limits, and size of the pocket to avoid postoperative malposition and firmness are paramount.
>
> The implants help not only to correct flaccid and mild ptotic buttocks, but also the lateral depression between hips and thighs. The overall better contour and harmony makes in some cases unnecessary the use of suction lipoplasty in these two areas. According to the body frame and height of the patients, the size of the implants vary between 200 and 275 cc. The patients are up and around the next day after surgery, and their happiness with the new roundness and fullness of the buttocks way outscores any discomfort they might experience.

SUGGESTED READING

Lemperle G, Nievergelt J: Plastic and Reconstructive Breast Surgery. Springer-Verlag, New York, 1991.

Gasparotti, Lewis, Toledo: Superficial Liposculpture: Manual of Technology. Springer-Verlag, New York, 1993.

McKinney P, Cunningham BL: Aesthetic Facial Surgery. Churchill Livingstone, New York, 1992.

Pitman GH: Liposuction and Aesthetic Surgery. Quality Medical Publishing, St. Louis, 1993.

Index

MIX
Papier aus verantwortungsvollen Quellen
Paper from responsible sources
FSC® C105338

If you have any concerns about our products,
you can contact us on
ProductSafety@springernature.com

In case Publisher is established outside the EU,
the EU authorized representative is:
Springer Nature Customer Service Center GmbH
Europaplatz 3, 69115 Heidelberg, Germany

Printed by Libri Plureos GmbH
in Hamburg, Germany